EARLY CHINESE MEDICAL LITERATURE

THE SIR HENRY WELLCOME ASIAN SERIES

Already Published

Ibn al-Jazzār on Forgetfulness and its Treatment: Gerrit Bos

Early Chinese Medical Literature: Donald J. Harper

Forthcoming

Ibn al-Jazzār on Sexual Diseases and their Treatment: Gerrit Bos

Al-Kindī on Weather-Forecasting: Gerrit Bos and Charles Burnett

A Soup for the Qan: Paul D. Buell and Eugene N. Anderson

Ibn al-Jazzār on Fevers: Gerrit Bos

馬王堆醫書譯注

EARLY CHINESE MEDICAL LITERATURE

The Mawangdui Medical Manuscripts

Translation and Study
by
DONALD J. HARPER

KEGAN PAUL INTERNATIONAL
London and New York

First published in 1998 by
Kegan Paul International
UK: P.O. Box 256, London WC1B 3SW, England
Tel: (0171) 580 5511 Fax: (0171) 436 0899
E-mail: books@keganpau.demon.co.uk
Internet: http://www.demon.co.uk/keganpaul/
USA: 562 West 113th Street, New York, NY, 10025, USA
Tel: (212) 666 1000 Fax: (212) 316 3100

Distributed by
John Wiley & Sons Ltd
Southern Cross Trading Estate
1 Oldlands Way, Bognor Regis
West Sussex, PO22 9SA, England
Tel: (01243) 779 777 Fax: (01243) 820 250

Columbia University Press
562 West 113th Street
New York, NY 10025. USA
Tel: (212) 666 1000 Fax: (212) 316 3100

The publishers wish to acknowledge the generous support provided for this series by The Wellcome Institute for the History of Medicine, London, and the Institut für Geschichte der Medizin der Ludwig-Maximilians-Universität, Munich.

Printed in Great Britain

British Library Cataloguing in Publication Data
Harper, Donald J.
Early Chinese medical literature : the Mawangdui medical manuscripts. - (Sir Henry Wellcome Asian series)
1.Medicine, Chinese
I.Title
610.9'51

ISBN 0710305826

Library of Congress Cataloging-in-Publication Data
Harper, Donald John
Early Chinese medical literature : the Mawangdui medical manuscripts / translation and study by Donald Harper.
p. cm. -- (Sir Henry Wellcome Asian series : v. 2)
Texts of medical manuscripts translated from Chinese
Includes bibliographical references and indexes.
ISBN 0-7103-0582-6 (alk. paper)
1. Medicine, Chinese--Early works to 1800. 2. Ma-wang-tui Site (China) 3. Manuscripts, Chinese. I. Title. II. Series.
R127.1.h37 1996
610'.951--dc21 96-47823
CIP

To the Memory of Edward H. Schafer (1913-1991)

CONTENTS

FIGURES

Preface

I began work on the Mawangdui 馬王堆 medical manuscripts in early 1977 when I examined partial transcriptions published in *Wenwu* 文物 1975.6 and 1975.9. My 1982 dissertation is the product of the first stage of my manuscript research. At that time a reproduction of the original manuscripts was not yet published, transcriptions of several texts had not yet appeared in print, and most of the published transcriptions used simplified graphs. *MWD*, vol. 4, published in Beijing in 1985, provided a photographic reproduction of the manuscripts and a transcription of all texts in modern *kaishu* 楷書 graphs. By 1986 I was gradually making my way through the as yet unseen texts and familiarizing myself with the original manuscripts (the physical relics as well as their script). While I was convinced that the manuscripts were a remarkable testament to early Chinese medicine, I was uncertain whether an annotated translation of the entire corpus would find a publisher. For a time I considered translating a selection of texts or writing a study based on the manuscripts. The decision to translate the entire corpus was made in the fall of 1990 while I was a guest at the Institute for the History of Medicine, Munich University. I am indebted to Professor Paul U. Unschuld, Director of the Institute, for encouraging me to undertake a complete translation; and for providing me with the ideal research environment in Munich as I began the task in earnest.

Professor Unschuld has continued to watch over the project at critical stages, from commenting on the work in progress to securing publication funds. I wish to offer heartfelt thanks to my friend and colleague for his enthusiastic and unstinting support. I am also grateful to Professor Li Xueqin, Director of the Institute of History, Chinese Academy of Social Sciences, Beijing. Professor Li is responsible for the final editing of the transcription in *MWD*, vol. 4, and has encouraged me to pursue research on the medical manuscripts since 1985 when we discussed the manuscripts in Beijing. At Professor Li's invitation I spent January to March 1993 at the Institute of History, during which time I consulted with Professor Li on matters related to the manuscripts. The memory of our meetings in his home—looking at the photographic reproduction of the manuscripts through a magnifying glass and weighing the evidence for determining the correct transcription—remains fresh. During these meetings I learned important lessons in manuscript studies and the art of transcription. Professor Li's generosity continued through the final stages of translation in letters responding to further questions concerning the manuscripts.

In addition, I wish to thank Professor Ma Jixing of the Academy of Traditional Chinese Medicine (who was a member of the editorial committee that produced *MWD*, vol. 4) and Professor Qiu Xigui of Peking University for their assistance during my 1993 stay in Beijing. Professor Ma kindly presented me with a publisher's advance copy of his own book on the Mawangdui medical manuscripts (Ma Jixing 1992) on the day before my departure from Beijing. A research fellowship from the Alexander von Humboldt Foundation and a Chiang Ching-kuo fellowship administered by the American Council of Learned Societies permitted me to spend most of the academic year 1990-91 in Munich. The Committee on Scholarly Communication with China awarded me a research grant to attend the International Symposium on Mawangdui Han Tombs in Changsha in August 1992 (at which time I was able to inspect the original medical manuscripts at the Hunan Provincial Museum) and to spend winter 1993 in Beijing. I thank the University of Arizona East Asian Studies Department for releasing me from teaching duties during Spring Semester 1993, permitting me to go to Beijing and then to make rapid progress on the translation after my return to Arizona. A grant from the University of Arizona College of Humanities enabled me to engage the services of Mr. Xu Datong, a graduate student at the University, to produce the excellent facsimiles of the manuscripts which appear in this book. Mr. Xu also wrote the Chinese title on the title page in script based on the Mawangdui medical manuscripts. The Alexander von Humboldt Foundation provided a publication grant for the preparation of the electronic layout, which has been skillfully executed by Bo and Christine Hu of Munich.

D.H.
June 1996

PROLEGOMENA

INTRODUCTION

Since the 1970s there has been a succession of manuscript discoveries in late-fourth to second century B.C. tombs in several regions of China, the provinces of Hubei and Hunan being particularly fertile ground for manuscripts. Han manuscripts later than the second century B.C. have also been discovered, but Warring States, Qin, and early Han manuscripts have been more numerous. It is evident that the manuscripts were selected from the book collections of the well-to-do tomb occupants; that is, they were not prepared solely as burial goods. Contemporary records are silent on the custom of book burial. Perhaps manuscripts were placed in tombs because they were intrinsically valuable objects that bespoke expertise and status, or because they were imbued with a magical efficacy that suited the underworld environment.[1] Whatever the rationale was at the time, the modern consequence is the recovery of manuscripts from the very period when books and book collecting first became popular in China. The spread of literacy and the transmission of books were themselves manifestations of intellectual ferment, which reached a high point by the third century B.C. Each tomb has yielded a unique collection of manuscripts—no doubt a reflection of their owner's avocations—all of them containing editions of texts that circulated in the Warring States, Qin, and early Han periods. While some of the texts have been preserved in received literature, most are lost works.[2] Collectively, the excavated manuscripts shed new light on a pivotal period in Chinese civilization. They may contain lacunae due to rotted bamboo, wood, or silk (the ma-

[1] Harper (forthcoming) speculates on the magical properties attributed to manuscripts. Before the 1970s the bulk of early manuscript material consisted of Han administrative documents, which were often excavated at the remains of fortifications in several northwestern provinces (Tsien 1962: 90-102; Loewe 1967). The tomb manuscript discoveries which include an array of literature have mostly occurred since 1972 (Loewe 1977; Shaughnessy forthcoming).

[2] I follow the definitions of text and edition proposed by Roth (1993: 227): "A *text* is the unique complex and expression of ideas of an author or authors, an *edition* is a distinct record containing a unique state of a text." An edition of a text exists on a manuscript, which is the physical object. My application of Roth's definition of "text" to the excavated manuscripts is discussed more fully in Section One. In addition to the meaning given, I also refer to "text" in the ordinary sense of the words of something written.

terials used for manuscripts), but the manuscripts have experienced none of the vicissitudes of transmission that led to the loss of most ancient literature, or that recast the original form and content of a book in a new edition. When the manuscripts restore texts that were either lost or significantly altered in the course of transmission, their importance for new interpretations of early Chinese civilization is particularly great.

Such is the case with the Mawangdui medical manuscripts. The medical manuscripts are part of a large cache of manuscripts discovered in 1973 in Mawangdui 馬王堆 tomb 3, situated in the northeastern part of the city of Changsha 長沙, Hunan. Other Mawangdui manuscripts contain philosophical writings and historical anecdotes as well as works on calendrics, astrology, divination, and related occult subjects. The man buried in the tomb was a member of the locally prominent Li 利 family. Skeletal remains indicate that he was about thirty years old when he died; a wooden tablet placed in the tomb gives a burial date corresponding to 168 B.C.[1] This date provides a firm *terminus ante quem* for the excavated manuscripts. From analysis of the script and other textual evidence we know that some manuscripts were already over forty years old at the time of burial, while others were copied during the decade preceding the man's death. Most of the medical manuscripts are thought to have been copied nearer to 200 B.C. than to the date of burial. Earlier editions of the texts written on them must have circulated in the third century B.C.; some were surely well known.

Several texts contain material that is related to but older than textual parallels in the oldest received classic of medical theory, the *Huangdi neijing* 黄帝内經 (Inner canon of the Yellow Thearch; ca. first century B.C.), which is extant in three medieval recensions: the *Suwen* 素問, *Lingshu* 靈樞, and *Taisu* 太素.[2] The Mawangdui texts provide evidence

---

[1]The tablet is reproduced in Fu and Chen 1992: 37. Chen Songchang convincingly argues that the inscription on the tablet concerns the official delivery of burial goods to the tomb on the burial date; and that it is not like the documents addressed to the underworld found in other second century B.C. tombs (1994: 64-69; Harper 1994:17-18).

[2]The *Huangdi neijing* in eighteen *juan* 卷 (rolls) is listed in the division of medical literature in the *Hanshu* bibliographic treatise (*Hanshu*, 30.78b), meaning that a fair copy of the text was prepared and deposited in the Han court library sometime after 26 B.C. as part of the bibliographic project directed by Liu Xiang 劉向 and Liu Xin 歆 (Tsien 1962: 14). The fate of this edition is not known. While there are differences of opinion regarding the priority of the three medieval recensions, which vary considerably from one to the other, there is a general consensus among modern scholars that the *Huangdi neijing* was compiled during the Former Han period from a variety of textual sources (see Sivin 1993). Two recent studies approach the problem of the original compila-

of an earlier stage in the formation of the physiological and pathological theories that support acupuncture therapy in the *Huangdi neijing*. In the manuscript texts there are eleven *mai* 脈 (vessels) in the body that contain *qi* 氣 (vapor), one less than the twelve vessels of the *Huangdi neijing*. The vessels are divided into Yin and Yang categories, but the theoretical conception of the system of vessels is less elaborate than the *Huangdi neijing*. The manuscript texts attribute illness to pathogenic conditions of vapor in the vessels, associate the occurrence of certain ailments with particular vessels, describe how to diagnose illness in the vessels, and recommend cauterizing the vessels to cure ailments.[1] Acupuncture is not mentioned, nor is the therapy attested elsewhere in the Mawangdui medical manuscripts.[2]

In addition to this type of theoretical writing, there are texts representing a broad range of lost medical literature. Recipe literature predominates. In their current state of preservation, five texts contain between them over 425 recipes. One long recipe manual deals exclusively with the treatment of ailments. It provides detailed instructions for a variety of remedies, among them: drugs, several forms of heat therapy including

---

tion and subsequent history of the text differently. Yamada attributes the composite nature of the *Huangdi neijing* to the influence of schools of Han physicians whose theoretical differences are preserved in the *Huangdi neijing*; and he regards the *Taisu* as closest to the original text (1979: 67-68, 86-89). Keegan, in contrast, argues that the *Huangdi neijing* came into being as a consequence of an ongoing process of physicians transmitting medical literature; pieces of medical texts were combined and recombined, and were transmitted as a corpus that came to be known as *Huangdi neijing*. According to Keegan, each of the medieval recensions is a reflection of one of the forms of this corpus; and it is impossible to say that one of them is closest to the original text, or indeed that an original text ever existed in the sense of a first recension produced by a single editor or editors (1988: 249-59).

[1]Cauterization therapy in the Mawangdui medical manuscripts is not solely practiced in conjunction with vessel theory; and several materials are used to cause the burn (see Section Three, "Therapy"). One of the materials is *ai* 艾 (mugwort), but the use of mugwort tinder (moxa) is not attested. Thus, it is anachronistic to refer to cauterization therapy in the medical manuscripts as moxibustion.

[2]Acupuncture is a therapy that treats pathogenic conditions of vapor in the body by pricking the vessels with needles in accordance with theories related to the vessels and vapor. I follow Unschuld (1985: 92-99) in distinguishing between the use of lancing instruments for draining pus from purulent swellings and acupuncture. The therapeutic paradigm established first for vessel cauterization was the crucial precedent for the emergence of acupuncture; lancing alone cannot have led directly to acupuncture. The earliest documentation of acupuncture is in second to first century B.C. sources (for similar judgments, see Liao Yuqun 1991: 272-74; and Yamada 1985a: 3-19, 57-72). I take exception to the views of Lu and Needham (1980: 69-88), who tend to equate medical lancing with acupuncture and read early references to lancing as evidence of acupuncture (even speculating that acupuncture might already have been known in Shang times).

cauterization, surgical procedures, exorcistic incantations, and other magico-religious operations. The recipes in two of the texts focus on macrobiotic hygiene (which encompasses dietetics, breath cultivation, exercise, and sexual cultivation) with many recipes for tonics and aphrodisiacs. A text that describes gestation concludes with recipes related to childbirth. The shortest recipe text concerns philters and miscellaneous charms. The subject of the remaining texts is macrobiotic hygiene. One text is composed of ten dialogues in which different macrobiotic specialists respond to questions (the questioner in the first four dialogues is the Yellow Thearch, who plays the same role in much of the *Huangdi neijing*). The specialists expound teachings that include instructions for cultivation techniques. There is a breath cultivation text on the technique of ingesting vapor from the external atmosphere while abstaining from regular food; and on the same manuscript, a text with drawings of exercises used both to treat ailments and to cultivate the body. Two texts focus on the techniques of sexual cultivation. All of the material on macrobiotic hygiene belongs to a medical tradition of *yangsheng* 養生 (nurturing life), but neither this term nor several related terms in received literature occur in the manuscripts.[1]

We always knew that these types of medical literature existed. Newly copied editions of thirty-six medical books were deposited in the Han court library at Chang'an around the end of the first century B.C.; only the *Huangdi neijing* survives in truncated form. We know the other titles from the *Hanshu* bibliographic treatise, which reproduces the general scheme of Liu Xin's 劉歆 now lost catalogue of the library (Tsien 1962: 14). The division of medical literature, entitled "Fangji" 方技 (Recipes and techniques), lists the thirty-six books in four sub-categories (*Hanshu*, 30.78b): "Yijing" 醫經 (Physicians' canons; medical theory as represented by works like the *Huangdi neijing*, which is listed first); "Jingfang" 經方 (Canonical recipes; as is clear from the titles listed, collections of recipes to treat ailments); "Fangzhong" 房中 (Intra-chamber; sexual cultivation); and "Shenxian" 神僊 (Spirit transcendence; other types of macrobiotic hygiene). The classification no doubt reflects a physician's conception of medicine and medical literature in the first century B.C.: the physicians' canons, which ground the practice of medicine in theories of the vessels

[1]The most prominent occurrence of *yangsheng* in early literature is undoubtedly in the section title and text of *Zhuangzi* 3, 54. Differences between the medical tradition of macrobiotic hygiene and Daoist thought are discussed in Section Four, "Intellectual Background."

and vapor, are placed first; the diffuse recipe literature, which collects a wealth of medical knowledge that does not necessarily conform to theory, comes next; private hygienic practices are last, and macrobiotic hygiene is identified with the immortality beliefs of the *xian* 仙 (transcendent) cult.[1] While the classification and its medical assumptions post-date the Mawangdui medical manuscripts, we may surmise that the contents of the manuscripts typify early Chinese medical literature—albeit in capsule form.

Manuscripts from tombs present problems not so different from the problems of interpreting other excavated artifacts; and many questions concerning the Mawangdui medical manuscripts must be answered with a judicious conjecture. On balance, however, the manuscripts provide a new foundation for the history of early Chinese medicine and medical literature. They are older than the *Huangdi neijing*; and they reveal more of what medicine was like than the *Huangdi neijing*, the contents of which center on the new, universal model of illness based on vessel theory along with the methods of diagnosis and treatment that accompany it. The only received medical literature that dates roughly to the time of the tomb 3 burial (168 B.C.) are selected writings of the physician Chunyu Yi 淳于意 (216–ca. 150 B.C.) quoted in chapter 105 of Sima Qian's 司馬遷 (ca. 145–ca. 86 B.C.) *Shiji* 史記. They consist of twenty-five medical case histories, eight explanations of his medical practice, and a personal history of his medical training. Chunyu Yi, who practiced medicine in Qi 齊 (present-day Shandong), originally submitted these writings to the Han court at Chang'an around 154 B.C. in order to vindicate his medical reputation. Like the *Huangdi neijing*, Chunyu Yi's writings dwell on etiology, diagnosis, and treatment (however, his understanding of vessel theory is not identical to the *Huangdi neijing*, and he favors drug treatments over cauterization or acupuncture).[2] There are, of course, references to medi-

[1]Ideas of health and longevity in the Mawangdui medical manuscripts appear to represent a tradition of macrobiotic hygiene that was older than the *xian* cult, which became prominent in the late third century B.C. Cross-fertilization between macrobiotic hygiene and the *xian* cult is well documented in Former Han sources, hence their fusion in the bibliographic classification. The classification may have been devised by Li Zhuguo 李柱國, the physician who was assigned the task of editing the medical books in the court library (*Hanshu*, 30.1b).

[2]Bridgman (1952–55) translates the *Shiji* account of Chunyu Yi and discusses its significance for the study of early Chinese medicine; see also, Lu and Needham 1980: 106–110. The same chapter of the *Shiji* opens with an account of the legendary physician Bian Que 扁鵲 (whose historical existence during the Warring States period is doubtful). Yamada (1988) has shown that Sima Qian fashioned the account of Bian Que from earlier anecdotal literature and tailored it to better reflect

cine in historical and philosophical texts as well as in belles lettres, but this material is mostly anecdotal and is not itself medical literature.[1]

There is an important difference between Chunyu Yi's writings and the Mawangdui medical manuscripts. In his personal history, Chunyu Yi names the medical books that were transmitted to him by his teacher Yang Qing 陽慶 in 180 B.C., which he states were the foundation of his medical practice (*Shiji*, 105.8b; Bridgman 1952–55: 26). Except for occasional quotations from a *Maifa* 脈法 (Model of the vessels) in the medical case histories, Chunyu Yi's writings concern his own medical practice; that is, we know virtually nothing about his collection of medical books other than their titles. With the Mawangdui manuscripts, we have examples of third to early-second century B.C. medical books. Considering the other manuscripts on philosophy, calendrics, astrology, and divination, the man buried in tomb 3 was an avid book collector who patronized specialists in several fields of knowledge including medicine. He need not have been a physician to collect literature on medicine, nor have been an astrologer or diviner. His manuscripts reflect the same range of subject matter as the *Hanshu* bibliographic treatise, which lists works on calendrics and the other subjects in a separate division—"Shushu" 數術 (Calculations and arts; *Hanshu*, 30.65a). Tomb 3 reveals that the pattern of book collecting exemplified in the *Hanshu* bibliographic treatise was maintained by private individuals as well as by the Han thearchs.

The combined literature in the "Shushu" and "Fangji" divisions of the bibliographic treatise falls broadly into fields of knowledge that I identify as natural philosophy and occult thought. I refer to the literature itself as "*fang*-literature," based on the significance of the concept of *fang* 方 (recipe) in defining natural philosophy and occult thought. These matters are discussed in Section Two ("Recipes, Techniques, Calculations, Arts"), but it would be wise to broach now the subject of early Chinese medicine and other fields of knowledge that come within the purview of the modern discipline of history of science. The history of science has long since moved beyond the stage of vetting ancient knowledge of nature to separate the rational from the irrational and the science from the superstition. Lively debate continues to focus on the relation between science, magic,

---

the image of Bian Que as a patron of certain medical arts (including acupuncture) in Sima Qian's own time. It is an important document, but is not an example of medical literature.

[1]See Bridgman 1952–55: 6–17, for a survey of some of the pre-Han and Han literature that refers to medicine.

and religion in a premodern context and on the question of what constitutes rationality. A number of earlier theories and interpretations have been put to rest, among them: that magic and religion are fundamentally different; that magic is failed science; and that scientific "progress" already separated science from magic in ancient times (Tambiah 1990; Vickers 1984; Lloyd 1979). The term "science" itself is part of the problem of defining the quiddities under investigation, because it assumes certain categorizations of knowledge that were not acknowledged in the past. "Natural philosophy," in the sense of systems of thought that take nature as their primary object of investigation and that develop theories to explain phenomena in terms of perceived regularities in the operation of nature itself, is gaining currency among English writers (Lindberg 1992: 1-4). However, "natural philosophy" has a long history in the Western intellectual tradition; from the standpoint of current research in the history of science, the term leaves open the question of the evident interpenetration of natural philosophy, magico-religious belief, and other forms of occult thought. It seems that we must speak dually of "natural philosophy" and "occult thought" in order to refer to something that was undivided or was divided differently in either the ancient Mediterranean world or early China.[1]

When we look for an identifiable Chinese natural philosophy what we find are principally the theories of vapor, of Yin and Yang, and of the Five Agents (*wuxing* 五行), which arose during the Warring States period and by the end of the third century B.C. coalesced into the system of thought that Graham refers to as "correlative cosmology"—a cosmology that establishes elaborate correspondences between nature, the individual human being, and society (1986; 1989: 313-70). Graham identifies the earliest exponents of cosmology as "court historiographers, astronomers, diviners, physicians, and musicmasters" (1989: 325); that is, what I tentatively call Warring States natural philosophy was originally the province of the practitioners of technical arts like calendrics, astrology, divination, and medicine.[2] Calendrics, astrology, and divination appear to have been most influential in the new rationalization of nature; medicine, while offering

[1]The question of magic is discussed further in Section Five.

[2]Kalinowski is in basic agreement with Graham: "The doctrine of the Five Agents matured from the contacts between religious, philosophical, and scientific conceptions of the end of the Warring States and the Former Han. Spilling over from the context of divinatory practices, it very quickly attained a sufficient degree of generality to become the conceptual basis for all activity" (1991: 47).

physiological and etiological theories that made the body a microcosm of the cosmos, was incorporating Yin Yang and Five Agent theories in stages. There is scant evidence of the theories in the Mawangdui medical manuscripts, whereas by the time of the *Huangdi neijing* (ca. first century B.C.) they have been assimilated; even then, assimilation was not absolute nor did it become so during the Han. Nevertheless, physicians (which translates *yi* 醫) were clearly active in the same social and intellectual milieu as the diviners and other specialists, all of whom shared a common interest in understanding natural phenomena and their consequences for humankind.

This account of the genesis of Warring States natural philosophy stands in contrast to the Greek pattern, where it was philosophers who developed universal theories of nature and change, from which they fashioned an understandable cosmos; and practitioners (like physicians) who applied the philosophers' theories to their craft. The "masters" (*zi* 子) of Warring States philosophy did not ignore nature entirely, but politics and ethics were their main concern. The extant writings of the masters of philosophy rarely exhibit an interest in nature outside of its utility as an analogy for their particular philosophical argument.[1] To be sure, nature-based political models figured prominently in philosophy by the third century B.C., and philosophical argumentation on *dao* 道 (way) as an ultimate organizing structure both in nature and in human society became quite sophisticated. Moreover, the humanistic orientation of the philosophers undeniably contributed to the rationalizing of nature and to skepticism of magico-religious conceptions. But natural philosophy as such was not their invention.[2]

Knowledge of nature during this age of intellectual ferment obviously encompassed more than what was channeled into Yin Yang and Five Agent theories. In the case of medicine, popular lore (much of it based on magico-religious beliefs), practical experiences, and competition between several kinds of medical practitioners brought forth a diversity of data and viewpoints—all of them drawn upon in the formation of a learned medicine. Just as clearly, the medicine of Chunyu Yi and the *Huangdi neijing*

[1]The exception were the Mohists, who for a brief time moved in the direction of causal explanations of natural phenomena (Graham 1989: 160-66).

[2]Sivin's review of Graham 1989 makes a spirited counter-argument that "cosmology entered the technical world from philosophy, not vice versa" (1992: 23). Sivin links the genesis of cosmology to the political theories of philosophers seeking to prove that "the state was natural" (1992: 24-25). On balance I think Graham's argument still stands.

shows that some physicians were using Yin Yang and Five Agent theories to establish a medicine that in principle adhered to naturalistic theories and rejected the influence of spirits and the use of magic. It is significant, however, that despite a kind of rationalistic skepticism which accompanied Yin Yang and Five Agent theories in various fields of knowledge, the theories themselves were not like laws of nature; and there was not a clear break with magico-religious conceptions. A wholly naturalistic explanation of phenomena was, therefore, a relative interpretation made by the person applying the theories; the theories themselves did not exclude occult interpretation. In short, Yin Yang and Five Agent theories did not constitute a "natural philosophy" that was opposed to "occult thought."[1]

A single term for the whole enterprise of investigating nature (and not just Yin Yang and Five Agent theories) is needed—one that might serve to differentiate between this enterprise and that of the Warring States philosophers, while not excluding occult thought. My use of "natural philosophy" and "occult thought" (or "occult knowledge"), either singly or as a pair, is a heuristic device. The reader should understand that the usage is intended to facilitate the discussion of early Chinese medicine, and that the two terms do not define opposite categories in the early Chinese conception.

This translation of the Mawangdui medical manuscripts is the first complete translation in any language; it is based on the transcription and photographic reproduction of the original manuscripts in *MWD*, vol. 4. Translation assumes the existence of a critical edition of the text to be translated. In working with lost texts copied on excavated manuscripts, I have been mindful of the principles of textual criticism. I offer a number of revisions of the transcription of individual graphs in *MWD*, vol. 4, which are recorded in the Translation notes and listed in Appendix 2. In addition, editions of three of the medical texts were discovered in a manuscript excavated from Zhangjiashan 張家山 tomb 247, Hubei, in 1983 (burial dated to mid-second century B.C.); these editions were still unavailable when *MWD*, vol. 4, was published. I have used the Zhangjiashan editions to prepare a new transcription of the Mawangdui texts,

---

[1]Kalinowski compares Yin Yang and Five Agent theories to the hermetic traditions of Greco-Roman times, and rejects the label "natural philosohpy": "To reduce this to a system of natural philosophy does not take account of the extreme diversity of the elements of which it is composed and of its multiple applications not only in the realm of the investigation of things in general, but also in that of politics, religion, and the arts" (1991: 47).

which appears in Appendix 1. The Translation notes also record other instances where my textual research has led to judgments that differ with *MWD*, vol. 4. Thus, while I have not prepared a new transcription of the entire corpus, the Translation provides a necessary text-critical supplement to the transcription of the texts in *MWD*, vol. 4.

The Introduction to the Translation reviews the conventions adopted in the translation. Interpretations and supporting documentation are set forth in the Translation notes. The Prolegomena situate the Mawangdui medical manuscripts in their social and intellectual context, with the aim of identifying their place in the history of medicine and in the history of ideas. Sections are devoted to: (1) the discovery of the manuscripts, contents, dating, and hermeneutic issues; (2) the manuscripts as *fang*-literature, readership, and transmission; (3) medical ideas and practices; (4) macrobiotic hygiene; and (5) magic.

Manuscripts from several tombs in addition to Mawangdui tomb 3 are providing us with our first look at the early texts of Chinese natural philosophy and occult thought. This kind of *fang*-literature probably began to circulate in the fourth century B.C. at the same time as philosophical literature burgeoned. Beyond the circle of specialists, the existence of a literate elite who collected books must have increased the demand for *fang*-literature. As transcriptions and reproductions of the manuscripts are published and research on them progresses, we will gain a far better understanding of the traditions they represent than could have been imagined only several decades ago; and our view of early Chinese civilization as a whole will be changed by them.[1] I must confess that I sometimes wish I might delay publication of my translation of the Mawangdui medical manuscripts until every textual problem is solved to my complete satisfaction and every interpretation offered with certitude. The discovery of the Zhangjiashan medical manuscripts alone has shed much light on the Mawangdui medical manuscripts, rendering lucid what was previously unclear. Given the record of the last two decades, new manuscript discoveries seem inevitable. One thought that recurs is how much more I will know about the Mawangdui medical manuscripts and early medicine in a decade's time. Despite its imperfections, I hope this translation of the medical manuscripts stimulates research in the history of Chinese medi-

[1] See Harper forthcoming for a survey of these manuscripts.

cine and helps to build a critical mass of scholarly research on excavated manuscripts related broadly to natural philosophy and occult thought.

SECTION ONE
MAWANGDUI MEDICAL MANUSCRIPTS

MANUSCRIPT DISCOVERY

Mawangdui tomb 3 was excavated during November and December 1973, followed by the excavation of tomb 2 (which continued into January 1974). Mawangdui tomb 1 was excavated in 1972. All three tombs were of the vertical-pit type. In tomb 3 the pit was 17.7 meters deep. A wooden burial-chamber had been built at the bottom of the pit with a central area to hold the three internested coffins and with four surrounding storage areas containing the burial goods. There is a full archaeological excavation report for Mawangdui tomb 1 (Hunan sheng bowuguan and Zhongguo kexueyuan kaogu yanjiusuo 1973), but not yet for tombs 2 and 3. Although basic facts about the latter tombs have been published, the information available is often not as specific as one would like. In addition to a wealth of burial goods, tomb 1 yielded the well preserved corpse of a woman—about fifty years old at the time of death—who has been determined to be the wife of Li Cang 利 蒼, the occupant of tomb 2. Three seals discovered in tomb 2 (two of bronze and one of jade) confirm the identity of the occupant as Li Cang, who held the aristocratic rank of Lord of Dai 軑 侯 and was also a chancellor in the Kingdom of Changsha 長 沙 國. According to the *Shiji* and *Hanshu*, Li Cang was installed as Lord of Dai in 193 and died in 186 B.C. It is presumed that the roughly thirty-year-old man buried in 168 B.C. in tomb 3 was the son of Li Cang and the wife in tomb 1. Because the construction of tomb 1 damaged tombs 2 and 3, Li Cang's wife died last; she was probably buried not long after 168 B.C. Opinion differs over whether the son was Li Xi 豨, who succeeded Cang as the second Lord of Dai (the *Shiji* and *Hanshu* state that Xi died in 165 B.C.), or was another son who may have held a military position in the region of Changsha (as suggested by weapons and other artifacts related to military activity among the grave goods). The Li family continued to be prominent in the region at least until 110 B.C. when their aristocratic entitlement was eliminated by Thearch Wu 武帝 (r. 141-87 B.C.).[1]

All of the tomb 3 manuscripts were found inside a rectangular lacquer box with a roof-shaped lid (sixty centimeters long, thirty centimeters wide, and twenty centimeters high) that lay in the storage area on the east side of the coffins. The majority of manuscripts are on sheets of silk of two widths: either approximately fifty centimeters wide (somewhat over two *chi* in Qin and Han measurements), or twenty-four centimeters (just over one *chi*). Of various lengths, most of the silk manuscripts had been folded and placed in a large rectangular compartment (one of five compartments inside the box). The silk had rotted at the creases, resulting in stacks of leaves that the restorers pieced back together. At least one silk manuscript (twenty-four centimeter width) was rolled around a wooden slat (three centimeters wide) and had been placed in the narrow compartment running the length of one side of the box. Another folded silk manuscript (*MS*II of the medical manuscripts) was also found in the side-compartment. On top of these silk manuscripts in the side-compartment were one manuscript of bamboo slips and another of bamboo and wooden slips (*MS*VI and *MS*VII of the medical manuscripts). The original binding cords were disintegrated. The slips of *MS*VI are twenty-three centimeters long (one *chi*); the wooden slips of *MS*VII are twenty-three centimeters, the bamboo slips are twenty-eight centimeters. *MS*VII had been rolled around a core of two bamboo flutes. There are other sizes of silk manuscripts, mostly containing maps, diagrams, and pictures. The largest manuscripts found in the box are two maps, one a square of silk ninety-six centimeters on a side and the other a rectangle seventy-eight centimeters wide and ninety-eight centimeters long. At present we lack a detailed record of the exact position of every manuscript in the lacquer

[1]During the first half of the second century B.C. the Kingdom of Changsha belonged to Wu Rui 吳芮 and his descendants (Twitchett and Loewe 1986: 124). The three seals from tomb 2 are reproduced in Fu and Chen 1992: 40. Hunan sheng bowuguan and Zhongguo kexueyuan kaogu yanjiusuo 1973, vol. 1: 157, gives the succession of the Lords of Dai based on the *Shiji* and *Hanshu*. Riegel (1975) summarizes the information on tombs 2 and 3 in the early archaeological reports published in Chinese journals. Initially, Li Xi's death date in the historical records was judged to eliminate him as the occupant of tomb 3. Fu Juyou (1983) offers a counter-argument that tomb 3 could only be that of the second Lord of Dai, and that the records of his death in 165 B.C. may be in error. Arguments for and against Li Xi continue to be made. Some scholars identify a commander named Sima De 司馬得 in a military garrison map found among the tomb 3 manuscripts as the tomb 3 occupant, reading Sima as an official title not as De's surname; others reject the identification. See Liu Xiaolu (1994), who favors Li Xi.

box at the time of excavation (one hopes that when the official excavation report for tomb 3 is published it will include this information). It is evident that the medical manuscripts were not all placed in the same compartment, but were divided between the side-compartment and the larger rectangular compartment which held most of the manuscripts.[1]

The original manuscripts are deposited in the Hunan Provincial Museum in Changsha. Shortly after excavation, the manuscripts were divided into categories by content and editorial committees were formed to restore and transcribe the manuscripts in each category. The work of transcription was—and is—done primarily with photographic reproductions.[2] Some transcriptions, usually in simplified graphs and not accompanied by reproductions of the manuscripts, were published relatively early in *Wenwu* and elsewhere. Full reproductions and transcriptions in modern ***kaishu*** 楷書 graphs are being published in individual volumes in *MWD*. These volumes provide a standard edition of the manuscripts for scholarly research. Publication has been gradual, leaving many manuscripts either inadequately represented or unpublished in any form.[3]

Because work on several categories of manuscripts is still on-going, it is possible that published figures for the number of manuscripts discovered and the total number of texts contained in them will be revised. According to current accounts, the manuscript corpus comprises thirty manuscripts and forty-five texts (including maps, diagrams, and pictures in the count). Some manuscripts contain only one text; others several. Several texts occur in two editions on separate silk manuscripts, most famously the

---

[1]My account of the manuscript discovery is necessarily provisional. There are contradictions in published accounts (Hunan sheng bowuguan and Zhongguo kexueyuan kaogu yanjiusuo 1974; Xiao Han 1974; Wang Shimin 1986). I am indebted to Li Xueqin (private communication) for providing me with the information he acquired from those directly involved in the excavation of the manuscripts. In identifying the manuscripts I exclude a bamboo-slip manuscript that inventories the burial goods in the tomb (it is worth noting that the inventory does not list the lacquer box containing manuscripts). The inventory, which was placed in the storage area on the west side of the coffins, is a type of burial document prepared specifically for the tomb. In contrast, the manuscripts in the box represent items that we may presume to have been selected from an even larger collection of manuscripts possessed by the occupant of tomb 3 during his life. I also exclude three paintings on silk: one draped over the innermost coffin and related to burial custom; and two paintings that were positioned on the eastern and western walls of the burial chamber (Fu and Chen 1992: 22-34).

[2]Li Xueqin and Ma Jixing, both members of the medical manuscript committee responsible for *MWD*, vol. 4, described to me the working procedures of that committee in conversations in Beijing in winter 1993.

[3]Excellent reproductions of some manuscripts as yet unpublished in *MWD* appear in Fu and Chen 1992.

two editions of the *Laozi* 老子. Only three texts are known in received literature: the *Laozi*; an edition of the hexagram text of the *Yijing* 易經; and an edition of the "Xici zhuan" 繫辭傳, the cosmological commentary on the hexagrams which forms part of the received text of the *Yijing*.[1] The medical manuscripts account for a sizeable portion of the corpus: seven medical manuscripts contain fourteen texts (one text occurs in two editions on separate silk manuscripts) with roughly 22,000 extant graphs—about eighteen percent of the extant graph count for the whole corpus, which I estimate to be 125,000.[2]

Having stated that there are forty-five texts on thirty manuscripts in the Mawangdui manuscript corpus, I should explain my use of the term "text." First, "text" corresponds to *pian* 篇 (roughly, "piece of writing"), which is the term used by the Mawangdui manuscript editorial committees when identifying the distinct "pieces of writing" on a particular manuscript. Second, I follow Roth's definition of a "text" as the "unique complex and expression of ideas of an author or authors" (1993: 227). The editorial committees base the identification of *pian* on identity with a received text (like the *Laozi*), on titles that occasionally appear in a manuscript, on obvious divisions in the layout of a manuscript, or on a change of subject that warrants distinguishing one "piece of writing" from another. Taking the manuscript with the second *Laozi* edition as an example, the *Laozi* is preceded on the manuscript by four writings each of which has a title. Perhaps these four *pian* should be grouped together and identified as one "text" on the assumption that they are inseparable parts of a single work like the *Laozi*. But without the additional testimony of other editions of the four *pian* as a single work, it is equally probable that the four *pian* circulated separately—or perhaps each *pian* is an extract from

[1]My figures for the Mawangdui manuscript corpus are derived from Wang Shimin's enumeration of the silk manuscripts and texts (1986), to which I add the two manuscripts written on bamboo and wooden slips that contain four texts. The two manuscripts containing *Laozi* editions and several lost philosophical texts are published in *MWD*, vol. 1. Reproductions of the *Yijing* hexagram text and the "Xici zhuan" are in Fu and Chen 1992: 106-26.

[2]It should be emphasized that the extant graph counts are rough estimates only, and are not based on my own research. Wang Shimin gives 120,000 for the whole corpus (1986: 307), but he does not include the two medical manuscripts on bamboo and wooden slips. The table in Ma Jixing 1992: 4-5, counts 4,616 extant graphs in these manuscripts; and the extant graphs in all the medical manuscripts add up to 22,314 (Ma's total of 23,707 includes editions of three Mawangdui medical texts written on one of the Zhangjiashan tomb 247 manuscripts—discussed below—which I omit). Ma estimates extant graphs in the whole corpus to be 130,000 versus my 125,000 (1992: 1). Allowing for imprecision in both estimates, the figure of eighteen percent is still a fair representation of the amount of medical literature in the corpus as a whole.

other lost works unknown to us. Given our lack of knowledge of authorship and manuscript transmission before the editorial project carried out by Liu Xiang 劉向 and Liu Xin 歆 in the first century B.C. (Tsien 1962: 14), I advise caution when dealing with lost literature on the manuscripts. Treating each *pian* of the editorial committees as a "text" establishes a minimal identification, which can always be revised if new manuscript discoveries prove that several *pian* form one text. In the case of the medical texts, the minimal identification—even when it results in texts of only several hundred graphs—accurately reflects how medical literature and *fang*-literature in general were composed. Teachings and recipes belonged to a common pool of medical literature (with oral material being continually introduced); any one medical manuscript might have made a different selection of short texts from the available literature, creating what could be called a "composite text" out of "text components." One of the Zhangjiashan 張家山 medical manuscripts illustrates this phenomenon well, containing editions of Mawangdui texts in combination with other texts not found in the Mawangdui medical manuscripts (see "Other Excavated Manuscripts Related to Medicine" below).[1]

Twenty-eight of the thirty Mawangdui manuscripts are written on silk; excluding the famous Chu silk manuscript (ca. 300 B.C.), unearthed in the vicinity of Changsha in 1942, there have been no other discoveries of silk manuscripts in the recent spate of manuscript discoveries.[2] Silk was a more costly book material than wood or bamboo. Silk also required greater care from the scribe. A miswritten graph or wrong phrase could always be scraped off a bamboo or wooden slip, and individual slips could be replaced, but once the ink saturated the silk the scribe could only blot out errors and proceed (as is evidenced in the Mawangdui manuscripts). Silk, of course, offered advantages. It was not bulky like wood or bamboo, and text and illustrations could be combined easily on the smooth surface. The Mawangdui manuscripts show how the format of bound-slip books continued to influence silk books. Many of the silk manuscripts are ruled with vertical lines in red ink to form columns that imitate the book-mat formed from bound slips of wood or bamboo; the graphs in black ink fill

[1]Keegan argues that the extant recensions of the *Huangdi neijing* are basically compilations of composite texts fashioned from what he calls "primary texts" (1988: 252-54).

[2]See Tsien 1962: 116-30, on silk as a material for written documents in early China, which began to be used around the fifth century B.C. Bamboo and wood were used as early as the Shang. The most recent monograph on the Chu silk manuscript is Li Ling 1985.

each column like one slip of a bound-slip book (in some cases extra ruled columns have been left blank). The two widths of silk used for most of the Mawangdui silk manuscripts are probably also related to book dimensions established for slips. The narrower width (twenty-four centimeters) corresponds to a common length of twenty-three to twenty-four centimeters for excavated Qin and Han slips, which in turn reflects a standard slip-length of one *chi* (23.1 centimeters) mentioned in Han sources (Tsien 1962: 105; Sun Ji 1991: 281-85).[1] The wider silk (fifty centimeters) probably corresponds to the two-*chi* slips mentioned in Han sources (Tsien 1962: 105).[2] Han sources associate the larger and smaller sizes of books with writings of greater or lesser importance. Considering the Mawangdui manuscript corpus as a whole, there is not a consistent correlation between the size of the manuscript and the relative significance of its contents. The choice of wider silk for two of the five medical manuscripts on silk was evidently to better accommodate the drawings included on those manuscripts.

The graphs in the Mawangdui manuscripts can be classified as either seal script (*zhuanshu* 篆書) or clerical script (*lishu* 隸書), or a hybrid in between; that is, the scribes wrote in the scripts used in Qin during the Warring States and promulgated as the standard for all regions of China following the Qin unification of 221 B.C. By Han times the script reform was complete and the different scripts that had been in use in feudal states like Chu 楚 and Qi 齊 were virtually forgotten.[3] The oldest Mawangdui manuscripts are those written in script which is predominately seal or in a hybrid of seal and clerical script. They were probably copied ca. 220-190

[1]Another standard slip-length is one *chi* two *cun*, represented in excavated slips by roughly twenty-eight centimeter slips like the bamboo slips in *MSVII*.

[2]Two *chi* four *cun* slips (just over fifty-five centimeters, double the length of one *chi* two *cun*) were also used. At fifty centimeters, it is also possible that the wider silk represents a standard width for silk used as a commodity of exchange. The Qin administrative documents from Shuihudi 睡虎地 tomb 11 (see below) stipulate a width of two *chi* five *cun* (just under fifty-eight centimeters) for cloth, while Han sources give two *chi* two *cun* (just under fifty-one centimeters; *SHD*: 36).

[3]Qiu Xigui provides an excellent overview of Qin to Han seal script and clerical script, including relevant paleographic evidence (1990: 59-72). Seal script was regarded in Qin as more formal—the appropriate script for inscriptions—whereas clerical script was a more convenient script for everyday use. Paleographic evidence indicates that clerical script was already developing in Qin in the fourth century B.C., contrary to received accounts that associate the invention of clerical script with the Qin unification.

B.C. The youngest manuscripts are in Han clerical script, and of course can be no younger than 168 B.C. (the burial date).[1]

Occasionally a manuscript avoids a graph that is the personal name of a Qin or early Han thearch. This evidence can sometimes supplement script analysis in dating a manuscript. For example, in one of the medical manuscripts the graph *chang* 常 replaces *heng* 恒, the latter graph being the personal name of Liu Heng 劉恒, Thearch Wen 文帝 (r. 180–157 B.C.). The manuscript must have been copied sometime after 180 and before 168 B.C. (see *MS*VI.B in the "List of Mawangdui Medical Manuscripts and Texts" below). However, evidence of name avoidance or the lack of it is often inconclusive. The manuscript containing the second *Laozi* edition avoids *bang* 邦, the personal name of the Han founder Liu Bang 劉邦 (the High Thearch 高帝, r. 202–195 B.C.), replacing it with *guo* 國. But the calligraphy looks identical to an astrological manuscript that refers to a date in the reign of Thearch Wen; both manuscripts were probably copied by a single scribe in the period 180–168 B.C. (*MWD*, vol. 1: "Chuban shuoming"). Curiously, the second *Laozi* edition does not avoid Thearch Wen's personal name; yet the medical manuscript (*MS*VI.B), copied during the same period of years, does. We do not have any contemporary accounts of the rules governing name avoidance in Qin and early Han times. The assumption has been that the use of the graph was prohibited during the reign of the thearch in question and perhaps for some time after the reign ended. This is borne out in the case of the medical manuscript (the reigning thearch's personal name is avoided), while the *Laozi* edition offers a counter-example. It is difficult to guess the factors that determined why one scribe observed the prohibition and another did not. And the example underscores the difficulty of relying on

---

[1]Discussions on dating the manuscripts tend to speak of Qin, late Qin, end of Qin and beginning of Han, early Han, etc. I find it more convenient to give approximate dates using multiples of five and ten years to replace the rough period designations.

name avoidance to date any of the Mawangdui manuscripts copied before Thearch Wen's reign.[1]

Examples of old Chu graphs in several manuscripts indicate that those manuscripts could only have been copied by scribes educated in the Chu tradition (Qiu Xigui 1990: 66; Li Xueqin 1981: 36-37). Changsha was politically attached to Chu before the Qin conquest and also participated in Chu culture. Simply based on the circumstances of the tomb, we might have surmised that the Mawangdui manuscripts were copied locally; the script evidence reinforces the surmise. There is also good evidence that some of the manuscripts were copied by a single scribe employed by Li fils. Five manuscripts in what appears to be the same calligraphy, a form of Han clerical script, can be dated to ca. 175 B.C.: the manuscript containing the second edition of the *Laozi*, the *Yijing* manuscript, a manuscript on physiognomizing horses, and two astrological manuscripts. Some common errors in writing graphs also run through all five manuscripts.[2] As for the medical manuscripts, some are older by virtue of their script and no two manuscripts are in the calligraphy of the same scribe; several contain the calligraphy of a second scribe. The majority of medical manuscripts were copied either before Li fils was born or during his infancy (assuming that he was about thirty when he was buried in 168 B.C.); either he collected old medical manuscripts himself or perhaps the manuscripts were part of an inherited family collection. Of course, dating the medical texts copied on the manuscripts is a separate problem from dating the manuscripts. In my judgment the medical texts are no earlier than third century B.C., and the Mawangdui manuscript editions of them may be fairly close in time to the original editions (see "Provenance and Hermeneutic Issues" below).

---

[1]The argument has also been made that avoidance of a thearch's personal name was observed after the reign ended, not during (Mansvelt Beck 1987: 68-76). But *MS*VI.B could only have been copied during Thearch Wen's reign (which ended after Li fils was buried). Lacking contemporary documentation of name-avoidance rules, it is best to approach all cases of name avoidance with caution and to consider this evidence in conjunction with other evidence for dating one of the manuscripts.

[2]One of the astrological manuscripts was used as evidence for dating the *Laozi* manuscript to the period 180-168 B.C. (*MWD*, vol. 1: "Chuban shuoming"). Li Xueqin identified the group of five manuscripts in private conversation in Beijing in winter 1993, judging them to have been written by the same scribe. Not all of the manuscripts have been published. For partial comparisons, see Fu and Chen 1992: 106 (*Yijing* hexagram text), 130 (second *Laozi* edition), and 132 (astrological manuscript).

LIST OF MAWANGDUI MEDICAL MANUSCRIPTS AND TEXTS

Five of the seven medical manuscripts are silk manuscripts; one consists of two sets of bamboo-slips, bound separately and rolled together in a single bundle; one consists of a set of wooden slips and a set of bamboo slips, bound separately and rolled together. The manuscripts do not include general titles for a whole manuscript nor do they provide titles for any of the texts within a manuscript. *MWD*, vol. 4, arranges the manuscripts in a sequence beginning with the longest silk manuscript and concluding with the two bamboo- and wooden-slip manuscripts; and assigns titles to the texts on each manuscript. The list of manuscripts and texts below follows the sequence of manuscripts in *MWD*, vol. 4, and identifies the assigned titles. To facilitate citation, I assign roman numerals I-VII to the manuscripts. When a manuscript contains a single text, no further indication is given; multiple texts on a manuscript are assigned letters. This form of identification is followed in the Translation, with the addition of arabic numerals to identify subdivisions of the texts in the translation (based on subdivisions in the original texts, like individual recipes in a recipe text). All references to the medical texts in the Prolegomena and Translation are in this citation style. Following the listing of each manuscript are data on its physical appearance, script, and date; and a brief description of the contents of each text.[1]

*MS*I

*MS*I.A "Zubi shiyi mai jiujing" 足臂十一脈灸經 (Cauterization canon of the eleven vessels of the foot and forearm)

*MS*I.B "Yin Yang shiyi mai jiujing," *jiaben* 陰陽十一脈灸經, 甲本 (Cauterization canon of the eleven Yin and Yang vessels, ed. A)

[1]Information on physical appearance, script, and dating is mostly taken from Ma Jixing 1992: 2-5, 8-11; and *MWD*, vol. 4: "Chuban shuoming." The photographic reproduction of the medical manuscripts in *MWD*, vol. 4, maintains the original size with the exception of *MS*II, which is approximately sixty percent of original size. Emura et al. 1987 is an index of the graphs in the medical manuscripts. The index reproduces different forms of the graphs as they appear in the seven manuscripts, which greatly facilitates study of the script and calligraphy. The exact location of each manuscript inside the lacquer box has been identified only for *MS*II, *MS*VI, and *MS*VII, which were in the long side-compartment. I presume that the other manuscripts (all silk) were folded and placed in the rectangular compartment.

MSI.C "Maifa" 脈法 (Model of the vessels)
MSI.D "Yin Yang mai sihou" 陰陽脈死候 (Death signs of the Yin and Yang vessels)
MSI.E "Wushier bingfang" 五十二病方 (Recipes for fifty-two ailments)

MSI is a silk manuscript approximately twenty-four centimeters wide and 450 centimeters long. The silk had been folded; when excavated, the silk at the creases had rotted, leaving a stack of over thirty leaves. *MSI*.E, with roughly 9,950 extant graphs, is the longest text on the manuscript and in the entire medical manuscript corpus.[1] It occupies approximately five sixths of *MSI*. The entire manuscript is in the calligraphy of the same scribe, with the exception of some text added at the end of *MSI*.E by a second scribe at a later date (*MSI*.E.283, and some fragments). The script used by the first scribe is a form of seal script that is older than the seal and clerical hybrid used in the manuscript containing the first edition of the *Laozi*. The script of the second scribe is similar to the script of the latter manuscript. The major portion of *MSI* in seal script was probably copied during the Qin, ca. 215 B.C.; and the addition by the second scribe probably dates to ca. 205–195 B.C.

MSI.A–B both describe the paths of eleven *mai* 脈 (vessels) inside the body; each vessel description is followed by a list of ailments associated with that vessel. There are six leg vessels and five arm vessels, which occur symmetrically on the left and right side of the body to give a total of twenty-two vessels (the Ceasing Yin vessel of the arm attested in the *Huangdi neijing* is absent). The arrangement of vessels in *MSI*.A is leg vessels first followed by arm vessels; each group is further subdivided into Yang and Yin vessels. *MSI*.B arranges the Yang vessels first and the Yin vessels second; within each group the leg vessels come before the arm vessels (the Yang arm-vessel names are "shoulder vessel," "ear vessel," and "tooth vessel," not the three technical names for the Yang vessels used elsewhere in *MSI*.A–B). Cauterization (*jiu* 灸) is the only therapy mentioned in both texts (at the end of every vessel entry in *MSI*.A, and once in *MSI*.B.9). The vessel descriptions in *MSI*.A are briefer and the listing of

---

[1]See Ma Jixing 1992: 4–5. Ma provides three graph-count estimates for the texts: extant graphs, graphs that can be added to fill lacunae, and the original number of graphs in each text (a judicious surmise). All three figures represent his editorial judgment, with which I am not always in agreement. However, his estimate of extant graphs is a useful indicator of the length of the texts relative to one another. I occasionally cite his estimates (especially for longer texts), but do not treat them as absolute figures.

ailments is less elaborate than in *MS*I.B. Also, *MS*I.B contains more text parallels with the enumeration of vessels and ailments in the *Lingshu* 10 essay entitled "Jingmai" 經脈 (Conduit vessels). *MS*II.B is another edition of *MS*I.B. A third edition of *MS*I.B occurs in the Zhangjiashan 張家山 manuscript *Maishu* 脈書 (Vessel book; see below). The *Maishu* edition is the best preserved of the three.

*MS*I.C is a brief discussion of vessel theory in three parts: the first discusses pathogenic conditions of *qi* 氣 (vapor) in the vessels and cauterization, concluding with a reference to cutting vessels open with a lancing-stone; the second concerns lancing technique, using the draining of pus from abscesses with lancing-stones as a model for how to open vessels; the third discusses vessel diagnosis, performed at the ankle. *MS*I.C was so severely damaged that it was largely unreadable before the discovery of a second edition in the Zhangjiashan *Maishu*.

*MS*I.D is the shortest text on the manuscript (approximately eighty-nine extant graphs). It concerns fatal signs associated with the Yin and Yang vessels as well as with five body constituents: flesh, bone, vapor, blood, and muscle. A second edition occurs in the *Maishu*.

*MS*I.E is a manual of recipes to treat ailments, arranged by categories of ailment. A list of the ailment categories at the beginning of the text gives fifty-two names. At the end of the text the second scribe added recipes for several more ailments which are not indicated in the original list. In its current state of preservation there are 283 recipes (nineteen fragments from the left end of *MS*I are transcribed in *MWD*, vol. 4: 76-82, but I do not translate them and do not include them in the recipe count). The ailments range from flesh wounds and warts to hemorrhoids, snake bites, and child sprites (a demonic affliction). The recipes sometimes are a brief sentence (to treat a snake bite, "daub mulberry liquid on it"), and sometimes include detailed descriptions of symptoms, drug preparation, and therapy. Nearly forty recipes detail exorcistic incantations and magico-religious operations; and they are interspersed among recipes for the same ailments which use drugs and other therapies.

*MS*II

*MS*II.A "Quegu shiqi" 却穀食氣 (Eliminating grain and eating vapor)

*MS*II.B "Yin Yang shiyi mai jiujing," *yiben* 陰陽十一脈灸經，乙本 (Cauterization canon of the eleven Yin and Yang vessels, ed. B)

*MS*II.C "Daoyin tu" 導引圖 (Drawings of guiding and pulling)

*MS*II is a silk manuscript forty-nine to fifty centimeters wide and 110 centimeters long. The manuscript was found beneath *MS*VI and *MS*VII in the side-compartment of the lacquer box. *MS*II.A-B occupy roughly eighteen centimeters at the front of the manuscript, written on twenty-six columns ruled in red ink. Another twenty ruled columns which are blank follow (evidently more texts were planned for the manuscript than were actually copied onto it). The *MS*II.C drawings begin immediately after the blank columns. *MS*II.A-B are in the calligraphy of a single scribe; the script is a hybrid of seal and clerical. The manuscript was probably copied ca. 205–195 B.C.

*MS*II.A concerns dietetics and breath cultivation in macrobiotic hygiene. The first part of the text discusses the technique of "eliminating grain" (*quegu* 却穀; that is, eliminating ordinary foodstuffs) by consuming the herb *shiwei* 石韋 (pyrrosia) and by performing breathing exercises in the morning and evening. The second part discusses a seasonal regimen of breath cultivation, identifying five vapors in the external atmosphere to be avoided and six to be consumed by the practitioner. Seasonal cultivation of the "six vapors" is similar but not identical to breath cultivation in the lost *Lingyang Ziming jing* 陵陽子明經, fragments of which are preserved in early commentaries. *MS*II.B is another edition of *MS*I.B, probably included in *MS*II because of the importance of vessel theory for macrobiotic hygiene (I do not translate *MS*II.B).

*MS*II.C consists of forty-four drawings of human figures performing exercises. Many of the drawings are damaged and most of the original captions with the names of the exercises are missing. The extant names indicate that some exercises are intended to treat ailments while others are part of a program of hygienic cultivation. One or two of the exercise names are attested in received literature. The Zhangjiashan manuscript *Yinshu* 引書 (Pulling book; see below) provides written descriptions of many exercises, some of which have the same name as drawings in *MS*II.C. However, the *Yinshu* descriptions mostly do not match the *MS*II.C drawings. *Yinshu* and *MS*II.C both exemplify the hygienic exercise tradition known as *daoyin* 導引 (guiding and pulling) in early sources.

*MS*III

*MS*III "Yangsheng fang" 養生方 (Recipes for nurturing life)

*MS*III is a silk manuscript approximately twenty-four centimeters wide. The silk is severely damaged, making it impossible to accurately estimate the length (the extant pieces in the reproduction measure roughly 140 centimeters). The script is a hybrid of seal and clerical similar to *MS*II (the calligraphy is not identical); *MS*III was probably also copied ca. 205–195 B.C.

*MS*III is basically a recipe manual for macrobiotic hygiene. In its present state of preservation there are eighty-seven recipes, followed by several entries related to sexual cultivation and exercise. There is a list of recipe categories at the end. Recipes for tonic drugs, foods, and beverages occur throughout the text. Aphrodisiacs for men and women are grouped in the first half of the text, interspersed with other types of recipes. Two recipe categories near the end of the text concern travel, including recipes for increasing one's speed on the road. The travel recipes are about evenly divided between drugs and magical operations. The final entries related to sexual cultivation and exercise include several text parallels with *MS*VI.A–B and *MS*VII.B. *MS*III.91 is a labeled diagram of the female genitals.

*MS*IV

*MS*IV "Zaliao fang" 雜療方 (Recipes for various cures)

*MS*IV is a silk manuscript approximately twenty-four centimeters wide. The silk is severely damaged (the extant pieces in the reproduction measure sixty-five centimeters). Following *MS*IV.25 there are about six blank ruled columns before a major gap in the manuscript. The script of *MS*IV.1–25 and *MS*IV.26–42 (after the blank columns and gap) is similar—a seal script reminiscent of *MS*I. However, the calligraphy of *MS*IV.26–42 does not match *MS*IV.1–25. The two sections were evidently copied by different scribes. The contents of the two sections are also sufficiently different to warrant identifying *MS*IV.1–25 and *MS*IV.26–42 as distinct texts on the manuscript. The title assigned to the whole manuscript in *MWD*, vol. 4, reflects a judgment that the two sections constitute a single text of mixed content. While the grounds for a formal division into two texts are strong (especially the occurrence of blank columns separating the two sections), I refrain from altering the identification of *pian* given in *MWD*, vol. 4.[1] Based on the similarity between the script of *MS*I and *MS*IV, *MS*IV was probably copied ca. 215–205 B.C.

Most of the recipes in *MS*IV.1–25 are similar to the aphrodisiacs and tonics of *MS*III. *MS*IV.22–23 concern burial of the afterbirth to ensure the well-being of the newborn infant. *MS*IV.28–35 are recipes for venomous bites, in particular attacks by a deadly southern water creature named *yu* 蜮 (*yu* lore is well represented in received sources, but the biological identity of the creature is unknown). Most of these recipes are magical.

MSV

*MS*V "Taichan shu" 胎 産 書 (Book of the generation of the fetus)

*MS*V is a silk manuscript approximately forty-nine centimeters wide and forty-nine centimeters long. It was folded into quarters. The script is similar to the Qin clerical script of the Shuihudi 睡 虎 地 tomb 11 manuscripts (burial dated ca. 217 B.C.). The graph *zhi* 雉 occurs in the text, which is the personal name of Dowager Lü 呂 太 后. Dowager Lü was the de facto ruler of the Han realm from 188–180 B.C. (Twitchett and Loewe 1986: 135–36). Both the type of clerical script and the lack of name avoidance suggest a date before 188 B.C. for *MS*V, perhaps as much as several decades before.

The contents of *MS*V all concern childbirth. The top half contains two drawings. The first drawing represents a technique for predicting the child's fortune at birth by consulting two human figures surrounded by the twelve Branch signs. The same drawing occurs in the first Shuihudi hemerological manuscript, which includes text to explain its use (see "Other Excavated Manuscripts Related to Medicine" below). The second drawing is a chart used to determine the most auspicious burial site for the afterbirth; the use of the chart is explained in *MS*IV.22. *MS*V.3 is a description of gestation with instructions for the care of the fetus during pregnancy. There are extensive text parallels in the medieval *Zhubing yuanhoulun* 諸 病 源 候 論, "Renzhen hou" 妊 娠 候; and *Qianjin yao-*

[1] Emura et al. also note the calligraphic differences between the two sections of *MS*IV and suggest that they are two *pian* rather than one (1987: v).

fang 千金要方, "Xu Zhicai zhuyue yangtai fang" 徐之才逐月養胎方 (both texts are reproduced in *MWD*, vol. 4: 140–41). *MS*V.3 is clearly the textual antecedent of the medieval accounts of gestation. *MS*V concludes with recipes for afterbirth burial, child conception, gender fixing, easing birth, and ensuring the child's vigor.

*MS*VI

*MS*VI.A "Shiwen" 十問 (Ten questions)
*MS*VI.B "He Yin Yang" 合陰陽 (Conjoining Yin and Yang)

The 101 bamboo slips of *MS*VI.A are approximately twenty-three centimeters long and .8 centimeters wide; the thirty-two bamboo slips of *MS*VI.B are approximately twenty-three centimeters long and one centimeter wide. The two sets of slips were originally bound separately. *MS*VI.A had been rolled first and *MS*VI.B was rolled around the outside of *MS*VI.A. The bundle was set on top of the silk manuscripts in the side-compartment of the lacquer box. The binding cords were disintegrated and the slips slightly jumbled. The exact position of each slip at the time of excavation and the contents of the texts were used to restore the correct sequence of slips (I differ with *MWD*, vol. 4, over the sequence of slips in *MS*VI.A). The script in both texts is Han clerical with a cursive quality to it; however, the calligraphy in each belongs to a different scribe (*MS*VI.B is more cursive than *MS*VI.A). Perhaps these texts written by different scribes on separate sets of bound bamboo-slips were always kept as a single manuscript in Li fils' book collection; but it is also possible that they were first rolled together when they were placed in the lacquer box. In the case of *MS*VII, it is very unlikely that the wooden and bamboo slips of *MS*VII.A-B were kept as a single manuscript prior to being placed in the box. However, rolling two sets of bound slips—each containing a different text—into a single bundle may have been a common practice when storing bound-slip books. Thus I concur with *MWD*, vol. 4, which treats the two bundles of slips as two manuscripts (*MS*VI and *MS*VII) with two texts each rather than break the two bundles into four separate manuscripts. *MS*VI.B writes the name of Constancy Mountain (the northern of the five sacred peaks) as 常山, replacing the original graph *heng* 恒 in the name of the mountain with *chang* 常 to avoid the personal name of Thearch Wen (the fact that *chang* was first used in the mountain name because of Thearch Wen is well documented). It must be post-180 B.C. *MS*VI.A is probably no older.

*MS*VI.A contains ten dialogues in which ten macrobiotic specialists respond to questions. The Yellow Thearch is the questioner in the first four dialogues, a reflection of his role as a student of esoteric knowledge in third to first century B.C. literature (the *Huangdi neijing* is the most notable example of the dialogue genre featuring the Yellow Thearch; Seidel 1969: 50-51). Rong Cheng 容成 and Ancestor Peng 彭祖, well-known exponents of macrobiotic hygiene in received literature, are among the specialists. The teachings include instructions for executing cultivation techniques, often describing the process in esoteric and metaphoric language. There are a number of text parallels with the sexual cultivation techniques in *MS*VI.B and *MS*VII.B.

*MS*VI.B focuses on sexual cultivation. The text opens with an esoteric poem summarizing intercourse from foreplay to achieving the goal of sexual cultivation. Subsequent sections of the text analyze the sex act and classify its essential parts in order to make intercourse conform to a macrobiotic regimen. Both *MS*VI.B and *MS*VII.B are the textual antecedents of the medieval sex manuals preserved in chapter 28 of the tenth century Japanese medical compendium *Ishinpô* 醫心方.

*MS*VII

*MS*VII.A "Zajin fang" 雜禁方 (Recipes for various charms)

*MS*VII.B "Tianxia zhidao tan" 天下至道談 (Discussion of the culminant way in Under-heaven)

The eleven wooden slips of *MS*VII.A are approximately twenty-three centimeters long and 1.2 centimeters wide; the fifty-six bamboo slips of *MS*VII.B are approximately twenty-eight centimeters long and .5 centimeters wide. The two sets of slips were originally bound separately. *MS*VII.B was rolled around two bamboo flutes (one about twenty-five centimeters long, the other about twenty-one centimeters) and *MS*VII.A was rolled around the outside of *MS*VII.B. The bundle was placed beside *MS*VI in the side-compartment. As with *MS*VI, the sequence of the loose slips was reconstructed based on their position at the time of excavation and on the contents of the texts (I differ with *MWD*, vol. 4, over the sequence of slips in *MS*VII.A). The script in *MS*VII.A is highly cursive Han clerical; *MS*VII.B is written in a more regular Han clerical. Both texts were probably copied within a period of one or two decades before Li fils' burial.

The charms and philters in *MS*VII.A reflect popular magic of the times. Crying infants and marital disharmony are among the daily problems that can be stopped by spreading a five-*chi* band of mud at specified places. An opponent in a suit will be magically trampled if you write the person's name and put it in your shoe. Three of the four philter recipes are to seduce the object of desire; one is to split apart a married couple. This type of popular magic also occurs in medieval literature, as attested both in chapter 26 of the *Ishinpô* and in the demonography *Baizetu* 白 澤 圖.

*MS*VII.B concerns primarily, but not exclusively, sexual cultivation. Numerous text parallels with *MS*VI.B suggest that the contents of both texts were drawn from a common body of macrobiotic literature (which also accounts for the text parallels in *MS*III and *MS*VI.A). In addition to sections which classify parts of the sex act like *MS*VI.B, there are several sections with brief essays that are unique to *MS*VII.B. The assigned title in *MWD*, vol. 4, is taken from a heading written on a separate slip at the beginning of *MS*VII.B.3.

OTHER EXCAVATED MANUSCRIPTS RELATED TO MEDICINE

The Mawangdui medical manuscripts remain the largest single collection of third to second century B.C. medical literature currently known to us. However, bamboo- and wooden-slip manuscripts from five additional tombs (the earliest is ca. 230–220 B.C.; the latest is first century A.D.) supplement the Mawangdui medical manuscripts and broaden our knowledge of early Chinese medicine. Not all of them are exclusively medical manuscripts, but all fall within the category of *fang*-literature. Still other tombs have yielded exemplars of *fang*-literature exclusive of medical contents. Even these discoveries are significant because they testify to the dissemination of *fang*-literature across the several geographical and cultural regions of ancient China. While we still cannot quantify exactly how popular *fang*-literature was among the elite, we at least know that the Mawangdui collection of *fang*-literature is not an isolated phenomenon.

Two medical manuscripts from Zhangjiashan 張 家 山 tomb 247 in Jiangling 江 陵, Hubei, are particularly important. The tomb, which was excavated in late 1983, dates to no later than the mid-second century B.C. The tomb is near in date to Mawangdui tomb 3 and is also situated in the old land of Chu. In addition to the medical manuscripts, tomb 247 contained judicial and administrative documents as well as works on military strategy and mathematical calculations. All of the manuscripts are written in Han clerical script.[1] Titles written on the back side of the first slip of each manuscript are in the calligraphy of a single scribe, suggesting that the titles were not original but were added to the manuscripts as a group afterwards. Whether the titles represent the generally acknowledged name for the text(s) placed on a particular manuscript, whether the scribe added descriptive titles under instructions from the man buried in tomb 247, or whether the titles were added after his death when these manuscripts were selected as burial goods from his book collection is not certain.[2]

The medical manuscripts are titled *Maishu* 脈書 (Vessel book) and *Yinshu* 引書 (Pulling book).[3] *Maishu* contains six texts for which I assign titles as follows: "Ailment List" (SS1-15); "Eleven Vessels" (SS16-47; another edition of *MSI*.B); "Five Signs of Death" (SS48-51; another edition of *MSI*.D); "Care of the Body" (SS51-52); "Six Constituents" (SS53-55); and "Vessels and Vapor" (SS55-65; another edition of *MSI*.C). "Ailment List" contains sixty-seven ailment names, sometimes with a few phrases on the symptoms of an ailment (five of the ailment names are lost because of lacunae). Most of the list is arranged anatomically: beginning at the head and ending at the feet, fifty-seven ailments are associated with a specific part of the body. Ten additional ailments that are not readily attached to a single region of the body conclude the list. "Ailment List"

---

[1]See Zhangjiashan Han mu zhujian zhengli xiaozu 1985. An inventory of burial goods includes the manuscripts in the list, which is the earliest example of manuscripts being included in an inventory (the Mawangdui tomb 3 inventory does not mention manuscripts).

[2]I am indebted to Li Xueqin for information regarding the manuscript titles. The work of editing the Zhangjiashan manuscripts is not yet finished, and only selected transcriptions have appeared in simplified graphs in *Wenwu*.

[3]*Maishu* contains sixty-five bamboo slips; it is transcribed in simplified graphs in *MSSW* (the original slips are not reproduced). *Yinshu* contains 113 slips; it is transcribed in simplified graphs in *YSSW* (slips not reproduced). The transcriptions mark the end of each slip but do not number them. Printing errors in *MSSW* affect both the identification of the individual slips and several graphs. I am indebted to Li Xueqin, one of the editors of the Zhangjiashan manuscripts, for re-checking the photographic reproduction of *Maishu* kept at the Bureau of Cultural Relics in Beijing and providing me with corrections to *MSSW* (Professor Li's corrections have been incorporated in the transcription of *MSI*.B, *MSI*.C, and *MSI*.D in Appendix 1). I am not aware of errors in *YSSW*. However, it is best to regard both transcriptions as provisional until reproductions of the manuscripts have been published. I have assigned the slip numbers which I use to identify the separate texts contained in the two manuscripts. Lian Shaoming (1989) and Ma Jixing (1992: 158-72) examine the contents of *Maishu*; Peng Hao (1990), Li Xueqin (1991), and Li Ling (1993: 335-46) do the same for *Yinshu*.

includes ailment names that are attested in received literature as well as names that were previously known only in the Mawangdui medical manuscripts. Vessel theory pathology does not enter into the identification of ailments in "Ailment List." Thus I cite it whenever possible to identify ailments in the Mawangdui medical manuscripts; and I correspondingly avoid relying on the understanding of a particular ailment in the *Huangdi neijing*, which represents a later understanding grounded in vessel theory.

There are minor differences between *MS*I.B and "Eleven Vessels," which I attribute to the fact that "Eleven Vessels" is a younger edition. Several differences between *MS*I.B and *MS*II.B suggest to me that *MS*I.B and "Eleven Vessels" are more closely related, while *MS*II.B may represent a different line of transmission (see Appendix 1). "Care of the Body" begins without interruption following "Five Signs of Death" in S51. It is a short statement on macrobiotic hygiene and the vessels. "Six Constituents" is an account of the six basic constituents of the body: bone, muscle, blood, vessel, flesh, and vapor. Each constituent exhibits a characteristic form of pain; and pain is a forewarning of physical breakdown. Following "Six Constituents," "Vessels and Vapor" begins without interruption in the bottom of S55 and continues to the end of the manuscript. The manuscript itself does not indicate any division between the end of "Five Signs of Death" and the beginning of "Care of the Body," nor between "Six Constituents" and "Vessels and Vapor."

With the discovery of *Maishu* we have confirmation that three of the texts on *MS*I circulated among physicians and the elite during the second century B.C. (recall that *MS*I was probably copied before the end of the third century B.C.). While the two manuscripts share three texts in common, they have selected differently from the pool of written medical knowledge for their remaining texts. The combining of "Five Signs of Death" with "Care of the Body," and of "Six Constituents" with "Vessels and Vapor" in *Maishu* is noteworthy for placing a greater emphasis on macrobiotic hygiene than is evident in *MS*I. I view the combination of texts in *Maishu* as indicative of the influence of macrobiotic hygiene in the development of vessel theory (see Section Three, "Physiology").

The entirety of *Yinshu* may be a single text devoted to exercise theory and practice within macrobiotic hygiene.[1] I divide the manuscript into three texts, partly to facilitate reference to it and partly because it seems

[1] Li Xueqin treats *Yinshu* as one text whose contents he divides into six sections (1991: 8).

possible that these three portions of the manuscript could have been combined with different works to fashion other manuscripts. The texts, with my assigned titles, are: "Seasonal Regimen" (SS1-7); "Exercises" (SS8-103); and "Cultivation of the Body" (SS104-113). "Seasonal Regimen" concerns the hygienic activity appropriate for each season, including the morning wake-up routine and the times of the day when sexual intercourse is permitted. The text is introduced as the way of Ancestor Peng. "Exercises" begins with basic exercise movements, most of which have names ("measuring worm," "tiger pulling," "pulling Yang," etc.). Next are descriptions of exercise routines used for specific conditions—mostly ailments with some hygiene mixed in. Breathing is an integral part of the exercise routines. "Exercises" ends with a list of exercises and the parts of the body each exercise benefits. "Cultivation of the Body" concerns hygienic theory and the nature of illness.

Shuanggudui 雙古堆 tomb 1 in Fuyang 阜陽, Anhui, is the burial of Xiahou Zao 夏侯竈, the second Lord of Ruyin 汝陰侯, who died in 165 B.C. according to historical records. The tomb was excavated in 1977. The bamboo and wooden slips of the manuscripts were not well preserved, thus the greater part of the texts is lost. Among the texts identified are fragments of the *Shijing* 詩經, *Yijing* 易經, and *Chuci* 楚辭. There are also texts on physiognomizing dogs, astrology, and hemerology. Among literature related to medicine, little remains of a text on breath cultivation, which is unfortunate because it might have supplemented *Yinshu* and the Mawangdui macrobiotic hygiene texts. However, another manuscript is a unique discovery for early Chinese medicine. The contents are not strictly medical. The manuscript lists various substances, and for each identifies its applications (Fuyang Han jian zhenglizu 1983).

The title *Wanwu* 萬物 (Myriad things) has been assigned to the manuscript, based on a reference to the necessity of "investigating the myriad things" on the first slip (Fuyang Han jian zhenglizu 1988; Hu and Han 1988). *Wanwu* catalogues human curiosity about the products of nature: a horse-gullet tube can be used to breathe under water; metal from Yue 越 is best for working with jade; *banxia* 半夏 (pinellia) fattens pigs; alkaline soil prevents drowsiness; *shiwei* 石韋 (pyrrosia) cures urine retention. *Wanwu* represents a type of *fang*-literature similar to the *Huainan wanbishu* 淮南萬畢術 (ca. first century B.C.) and to passages in the *Shanhaijing* 山海經 (ca. fourth century B.C.) which enumerate substances and their uses, including drugs used to cure ailments or to enhance physical well-being.[1] *Wanwu* lists many drugs used for ailments or for hygienic cultivation. Moreover, it shares drug and ailment names in common with the Mawangdui medical manuscripts; and the specific applications of some drugs to either an ailment or a cultivation technique also match. Thus, we now know that the drug knowledge implicit in many of the Mawangdui recipes was being disseminated in digests like *Wanwu* (and the site of Shuanggudui tomb 1 extends the range of dissemination beyond Chu and into the Yellow River region). *Wanwu* provides a clear antecedent to the genre of materia medica, the oldest received text being the *Shennong bencaojing* 神農本草經 (Divine Agrarian's canon of materia medica) from the first or second century A.D. (the term *bencao* 本草 denoting knowledge of materia medica is not attested before the second half of the first century B.C.).[2]

Another type of early *fang*-literature are compilations combining astrology and hemerology with an assortment of material related to divination and magic. Two such third century B.C. manuscripts were excavated from Shuihudi 睡虎地 tomb 11 at Yunmeng 雲夢, Hubei, in 1977. The tomb dates to ca. 217 B.C., and is the site more often noted for the discovery of Qin judicial and administrative manuscripts (Hulsewé 1985). The second manuscript bears the title *Rishu* 日書 (Day book) at the end, referring to hemerological arts. Han accounts attest to the popularity of hemerological treatises among the elite. They were one of the vehicles for the dissemination of Yin Yang and Five Agent theories, whose correlations lay at the base of many of the numerological systems that determined whether a particular time or location was lucky or unlucky. As evidenced by the Shuihudi hemerological manuscripts, they were also a grab bag of miscellaneous occult knowledge (Harper 1985: 462–70). Hemerological texts have been recovered from other third and second century B.C. tombs, most recently in 1986 from Fangmatan 放馬灘 tomb 1 at Tianshui 天水, Gansu—a tomb that probably dates to ca. 230–220 B.C.[3]

---

[1]The *Huainan wanbishu* (current editions are reconstructions based on preserved quotations) is associated with the *fangshi* 方士 (recipe gentlemen) at the Huainan court of Liu An 劉安 in the second century B.C. (Kusuyama 1987). Drugs and their uses in the *Shanhaijing*, a work replete with magico-religious lore, are itemized in Zhao Pushan 1986.

[2]See the discussion of *bencao* in Unschuld 1986a: 11–16. Unschuld does not refer to *Wanwu* because he was writing before the transcription was published.

[3]Transcriptions and reproductions of the two Shuihudi hemerological manuscripts are in *SHD*. The contents of the two Fangmatan manuscripts are described in He Shuangquan 1989a and 1989b; a transcription in simplified graphs of the first manuscript (without reproduction) is in Qin

Sections on iatromancy in the Shuihudi and Fangmatan hemerological treatises suggest cross-influences between iatromantic prediction of the cause and course of an ailment and the vessel-based diagnosis performed by physicians like those whose ideas are contained in the *Huangdi neijing*. Perhaps the iatromantic systems—which utilize Yin Yang and Five Agent theories—preceded vessel-based diagnosis, which for the first time incorporated Yin Yang and Five Agent ideas into medical diagnosis.[1] Iatromantic ideas are not evident in the Mawangdui medical manuscripts. However, other kinds of sharing between the Shuihudi and Mawangdui manuscripts are in evidence. The method for predicting the fortune of a child based on the Branch sign of the date of birth in the first Shuihudi hemerological manuscript (*SHD*: 206) occurs in *MSV*.1. The belief that demons cause ailments, which are cured by exorcising the demons, is documented in a short demonography entitled "Jie" 詰 (Spellbinding) in the first hemerological manuscript; the same conception underlies the magical recipes in *MSI*.E (*SHD*: 212-16; Harper 1985; Harper 1990: 217-25). And scattered throughout the Shuihudi and Fangmatan hemerological manuscripts is evidence of magic—incantations and other magico-religious acts—that has exact counterparts in the Mawangdui medical manuscripts. Thus, the hemerological manuscripts provide yet another context for occult knowledge which in the Mawangdui manuscripts is presented in a primarily medical context (see Section Five, "Magical Recipes" and "Varieties of Magic"). Evidently by the third century B.C. this kind of occult knowledge was being widely disseminated in *fang*-literature, be it in medical books or in hemerological treatises. The geographic distribution of the excavated hemerological manuscripts from the north to the south once again attests to the broad dispersion of the knowledge contained in *fang*-literature.

---

jian zhengli xiaozu 1989. I follow Li Xueqin's judgment on the dating of the Fangmatan tomb (1990). To date, none of the second century B.C. hemerological treatises have been published.

[1]For iatromancy in the Shuihudi hemerological manuscripts, see *SHD*: 193, 245-46. The passages identify the demonic origin of an ailment and predict its course based on the conquest sequence of the Five Agents. I am currently preparing a study of the relation between the Shuihudi iatromantic passages and prognosis in the *Huangdi neijing*. Yamada (1980) has already demonstrated the influence of wind divination involving the deity Taiyi 太一 in the *Huangdi neijing* (cf. Unschuld 1982a; Unschuld 1985: 68-71). The occult, hemerological elements are eliminated or marginalized in the *Huangdi neijing*. He Shuangquan (1989a: 27) refers briefly to the Fangmatan treatise with iatromantic material, but the manuscript is not yet published.

The final site to yield manuscripts related to medicine is a tomb near Wuwei 武威, Gansu, excavated in 1972. The tomb dates to sometime in the first century A.D. Two sets of wooden slips were discovered—a total of seventy-eight slips—containing recipes to treat ailments. The binding cords had disintegrated; while it is not possible to reconstruct the original sequence of the slips in each set, the several slips recording a single recipe can be grouped together by context. Another fourteen wooden tablets were also discovered, most of which had several columns of text written on both surfaces of the tablet. One tablet concerns hemerological prohibitions related to medical treatment; one concerns astrology; and one is a drug price list. The remaining eleven tablets contain recipes similar to those in the wooden slips. The drugs, ailments, and treatments in the Wuwei recipes are quite similar to the Mawangdui recipes texts, in particular *MSI.E*. In tracing developments in early Chinese medicine, the Wuwei medical manuscripts provide an important bridge between the Mawangdui medical manuscripts and later received medical literature.[1] There have been other discoveries in the northwest of Later Han wooden slips and tablets with medical contents, but none comparable to the Wuwei manuscripts (Unschuld 1986a: 15).

PROVENANCE AND HERMENEUTIC ISSUES

In order to better situate the Mawangdui medical manuscripts in the overall scheme of early medicine and medical literature one would like to know much more about their history before the manuscripts were packed in the lacquer box and buried. Speculation on the intellectual and social milieu in which medical and other manuscripts related to natural philosophy and occult thought circulated will occupy us in Section Two. The contents of the Mawangdui medical manuscripts are surveyed in the subsequent three sections. My purpose here is to raise briefly several textual questions concerning the manuscripts. How old are the texts? Who were the authors, the scribes, the collectors? Are the manuscripts representative of third to second century B.C. medical literature? What sort of interpretive principles are best applied to the manuscripts? There are, of course, no absolute answers to the questions, yet addressing them brings some clarity to the evaluation of the medical manuscripts.

---

[1] *WWYJ* provides a photographic reproduction, facsimile, and transcription; *KGS*, vol. 1: 363-404, gives a transcription and Japanese translation.

For reasons discussed in Section Two I assume that physicians were primarily responsible for medical literature, of which the earliest examples are now the Mawangdui medical manuscripts. At the same time, the elite participated in medicine, and the probability is great that the elite contributed to the production and dispersion of medical literature. Moreover, oral medical knowledge of both the popular and esoteric varieties was being continually committed to writing in ways that we cannot trace exactly. Pronouncing final judgment on the provenance of the Mawangdui medical manuscripts is not feasible. But as indicated in the listing of the fourteen medical texts and in the survey of other excavated manuscripts above, the Mawangdui manuscripts exhibit a range of textual relations not only with the other manuscripts but also with later received medical literature. This alone justifies a presumption of representativeness for them.

Who copied the medical manuscripts and how they were acquired are matters for conjecture. Li fils' manuscript corpus includes many examples of *fang*-literature in addition to the medical manuscripts. Other members of the Li family may have preceded Li fils in collecting *fang*-literature. He himself no doubt patronized specialists in natural philosophy and occult knowledge. Perhaps the very specialists he patronized were the scribes of his manuscripts; he even might have copied several himself (the transmission of *fang*-literature and elite patronage are examined in Section Two, "Readership and Transmission"). We also know that in the second century B.C. men of education were employed to "copy books" (*xieshu* 寫書) for others. Thearch Wu established an office for "copying books" to supply his library with fair editions of all works of literature, presumably employing as scribes the same men who filled other positions in the bureaucracy by virtue of their literacy (*Hanshu*, 30.1b). The ruling family in the second century B.C. included several prominent book collectors. Liu De 劉德, the King of Hejian 河間王 (r. 155-129 B.C.), acquired many valuable old manuscripts by offering rewards and promising to provide the donor with a "fair copy" 好寫. He obviously maintained a staff of scribes. Liu An 劉安 (179-122 B.C.), the King of Huainan 淮南王, was also "fond of books" and must have kept a staff of scribes to copy the *fang*-literature for which he was renowned (*Hanshu*, 53.1b). In Li fils we witness the bibliophilia of a broader spectrum of the elite (silk manuscripts were a luxury). In any case, in the second century B.C. it is too early to speak of a commercial book trade (the earliest reference to something we might call a bookshop where books were sold is first century A.D.; Tsien 1962: 15).

Turning to the question of the age of the medical texts, one must keep in mind that private literature did not exist before the fifth century B.C. Earlier writing consisted primarily of official records and collections like the *Shijing*, which by the age of Confucius were revered as canons (Tsien 1962: 9–11). The Warring States was a watershed for the rise of private literature, the most prominent received examples being the books of the philosophers. *Fang*-literature surely circulated in the fourth century B.C., however I regard the third century B.C. as the upper limit for the Mawangdui medical texts (some must be early second century B.C.). My judgment is influenced both by simple skepticism and by the contents of the Mawangdui texts. The third century B.C. saw the rapid development of medical ideas (including ideas about macrobiotic hygiene) and of natural philosophy in general. For vessel theory texts like *MS*I.A–B to be relevant to medicine in the early second century B.C., I doubt that they would not reflect third century B.C. developments. Macrobiotic teachings in *MS*VI.A.9–10 are attributed to two physicians who flourished in the late-fourth and early-third centuries B.C. The teachings themselves were probably recorded somewhat later; and the entirety of *MS*VI.A with its full cast of legendary specialists is best treated as third century B.C. The composition of the recipe texts would have been especially fluid, since any one text might have drawn its collection of recipes from a variety of written and oral sources. There is certainly old medical knowledge in the recipes of *MS*I.E, but lacking clear textual evidence of their antiquity I do not think we are justified in dating the text earlier than the third century B.C.

My assessment might change were fourth century B.C. tombs to yield comparable texts, but to date manuscripts from the late fourth century have been markedly more lapidary than third and second century B.C. manuscripts. A prime example of what could be called *fang*-literature is the divination manuscript from Baoshan 包山 tomb 2, Hubei, excavated in 1987. Written in Chu script in a terse, hieratic style, the manuscript is a personal record of turtle-shell divination and hexagram divination performed for the benefit of the tomb occupant during his lifetime (Hubei sheng Jing Sha tielu kaogudui 1991: 32–37). The world of divination and religion reflected in the text belongs to a time preceding the pervasive influence of correlative cosmology reflected in the third century B.C.

Fangmatan and Shuihudi hemerological manuscripts. To generalize from a single example is incautious, but significant spiritual and intellectual changes were clearly underway between the fourth and third centuries B.C. The changes produced a flowering of specialists in natural philosophy and occult knowledge in the third century B.C., as well as an explosion of *fang*-literature. The Mawangdui medical texts belong to the third century B.C. explosion along with the hemerological literature.

Where are we to place the Mawangdui medical texts in relation to Chunyu Yi's 淳于意 medical writings and the *Huangdi neijing*? The simple answer is "before." Complications immediately arise. Certainly the vessel theory texts in *MSI* reflect an earlier theoretical stage than the *Lingshu* 10 essay and other writings on vessel theory in the *Huangdi neijing*. Placing the *Huangdi neijing* after the Mawangdui texts makes sense, and for a variety of reasons the first century B.C. represents the best date for its composition. Yet Chunyu Yi's career in medicine overlapped the life of Li fils. His medical writings reflect an understanding of vessel theory different from the *Huangdi neijing*, but definitely more theoretically elaborate than the Mawangdui texts. Moreover, while Chunyu Yi used acupuncture infrequently, he did know the therapy. How are we to explain the contemporaneous Mawangdui texts (and Zhangjiashan editions) which do not know acupuncture?

One could propose several explanations—differences between medicine in the south (Chu 楚) and northeast (Qi 齊), Chunyu Yi's superior medical knowledge, etc. I think this is not the best approach to take to the problem. Ultimately, between the Mawangdui texts, Chunyu Yi's writings, and the *Huangdi neijing*, we still lack sufficient evidence to fashion a complete, diachronic account of the development of medicine from the Warring States to the Han. A synchronic account of medicine in the third and early-second centuries B.C. based on the Mawangdui texts would also be seriously flawed. The texts are representative of medicine at that time, but one cannot claim they are the totality of medicine—and except for the Zhangjiashan manuscripts, there is as yet no other evidence. If the texts do not directly explain the genesis of acupuncture and of *Huangdi neijing* medicine, they are nevertheless examples of medical literature before the *Huangdi neijing*. They are an embarrassment of riches; they are invaluable historical documents. The factual information contained in the Mawangdui medical manuscripts—which was unknown before their discovery—restores a picture of early Chinese medicine that had vanished from the received tradition. The manuscripts provide the basis for investigating a broader range of issues in early Chinese medicine than was possible in the past.

As a collection of texts unedited since burial in 168 B.C., the Mawangdui medical manuscripts present interpretive difficulties. The texts predate script normalization which tended to designate specific graphs as the standard graphs for specific words; in numerous instances the words and meanings intended by the graphs written in the texts are not obvious. Vocabulary can be technical and arcane, some of it obsolete and unattested outside of the manuscripts. And the idiom is sometimes puzzling. In received texts many of these difficulties have been smoothed out over the centuries in editions which use standard graphs and in commentaries which intend to make the meaning of the old texts plain. Indeed, we are accustomed to viewing ancient literature through the hermeneutic lens of editors and commentators (often the same individual). Already accorded canonical status in Han times, the subsequent history of the *Huangdi neijing* wedded the original text to the hermeneutic endeavors of its editors and commentators.

Huangdi neijing hermeneutics is a complex subject that cannot be investigated here. I raise it because of a tendency among some scholars working on the Mawangdui medical manuscripts to rely overmuch on the *Huangdi neijing* to interpret the Mawangdui texts; and to adopt the *Huangdi neijing* as the standard against which the Mawangdui texts are to be judged. Unattested anatomical terms are sometimes identified by reading the graphs as equivalent to graphs used to name acupuncture points (even though the Mawangdui texts predate the existence of a system of named acupuncture points). Ailments may be explained according to *Huangdi neijing* etiology; *Huangdi neijing* theory read into passages in the Mawangdui texts; and *Huangdi neijing* parallels used to edit (and "correct") the Mawangdui passage. I advocate extreme caution when comparing the Mawangdui medical manuscripts to the *Huangdi neijing*, lest interpretation of the manuscripts become attached to *Huangdi neijing* interpretation.

Of course the *Huangdi neijing* must be consulted. It is a rich resource; and it is medical literature. We would be at an even greater loss to explain the Mawangdui texts without it. And I do not mean to slight the honest efforts of scholars to devise an interpretive framework for the Mawangdui medical texts. We are all finding our way hermeneutically in uncharted territory. My own working method has chiefly entailed continuous evaluation of my contextual reading of a passage in one of the Mawangdui medical texts while casting about widely for pieces of evidence to solve textual puzzles. At times the *Huangdi neijing* provided the solution; at times the solution came from unexpected sources. The best claim I can make for the rightness of my solutions is that they appear most suited to the context; a subjective claim to be sure, but one that I think holds up under critical scrutiny. Naturally other scholars have eased my work. The transcription notes in *MWD*, vol. 4, are always insightful. *KGS*, vol. 1, does not include all of the texts since it is based on transcriptions published before *MWD*, vol. 4, but the notes and Japanese translation are of high quality. Among the Chinese scholars working on Mawangdui medical manuscripts, Ma Jixing has written an encyclopedic book that exhibits both his philological expertise and his erudition as a medical historian (1992). Other major contributions to Mawangdui medical manuscript studies are Zhou and Xiao (1988); Wei and Hu (1992); and Li Ling (1993: 281-402). I have also benefited from Wile's translation and study of Chinese sexual cultivation literature (which includes a translation of *MS*VI.B and *MS*VII.B; 1992); from Li and McMahon's study of the Mawangdui sexual cultivation texts (1992); and from Qiu Xigui's critical review of *MWD*, vol. 4 (1992). I have learned from them all even if I do not always agree with them.

SECTION TWO
MEDICINE, MEDICAL LITERATURE, MEDICAL MEN

*MS*VI.A.9 offers a vignette of a physician at court in the second half of the fourth century B.C. The physician is Wen Zhi 文 摯, known in the *Lüshi chunqiu* as the physician from Song 宋 who cured King Min of Qi 齊 湣 王 (r. 300–284 B.C.) at the cost of his life (causing the ruler to explode with anger was the only treatment; and King Min would not forgive the physician's offensive behavior, which was calculated to cure him). *MS*VI.A.9 finds Wen Zhi in better times advising King Min's predecessor King Wei 威 王 (r. 357–320 B.C.), eminent patron of learning and founder of the Jixia 稷 下 Academy. King Wei would like to hear just "two or three words" summarizing the physician's "way." Wen Zhi responds, "Your Servant's practice of the way consists of three hundred fascicles, but sleep is foremost." Thus begins a discussion of physical regimen, diet, drugs, and health with King Wei an active participant (at one point the ruler demands explanation of a seeming inconsistency in the physician's teaching). The interview is idealized, but no more so than interviews between Mencius and King Xuan of Qi 齊 宣 王 (r. 319–301 B.C.) which figure prominently in the *Mengzi* (Graham 1989: 112). Much of Warring States philosophical literature records the philosophers' speeches, and the dialogue between a philosopher and a ruler is conventional. The written rendition of a given interview may be suspect as a historical record—its purpose, after all, is to formalize the teaching for the philosopher's partisans (and his disciples probably composed the text)—but the depiction of rulers questioning and listening to the philosophers accurately reflects a prominent feature of Warring States intellectual history.

Wen Zhi's interview with King Wei bears witness to a state of medicine and medical men which crystallized during the Warring States. Like the philosophers, the physician (*yi* 醫) possessed a way (*dao* 道); this way was recorded in his medical books (Wen Zhi's "three hundred fascicles" is self-advertisement and signifies that the written record of his way of medicine is "complete"). To teach medicine was to give verbal amplification of the books. Medical literature proliferated in the fourth to third centuries B.C. as new ideas arose and the impetus for committing knowledge to writing grew. The transformation of medicine from an archaic craft dominated by magico-religious belief and practice into a theoretically-grounded discipline was as much a function of the new literacy as it was of the rationalizing tendencies in thought. Medicine became one of many fields of natural philosophy that were defined by the books the specialists transmitted. Of course, the knowledge committed to writing was diverse. As documented in the Mawangdui medical manuscripts, incantations and magico-religious operations were collected together with other medical recipes. If such practices had once been the preserve of religious officiants and shamans (*wu* 巫), or formed part of oral folklore, they acquired a new kind of prestige as they were incorporated into the books of specialists in natural philosophy and occult knowledge. Magic became a technique to be taught and transmitted in books along with other techniques; it became a segment of occult thought.

I attribute the emergence of a learned and literate medicine between the fourth and first centuries B.C. to the *yi* 醫, the word I translate as "physician." The word antedates the Warring States; etymologically, *yi* is related to words for exorcism in Shang inscriptions (see Section Five, "Varieties of Magic"). The notion of *yi* as originally a medicine man is also evident in the Warring States legend that credits Shaman Peng 巫彭 with creating the profession of physician in antiquity. Even during the Warring States and through the Han, the compound *wuyi* 巫醫 sometimes meant shamans and physicians collectively and sometimes was an epithet for a "shaman-physician." Received sources often contrast the methods of the *wu* with those of the *yi*, the former specializing in incantation and ritual and the latter in drugs and other therapies. The contrast is sometimes pejorative, but not always; that is, patients continued to believe in the efficacy of shamanic medicine, and physicians did not uniformly eschew magic (Harper 1982: 42-47). Despite the flexible attitudes, by Warring States times physicians participated in the new text-based alignment of knowledge, which distanced them socially and intellectually from shamans who formed part of the substratum of a popular religion about which we know little.[1] Moreover, magico-religious skills were now part

[1]The question of the *wu* tradition is addressed in Section Five, "Magical Recipes."

of an occult tradition; books of incantations and demonological lore circulated. Parallels between the forms of magic in the Mawangdui medical manuscripts and in the Shuihudi hemerological manuscripts suggest that in both cases the source of much of the magical lore was textual (Harper 1985; Harper 1990; Harper forthcoming). Occult literature certainly drew upon oral traditions of popular and shamanic religion; but it also changed the perception of magic among the elite and connected magic to natural philosophy.

Medicine was practiced by others besides physicians. Some participated in the same text-based traditions as the physicians. Diviners and astrologers practiced iatromancy; and popular iatromancy is recorded in the Shuihudi hemerological manuscripts (*SHD*: 193, 246). Macrobiotic hygiene was among the many specialties of the recipe gentlemen (*fangshi* 方士). Cross-fertilization between medicine and other branches of natural philosophy led as well to the assimilation of Yin Yang and Five Agent theories. Oral medical traditions were probably transmitted not only by shamans, but also by drug gatherers,[1] midwives,[2] and wet nurses. No doubt some of the material in the Mawangdui medical manuscripts should be attributed ultimately to such sources. However, the formation of the discipline of medicine backed by medical literature was accomplished by physicians. By the fourth century B.C. physicians were transmitting a written "way" of medicine. Their organization placed them in a relationship with other specialists in natural philosophy and occult knowledge as well as with the philosophers. A physician taught his way to select disciples, to whom he also transmitted his books. And the elite were not simply patients; they patronized physicians and collected their books.

The Mawangdui medical manuscripts belonged to this social and intellectual milieu. The following account of medicine, physicians, and their literature is an attempt to reconstruct the world in which the manuscripts

---

[1]Several of the *xian* adepts whose lives are recounted in the *Liexian zhuan* sold drugs, which they probably also gathered (Kaltenmark 1953: 116, 120).

[2]The Shuihudi text *Fengzhenshi* 封診式 refers to an official dispatching a woman "who has given birth several times" to examine a woman who has aborted (*SHD*: 161; Hulsewé 1985: 205). No doubt such women also participated in childbirth.

were produced. I begin with the concepts that defined medicine as a field of knowledge and linked medicine to other fields. Then I discuss the readership for and transmission of medical literature.

RECIPES, TECHNIQUES, CALCULATIONS, ARTS

Yi 醫 can denote the field of medicine. When the First Qin Thearch 秦始皇帝 banned literature in 213 B.C., books on *yi* (medicine) and *yao* 藥 (drugs) were exempted (*Shiji*, 6.22b). Chunyu Yi 淳于意 also writes of "medicine and drugs" (*Shiji*, 105.8b), but usually he refers to the practice of medicine using terms which emphasize medicine as a technical skill. *Fang* 方, a word that refers to "methods" for carrying out a procedure and to "written recipes," is ubiquitous in his writings.[1] To practice medicine is to "practice recipes" (*wei fang* 爲方; *Shiji*, 105.23a); medical books are "recipe books" (*fangshu* 方書; *Shiji*, 105.8b). One learns medicine by studying a physician's recipe books—which are "prohibited" (*jin* 禁), meaning they are secret (*Shiji*, 105.9a). Given Chunyu Yi's usage, the title of the division of medical literature in the *Hanshu* bibliographic treatise clearly represents a label that physicians themselves would have applied to medicine. "Fangji" 方技 (Recipes and techniques) pairs the "recipes" which are the core of medicine with a standard word for skillful "technique" in any endeavor.[2]

If recipes and techniques were what defined medicine for physicians, they were also what connected physicians to other specialists in natural philosophy and occult thought. The division in the *Hanshu* bibliographic treatise entitled "Shushu" 數術 (Calculations and arts) parallels "Fangji" (*Hanshu*, 30.78b). *Shu* 數 must refer in part to cosmological "calculations," since "Shushu" is the location of books on astrology, the calendar and hemerology, and Yin Yang and Five Agent correlations; *shu* "art" is the most common term for technical skill. At the same time, "Shushu" is a grab bag of occult literature, including divination, demonology, and incantation. What appears to be a heterogeneous mixture makes sense when one realizes the chief criterion for classifying these books in the same division: they all concern techniques applied to dealing

[1] *Fang* has other meanings, but these are the meanings relevant to medicine as a skill. Harper 1982: 54–55, provides text citations, especially for the meaning "written recipe."

[2] *Hanshu*, 30.82b. Cf. Harper 1982: 52–54.

with particular areas of the natural world and spirit world. Thus the specialists in various fields of natural philosophy and occult knowledge were appreciated above all for the results of their *shu* "calculations" and *shu* "arts"; simultaneously, physicians were known by their *fang* "recipes" and *ji* "techniques."

The picture that emerges of medicine in relation to natural philosophy and occult thought has several important features. To begin, physicians regarded themselves as part of a text- and technique-based tradition that extended to many kinds of specialists. Before the Warring States, the practice of medicine, astrology, or divination was often inherited within a family tradition.[1] By the Warring States, medicine had become a field of knowledge alongside other fields. And general interest in techniques crossed the boundaries between fields. Although Chunyu Yi lived in the second century B.C., his experiences must have represented a common pattern for physicians by the third century B.C. Chunyu Yi did not come from a family of physicians. He was drawn to medicine because as a boy he "liked all matters related to recipes." Even before being accepted as a disciple by his first teacher Gongsun Guang 公孫光, Chunyu Yi had been collecting whatever recipes he could obtain and testing them (*Shiji*, 105.23a). One wonders whether the recipes were necessarily all medical. Perhaps his youthful curiosity was drawn to the myriad phenomena of the sort recorded in the Shuanggudui manuscript *Wanwu*. Later, when Gongsun Guang recommended Chunyu Yi to the son of his future teacher Yang Qing 陽慶, he characterized Chunyu Yi as "fond of calculations" (*Shiji*, 105.24a). No doubt the phrase praises his talent for medical study; it also reflects the easy communication between the fields of natural philosophy and occult knowledge.

Ideas arise in an environment. Was it common interests and communication among physicians and the other specialists that produced theories of nature? If so, where are the Warring States philosophers in the picture of early Chinese natural philosophy and occult thought? By the third century B.C. the belief that all knowledge and action could be formulated as a technique was widespread, and the philosophers also used the vocabulary of "recipes" and "arts" to designate the techniques of statecraft, rhetoric, mind cultivation—virtually any significant activity had a skill particular to

---

[1] *Liji*, 5.6b, cautions against taking the drugs of a physician who is not at least the third generation descendant of a physician; no doubt in Han times the idea that physicians who inherited the occupation were more trustworthy was still current.

it.[1] To be sure, *dao* "way" as a central idea in philosophy was always more concerned with patterns of human behavior than with abstract questions of truth and reality; the aim of philosophy beginning with Confucius was to present a course for humans to follow.[2] But the Warring States emphasis on defining techniques to quantify *dao* reflects both rationalizing tendencies in thought and the increasing specialization of knowledge. The trend had its critics. A *Zhuangzi* passage that is probably mid-second century B.C. assesses five groups of philosophers, opening with the statement: "Those who cultivate *fangshu* 方 術 (recipe-art) have become numerous . . . but where can be found what of old was called *daoshu* 道 術 (way-art)."[3] Interestingly, all philosophy is assumed to be an art. The subsequent passage decries the fragmentation of *dao* into the many *fang* of the philosophers, who are treated as recipe peddlers (*fangshu* and *daoshu* occur as synonyms for skillful knowledge in other philosophical writings, thus the pointed contrast between the philosophers' fragmented "recipes" and the undivided "way" in the *Zhuangzi* was not the common understanding).[4]

The question remains, did the recipes or arts of the Warring States philosophers include the investigation of nature; did they have a hand in the development of Yin Yang and Five Agent theories which became the basis for what Graham calls correlative cosmology? First, we need to know who were recognized as philosophers in Warring States times. There are two sources of evidence: references to other philosophers and their followers in well-known Warring States philosophical books like *Mengzi*, *Zhuangzi*, *Xunzi*, and *Hanfeizi*; and retrospective classifications of philosophical traditions in Han literature, in particular the "Zhuzi" 諸 子 (The masters) division of the *Hanshu* bibliographic treatise (*Hanshu*, 30.27b-52a). Being known as *zi* "master" was one criterion for philosopher status, whence the division title in the bibliographic treatise. "Zhuzi" includes a category for "Yin Yang jia" 陰 陽 家 (Yin Yang specialists)

---

[1] The emphasis on *shu* "art" in philosophy is traceable to fourth century B.C. theories of statecraft (Graham 1989: 268).

[2] Graham touches on this aspect of *dao* when he states: "Chinese thinkers want to know how to live, how to organize community and, at the very end of the pre-Han period, how to relate community to cosmos. As for what is real, what exists, visible to the eye, audible to the ear, solid to the touch, what questions does it raise? From the Western viewpoint, pre-Buddhist Chinese philosophy is epistemologically naive" (1989: 222-23).

[3] *Zhuangzi* 33, 461. I accept Graham's dating (1989: 374-76).

[4] See Chen Pan 1948: 17-18, for examples of synonymy between *fangshu* and *daoshu*.

which lists the writings of Zou Yan 騶衍, the early third century B.C. man reputed to have explained change in nature according to cycles of Yin Yang and the Five Agents in order to predict the political fortunes of rulers (Graham 1986: 70-92; Graham 1989: 325-30). Graham notes that despite the listing in the bibliographic treatise and another Han reference to "Yin Yang specialists" in Sima Tan's 司馬談 (d. 110 B.C.) classification of philosophy, Zou Yan is ignored in the enumerations of philosophers in third and second century B.C. books of philosophy like *Xunzi*, *Zhuangzi*, *Lüshi chunqiu*, and *Huainanzi* (1989: 328-29). Zou Yan may have been what we would call a cosmologer, but it appears that in the third century B.C. Zou Yan and other Yin Yang specialists were not among the masters of philosophy; inclusion of Yin Yang specialists among the masters was first recognized in Han times, after the assimilation of cosmology into philosophy was an accomplished fact. Graham's judgment that down to the mid-third century B.C. "cosmological speculation . . . belongs to a world right outside the philosophical schools," and that Zou Yan "belongs to the world not of philosophers but of the court diviners and physicians" has justice (1989: 325, 328). The masters of philosophy knew of the theories about nature—at the courts of Warring States rulers they shared the stage with physicians like Wen Zhi and the other specialists—but they did not mastermind them.

It should be evident that in the Warring States the categories of master of philosophy on the one hand and physician, to name just one specialty, on the other do not correspond precisely to the division between philosophy and craft in Greek civilization.[1] Unlike the Greek philosophers, speculation on natural phenomena was tangential to the way of the masters of philosophy until a late date. For physicians and the other specialists, interest in natural phenomena in general was a function of the specialties (frequently overlapping) they practiced; they shared text- and technique-based traditions; and theories developed among them without direction from the philosophers. With Zou Yan we appear to have a generalist—a cosmologer who formulated a body of theory, demonstrated its relevance to the state and the individual, and thereby made natural philosophy indispensable to all.

Yin Yang is one term for Zou Yan's kind of natural philosophy in Han literature, but terms like *fangshu* or *daoshu* and a variety of related com-

[1]Edelstein's statement of the influence of Greek philosophy on the craft of medicine is classic (1987: 349-66).

pounds which refer broadly to natural philosophy and occult thought are more common (Chen Pan 1948). The same vocabulary continues to be used for other erudite skills; for example, the Han socio-intellectual orthodoxy grounded in canonical books like the *Yijing* and *Shijing* is termed *jingshu* 經術 (canonical art), which is sometimes contrasted with the dubious moral guidance provided by the books of the Warring States masters of philosophy.[1] The multiple usages of the vocabulary of recipes and arts indicate that within the intellectual tradition no one attempted to formulate a restrictive concept of skill itself so as to privilege only certain types of knowledge and to exclude knowledge that failed to satisfy the definition of skill. Thus, fundamental ambiguities regarding recipes and arts remained unresolved: were they genuine or spurious; were they ethical or did they aim to deceive and mislead; did they appeal to rationalized principles or claim magical power? Suspicions and accusations were commonplace, especially by the arbiters of Han socio-intellectual orthodoxy against those whose ideas and activities did not conform, but their arguments were more *ad hominem* attacks than reasoned critiques of the conceptual issues.[2] In the area of natural philosophy and occult thought, where the vocabulary of skill was most frequently applied, there were skeptics for whom rationalized models replaced magic. In medicine, Chunyu Yi and the physicians whose views are represented in the *Huangdi neijing* maintained a rationalistic skepticism in their application of Yin Yang and Five Agent theories to the understanding and treatment of illness. But it is evident from the magical contents of the Mawangdui medical manuscripts that there was not a dichotomy between natural philosophy and occult thought; the medical manuscripts simply bear out the evidence of the division "Shushu" in the *Hanshu* bibliographic treatise.[3]

[1]Thearch Cheng 成帝 (r. 33-7 B.C.) refused an uncle's request to be given copies of the books of the masters of philosophy and Sima Qian's *Shiji* after a court official warned him that such books were dangerous and inimical to "canonical art" (*Hanshu*, 80.8a).

[2]Cf. Ngo 1976: 64-66, for observations on differences between the Han *ru* 儒 tradition (so-called Confucian orthodoxy) and the *fangshi* 方士 (recipe gentlemen).

[3]Harper 1990: 211, cites several passages from the *Huangdi neijing* which explicitly reject the belief in demons and spirits as the cause of illness (without, however, denying their existence). The *Lunheng* 論衡 is remarkable for its skeptical scrutiny of all manner of ideas that Wang Chong 王充 (A.D. 27-ca. 100) finds illogical (including the politics and ethics of the pre-Han philosophers). He lambasts what to him are superstitious ideas concerning Yin Yang and Five Agent theories as well as other occult beliefs. His own arguments, however, often rely on Yin Yang and Five Agent theories to explain phenomena that others would have believed to be magic; for example, Wang

I have referred to Zou Yan as a generalist and a cosmologer. Based on the record of the *Shiji*, *fangshi* 方 士 (recipe gentlemen) appeared near the end of the third century B.C., claiming to be followers of Zou Yan. The idea that Zou Yan spawned a new kind of practitioner in natural philosophy and occult knowledge is plausible. Perhaps in the context of third century B.C. natural philosophy and occult thought, Zou Yan stood out as master of the ultimate secrets of the cosmos. In addition to correlative cosmology, the *xian* 仙 cult (which promised immortal life as a transcendent being) swept late third century B.C. elite society, adding yet another element to the already varied mixture of natural philosophy and occult thought. The recipe gentlemen described in the *Shiji* catered to the demand for esoteric knowledge in these areas—magic, macrobiotics, alchemy, and *xian* transformation their strong suit. The *Shiji* first uses the title *fangshi* for men who arrived at the court of the First Qin Thearch with recipes (*fang*) for "the way of transcendence (*xian* 仙), release of the form, and fluxing transformation."[1] They were, according to the *Shiji*, mountebanks who "exploited demons and spirits":

> Zou Yan gained fame with The Lords for the cycles of domination of Yin and Yang. The recipe gentlemen of Yan 燕 and Qi 齊 and along the sea transmitted his arts without being able to penetrate them; and thus there arose at this time the uncounted followers who mislead with marvels, toady, and connive. (*Shiji*, 28.10b.)

Similar recipe gentlemen continued to flourish through the second and first centuries B.C., finding in Thearch Wu 武 帝 (r. 141–87 B.C.) an enthusiastic patron. Li Shaojun 李 少 君 gained Thearch Wu's favor with "recipes for worship of the stove, the way of grain, and repelling age"; that is, he taught alchemy, dietetics, and longevity techniques. Even before arriving at Thearch Wu's court, Li Shaojun had made a circuit of the households of the elite with his recipes:

> When people heard that he was able to command spirit beings and to not die, they every time fed and begifted him. He always possessed a surfeit of gold, cash, clothing, and food. People all thought that he did not engage in an occupation

---

Chong argues that the correlation between the agent Fire and speech explains why incantations work (see Section Five, "Varieties of Magic").

[1] *Shiji*, 28.10b. The *xian* cult and the concept of "release of the form" are discussed in Section Four, "Intellectual Background" and "Body and Spirit."

> and yet he was richly provided for. Moreover, because they did not know where he came from their faith was all the greater and they vied to serve him. (*Shiji*, 28.21a.)

The *Shiji* is a hostile witness, but revealing nonetheless. Unlike physicians and others who practiced recognized occupations, Li Shaojun increased his appeal to the elite by cultivating a mystique. Their generous contributions were intended to secure his agreement to teach them his secrets (by accepting them as disciples in his service).

Li Shaojun and the others mentioned in the *Shiji* probably would have referred to themselves as *fangshi*, but the title need not have applied exclusively to their kind of occult practitioner. According to the *Hanshu*, the southern court of Liu An 劉安 (179-122 B.C.) at Huainan 淮南 was renowned for its assembly of several thousand "guests-in-residence" 賓客 and "recipe-and-art gentlemen" 方術之士. The latter title is usually equated with *fangshi*. These men participated in the compilation of the *Huainanzi* 淮南子 with its several chapters devoted to cosmology, astrology, geography, and the human body. In addition to the *Huainanzi*—the "inner book" 內書 produced at Huainan—there were also a voluminous "outer book" 外書 and the "middle fascicles" 中篇, both now lost. The latter work comprised over 200,000 graphs and dealt with "spirit transcendence and the art of yellow and white."[1] As a book of natural philosophy, the *Huainanzi* undoubtedly distills the knowledge of Liu An's recipe-and-art gentlemen. And they must have been responsible for the clearly occult "middle fascicles," which was perhaps similar to the *Huainan wanbishu* 淮南萬畢術 (Kusuyama 1987). These scholars of natural philosophy and occult knowledge were a different sort than the itinerant wonderworkers called recipe gentlemen in the *Shiji*.

The title *fangshi* even occurs twice in the *Huangdi neijing* denoting physicians (*Suwen* 11, 3.13b; 74, 22.24b). The physician-authors of the *Huangdi neijing* obviously knew the association of the title with men like Li Shaojun. Did they borrow the title? I think not. More likely, *fangshi* was a generic title appropriate for anyone whose knowledge centered on his *fang* "recipes." In short, even though historical records dwell on the notoriety of a certain group of recipe gentlemen whose exploits also serve

[1] *Hanshu*, 44.8b. Cf. Roth 1992: 12-26. The reference to "yellow and white" is alchemical, with significance for *xian* transformation as well.

the purposes of historiography, the title *fangshi* itself covered a range of specialists in natural philosophy and occult knowledge.[1]

The chief attribute of *fangshi* is the possession of *fang*—specifically the books that contain both their knowledge and their techniques. I adopt the term "*fang*-literature" to refer to all literature produced in the milieu of the specialists in natural philosophy and occult knowledge during the Warring States, Qin, and Han. The amount of *fang*-literature in circulation by the first century B.C.—both among the specialists and the elite—was considerable. The divisions "Shushu" and "Fangji" in the *Hanshu* bibliographic treatise contain roughly one third of the books in the whole treatise, and these books account for one fourth of the total amount of literature calculated in number of *juan* 卷 (rolls) or *pian* 篇 (fascicles).[2] There was undoubtedly more literature in circulation than recorded in the bibliographic treatise, all of it virtually lost before the manuscript discoveries of the last several decades.[3]

There are parallels between the ideas that grew around the terms *fang* "recipe," *ji* "technique," *shu* "calculation," and *shu* "art" and arguments about *techne* in Greek civilization. Originally *techne* meant the skill of an artisan. By the fifth century B.C. it also denoted a "rational discipline." Gorgias introduced the idea of magic as a *techne* into his theory of rhetoric and the power of words to influence human behavior, treating magic as a technique to be learned and thus "rationalizing" the "irrational" (Romilly 1975: 20-21). At roughly the same time, medicine was established as the *techne iatriche* as reflected in the eponymous essay in the Hippocratic Corpus (Lloyd 1983: 12-14).[4] For the Hippocratic writers their *techne* left no place for supernatural explanation, while in the culture at large magical

[1]The origin and application of the title *fangshi* await definitive treatment. Chen Pan's classic study has not been surpassed (1948). In my judgment, Chen places too much emphasis on the philosophers and not enough on the tradition of natural philosophy and occult thought, even though the title itself seems to have mostly been significant in the latter tradition.

[2]The statistics are based on Gu Shi, who counts 226 titles in "Shushu" and "Fangji" out of a total of 677 in the bibliographic treatise; and 3,420 *juan/pian* out of a total of 13,201. "Zhuzi" contains fewer titles (189) but more *juan/pian* (4,541; 1924: 95, 173, 196, 213, 243, 254).

[3]There are received texts of two books in "Shushu" and "Fangji": the *Shanhaijing* (*Hanshu*, 30.77a) and the *Huangdi neijing* (*Hanshu*, 30.78b). Text parallels between excavated *fang*-literature of Han and earlier date and medieval manuscripts from Dunhuang 敦煌 confirm that old *fang*-literature continued to be transmitted sub rosa without being recorded in bibliographies (see Harper 1988).

[4]*Techne* is usually translated as "skill," "art," or "science." Which translation is chosen often depends on the modern interpretation of the context in which *techne* occurs, hence I refrain from translation.

attitudes persisted.[1] The fourth century B.C. witnessed philosophical debate over genuine and spurious *techne*. Plato, for example, reasoned that medicine was a genuine *techne* because it concerned health, whereas the *techne* of cooking—which aimed at pleasure not health—was spurious.[2] After Plato and Aristotle, the philosophers' definition of *techne* set its "rational discipline" apart from ordinary skill on the one hand and occult thought on the other.

To the extent that *techne* in philosophy formally excluded occult thought from the realm of natural philosophy, the Greek term differs from Chinese ideas about "recipes" and "arts." However, occult thought and literature in the Greco-Roman world was nowise less flourishing than in Warring States, Qin, and Han China. The so-called Hermetic texts of late Hellenistic and Roman date bear witness to the vitality of the occult tradition (Scarborough 1988). Greek and Demotic magical papyri excavated in Egypt in the nineteenth and twentieth centuries have restored original fragments of magic handbooks and inscribed amulets of comparable date (Betz 1986; Faraone and Obbink 1991; Brashear 1992). Inscribed amulets of lead, silver, and gold unearthed around the Mediterranean, dating from the fourth century B.C. through Roman times, are yet another addition to the evidence for the occult tradition in Greco-Roman civilization (Kotansky 1991). Magical medicine is common in all of these materials. Studies of Greek and Roman medical literature are beginning to delineate the influence of occult thought on physicians as they formulated their *techne*; older arguments that neatly separated Greek and Roman medicine into the scientific tradition of the physicians and a popular occult tradition have given way to an awareness of a complex pattern of mingling between the two traditions.[3]

The conception of *fang*-literature facilitated exchange between the literatures of natural philosophy and occult knowledge. Imagine combining parts of the Hippocratic Corpus with Hermetic texts and magical papyri and you would have something like the syncretic mixture of the Mawangdui medical manuscripts. The emphasis on texts over oral traditions—the expectation of mastering an esoteric specialty by receiving

[1]Lloyd 1979: 10-58, examines the Hippocratic criticism of magic.
[2]Romilly 1975: 48. Romilly describes in detail the fourth century B.C. debate over *techne*, especially in connection with the status of rhetoric (1975: 47-66).
[3]Cf. Lloyd 1979. Scarborough (1991: 150-51) incisively critiques Edelstein's earlier arguments concerning Greek medicine and magic (1987: 205-46).

written *fang* from a teacher and the popularity of *fang*-literature among the elite—also seems more prominent in early China than in the Greco-Roman world. In regard to its popularity and its focus on recipes and arts, I am inclined to compare *fang*-literature to the abundant *artes*-literature of medieval Europe, which encompassed books in three categories of the medieval arts: liberal arts (including arithmetic and astrology), mechanical arts (including medicine), and occult arts (magic, divination, and the like).[1]

The characteristics of *artes*-literature are exemplified by the *Secretum secretorum* (Secret of secrets), which enjoyed wide circulation in Europe from the tenth to the seventeenth century. Translated into Latin from an Arabic original, the *Secretum secretorum* purports to be the wisdom imparted by Aristotle to Alexander the Great; its contents range from statecraft to astrology, alchemy, divination, magic, and medicine—in short, it is an arcane miscellany whose attractiveness to medieval intellectuals lay in its claim to antique wisdom (Ryan and Schmitt 1982; Eamon 1990: 335-36). Similar miscellanies are common in *artes*-literature, compiled with the intent of recording the secrets of nature. In fact, the secrets are often recipes and formulas collected from medicine and other crafts to serve everyday needs; miracles and home remedies share the quality of being secrets. And *artes*-literature is the repository of oral traditions which would not have been admitted into the more theoretically-oriented books of natural philosophy.[2] The Mawangdui medical manuscripts and Mawangdui manuscripts of literature classified in the "Shushu" division of the *Hanshu* bibliographic treatise would fit nicely into the genre of *artes*-literature.

---

[1]The term *artes*-literature and its denotation derive from the German discipline of *Fachprosaforschung* as formulated by Eis (1967: 1). Major studies of medieval *artes*-literature include Keil et al. 1968; Keil and Assion 1974; and Keil 1982.

[2]See Follan 1968 for a description of the contents of a popular German miscellany. Eamon characterizes the "books of secrets" in sixteenth century Italy as "technical 'how-to' books rather than works of theoretical science," and notes the source of many of the secrets in knowledge normally communicated orally (1985: 473).

READERSHIP AND TRANSMISSION

MSI.C concludes with an exhortation:[1] "The vessel connections—let it be written and thoroughly studied. Pupils, be devoted and respectful. Study [4] {4} [6] words, it is imperative to investigate them." The only explicit reference to medical training in the Mawangdui medical manuscripts, it captures the relationship between physician and disciple; and it enunciates the first task in medicine—"let it be written." Most likely Li fils was an elite aficionado of medical books and other *fang*-literature (as was the man buried in the Zhangjiashan tomb) and never served a physician as disciple. In *MSI*.C and the other vessel theory texts on *MSI*, we have evidence that the elite read books on diagnosing vessels and appropriate therapy which formed part of the curriculum of the relatively new vessel-theory based medicine being taught by physicians like Chunyu Yi. Editions of *MSI*.B, *MSI*.C, and *MSI*.D in the Zhangjiashan *Maishu* show that the same texts circulated among physicians and the elite across geographical regions, with later parallels in the *Huangdi neijing*. Thus we can now trace the growth of vessel theory within the larger community of physicians and simultaneously observe its spread to an elite readership.

Chunyu Yi's medical writings and passages in the *Huangdi neijing* treat disciples as the principal readership for medical literature, the assumption being that the physicians' books contain the crux of their "way"; the books introduce disciples to the profession and are the foundation of medical practice. Text-transmission customs observed by physicians are discussed below. The event of receiving medical books constituted an initiation which bound the disciple to the physician and sanctified the books, confirming the exclusiveness of the knowledge they contained. Like all *fang*-literature, medical *fang* were idealized as secrets intended for the enlightened few. It is clear from the Mawangdui medical manuscripts that the elite readership was perhaps equally influential in shaping the contents of medical literature; they also participated in its dispersion. Besides the elite's understandable concern over illness and the esoteric appeal of medicine, physicians possessed knowledge of many matters vital to their well-being: hygiene was foremost, followed by childbirth, relations between the sexes, everyday hazards, and the like. Medical literature addressed these subjects, much of it written expressly for the elite. They

---

[1]See the Introduction to the Translation for the use of brackets and braces to represent lacunae and untranslatable graphs.

participated as well in the culture of secrecy created by specialists in natural philosophy and occult knowledge.

Let me illustrate some of the characteristics of the elite readership for medical literature with a brief review of the Mawangdui medical texts. Li fils probably did not diagnose vessels himself or cauterize them, but by reading the four vessel theory texts on *MS*I he would have been more keenly aware of his own physical condition—especially when bothered by an ailment—and he would have had a standard for judging the physicians he consulted. Simply owning their theoretical texts identified him as a participant in their secrets. The only other text to deal extensively with illness is *MS*I.E, the ailment recipe manual. *MS*I.E contains rich detail on drugs and therapies, but is virtually unaffected by vessel theory; its conception of the ailments for which it provides treatments derives from older ontological ideas, which continued to exist alongside the physiological ideas derived from vessel theory even after the Han (see Section Three, "Illness"). A number of the recipes are simple to execute. However, the complicated technique for the surgical removal of an anal fistula (*MS*I.E.153) is but one of many recipes which reflect the skill of a physician. I doubt that Li fils would have attempted it.

But I see no reason why he would not have chanted the incantations and performed the exorcistic rituals described in some of the recipes. Magical operations in other Mawangdui medical manuscripts and in the Shuihudi and Fangmatan hemerological manuscripts indicate that these activities were customary for the elite (see Section Five, "Magical Recipes" and "Varieties of Magic"). By following the four vessel theory texts on the same sheet of silk, *MS*I.E presents itself as yet another source of expertise for the treatment of ailments. The magical contents, including exact wording for incantations and instructions for exorcistic rituals, exemplify the sophisticated treatment of magic within the occult tradition; occult books with identical or similar contents must have circulated. Once again, the air of secrecy is manifest.

Macrobiotic hygiene was a drawing card for physicians by the third century B.C. All seven hygiene texts assume an elite readership, idealized in the figures of rulers like King Wei of Qi or the more archetypal Yellow Thearch. The aspect of these texts that warrants emphasis in the present context is the esoteric quality of the language, best illustrated by the many metaphors in which cultivation techniques are couched. The breath cultivation technique in *MS*VI.A.1 instructs a person to "still your spirit wind" and "make fast your two racks," which will produce the "dark winepot." None of the terms are attested in a physiological denotation in received literature. The "two racks" might be the ribcage. "Dark winepot" is attested in the *Lüshi chunqiu* as the name of a liquid used in religious worship; in *MS*VI.A.1 it must be saliva. A sequence of metaphors for parts of the female anatomy in *MS*VI.B.1 forms a coded description of intercourse. The denotation of the majority of the metaphors is unknown (although judicious guesswork is possible). Clearly in order to practice these techniques one must be taught the meanings of the metaphors, which constitute a secret language. Thus, through the practice of macrobiotic hygiene the elite were significant participants in the culture of secrecy and privileged knowledge.

Perhaps the charms for everyday use in *MS*VII.A.1 will suffice to round out a picture of the Mawangdui medical texts as a mixture of home remedies, physicians' theories and skillful techniques, and knowledge both arcane and occult—all constituting varieties of *fang*-literature transmitted within the field of medicine. Like medieval European *artes*-literature, medical books and other *fang*-literature attracted an elite readership with a promise of secret knowledge, even though the contents were not necessarily arcane.

The amount of *fang*-literature recorded in the "Shushu" 數 術 and "Fangji" 方 技 divisions of the *Hanshu* bibliographic treatise and unearthed from elite tombs suggests that anyone who could afford to own books would have been able to collect it. Exactly how they collected it is more problematic. Presumably elite patronage of men of learning (including philosophers and physicians), who provided patrons with knowledge and books in exchange for support, was the chief mechanism. However, the text-transmission customs of specialists and their disciples described in Han sources give the appearance of excluding anyone outside that relationship. The obvious question to consider here is whether medical literature transmitted between a physician and a disciple differed in kind and quality from what the elite could acquire. There is also the question of how freely medical literature circulated—how popular was it, really?

The Han accounts of text transmission between physicians and disciples are the best evidence we have for addressing both questions. By examining how the community of physicians was organized and the role of medical books, we can perhaps identify several motifs that also apply to the elite readership. Some of the accounts contain miraculous elements—as in the case of the legendary physician Bian Que 扁 鵲, who is said to have received his secret medical books from a spirit.[1] Chunyu Yi's medical writings and passages in the *Huangdi neijing* provide a more certain gauge of the physician/disciple relationship in connection with medical literature and secrecy.

Chunyu Yi describes his introduction to medical literature and medicine in three separate passages: twice in response to questions asking him to explain what he knows about the source of Yang Qing's medical knowledge, and why Yang Qing selected Chunyi Yi as the recipient of it; and once in his personal history of his medical training. I begin with the two questions and Chunyu Yi's explanations:

> (1) Your servant Yi is asked: How did Teacher Qing receive it; was he renowned among the noble households of Qi or not? The response: (Yi) does not know from what teacher Qing received it. Qing's family was wealthy. Skilled in the practice of medicine, he was unwilling to treat ailments for other people. It must be for this reason that he was not renowned. Moreover, Qing instructed your servant Yi, "Be careful to not allow my sons and grandsons to know that you are studying my recipes."
>
> (2) Your servant Yi is asked: What did Teacher Qing see in Yi that made him love Yi and want to teach Yi all of his recipes? The response: Your servant Yi had not heard that Teacher Qing was skilled in the practice of recipes. Yi came to know Qing because when Yi was young he liked all matters related to recipes. When your servant Yi tested the recipes the majority produced results which were truly excellent. Your servant Yi heard that Gongsun Guang of Tang Village in Zichuan 菑 川 was skilled in the practice of old transmitted recipes. Your servant Yi immediately went to visit him and was able to have an interview and serve him, receiving recipes for the transformations of Yin and Yang as well as the models of transmitted speech.[2] Your servant Yi received them all and copied them. When your servant Yi wanted to

---

[1] The *Shiji* account of Bian Que and several other accounts of divine transmission are translated and discussed in Harper 1982: 59-62.

[2] "Models of transmitted speech" translates 傳 語 法, possibly referring to written records of oral instructions.

receive all of the other fine recipes, Gongsun Guang said, "My recipes are exhausted with these. It is not that I am stingy with you sire. My body is already in decline and I have no means to once again serve (a teacher). These are the marvelous recipes which I received in my youth. I have given them all to you sire; do not teach them to others." Your servant Yi said, "To have been able to see and serve you sire, and obtain all the prohibited recipes, has been my great good fortune. Were Yi to die he would not dare recklessly transmit them to others." Some time later when Gongsun Guang was in his private chamber your servant Yi discussed the recipes in depth, speaking the finest words for a hundred generations. Teacher Guang was delighted and said, "You sire are certain to become a state craftsman. There are some whom I regard as skilled, but all are crude (compared to you). In my birthplace Linzi 臨 菑 there is someone skilled in the practice of recipes with whom I cannot compare. His recipes are very extraordinary—like nothing the world has heard of. In my middle years I once wanted to receive his recipes, but Yang Zhongqian[1] was unwilling and said 'You are the wrong person.' I must go with you sire to see him. He ought to know that you sire delight in recipes. This man is also old now, and his family is furnished with wealth." We had not yet gone when just at that time Qing's son Yin arrived to offer a horse to the court. Through the assistance of Teacher Guang he presented the horse at the King's place.[2] Thus Yi was able to become friendly with Yin. Moreover, Guang entrusted Yi to Yin saying, "Yi is fond of calculations. You sire should treat him with respect. This man is a sage *ru*."[3] Then he wrote a letter entrusting Yi to Yang Qing, which is how I came to know Qing. Your servant Yi served Qing respectfully, which is why he loved Yi. (*Shiji*, 105.23a.)

---

[1]I.e. Yang Qing.

[2]It is not certain at whose court the horse was presented. According to historical records, Zichuan did not become a kingdom until sometime during Thearch Wen's 文 帝 reign (180-157 B.C.), after the events described by Chunyu Yi.

[3]The exact sense of *ru* 儒 is uncertain. *SW*, 8A.3b-4a, identifies *ru* as a title for an "art-gentleman" 術 士. Despite Chen Pan's lengthy argument linking the name for followers of Confucius with the notion of skillful techniques (1948: 33-40), the evidence for equating *ru* with "art-gentleman" before the Han is not convincing. Gongsun Guang may be praising Chunyu Yi as "scholarly" in the manner of the *ru* tradition.

The additional information in Chunyu Yi's personal history can be summarized briefly. Having been accepted as a disciple by Yang Qing, Yang Qing ordered him to "get rid of the entire lot of your recipe books, for they are incorrect." Yang Qing then promised to transmit to Chunyu Yi all of his "prohibited recipe books," which included the "vessel books of the Yellow Thearch and Bian Que." There followed a three year training period consisting of text recitation and explication as well as practical experience, after which Chunyu Yi "treated other people—examining ailments, judging death and life, and obtaining truly excellent results" (*Shiji*, 105.8b-9a).

Chunyu Yi's account offers remarkable details concerning three late-third to second century B.C. physicians and how they acquired their knowledge. First, Yang Qing did not even practice medicine as an occupation; family wealth made the "practice of recipes" unnecessary and undesirable. It appears that Yang Qing did not inherit his knowledge in a family tradition; if hereditary practice of medicine had been the source of family wealth he would have been less likely to transmit his books to an outsider. Although Yang Qing possessed many medical books, including vessel books attributed to the Yellow Thearch and Bian Que, Chunyu Yi does not know who Yang Qing's teacher was. Someone gave Yang Qing his books and taught him, but he did not identify a text or teacher lineage to Chunyu Yi. Gongsun Guang also did not name his teacher when he told Chunyu Yi that his medical skill was based on "marvelous recipes which I received in my youth." And like Chunyu Yi, Gongsun Guang studied medicine out of youthful curiosity. Three men—not one a hereditary physician, not one identified with a specific lineage of texts or teachers extending over several generations.

Apart from the importance both of texts and of the relationship between teacher and disciple, there is little evidence in Chunyu Yi's account of a larger organization binding physicians into exclusive brotherhoods. I suspect that the pattern for physicians and other specialists in natural philosophy and occult knowledge was similar to the philosophers. While we have good evidence of a type of school organization for followers of Confucius (the *ru*) and the Mohists, other philosophers and their philosophies cannot be said to represent schools. Equating the classification of books in the "Zhuzi" 諸子 division of the *Hanshu* bibliographic treatise with schools of philosophy is by now a well-known fallacy (Twitchett and Loewe 1986: 651-52; Graham 1989: 379-81). To be sure, certain books can be grouped together based on shared philosophical viewpoints, but the authors of the books did not see themselves as members of a school.

One should be equally cautious in considering whether there were medical schools between the fourth and first centuries B.C.; and if they existed, what the nature of their organization was. Yamada speculates that there were two kinds of physician: one a physician whose practice was hereditary and tied to the family's place of residence; and the other an itinerant physician who learned medicine from a teacher and then sought clients in various regions (similar to the philosophers and recipe gentlemen). According to Yamada, text and school lineages formed among the itinerant physicians, which by Han times influenced all of medicine. Thus the Bian Que school specialized in vessel diagnosis in the third and second centuries B.C., with theories paralleling the Yellow Thearch school; by the first century B.C. the texts of several branches of the Yellow Thearch school were combined in the *Huangdi neijing* (1979: 87-89; 1988: 120-29; 1990). In all, Yamada identifies three major Han medical schools on the basis of three book titles in the "Yijing" 醫經 category of the "Fangji" 方技 division of the *Hanshu* bibliographic treatise (one of which is the *Huangdi neijing*; 1979: 67; 1990: 66-67).

Insofar as Yamada associates physicians with text-based traditions similar to those of the other specialists in philosophy, natural philosophy, and occult knowledge, I am in basic agreement. But his argument regarding medical schools, which relies on the assumption that a book like the *Huangdi neijing* was composed within a Yellow Thearch school, is no more certain than the assumption of philosophical schools.[1] Between the fourth and first centuries B.C. the Yellow Thearch became prominent among specialists in natural philosophy and occult knowledge as well as among philosophers. He was the archetypal disciple to whom esoteric teachers revealed the secrets of the cosmos; books in the "Zhuzi," "Shushu," and "Fangji" divisions of the *Hanshu* bibliographic treatise are

[1]Explanations have been proposed for the composite nature of the *Huangdi neijing* which do not assume the existence of various Yellow Thearch schools (Keegan 1988: 249-59). Yamada also bases his argument for medical schools on the speculation that the so-called itinerant physicians still associated their occupation with *wu* 巫 (shaman) traditions and that schools of itinerant physicians preserved elements of *wu*-style social organization which included rituals for transmitting the secrets of the group. Thus, as medicine went from magico-religious origins to become a field of natural philosophy, medical schools developed out of earlier *wu* groups (1990: 62-64). I reject the sociological schema that equates Warring States specialists in natural philosophy and occult knowledge with shamans for reasons discussed in Section Five, "Magical Recipes," and thus do not find Yamada's speculation convincing.

attributed to him (Seidel 1969: 21-23, 50-52; Harper forthcoming). If we are going to equate books with schools, we find ourselves in the awkward position of supposing either that each set of Yellow Thearch books signifies yet another school which adopted the Yellow Thearch as school patriarch or that all the books together represent sub-groups of a single, large Yellow Thearch movement. It is more likely that the Yellow Thearch had become a legendary spokesman for a variety of esoteric knowledge, leading to a diverse body of literature attributed to him. As medical theory grew, physicians could have attributed many teachings and texts to both the Yellow Thearch and Bian Que. The formation of a Yellow Thearch or Bian Que medical literature would then have been the outcome of physicians sharing text traditions, not of medical schools with different legendary patriarchs.[1]

With a premium placed on "old transmitted recipes" and new medical texts continually appearing, the transmission of medical literature was probably more random than would be the case if the core medical literature were in the hands of schools. There was surely an element of chance in the selection of medical literature owned by any one physician. It was Chunyu Yi's "great good fortune" to have first served Gongsun Guang and under his auspices to have received superior books and instruction from Yang Qing. Chunyu Yi dates the beginning of his career as a practicing physician to after his tutelage under Yang Qing, as if his earlier study had been at the level of talented amateur. Chunyu Yi's experience was probably repeated many times over in different regions. The Mawangdui medical manuscripts give us a selection of the medical literature available in Changsha at roughly the same time.

Chunyu Yi's descriptions of the event of receiving medical books from his two teachers include several details concerning transmission etiquette and secrecy. A would-be disciple must first be accepted by (or allowed to

[1] I should note that many historians of Chinese medicine share Yamada's basic identification of the *Huangdi neijing* with a Yellow Thearch school. Liu Zonghan further identifies this Yellow Thearch school with the political philosophy known as Huang Lao 黄老 (i.e. the Yellow Thearch and Laozi), citing those parts of the *Huangdi neijing* which present the Yellow Thearch in his cosmo-political role (1992a: 97). Sivin similarly suggests that the use of Yin Yang theory in connection with macrobiotic hygiene in *MSVI.A* appears to be associated with "Huang-Lao ideology" (1992: 23). To be sure, intellectual developments in the third century B.C. brought physicians into contact with political theory, and there are significant political elements in the *Huangdi neijing*; but evidence of cross-fertilization between medicine and politics does not support the hypothesis that either a school of medicine or of hygiene as a separate specialty grew under the aegis of "Huang-Lao ideology."

serve) the physician. Having received Gongsun Guang's recipes, Chunyu Yi made his own copies of them. The verbal exchange between the two men after Chunyu Yi requested still more recipes should be read as part of the same event. It represents a formal vow: Gongsun Guang instructs Chunyu Yi to "not teach them to others"; Chunyu Yi, in possession of the "prohibited recipes" promises that "were Yi to die he would not dare recklessly transmit them to others." The source of Chunyu Yi's statement that Yang Qing instructed him to "not allow my sons and grandsons to know that you are studying my recipes" must be the time when he received Yang Qing's "prohibited recipes books." A physician could also refuse to teach a would-be disciple, as Yang Qing did when he stated that Gongsun Guang "was the wrong person" 非其人.

The vow of secrecy must have been common to all specialists in natural philosophy and occult knowledge when transmitting *fang*-literature to disciples. The vow was the centerpiece of the initiation rite binding the disciple to the teacher. The best statement of the principle of secrecy occurs in the *Huangdi neijing*. In the words of the Yellow Thearch, "to obtain the right person and not teach him is called losing the way; to transmit (the way) to the wrong person is to wantonly divulge heaven's treasure" (*Suwen* 69, 20.1b). Other passages give evidence of precautions observed when handling medical books lest their privileged contents be abused (Harper 1982: 63). A model for a text-transmission rite is described in the *Lingshu*. The Yellow Thearch guides Thunder Sire 雷公 through the rite, which begins with three days of ritual purification:

> The Yellow Thearch then entered the purification chamber with him. They cut their forearms and smeared the blood on their mouths. The Yellow Thearch chanted this incantation: "Today is True Yang. Smearing the blood I transmit the recipes. He who dares to turn his back on these words will himself receive the misfortune." Thunder Sire bowed twice and said: "The little son receives them." The Yellow Thearch then with the left hand gripped his hand and with the right hand gave him the books, saying: "Take caution, take caution. I will explain it to you. . . ." (*Lingshu* 48, 8.1a-b.)

The Yellow Thearch then lectures Thunder Sire on vessel theory and acupuncture.

Blood covenants (*xuemeng* 血盟) originated in Zhou religious and political life (Lewis 1990: 43-50). The Yellow Thearch's incantation includes a standard curse on the person who breaks the covenant. Yamada doubts that the *Huangdi neijing* passage can be read literally as evidence that Han physicians swore an oath in blood when transmitting books (1990: 83). However, in the fourth century A.D. blood oaths were still being used by Daoist adepts for oral transmission of secrets.[1] Han popular and shamanic religion probably used blood oaths and were one source for the Daoist custom, but I suspect that blood oaths exchanged among specialists in natural philosophy and occult knowledge were another source. The question is not whether physicians used blood oaths when transmitting medical books but which physicians used them.

The text-transmission customs described above reflect widespread ideas about the value of books. Notions of secrecy fueled Han bibliophilia in general; books were regarded as objects of power. In this environment the concern that books might be misused by the "wrong person" and the desire to possess them were equally matched.[2] Specialists and elite collectors like Li fils shared this mentality, which found concrete expression in the transmission customs for *fang*-literature. Without minimizing the significance of vows of secrecy and blood oaths, I am not so sure that they severely constrained the actual dispersion of *fang*-literature. Keep in mind that Chunyu Yi encountered no obstacles obtaining recipes as a youth, which led to more serious study with Gongsun Guang and Yang Qing. During his own career as a physician Chunyu Yi taught parts of his recipes to at least five pupils: two men from Linzi, one physician from the court of the King of Jibei 濟北, one physician from the court of the King of Zichuan, and a man from the household of the Lord of Gaoyong 高永 who "delighted in vessel (theory)." Chunyu Yi lists what each pupil studied and for how long: two studied for over a year, one for two years, and one did not complete his course of study (*Shiji*, 105.24a-b). The pupils seem to have been quasi-disciples in the sense that Chunyu Yi did not fully introduce them to the medical tradition he inherited from Yang Qing (there is no record whether near the end of his career Chunyu Yi

[1] See *Baopuzi*, 18.92, describing the oral transmision of secret names for the sacred One: "These things, then, are important to adepts of the Dao, who for generations have smeared their mouths with blood and orally transmitted the surnames and private names."

[2] See Harper forthcoming on the value attached to possessing books. See p. 49,n.1, above for an example of refusal to transmit philosophy books out of concern for potential misuse of their contents.

found the "right" disciple to whom he gave everything as Yang Qing did to him). Yet we have no reason to doubt that he transmitted medical books to them related to their studies, which they probably copied themselves; Yang Qing's "prohibited recipe books" were transmitted to appropriate pupils.[1]

Of course, Chunyu Yi and all of his pupils belonged to the literate elite, who constituted the chief pool for disciples. One wonders whether a great distinction was made between elite patrons and elite disciples. We have already seen that the recipe gentleman Li Shaojun cultivated a clientele who, desiring to learn his secrets of immortality, "vied to serve him" (see above, "Recipes, Techniques, Calculations, Arts"); that is, they served him in the manner of disciples while generously rewarding him for his knowledge. The elite demand for medical knowledge encouraged a similar market for medical books. Writing of the situation in the first century A.D., Wang Chong 王充 sardonically observed:

> At present among the recipe-and-technique books[2] written on bamboo and silk, if (a book) lacks attribution and provenance, those who see it dismiss it and waste no time on its remedies. But if (a book) bears the heading "so-and-so's recipes" or declares "already proven" and "previously tested,"[3] people vie to engrave and copy it, regarding it as something treasured and secret. It is memorialized to the state, reported to the commandery, and recommended with praise to gentlemen and officials. (*Lunheng*, "Xusong," 20.406.)

The size of the market for medical books in the third and second centuries B.C. was smaller than the first century A.D. (by which time books could be purchased at a shop; see Section One, "Provenance and Hermeneutic Issues"). But I expect that "vessel books of the Yellow Thearch and Bian Que" or Wen Zhi's macrobiotic recipes were being touted by physicians—with discretion of course, and in accordance with transmission etiquette, but touted nevertheless.

Prohibitions on transmitting a recipe are written at the end of several recipes in the Wuwei medical recipes, also first century A.D. Among the

[1] I do not accept Liu Zonghan's argument that Chunyu Yi taught parts of his medical knowledge to several pupils in order to prevent any one pupil from learning the whole of his medical secrets (1992b: 254).

[2] I.e. medical books.

[3] Both terms are used to evaluate recipes in *MSI*.E (see *MSI*.E.21, 197).

phrases are "take caution, do not permit it to be revealed" and "this ointment drug is extremely good—do not permit it to be transmitted."[1] The contents of the recipes with prohibitions are comparable to the other recipes. My impression is that the vow exchanged between physician and disciple has been popularized as a written formula attached to recipes which for various reasons were regarded as notable; that is, the prohibition on transmission identifies their excellence in the same way as phrases like "already proven" and "previously tested." This type of prohibition formula does not occur in the Mawangdui medical manuscripts; its use may have come later.[2] However, the convention of secrecy noted by Wang Chong and evident in the Wuwei medical manuscripts probably existed earlier.

A convention of secrecy does not in itself trivialize the status and allure of secrets. Transmission customs perpetuated a tradition of professional secrecy; surely physicians had secrets which they shared with select disciples (or never revealed). And in the elite quest for knowledge, secrecy bespoke significance. My interpretation of the evidence given above is that transmission customs observed by specialists and their disciples formed the background for a more popular participation in natural philosophy and occult knowledge by the elite. Physicians cultivated the elite readership; segments of medical literature were directed to the elite (macrobiotic hygiene being the prime example), who were also encouraged to acquire knowledge of other areas of medicine. I expect that some medical books came to be well known among the elite and circulated independently of physicians. What would have prevented Li fils, however he originally acquired his medical books, from permitting an acquaintance to copy them (after, no doubt, extracting a promise to treasure them and keep them secret)? Perhaps it was in this way that editions of *MSI*.B, *MSI*.C, and *MSI*.D were acquired by the man buried in the Zhangjiashan tomb.

In Section One ("Provenance and Hermeneutic Issues") I argued for treating the Mawangdui medical manuscripts as representative of third to early-second century B.C. medicine. Even though it is ultimately impossible to situate the manuscripts precisely in a synchronic or diachronic scheme, they belong ahead of the *Huangdi neijing* in any historical investi-

---

[1] *WWYJ*: 8a, 10a.

[2] Keegan misinterprets an incomplete phrase in *MSI*.E.238 concerning medical prohibitions to be observed during treatment of the ailment as evidence of the prohibition formula in the Mawangdui medical manuscripts (1988: 239).

gation of early Chinese medicine. One part of that argument is based on the presumption that Li fils and other elite collectors could acquire the kind of medical literature used by physicians. Obviously, my examination of transmission customs and secrecy is influenced by my judgment that the contents of the manuscripts correlate with contemporary medical ideas and practices. Nevertheless, judicious review of the evidence simply does not support Liu Zonghan's counter-argument that physicians like Chunyu Yi did in fact observe strict professional secrecy with respect to their knowledge and their books; and that comparison of the Mawangdui vessel theory texts to Chunyu Yi's writings shows the former to be texts of the sort belittled by better physicians who possessed better medical books (1992b: 252-54). In addition to having pupils, Chunyu Yi was prepared to debate medical theory with other physicians, as when he criticized Physician Sui's 醫遂 understanding of a homeopathic principle attributed to Bian Que: "Bian Que states 'treat Yin ailments with Yin minerals; treat Yang ailments with Yang minerals'" (*Shiji*, 105.19b). Both physicians knew and accepted the statement—it belonged to a common core of medical theory—but Chunyu Yi claimed that his interpretation was right and Physician Sui's was wrong. Medical discourse was not confined to confidences exchanged sub rosa.

Secrecy, disciples, debates over the interpretation of theory, derisive statements about the poor quality of others' books—all have a place in the social history of early Chinese medicine. I have not even discussed professional competition as a motive for physicians' conduct, and must leave it for future study (there are many relevant passages in the *Huangdi neijing*). In focusing on readership and transmission customs, I have aimed to underscore the dialogue that existed within the culture of secrecy in which physicians and elite participated. The Mawangdui medical manuscripts bear witness to this dialogue.

SECTION THREE
MEDICAL IDEAS AND PRACTICES

The discussions in Sections Three, Four, and Five present an overview of the main features of medicine as revealed in the Mawangdui medical manuscripts. My purpose is not to write a history of early Chinese medicine, nor do I propose to examine in detail the relation between the Mawangdui texts and received medical literature. I have chosen to survey the texts from three interrelated perspectives. Section Three deals with the basics of medicine: illness, physiology, therapy, and materia medica. Macrobiotic hygiene, which flourished as a consequence of physiological speculation, was no less basic in Warring States medicine. Indeed, the Mawangdui and Zhangjiashan medical manuscripts indicate that vessel theory may have developed first in connection with hygienic theories, and was then applied to pathology. This is but one of the bridges linking the discussion of macrobiotic hygiene in Section Four to Section Three. The evidence of magic in the Mawangdui manuscripts is the subject of Section Five.

Although the Mawangdui medical manuscripts do not require an apology, a reminder of the single-minded viewpoint of the physician-authors of the *Huangdi neijing*—for whom all of medicine depended on vessel theory—would not be out of place. Here is how the centrality of vessel theory in combination with acupuncture (as represented by the "nine needles" of acupuncture) is portrayed in the *Lingshu*:

> The Yellow Thearch said: "I have received the nine needles from the Master and privately examined the various recipes. Between guiding and pulling, circulating vapor, flexing and massage, cauterization and hot-pressing, needling and burning, and drinking drugs—is there perhaps just one which can be maintained singly, or should I practice them all?" Qi Bo said: "The various recipes are recipes for the masses. They are not all practiced by the singular man." The Yellow Thearch

> said: "This, then, is what is called 'guard the one without fail and the myriad things will be complete.'" (*Lingshu* 42, 7.2a.)

Among the "various recipes" listed, the first three belong to hygiene while the remaining therapies evidently lack the sanction of the "nine needle" acupuncture theorists, who "guard" their one theory. The "various recipes" depreciated in the *Huangdi neijing* are in some measure restored to us in the Mawangdui manuscripts.

ILLNESS

Every society constructs its own ideas of illness, health, and disease out of a mixture of bodily discomfort, observed phenomena, and shared cultural experience.[1] The idea that demons and the spirits of the dead sicken the living is in evidence in the earliest Chinese written records, the Shang inscriptions on bone and turtle shell (ca. thirteenth to eleventh century B.C.; Harper 1990). Demonic illness reflects the belief that something with an existence outside the body has relocated on or in the body; exorcism is a logical treatment. Warring States medicine added more agents and pathogens of a naturalistic origin, but the idea that an ailment was localized and attributable to an agent or agents was essentially the same. Stated in general terms, this represents an ontological explanation of illness—ailments are entities with an existence of their own (Unschuld 1987; Unschuld 1993: 21-22; Hudson 1993: 45-46).

Another explanation of illness emerged in tandem with the formulation of physiolgical theories. By the third century B.C., ideas concerning the *mai* 脈 (vessels) filled with blood and *qi* 氣 (vapor) inside the body dominated physiological speculation; one definition of health was the maintenance of a constant supply of free-flowing blood and vapor in the vessels. Thus in *MS*VI.A.8, the legendary flood-hero Yu 禹 is taught that "when blood and vapor ought to move yet do not move, this is called the calamity of blockage"; that is, stagnation in the vessels causes infirmity. As elaborated in the *Huangdi neijing*, vessel theory is the basis for a universal model of illness which explains illness as a dysfunction of the human organism within the system of vessels and internal organs. What is perceived as illness, or as nameable ailments, is the manifestation of that dysfunction; the goal of therapy—principally acupuncture—is to re-establish the har-

[1]Hudson (1993) offers a concise statement on the concepts of illness, health, and disease in a Western setting which covers the basic issues.

monious functioning of the organism, thereby eliminating the signs of illness. Unschuld describes this explanation of illness as "functional" (1987; 1993: 21); it is the Chinese counterpart to humoral pathology and other types of physiological explanation of illness in Western medicine (Hudson 1993).

The physiological explanation of illness based on vessel theory was championed earlier by Chunyu Yi, who claimed that vessel theory itself was created by ancient sages seeking to bring order to the identification of *bing* 病 (ailments):

> Ailment names are mostly alike and are unknowable. Thus the ancient sages created the model of the vessels (脈 法)[1] for them. . . . They differentiated the vessels in man and named each one. Matching with heaven and earth, (the vessels) combine in man to form a trinity. Thus they then differentiated the hundred ailments, distinguishing between them. (*Shiji*, 105.21b.)

According to Chunyu Yi's medical case histories, vessel diagnosis is the only accurate way to determine the nature of a patient's illness; treatment focuses on ameliorating the morbid condition exhibited by the vessels.

Despite the privileging of vessel theory and the physiological explanation of illness in Chunyu Yi's writings and the *Huangdi neijing*, ontological ideas were never supplanted in later Chinese medicine. In medieval recipe manuals and materia medica, ailments continued to be treated as localized entities which drugs and other therapies could control. As in *MSI*.E, demonic illness and magical treatment remained part of the medicine practiced by physicians, demonic agents being comparable to the other entities responsible for illness.[2] Moreover, medicine dealt with many matters besides the actual incidence of illness; the course of development in pharmacy and other medical practices was not determined solely by vessel theory and physiological pathology. Thus there is nothing unusual about the multifarious contents of the Mawangdui medical manuscripts. What is noteworthy about them is that the application of vessel theory to pathology is evidently at an early stage of development and is not yet established doctrine. It seems that in the second and first centuries B.C. Chunyu Yi and like-minded physicians were justifying a new understanding of illness

---

[1]The same term is used in *MSI*.C.

[2]Sun Simo's 孫 思 邈 (seventh century) *Qianjin yifang* 千 金 翼 方 is notable for its two final chapters devoted to magical medicine (*Qianjin yifang*, 29-30).

based on vessel theory. Ailments—the majority of which already had proper names in contemporary language—were being redefined according to physiological pathology; the physicians had to demonstrate that ailments did not exist as discrete entities, but were in fact manifestations of a deeper disturbance in the human organism.

The ailment *tui* 穨 (inguinal swelling) provides a convenient example. *Tui* means literally "drop down," and is first attested as a word for a fiery, descending wind in received literature; the Mawangdui medical manuscripts provide the earliest attestation of *tui* as a name for various kinds of swelling in the inguinal region, including hernias (Harper 1990: 219). The majority of recipes for *tui* in *MS*I.E.118-41 attribute the ailment to demonic agents who are exorcised; wind and vapor as pathogens may also be involved.[1] *MS*I.E.135 first recommends treating *tui* with a lancing-stone and cauterizing the lance wound, and then states, "for an easy cure, cauterize the Great Yin and Great Yang (vessels)." Among the examples of cauterization therapy in *MS*I.E, this is the only reference to cauterization in accordance with vessel theory, and is also the only indication of physiological pathology in the ailment recipe manual. However, *tui* is not listed under any vessel in *MS*I.A; in *MS*I.B it is listed under the leg Ceasing Yin vessel (*MS*I.B.8). Although Chunyu Yi credited sages with inventing vessel theory precisely to resolve doubts, pathological theory was still evolving.

The ascendancy of vessel theory and physiological pathology was driven by correlative cosmology. Vessel theory provided a basic structure for the application of Yin Yang and Five Agent theories to the human organism; it allowed physicians to precisely classify the human microcosm and link its operation to phenomenal processes in the macrocosm (which is the essential point in Chunyu Yi's statement on the "model of the vessels"). And it gave rise to a dual view of illness, with earlier ontological explanations overlaid by physiological explanations. I leave further discussion of vessel theory for "Physiology" below. In *MS*I.E we find evidence of the varied ontological pathology of third century B.C. medicine which preceded physiological pathology. Some ailment names in *MS*I.E are attested in received literature, others are not. References to ailments in other ex-

---

[1]Pathogenic *qi* represents ontological pathology, the vapor being the cause of a specific ailment rather than some other entity (Harper 1990: 217). On wind and vapor as pathogens, see Unschuld 1985: 67-73.

cavated manuscripts, including some of the same unattested names, add to the record of ontological pathology in early Chinese medicine.

"Conditions requiring medical attention" might be a better term than "ailments" for the categories of *MSI*.E. The recipe manual begins with seventeen recipes for flesh wounds, including techniques for staunching the flow of blood (in *MSI*.E.7, scalp hair is used; in *MSI*.E.9, an incantation) and relieving pain. Categories for burns (*MSI*.E.176-93) and animal bites (for example, dog bites and mad dog bites; *MSI*.E.28-33) are of a similar nature. However, the boundary between such conditions and ailments is slight. Immediately following the recipes for wounds are recipes for "rigidity due to a wound"; two recipes specify that wind entering the wound is the pathogen causing rigidity (*MSI*.E.19, 21). The third recipe category is a single recipe for rigidity in infants, perhaps associated with the wound created by cutting the umbilical cord (*MSI*.E.25). Throughout *MSI*.E there is a noticeable pattern in which conditions or ailments are treated as localized entities. Agents or pathogens may or may not be specified, and sometimes they are identical to the entity itself; that is, both conditions and ailments are given an ontological explanation.

Let me provide several examples. *MSI*.E.178 treats a burn (a condition) with a curse in which the burn is reified in the form of a demonic agent who is expelled in the curse (the curse addresses the agent directly as "you"). In several recipe categories concerning bites, the creature that bit is thought to lodge in the bite, which explains the curses for scorpions (*MSI*.E.48-49) and lizards (*MSI*.E.56, 60). The rash caused by working with raw lacquer is reified as the lacquer spirit (*MSI*.E.235); inguinal swelling is reified as misbegotten sons of perverse parents in one recipe (*MSI*.E.120) and blamed on a fox demon in another (*MSI*.E.124). I draw examples from magical recipes because they vividly illustrate ontological thinking about illness, but pathogens like wind or vapor—or unnamed pathogens in the ailment categories of *MSI*.E—are not unlike the demonic agents. The basic identity of an ailment as an entity permitted dual interpretation.[1]

The most common term denoting illness in the Mawangdui medical manuscripts is *bing* 病; I translate the verb as "ail" and the noun as "ailment." The word is classificatory; a morbid condition which can be

[1]The similarity between natural and demonic causes of illness in early Chinese belief is discussed in Harper 1990: 222-25.

given a name is a *bing*.[1] The origins of ailment names are as varied as the ailments themselves (and excavated manuscripts have increased the record of ailment nomenclature). Whatever their origins, we can safely say that before vessel theory and physiological pathology ailment names were devised under the influence of ontological ideas. One of the problems that physicians like Chunyu Yi had to confront was how to correlate the contemporary, multifarious ailment nomenclature with vessel theory; as Chunyu Yi phrased it, "ailment names are mostly alike and are unknowable." Part of the redefinition of illness was the "rectification" of ailment names in accordance with vessel theory. *MSI*.A and *MSI*.B bear witness to this process with their lists of ailments associated with each vessel. The kinds of ailments listed reflect a new sensitivity to somatic condition; most are pain felt in parts of the body along the path of a given vessel (the significance of pain is discussed in "Physiology" below). Only four of the names which appear in these lists also occur in *MSI*.E—*dian* 瘨 (seizure; *MSI*.A.1; *MSI*.E.71), *long* 癃 (urine retention; *MSI*.B.8; *MSI*.E.88-114), *tui* 穨 (inguinal swelling; *MSI*.B.8; *MSI*.E.118-41), *zhi* 痔 (hemorrhoids; *MSI*.A.1; *MSI*.B.1; *MSI*.E.142-54)—indicating gradual incorporation of traditional ailments coupled with elimination of ailments not susceptible to physiological explanation. The formula concluding each ailment list in *MSI*.A suggests a lingering association with ontological ideas: "In all cases of ailing from these things (*wu* 物; that is, the ailments listed), cauterize (the designated vessel)." By referring to ailments as *wu*, *MSI*.A perhaps comes closest to verbalizing the ontological explanation of ailments as entities that underlies *MSI*.E.

The majority of ailments in *MSI*.E are external. In addition to wounds and bites, there are numerous flesh ailments: warts (*MSI*.E.64-70), several skin afflictions of uncertain nature (*MSI*.E.34-35, 36, 73-75), two categories of abscesses (*MSI*.E.157-73, 225-32), scabies (*MSI*.E.200-223), itch (*MSI*.E.249-56), scabbing (*MSI*.E.257-70), and the like. Inguinal swelling and urine retention are among the few clearly internal ailments. References to the inside of the body are also scant: the bladder is mentioned twice in connection with urine retention (*MSI*.E.95, 101); the heart once, but only to designate that region of the exterior of the body (*MSI*.E.153); *shen* 腎 refers to testicles, not to the kidney (*MSI*.E.134, 137). Except for the lone mention of cauterizing the Great Yang and Great Yin vessels,

[1] Its classificatory usage is perhaps best attested in *SW*, 7B.26b-35b, which lists the names of ailments written with the signific 疒, many of which are simply identified as "a *bing*."

there is no evidence of Yin Yang and Five Agent theories; hemorrhoids are divided into "female" and "male" types using the older gender vocabulary *pin* 牝 and *mu* 牡. The greater attention paid to the exterior suggests a view of the body as the place where ailments lodge—a host to ailments—rather than as a functioning organism subject to physiological breakdown.

The contents of *MSI*.E must conform to a rubric shared with contemporary ailment recipe manuals: wounds come first, followed by wound-related rigidity; several categories of bites are grouped in sequence (*MSI*.E.44–63; but a single recipe for snake bite is placed near the end, *MSI*.E.224); urine retention, inguinal swelling, and hemorrhoids follow one another (*MSI*.E.88–154). One wonders why the two categories of abscesses are separated (*MSI*.E.157–73, 225–32), which reinforces the impression that an element of randomness is also involved in the organization of ailment categories. I doubt that the kinds of ailments treated and the sequence of the ailment categories in *MSI*.E are intended to communicate specific etiological or nosological ideas.[1] This does not mean that there is no evidence of etiological ideas. I have already mentioned demons, wind, and vapor. More prevalent than these are the many bugs associated with ailments. I use the word "bug" to refer to a category of creatures that includes, at minimum, insects and reptiles as well as all of their demonic variations in early Chinese belief. The breadth of the category is indicated in the earliest etymology of *hui* 虫, defined as a name for the viper and then explained as a general term for anything small that crawls or flies, is hairy or naked, or has shell-like plates or scales (*SW*, 13A.40b–41a). *Chong* 蟲 denotes bugs with legs, but also connotes an infestation of bugs (*SW*, 13B.4b).

Bugs as both natural and demonic agents of destruction can be traced to the Shang inscriptions, which provide the first attestation of *gu* 蠱 (pictographically a representation of bugs contained in a vessel). If later definitions of *gu* are applicable to Shang usage, the word refers to a demonic potion prepared from bugs which sickens select victims. By extension, *gu* refers to demonic evil and black magic in general. By Warring

---

[1]Yamada argues that there is an etiological and nosological plan in *MSI*.E, which he deduces by arranging the original fifty-two ailment categories into fourteen groups. He then identifies seven or eight combined groups within the fourteen, whose coherence he interprets in terms of four "images" of the body (1985b: 234–53). I am not convinced by Yamada's argument, especially given the uncertainty surrounding the identification of some of the ailment names and the ailments they designate.

States times *gu* was also applied to ailments involving infestations of bugs in the body. It has been hypothesized that *gu* denoted ailments like schistosomiasis, yet the underlying conception of the ailment cannot be separated from the magico-religious significance of a demonic bug-attack (Harper 1990: 225; see *MSI*.E.271).

Gu is one of eight ailments in *MSI*.E which can be classified as bug ailments simply on the basis of their names: *gu* (*MSI*.E.271-75), scorpion (*MSI*.E.44-49), leeches bite (*MSI*.E.50-51), lizard (*MSI*.E.52-63), *ming* 螟 (*MSI*.E.78), *quan* 蠸 (*MSI*.E.79), snake bite (*MSI*.E.224), and chewing by bugs (*MSI*.E.240-48). The presence of bugs is noted in other ailments, like female hemorrhoids (*MSI*.E.149) and scabies (*MSI*.E.208); bug etiologies for both ailments are documented in later medical literature. Chunyu Yi regards bugs in certain ailments as a secondary phenomenon arising from pathogenic wind and vapor, not as the first cause.[1] However, the ailment categories *ming* and chewing by bugs make bugs the primary agents of decayed flesh. *Ming* is only attested as an ailment name in *MSI*.E, where it is plausible to associate it with leprosy. In received literature *ming* is a crop pest regularly paired with *te* 蟘, which is the bug named in chewing by bugs as the cause of chewed flesh around the mouth and nose (*MSI*.E.244) and of tooth decay (*MSI*.E.248). In Han times it was believed that a plague of *ming* and *te* bugs was an omen of moral corruption in government; in *MSI*.E, both bugs plague the body, the ravages of the former more destructive than the latter. Although neither *ming* nor *te* occurs as an ailment name in received literature, there is ample testimony of the widespread fear of bugs and of their association with demonic activity and illness in Warring States, Qin, and Han times (Harper 1990: 225-30). The derivation of the ailment names *ming* and *te* is easy to trace. And the imprint of etiological ideas about bugs derived from ontological pathology in *MSI*.E is easy to detect.

The "Ailment List" in the Zhangjiashan *Maishu* represents an effort to bring nosological order to ailments from an ontological perspective. The body itself serves as the organizational principle. Beginning with the words, "when the ailment is located on the head," the text lists three head ailments, then continues downward to the bottom of the foot for a total of fifty-seven ailments. "Ailment List" concludes with ten ailments that affect the body generally (*MSSW*: 72). The text is notable for both the

[1] In diagnosing a case of intestinal parasites, Chunyu Yi argues that the pinworms are a natural transformation of cold, damp vapor (*Shiji*, 105.18a; pinworms are named in *MSI*.E.149).

precision with which it localizes ailments and the specificity of the ailment names. The first ten ailments listed are representative:

> When the ailment is located on the head and there is pus it is *qian* 𨍭; when there are sores it is *tu* 秃; when there is itching it is *qiang* 㿉. When (the ailment) is located on the eye and tears come out it is *qin* 浸; when a screen covers the pupil it is screen-*qin*. When (the ailment) is located on the canthii and spreads it is *fu* 㲴. When (the ailment) is located on the nose it is *qiu* 肍; when there are painful scabs it is *te* chewing. When (the ailment) is located on the ear it is *long* 聾; when pus comes out it is *jiao* 澆.

"Ailment List" includes a number of the ailments in *MSI*.E; for example, it provides a valuable second attestation of "*te* chewing," identified as painful scabs on the nose. Recall that "Ailment List" precedes the *Maishu* edition of *MSI*.B on the manuscript, thus both ontological and vessel-theory classifications of ailments are represented in *Maishu*.

Another example of ontological classification occurs in *Wanwu* (from Shuanggudui) in the form of ailments identified according to the drugs that cure them. Among the fragmentary slips there are over thirty such entries, including drugs used for the same ailment in *MSI*.E; for example, *shiwei* 石 韋 (pyrrosia) cures urine retention (Fuyang Hanjian zhenglizu 1988: 36; *MSI*.E.109; the importance of *Wanwu* as a drug list is discussed in "Materia Medica" below).

Between *MSI*.E, the *Maishu* "Ailment List," and *Wanwu*, we have evidence of refinements in ontological pathology which were contemporary with vessel theory and physiological pathology. Chunyu Yi's categorical statement that only vessel theory can explain illness and bring order to ailments is as much a criticism of ontological classifications like "Ailment List" as it is a paean to vessel theory. Because the *Huangdi neijing* has served to make vessel theory the standard for pathology in Chinese medicine, we tend to overlook the fact that in the third and second centuries B.C. it was still new; the excavated manuscripts allow us to see some of the alternatives to vessel theory and to speculate on the debate among physicians over the issue of illness.

PHYSIOLOGY

The earliest explicit statement in received literature of the idea that *qi* "vapor" flows along with blood through *mai* "vessels" inside the body occurs in the *Guanzi*, in an essay on water which probably dates to the first half of the third century B.C.: "Water is the blood and vapor of the earth—like what flows through the muscles and vessels."[1] The idea that *qi* and blood together are the essential components of human life is only reliably documented in fourth century B.C. sources, by which time *qi* already referred to the omnipresent "basic stuff" of the phenomenal world. And between them, *qi* was already seen to be more necessary to human existence than blood: it was the air man breathed, it was the nourishment extracted from food; it was what suffused the body and made man alive; it was what connected the human organism to the larger operations of nature. It is not clear whether *qi* originated as a word for atmospheric vapors (clouds, steam, etc.) which was generalized to encompass the source of human vitality and everything else; or whether *qi* was a term for the life-sustaining stuff received from food, drink, and air or breath, which was extended to the natural world. The graph 气, glossed as "cloud *qi*" 雲气 in *SW*, 1A.39a, suggests the former derivation; but the meaning is not attested in the oldest uses of this graph in Shang and Zhou inscriptions (where it means "beseech," "end," "food donation"). The graph 氣—which became the standard graph for the word in its generalized meaning—may have had earlier associations with food and breath, from which the concept of "stuff" in nature arose. By the fourth century B.C. the word was already a fixture in discourse on nature; barring new evidence, the question of etymological derivation is moot.[2]

My decision to translate *qi* as "vapor" is in part practical—why not translate such a basic concept in early Chinese thought, especially since modern use of the word *qi* both in Chinese and in English has colored its original meaning? "Vapor" avoids potentially misleading associations with

---

[1]*Guanzi* 39, 14.236. I concur with Graham's judgment that the essay pre-dates the crystallization of Yin Yang and Five Agent theories in the third century B.C. (1989: 356).

[2]The relevant etymological and textual evidence is conveniently summarized in Onozawa et al. 1978: 14-17, 30-34; see also Sivin 1987: 46-48. The compounds "blood and vapor" and "food vapor" occur in the *Lunyu* 論語, but in late chapters which are probably no earlier than fourth century B.C. Other occurrences in received literature also cannot be dated earlier than fourth century B.C.

"air" or "pneuma" in Western thought while retaining the sense of *qi* as something material but simultaneously volatile and pervasive. Its greatest flaw is old Western medical usage which applies "vapor" to injurious emanations of the internal organs; so long as one does not permit this denotation to intrude, the connotations of "vapor" are by and large transferable to *qi*. For those who believe that *qi* cannot or should not be translated, it is always possible to pronounce "vapor" as *qi*.

Physiological ideas proliferated during the fourth century B.C. This was the century when maintaining one's own physical existence became a philosophical issue (Yang Zhu 楊朱 is best known as the exponent of caring for life); and when the belief that the body was constituted of physical and spiritual/mental components led to a greater focus on the nature of the indwelling spirit. Building on ideas about vapor, it was thought possible to enhance physical and spiritual well-being through a program of cultivation. As evidenced in *Guanzi*, "Neiye" 内業, vapor was at the base of physio-spiritual transformations which concentrated *jing* 精 (essence) and *shen* 神 (spirit) inside the body to produce the physique of the sage (Graham 1989: 53-64, 100-105). The Mawangdui and Zhangjiashan medical manuscripts restore the earliest documentation of the physicians as exponents of physiological theory and macrobiotic hygiene. Cross-fertilization between the medical tradition of macrobiotic hygiene and philosophy is discussed in Section Four, "Intellectual Background." The following treatment of physiology considers primarily the evidence of vessel theory in the manuscripts.

Chunyu Yi gives us to think that physiological theory is vessel theory, that the vessels are the essential structure subsuming the other constituents of the body. This understanding of vessel theory is also characteristic of the *Huangdi neijing*. In contrast, there are two passages in the Mawangdui medical manuscripts that list five body constituents without naming vessel among them; a third passage in the Zhangjiashan *Maishu* lists vessel as one among six constituents of the body. For obvious reasons I do not accept Chunyu Yi's statement that "ancient sages created the model of the vessels." Physiological speculation between the fourth and first centuries B.C. moved gradually towards the view that vessel and vapor constituted the body's core, and that constituents like bone, muscle, and flesh were subsidiary. While we cannot determine whether the three passages antedate the vessel theory texts like *MS*I.A-B, they do document other physiological views and help to place vessel theory as described in the manuscripts in perspective.

The first passage occurs as part of the account of gestation in *MSV*.3 and is notable for including the only reference to Five Agent theory in the Mawangdui medical manuscripts. After three months during which the fetus settles into the womb, from the fourth through the eighth months the fetus develops five essential constituents: Water produces blood in the fourth month; Fire produces vapor in the fifth month; Metal produces muscle in the sixth month; Wood produces bone in the seventh month; Earth produces skin in the eighth month (the constituents are produced following the conquest sequence of the Five Agents). Notice that blood and vapor are the first constituents produced, but that vessel is not listed. Perhaps the existence of blood and vapor assumes that vessels are present in the fetus to hold them, perhaps not. A similar list of constituents occurs in *MSI*.D in connection with death. Five sets of physical symptoms signify that one of the constituents has "died first"; when all five sets of symptoms occur, the person cannot live. The constituents in the order listed in the text are: flesh, bone, vapor, blood, muscle.

Immediately preceding this passage in *MSI*.D is a passage on the Yang vessels (Great Yang, Minor Yang, Yang Brilliance) and Yin vessels (Great Yin, Minor Yin, Ceasing Yin); the latter are called the "vessels of death." Thus *MSI*.D presents two views of mortality: the first is based on disturbance in the Yin vessels; the second on failure of a body constituent. By virtue of their juxtaposition the two views are related, but there is no indication that the Yin vessels are to be correlated with the five constituents. The correlation of Yin vessels with body constituents first occurs in a parallel text in *Lingshu* 10. Five Yin vessels (the hand Ceasing Yin vessel is not included) are correlated with flesh, bone, hair, blood, and muscle; the failure of one of the constituents is attributed to the "severing of vapor" 氣 絕 in the vessel associated with it (*Lingshu* 10, 3.7a-b). Yamada explains the substitution of hair for vapor as evidence that vapor "is no longer regarded as one of the constituents of the body parallel with the flesh and other elements but rather as a more fundamental source power of life" (1979: 77). In the *Huangdi neijing*, body constituents are subsumed within vessel theory. *MSI*.D represents physiological ideas at a time when vapor was still listed among the body constituents, and before vessel theory's predominance. The constituents are the constituents produced during gestation in *MSV*.3 (associating flesh in *MSI*.D with skin in *MSV*.3), now observed in decay (note, however, that there is no evidence of Five Agent theory in *MS*I.D).

The *Maishu* "Six Constituents" similarly concerns signs of breakdown associated with body constituents. The constituents are identical to *MS*I.D with the addition of vessel as the sixth constituent. Each constituent serves a function; and each manifests a distinctive feeling of pain, which is bred in it:

> Now, bone is the pillar; muscle is the binding; blood is the moistener; vessel is the channel; flesh is the attachment; vapor is the exhalation. Thus, bone pain is like chopping; muscle pain is like binding; blood pain is like leaking; vessel pain is like flowing; flesh pain is like floating; when vapor moves there is anxiety.[1] Now, the six pains all exist in the body and no one knows how to treat them. Thus, if the gentleman becomes fat and loses the standard measure, this is called "muscle and bone do not succeed in their responsibilities." His vapor then becomes abundant; his blood then becomes uncontrolled. Blood and vapor putrefy and rot; the hundred joints all collapse. They clog the twenty extremities[2] and turn back, racing to the heart. If this is not treated in advance, one will hear the sound of weeping. (*MSSW*: 74.)

"Six Constituents" treats knowledge of pain in the constituents as the key to knowing the body; pain signifies a specific dysfunction which if not remedied leads to death. The "loss of the standard measure" due to obesity initiates a fatal scenario: muscle and bone are overtaxed (flesh, which is the "attachment," is too heavy for the bone "pillar" and muscle "binding" to support); blood and vapor are unleashed, causing general collapse throughout the body; and finally the blocked blood and vapor reverse their course and attack the heart.

"Care of the Body," the text preceding "Six Constituents" in *Maishu*, offers the teaching that only things which maintain regular movement do not stagnate. Stagnation inside the body causes "the vessels to rot and flesh to die." The words vapor and blood do not occur in the text (as they do in *MS*VI.A.8), but the conclusion implicitly understands either vapor alone or both: "When the vessels are brimful, drain them; when empty,

---

[1]"Move" translates *dong* 動, which here signifies disturbance. In other contexts *dong* can refer to the normal movement of blood and vapor in the vessels and to their pulse.

[2]Fingers and toes.

fill them; when still, stay in attendance on them" (*MSSW*: 74). In "Care of the Body" and "Six Constituents" it is evident that among the constituents the vessels and their contents are the focal point of physiology; and that physiology is oriented towards hygiene rather than pathology. This orientation is confirmed in the opening of "Vessels and Vapor," the *Maishu* edition of *MSI*.C, which follows "Six Constituents":[1]

> Now, the vessels are something the sage prizes. As for vapor, it benefits the lower part (of the body) and harms the upper part; it follows warmth and departs from coolness. Thus, the sage has a cold head and warm feet. To treat ailments, take away the surplus and increase what is insufficient. (*MSSW*: 74.)

To paraphrase, health depends on the condition of vapor in the vessels. Vapor should flow in a downward direction; upward movement is contrary movement and creates disturbance. The sage is the model of good hygiene; his cold head and warm feet ensure that vapor moves as it should. Applying the principles of hygiene to pathology, ailments can be treated by redistributing the vapor in the vessels; therapies designed to remove surplus and correct insufficiency are counterparts to the routine "draining" and "filling" of the vessels in hygiene. The remainder of both editions of *MSI*.C detail aspects of vessel theory in connection with illness, beginning with a description of cauterization to make vapor move downward in a vessel that has been diagnosed as having an excess of vapor.

Following the leads in the Mawangdui and Zhangjiashan medical manuscripts, we arrive once again at vessel and vapor as the core of physiology. But whereas Chunyu Yi proposes that "sages created the model of the vessels" in order to deal with human illness, the manuscripts present the vessels as idealized in the body of the sage; secondarily, they are the basis for diagnosing and treating illness. Formally, the evidence pits the word of Chunyu Yi and the *Huangdi neijing* against the manuscripts. However, there is logic in supposing that vessel theory began in connection with hygienic theory and practice, and over time became the basis for a new understanding of health and illness—at which point the significance of vessel and vapor in physiological pathology led vessel theory in a

[1]The two editions are slightly different. For example, *MSI*.C opens with the exhortation that the "model of the vessels be clearly taught," which is not included in the *Maishu* edition.

new direction. Once health was defined in terms of the circulation of blood and vapor in the body, maintaining health was essentially monitoring the condition of the vessels; transposing this scheme to illness and pathology would have been a small step to take. The *Maishu* "Six Constituents" suggests what the new index of illness was: pain. It is not coincidental that the great majority of ailments listed under each vessel in *MSI*.A and *MSI*.B (as well as in the parallels in *Lingshu* 10) are related to pain. The standard ailment name in these texts is a compound composed of *tong* 痛 (pain) and the name of the affected body part, which in almost every instance lies along the path of the vessel under discussion.

Hygiene is not ignored in the *Huangdi neijing*, but for reasons discussed in Section Four ("Intellectual Background") the *Huangdi neijing* affirms the ideal of health while at the same time insisting on the priority of vessel theory pathology and acupuncture; that is, the business of physicians is to treat illness, not to encourage their patients or patrons to undertake hygienic regimens. Chunyu Yi makes no references to hygiene at all. The Mawangdui and Zhangjiashan medical manuscripts present hygiene and pathology on more or less equal footing, and suggest historical priority for vessel theory in hygiene. Thus, there are two aspects to vessel theory to be considered: its continuing role in macrobiotic hygiene, and its development as part of pathology.

Keeping these two aspects in mind, let me turn to the question of how vessel theory developed from initial awareness of a physiological structure holding blood and vapor—and named *mai* 脈—to become the foundation of physiological theory. The conception of the vessels in the body and the meaning of the word *mai* were continually changing as physiological ideas flowered and interacted with correlative cosmology to produce a new image of the microcosmic body. Our knowledge of vessel theory before the *Huangdi neijing* is still rough, but the differences between vessel theory in the Mawangdui and Zhangjiashan medical manuscripts and in the *Huangdi neijing* shed light on a theory in the course of development.

Blood vessels are the obvious original referent of *mai* 脈. The earliest attestation of the word is fourth century B.C., in a *Zuozhuan* 左傳 description of a horse: "chaotic vapor, untamed, erupts; dark blood[1] springs forth, coursing; ridges of swollen vessels (*mai*) bulge" (*Zuozhuan*, Xi 15, 14.3a). Blood continues to be the defining feature of *mai* in the *SW* gloss,

[1]"Dark" translates *yin* 陰, which is not used in the technical sense of Yin here.

listed in the form 衇 with 脈 given as an orthographic variant: "The distribution network for blood which angles through the body" 血理分衺行體中者 (*SW*, 11B.6a). The graph is composed of two significs, 血 and *pai* 𠂢; the latter is the signific under which the *SW* classifies *mai* and it also serves as the phonetic of the graph.[1] Thus *pai* 𠂢 and its word family provide clues to the etymology of *mai* "vessel." As a graph, the *SW* identifies 𠂢 as the reverse image of the pictograph *yong* 永: the gloss of the former is "water angling and flowing separately" 水之衺流別也 (*SW*, 11B.6a); the latter is "water which is long; it depicts the long extension of the network of subterranean water-channels" 水長也象水巠理之長永也 (*SW*, 11B.5b).[2] The *SW* gloss of *jing* 巠 (subterranean channel) is necessary to round out the etymological evidence: "Water vessels 水衇. (The graph) is composed of 川 (stream) underneath 一, and 一 signifies earth; the phonetic is an abbreviation of 壬" (*SW*, 11B.3b).

Evidence from the *SW* must be weighed carefully—its etymologies do not invariably yield the original meaning of a word. However, even cautious evaluation of the evidence for *mai* would lead one to surmise that when the word was first adopted there already existed a conceptual correlation between the body and earth, and between blood vessels and streams. The idea of a "network" (*li* 理) of vessels is probably also significant in the original meaning of *mai*. I interpret two occurrences of *li* in the Mawangdui macrobiotic hygiene texts as allusions to the "network of vessels" (*MS*VI.A.9; *MS*VII.B.19). Given the plurality of blood vessels, it would have been logical to conceive of them as a system, even if the exact nature of the system was not determined.[3] The *Guanzi* analogy comparing water flowing through the earth to blood and vapor flowing through the muscles and vessels can be read as an expression of the meaning of *mai*.[4]

The transition from the old idea of blood vessels to a physiological theory whose main purpose was to explain the movement of vapor in the

---

[1]Phonetic contacts between words with initial **p*- and initial **m*- in Old Chinese are common.

[2]It is common to write *mai* "vessel" using 永 rather than 𠂢. The scribal variant 温 is used for *mai* in *MS*I.A, but it appears to be simply a variant and does not contribute to etymological analysis of the word *mai*.

[3]Liu Zonghan notes several occurrences of the compound *mai li* "vessel network" which are probably of Han date (1992b: 250).

[4]Yamada is skeptical of the *SW* etymological evidence and considers the *Guanzi* passage to be of Han date; he argues for a pristine idea of *mai* as vessels in animals (based on the *Zuozhuan* passage), which was extended to vessels in humans and only later acquired connotations relating blood vessels to streams in the earth (1985a: 64-67). I disagree with his argument and his dating of the *Guanzi* passage.

body directed attention away from the blood-vascular system *per se* and towards an idealized system which meshed with correlative cosmology. As vessel theory developed, what held vapor was not clearly distinguished from what held blood. *MS*I.C does pair vessel and vapor as the principal terms of vessel theory, and the same can be assumed for *MS*I.A and *MS*I.B; but there are enough occurrences of "blood and vapor" or "vapor and blood" in the macrobiotic hygiene texts to indicate that the substances are inside the same vessels (*MS*III.89, *MS*VI.A.8, *MS*VI.B.7, *MS*VII.B.4). This is also true in the *Huangdi neijing*, where the vessels contain both vapor and blood (Epler 1980: 339; Unschuld 1985: 74-76; Sivin 1987: 135-38).

Most attention has been given to comparing the system of vessels described in *MS*I.A and *MS*I.B with the *Huangdi neijing*, in particular with *Lingshu* 10. Both texts already know of the classification of the vessels into three types of Yang vessel and three types of Yin vessel; and each vessel has a name. Not enough attention has been paid to differences between the Mawangdui vessel theory texts and the macrobiotic hygiene texts. The hygiene texts understand that vapor circulates in the vessels; *MS*VI.A.8 includes one of several generic references to the "hundred vessels." References to cultivating vapor sometimes specify Yin vapor (Yang vapor is not specified). But there is no evidence of vessel nomenclature nor of a vessel classification scheme; and the concept of Yin and Yang is understood as a complementariness grounded in physiological correlates other than the vessels themselves. The evidence suggests to me that macrobiotic hygiene was not the source of vessel nomenclature and classification. Rather, the Yang and Yin classification of vessels and their names arose in the context of pathology (hence the Yin vessels are the "vessels of death" in *MS*I.D). This new elaboration of vessel theory probably explains Chunyu Yi's perception of it; and he is undoubtedly correct that "differentiating" and "naming" the vessels was accomplished as part of vessel-theory pathology.

Speculation on antecedents to vessel theory as presented in *MS*I.A and *MS*I.B is aided by intriguing evidence in the Zhangjiashan *Yinshu*. Although I still suspect that pathology had the greater influence, we may want to leave open questions regarding vessel classification and nomenclature. In an entry on exercises to treat *lou* 瘻 (neck lumps), "Exercises" classifies the neck muscles into two Yang and two Yin types; and identifies vessels where the neck lumps appear by naming the muscles to which the vessels are attached. At this point I must offer a belated comment on *jin* 筋 (muscle). The *SW* defines *jin* as "the strength of flesh" (*SW*, 4B.41a). There exists a separate word for "tendon" (*jian* 笏; *SW*, 4B.41a), but *jin* itself seems to have included any fibrous tissue binding flesh to bone and giving the body tensility. Muscles and vessels were associated; the *Guanzi* refers to "muscles and vessels" when describing the flow of blood and vapor. And the *Huangdi neijing* gives a separate classification of muscles which in its main features copies vessel classification (*Lingshu* 13, 4.1a). It has been thought that vessel theory combined ideas about muscles and blood vessels (and perhaps nerves) in producing an idealized vascular system (Yamada 1979: 80).

The neck muscles listed in *Yinshu* are: Constant Yang 恒 陽 (right and left),[1] Lateral Yang 側 陽 (right and left), Lateral Yin 側 陰 (right and left), and Front Yin 前 陰 (*YSSW*: 85). The vessels are identified as "vessel attached to the Lateral Yang muscle on the right," "vessel attached to the Lateral Yin muscle on the right," and so forth; the exception is the single Front Yin muscle which is itself the location of the neck lumps (and no vessel is mentioned). *SW*, 10B.14b, analyzes *gang* 亢 (throat) as a pictograph of the "form of the neck vessels." The most obvious blood vessels are the jugular veins, which do give the appearance of being attached to the sternocleidomastoid muscles. Given the conceptual pairing of muscles and vessels, whether the graph 亢 depicts vessels or muscles may be a moot question. The *Yinshu* classification of muscles seems to be old; otherwise one would expect to find the muscles classified in terms of the vessels (as occurs in the *Huangdi neijing*). Perhaps it represents early knowledge of the muscles in connection with hygienic exercises. Another *Yinshu* exercise to cure pain in the malleolus refers to Yin and Yang muscles in the thigh. Pulling the thigh Yin muscle cures pain in the inner malleolus, pulling the thigh Yang muscle cures the outer malleolus—Yin and Yang clearly designate inner and outer sides of the leg as they do in *MSI*.A and *MSI*.B (*YSSW*: 83).

Yinshu does not describe a system of muscles throughout the body, thus we do not know if the classification of neck muscles was applied generally. However, ideas about a physiological structure running from head to foot would be as likely to focus on muscles as on vessels. I presume that ideas about muscles and vessels and their functions are implicit in the ex-

[1]The word *jin* "muscle" is not written after the name Constant Yang, but based on the subsequent names it must have been omitted by mistake.

ercises described in *Yinshu* even though there are few direct references to them; and I suspect that the early conception of a system of vessels was influenced by a parallel conception of muscles which connected the two ends of the body. One mention of vessels is particularly suggestive. It occurs in a list of hygienic exercises and their benefits at the end of "Exercises": "Make a circuit in the vessels and follow along the skin's webbed pattern to benefit the heels and head" (*YSSW*: 85). Recall that *MSI*.C praises the sage's cold head and warm feet, which ensure that vapor travels in the proper downward direction. I submit that what is envisioned in *Yinshu* and in *MSI*.C is not a circulatory system in which vapor passes from one vessel to another in a single, continuous cycle. Rather, the vessels are individual channels (as stated in "Six Constituents") and the vapor circulates inside each channel. What is important is that "heels and head" are united as the result of vapor circulation, not that there is a centralized circulatory system.

This idea of vertical channels is in fact described in *MSI*.A: all three Yang vessels of the foot pass from the foot (more precisely, the Great Yang and Minor Yang vessels begin near the outer malleolus, the Yang Brilliance vessel begins somewhere in the shin) to the head (ending at the nose, eyes, and nose respectively). Of the Yin vessels, only the Minor Yin vessel passes from the inner malleolus to the tongue, while the Great Yin and Ceasing Yin vessels pass from the big toe to the thigh and mid-body region respectively. The vessels are parallel channels which do not communicate with one another. Perhaps the idea of "making a circuit in the vessels . . . to benefit the heels and head" in *Yinshu* centered on vessels which came to be classified as Yang vessels in *MSI*.A. Referring to *MSI*.B, which also represents the vessels as parallel channels, Unschuld suggests that the vessels may have been seen as "strings linking various sections of the body" (1986b: 283). The analogy is apt, and suggests the probable influence of muscles in the development of vessel theory.

Yamada concludes with good reason that vessel theory focused first on identifying and classifying the foot/leg vessels, and that the hand/arm vessels were added later (1985a: 69). The brevity of the accounts of the hand vessels in *MSI*.A and *MSI*.B and the absence of a twelfth hand Ceasing Yin vessel is evidence enough, not to mention the obvious priority of the vessels rising from the lower limbs as outlined above. The key difference between vessel theory in the manuscripts and in *Lingshu* 10 is in the basic structure of the system of vessels. In contrast to the parallel-channel system of vessels in *MSI*.A and *MSI*.B, *Lingshu* 10 describes an interconnected circulatory system. Each vessel is linked to one of the internal organs, whose physiological function influences the vessel.[1] The directionality of the vessels is no longer uniform as in *MSI*.A (according to which the hand vessels also extend upwards from the hand and forearm); in *Lingshu* 10 the twelve vessels are laid out so that they communicate with the organs and one another in a great, interconnected circuit. This interconnected circuit is the basis for applying a broad range of Yin Yang and Five Agent theories to physiology, as well as for applying the calendro-numerological correspondences which quantify correlative cosmology. Moreover, the *Huangdi neijing* vessels are identified as *jing* 經 (conduits), and these conduits are additionally linked by branch systems which contribute to the complexity of the overall system. There are holes (*xue* 穴) on the body located at precise points along the paths of the conduits which permit external access to them (chiefly using acupuncture). Vapor is also classified, with Yin and Yang among the several varieties. Some of these ideas were already known to Chunyu Yi; they represent a new level of theorization combined with idealization (Unschuld 1985: 73-91; Sivin 1987: 49-53, 117-39).

None of these ideas are present in the Mawangdui and Zhangjiashan medical manuscripts. The eleven vessels are not yet conceived as interconnected conduits; the five mentions of internal organs in describing the paths of the vessels in *MSI*.A and *MSI*.B do not indicate any theoretical relation between the vessels and the organs, nor are the organs physiologically significant anywhere in the vessel theory texts;[2] no vessel holes are identified; no varieties of vapor are described. In the absence of fuller theoretical explanations in the texts themselves, we are left to guess at their precise understanding of vessel theory and pathology. The following summary attempts to state what can be known from the texts. We clearly

---

[1]The organ forms part of the name of each vessel in *Lingshu* 10.

[2]*MSI*.A.4 mentions the liver in describing the path of the foot Minor Yin vessel; in *MSI*.A.7 the forearm Great Yin vessel ends at the heart; the kidney is on the path of the foot Minor Yin vessel in *MSI*.B.9, coincidentally the organ associated with the foot Minor Yin vessel in *Lingshu* 10; the forearm Great Yin and Minor Yin vessels both end at the heart in *MSI*.B.10-11. *MSI*.D contains the only reference to *zang* 臟 (depot): the Yin vessels "putrefy the depots," presumably the five depots (heart, kidney, liver, lung, spleen). Yamada sees significance in the fact that *MSI*.A and *MSI*.B only mention organs in connection with Yin vessels, perhaps reflecting the special pathology of the Yin vessels as stated in *MSI*.D (1979: 82). The macrobiotic hygiene texts do not mention specific organs other than the heart, but do include references to the five depots and six *fu* 腑 (cavities) as storage areas inside the body (see Section Four, "Body and Spirit").

know that a six-fold classification of vessels into Yin and Yang types has been achieved; and that the vessel names are the same as those in the *Huangdi neijing*. Notably, *MSI*.B does not use the names Great Yang, Minor Yang, and Yang Brilliance for the three hand Yang vessels, which instead are named shoulder vessel, ear vessel, and tooth vessel respectively. Whether these names represent the older anatomical names for the same vessels before Yin Yang classification, as has been generally thought, or whether the anatomical names are simply accepted alternate names of the hand Yang vessels is not certain (according to *MSI*.B.7, the foot Great Yin vessel is also called the stomach vessel). I am wary of assuming that a definite system of vessels was already identified prior to Yin Yang classification, which then simply imposed itself onto the pre-existing system. Perhaps the system as we see it in *MSI*.A and *MSI*.B crystallized because of the stimulus of Yin Yang theory and the need to classify which it created.[1]

The Yang vessels are associated with the "vapor of heaven" and their ailments are less likely to be fatal than those of the Yin vessels, which are associated with the "vapor of earth" and are the "vessels of death" (*MSI*.D). The lists of ailments associated with the vessels in *MSI*.A and *MSI*.B give nosological specificity to this basic principle of vessel theory pathology in the manuscripts.[2] Pathogenic conditions of vapor in the vessels take several forms: surplus or insufficiency (in which case the vessel must be drained or filled); vapor which moves in the wrong direction; and blockage.[3] Individual vessels can be diagnosed for signs of illness at the malleolus by applying pressure above the malleolus with the left hand and palpating it with the right hand (*MSI*.C).[4] Cauterization is the only ther-

---

[1]The muscle nomenclature in *Yinshu* also suggests that Yin Yang theory and correlative cosmology may have inspired systematic theorizing about physiology. This is not to say that there was no prior knowledge of muscles, but rather that the conception of a system of muscles may not have existed yet. My wariness may prove to be excessive if future manuscript discoveries clarify the issue.

[2]*MSI*.A.6 also associates ailments of the three foot Yin vessels with death. *MSI*.B.7-8 concur that the ailments of the foot Great Yin and Ceasing Yin vessels can be fatal.

[3]The first paragraph of *MSI*.C refers to surplus and insufficiency, as does the third paragraph which describes ailing vessels as being empty or as having excess (manifested in pathogenic movement of vapor). Vapor moving in the wrong direction is described in *MSI*.C when "vapor ascends and does not descend," and in the "reversal ailments" listed in *MSI*.B. Blockage is mentioned in the third paragraph of *MSI*.C.

[4]Diagnosis at the malleolus applies to the foot vessels. The *Maishu* edition of *MSI*.C concludes with several sentences, not found in *MSI*.C, which confirm that vessels are diagnosed individually: "The method for treating ailments. Discern which (vessel) erupted first and treat it. When several vessels

apy mentioned specifically in *MSI*.A, *MSI*.B, and *MSI*.C, although in an extreme situation a vessel can be lanced with a lancing-stone (see "Therapy" below).

The parallels shared between the vessel theory texts on *MSI* and the *Huangdi neijing* indicate a textual relation. The manuscript texts graphically confirm the hypothesis that the *Huangdi neijing* is a summation of written medical knowledge edited so as to reframe older recorded teachings in terms of theoretical innovations (thus the *Lingshu* 10 parallel to the account of the five constituents in *MSI*.D additionally correlates each constituent with one of five Yin vessels). Despite the formal text parallels, it is difficult to trace the historical growth of vessel theory from one text to the next. Ma Jixing is one of several scholars who have argued for a developmental progression of vessel theory with *MSI*.A representing the oldest attested stage and *MSI*.B as the immediate antecedent to *Lingshu* 10 (1992: 87-102). It is true that the vessel descriptions in *MSI*.B contain more anatomical detail than *MSI*.A; and the contents of the *MSI*.B ailment lists are quite close to *Lingshu* 10. However, Yamada and others have noted several features linking *MSI*.A and *Lingshu* 10 which are missing in *MSI*.B. For example, *MSI*.A consistently uses the technical names for all the vessels whereas *MSI*.B uses anatomical names for the three hand Yang vessels; and *MSI*.A describes branches of some vessels which relate well to the branches described in *Lingshu* 10, but branches are missing entirely from the *MSI*.B descriptions. The argument for a progression from *MSI*.A to *MSI*.B to *Lingshu* 10 is weakened on both points. Yamada prefers to identify *MSI*.B as the "direct archetype" of *Lingshu* 10 and *MSI*.A as the "collateral archetype" (1979: 72-73).[1]

Even speaking of both manuscript texts as archetypes of *Lingshu* 10 without implying historical progression is problematic. The essential feature of vessel theory in *Lingshu* 10 is the concept of a great circuit formed by twelve interconnected conduits, which is missing in *MSI*.A and *MSI*.B. Recall that *MSI*.A represents the eleven vessels as parallel channels which all extend upwards from the extremities. *MSI*.B is similar, except that two vessels extend in the opposite direction: the foot Great Yin vessel passes from the stomach down to the inner malleolus, and the shoulder

---

erupt in ailments together, pick the one that is most severe and treat it first" (*MSSW*: 74). There is no corresponding description of diagnosing vessels at the wrist.

[1] I should note that Yamada consistently refers to the *Taisu* edition of the vessel description text in *Lingshu* 10, which he regards as the older edition.

vessel (corresponding to the forearm Great Yang vessel in *MSI*.A) passes from the ear down to the back of the hand. A survey of the *Huangdi neijing* shows that it does not present a unified vessel theory in accordance with *Lingshu* 10. There are several references to eleven vessels (the hand Ceasing Yin vessel is regularly missing) and to vessel systems reminiscent of *MSI*.A and *MSI*.B. The directionality of the vessels in *Lingshu* 17, 4.7a, coincides exactly with *MSI*.A (Unschuld 1986b: 298-99). One might argue that the two vessels which extend downwards rather than upwards in *MSI*.B indicate a stage in the transition from the idea of parallel channels to an interconnected circuit, but other factors—like connecting the organs into the system—are more probable inspirations for the *Lingshu* 10 vessel system. Liu Zonghan argues convincingly that *MSI*.A and *MSI*.B are the prototypes of vessel theory not in *Lingshu* 10, but in the other *Huangdi neijing* passages which maintain older ideas; that is, the idea of an interconnected-circuit of conduits in *Lingshu* 10 was not derived directly from the kind of parallel-channel system described in *MSI*.A and *MSI*.B, hence its origin is not explained by the manuscript texts (1992a).

Yamada observes that knowledge of internal organs and other parts of the body in *Lingshu* 10 "clearly proves that there had been rapid development in anatomy" prior to its compilation (1979: 80). What we find in *MSI*.A and *MSI*.B is just as clearly a record of vessel theory pathology at a time when anatomical knowledge was more limited. Yet the idea of vessels which hold vapor has already resulted in a classified system of vessels, which serves as the basis for pathology. I find it noteworthy that so many theoretical pieces are already in place—in particular the detailed linkage between the vessels and ailments as indicated in the parallels between the vessel ailment lists in *MSI*.B and *Lingshu* 10. Speculation on the relation between physiology and illness was ahead of actual anatomical knowledge.

THERAPY

The main evidence of therapy is in *MSI*.E, whose basic view of illness is ontological not physiological. The only exception is the single inguinal swelling recipe in *MSI*.E.135. Internal and external uses of drugs predominate, and are discussed in "Materia Medica." Magical therapy (primarily exorcistic) is discussed in Section Five. Medical theory is not discussed in *MSI*.E, but there are examples of choosing drugs and applying therapy that reflect theoretical considerations, including: plants picked at the summer solstice or eggs collected in spring, which are understood to have solar, Yang potency (prior magico-religious belief regarding the solar virtues of drugs must also be taken into account); homeopathy;[1] and environmental factors affecting treatment.[2] In comparison with Chunyu Yi—who in his medical case histories only proceeds with treatment after diagnosing the vessels to determine the nature of the ailment—therapeutic principles in *MS*I.E are fashioned from a combination of practical experience, magical belief, and naturalistic reasoning.

The inclusion of *MS*II.B (the second edition of *MS*I.B) ahead of the hygienic exercises in *MS*II.C indicates a relation between the exercises used to cure ailments and vessel theory pathology. Of course the main evidence of therapy in combination with vessel theory pathology is in *MS*I.A, *MS*I.B, and *MS*I.C. *MS*I.A and *MS*I.B specify cauterization as the therapy used with vessel theory pathology. *MS*I.A concludes each vessel ailment list with the recommendation to treat the ailments by cauterizing the vessel. *MS*I.B does not include the formulaic recommendation of cauterization, but does mention some precautions for the patient when cauterizing the foot Minor Yin vessel (*MS*I.B.9). Neither text describes how cauterization is performed and exactly where on a vessel it is applied. *MS*I.C refers to cauterizing vessels near the waist; the actual technique is not described. The condition being treated is an excess of vapor in one of the vessels which causes "vapor to ascend and not descend." Cauterization near the waist is intended to redirect the vapor downwards (in the warm foot and cold head paradigm, vapor normally flows downwards in the vessels towards warmth). The condition is evidently serious, because the text recommends a second cauterization higher on the body than the first if the first cauterization is ineffective. Finally, if cauterization fails to work, it is necessary to cut open vessels at the elbow and knee with a lancing-stone (*bian* 砭) to release the vapor. As a rationale of lancing the vessels, *MS*I.C recounts the principles which apply to lancing abscesses and other swellings in order to drain pus.

---

[1]In *MS*I.E.267, chilblain is treated by steaming frozen earth and hot-pressing the chilblain with it. The homeopathic treatment of facial pustules in *MS*I.E.280 involves magical correspondence—the ailment name, *ma* 瘍, is written with the graph for horse inside, and horse cheekbone is the drug used to treat it.

[2]*MS*I.E.188 forbids exposure to the night sky while treating scars lest the stellar and lunar essences interfere with the treatment.

Both cauterization and lancing with a lancing-stone are included in *MSI*.E; that is, both are older therapies which *MSI*.C employs in the newer framework of vessel theory pathology. Before surveying therapy in *MSI*.E, let me first examine these two therapies from the perspective of the vessel theory texts. *MSI*.A clearly understands cauterization to be the ideal therapy for correcting pathogenic conditions of vapor in the vessels. Lancing, on the other hand, is still used primarily for draining pus; lancing vessels is an extreme measure, not the therapy of choice. The Mawangdui vessel theory texts confirm cauterization as the earlier therapy associated with vessel theory pathology. I concur with Yamada that the practice of cauterization contributed to the elaboration of vessel theory. Because cauterization applied externally affected the condition of vapor in the vessels internally, successful cauterization also confirmed the location of the vessels. And the knowledge that some places on the path of a vessel were more efficacious therapeutically than others certainly began with cauterization and culminated with the identification and naming of acupuncture pits (*xue* 穴) where needles were inserted. Yamada speculates that physicians began using metal needles (*zhen* 鍼) by the late third to early second century B.C., substituting the prick of a needle for the hot stimulus of cauterization. By the time of the *Huangdi neijing*, acupuncture overshadowed cauterization (Yamada 1985a: 70–73).

The use of the *bian* in *MSI*.C seems to be transitional. Chunyu Yi's writings combine the word *bian* for the lancing-stone in a compound with *jiu* 灸 for cauterization, understanding *bian jiu* to be the vessel-theory therapies "acupuncture and cauterization"; the lineage of the new acupuncture therapy is traced to the old lancing-stone (*Shiji*, 105.23a, 24b; Yamada 1985a: 37–39). We can be reasonably certain that Chunyu Yi pricked patients with metal needles (*zhen*), especially in the light of the gold and silver needles discovered in 1968 in the tomb of Liu Sheng 劉勝 (King of Zhongshan 中山王 from 154 B.C. to his death in 113 B.C.).[1] The same tomb also contained two small ax-shaped blades of rock crystal which are thought to be lancing-stones. The blades are well suited for lancing abscesses as detailed in *MSI*.C (Sun Ji 1991: 300). Which medical instrument—needle or blade—is understood in the *MSI*.C description of lancing vessels with a *bian*; and what is the significance of attaching the account of lancing abscesses to drain pus?

[1] Ma Jixing associates the excavated needles with the "nine needles" of the *Huangdi neijing* (1972).

Yamada characterizes the transition from cauterization to acupuncture as rapid, and speculates that early acupuncture needles imitated the forms of the older *bian*. The newer metal needles were also used for lancing abscesses, and—according to passages in the *Huangdi neijing*—for bloodletting, although these uses did not fit into the theoretical framework of vessel theory and were abandoned except for some simple bloodletting techniques (1985a: 70-71). Perhaps *bian* in *MSI*.C refers to a metal needle rather than a stone blade. But even if it is a needle, its use still does not constitute a formal therapy grounded in vessel theory, for which the earliest evidence is Chunyu Yi's writings. In short, acupuncture as a therapy still did not exist at the time *MSI*.C was composed.[1]

However, a parallel to the *MSI*.C account of lancing vessels in *Lingshu* 7 indicates that lancing abscesses was indeed one of the rationales of acupuncture which found its way into the *Huangdi neijing*. In the *Lingshu* 7 passage, which concerns the proper use of the nine needles of acupuncture, every occurrence of *bian* "lancing-stone" is replaced by *zhen* "needle"; and every reference to *nong* 膿 (pus) is replaced by *bing* 病 (ailment). The technique of using lancing-stones to rid an abscess of pus has been transferred to the technique of using acupuncture needles to rid the patient of an ailment (*Lingshu* 7, 2.5b; Yamada 1985a: 44). The central idea is that the needle, like the lancing-stone, opens the vessel to "release" the ailment; that is, to release the pathogenic vapor which is the counterpart to pus. This idea is present in *MSI*.C in embryonic form. Recall that the rationale for cauterization is the use of heat to correct the condition of pathogenic vapor inside the vessel. Lancing contributes a new element—the discharge of pathogenic vapor.

---

[1]Lu and Needham (1980: 77-88) state that acupuncture is attested for the sixth century B.C. in two passages in the *Zuozhuan* (whose information is best treated as fourth century B.C., the probable date of its compilation). They also conclude that the *Shiji* account of Bian Que documents knowledge of the *xue* "pits" in acupuncture theory by the fourth century B.C. Their interpretation of the *Zuozhuan* passages is inaccurate (cf. Unschuld 1985: 94, n. 64; and Yamada 1985a: 6-11); and imputing a fourth century B.C. date to Bian Que and his practice of acupuncture is not credible (cf. Yamada 1988). Moreover, Yamada has shown that the interpretation of the term 三陽五會 in the *Shiji* as the name of an acupuncture pit is doubtful (1988: 130-32). Perhaps this is the place to state once again that lancing is not acupuncture; the latter began when the use of needles was adopted as a therapy in vessel theory pathology (see the Introduction, p.5, n.2). Chinese scholars may be correct when they speculate that certain neolithic, Shang, and Zhou needle- and blade-like instruments are medical instruments (Ma Jixing and Zhou Shirong 1978), and when they propose interpreting certain Shang graphs as related to the medical use of such instruments (Hu Houxuan 1984). However, the use of these instruments does not constitute acupuncture.

Since Epler's study of bloodletting in the *Huangdi neijing* this practice has also been seen as belonging to the prehistory of acupuncture (1980). One of the problems with Epler's hypothesis is the lack of documentation of bloodletting in Chinese medicine before the *Huangdi neijing*; all references to *bian* in Warring States, Qin, and early Han sources consistently associate the lancing-stone with the treatment of abscesses and other purulent swellings. Even with the archaeological discovery of medical manuscripts we have not found a single reference to bloodletting.[1] The hypothesis remains plausible if only because of the importance of blood vessels in the development of vessel theory, and because bloodletting is known to have been practiced in other ancient cultures. However, one might argue that bloodletting as medical therapy in the *Huangdi neijing* arose simultaneously with acupuncture as physicians began to insert needles into vessels.[2] In any case, *MS*I.C does not corroborate the bloodletting hypothesis and suggests an alternative to it.

Despite the association between vessel theory and cauterization in the Mawangdui vessel theory texts, cauterization did not monopolize therapeutic practice in the third and second centuries B.C. even within vessel theory pathology. The applicability of the newer acupuncture therapy was of course still being established. Chunyu Yi's writings provide the clearest evidence. Chunyu Yi states categorically that when he treats patients, "I invariably press their vessels first and then treat them" (*Shiji*, 105.24b). Thus vessel diagnosis is indispensable. But of the eighteen instances of therapy administered by Chunyu Yi in the medical case histories, fourteen are drug therapy, two are cauterization of vessels, and two are acupuncture (Yamada 1985a: 37-38). The only traditional ailment treated with cauterization or acupuncture is a case of cauterization for dental decay.[3] Moreover, while Chunyu Yi uses both therapies, he explicitly cautions against using them when "according to the model one should not perform

[1]Epler (1980: 349) relies on Miyashita's conjecture regarding bloodletting in the Shang bone and shell inscriptions as proof of the antiquity of bloodletting in China (1959: 235). Miyashita's interpretation of the inscriptional evidence as bloodletting is uncertain; and it certainly cannot be used to prove the existence of bloodletting in Warring States medicine in the absence of any evidence.

[2]Chunyu Yi states in one of his medical case histories that after inserting acupuncture needles into three places on the patient's foot he pressed on the spots to prevent bleeding (*Shiji*, 105.15b).

[3]*Shiji*, 105.16a. The other ailments concern: disturbance in the foot Ceasing Yin vessel, requiring cauterization of the vessel (*Shiji*, 105.15a); heat reversal (*re jue* 熱 蹶), treated by pricking the feet with needles (*Shiji*, 105.15a); and ascending reversal (*jue shang* 蹶 上), treated by performing acupuncture on the foot Yang Brilliance vessel (*Shiji*, 105.17a). *Jue* "reversal" is the same condition described in *MS*I.C when vapor moves in the wrong direction.

acupuncture and cauterization" (*Shiji*, 105.23a); that is, after diagnosing the vessels a physician had to additionally determine if acupuncture and cauterization should or should not be administered. Based on the medical case histories, Chunyu Yi favored drugs.

Chunyu Yi's medical practice apparently combined the older tradition of drug therapy with the new vessel theory pathology; and also utilized cauterization and acupuncture in accordance with vessel theory. Chunyu Yi was surely not alone, but the promotion of acupuncture at the expense of other therapies in the *Huangdi neijing* suggests that many physicians ranked acupuncture well above the other therapies. Let me turn now to these other therapies (exclusive of drugs and magic) as represented in *MS*I.E.

Cauterization is one of five forms of heat therapy in *MS*I.E. In the first of two descriptions of the technique in *MS*I.E, a cord is ignited and pressed against a wart; once the wart is hot it is plucked off (*MS*I.E.64). In the second description (in *MS*I.E.127), inguinal swelling is treated by cauterizing the center of the crown of the patient's head with a kind of lit cigarette until it blisters. The cigarette wrapper is made of *ai* 艾 (mugwort) leaves, perhaps anticipating the later use of moxa (prepared mugwort leaves) for moxibustion. Cauterizing the center of the crown of the head has inspired conjectures about early knowledge of acupuncture pits, since it coincides with the location of the well-known *baihui* 百會 (hundred convergence) pit. However, the same spot is also where *ji* 薊 (thistle) is pressed to treat a lizard bite in *MS*I.E.53 (an example of counterirritation). The idea that therapy applied to one part of the body affects another part does not require an explanation based on vessel theory. Physicians probably discovered the therapeutic virtue of the crown of the head long before vessel theory.

The other four forms of heat therapy are: roasting (*zhi* 炙), literally roasting the affected part of the body over fire after first applying medicines to it; hot-pressing (*yun* 熨), most often pressing heated materials against the patient's body but there are variations; fumigation (*xun* 熏), in which heat and the steam or smoke of the fumigants play a role; and balneotherapy, immersing the affected part of the body in hot medicinal baths. The therapeutic use of heat in *MS*I.E is sophisticated, and surely bears witness to a naturalistic rationale of heat in ontological pathology. Nevertheless, heat therapy has older magico-religious associations which were still very much alive in the third and second centuries B.C. The heat of fire is transformational, exorcistic, and prophylactic. It is not coincidental that *jiu* "cauterize" is one of the verbs used to denote the act of thrusting the firebrand against the turtle shell to make it crack in the *SW* gloss of *bu* 卜 (pyro-plastromancy; *SW*, 3B.41b). The use of a burning cord or mugwort-wrapped cigarette in *MSI*.E is analogous to the divination technique. The demonography "Jie" in the first Shuihudi hemerological treatise prescribes holding a burning torch aloft to bar revenants from entering the home (*SHD*: 213). The affinity between medical cauterization and magico-religious acts may be overlaid by naturalistic ideas, but it is definitely present in *MSI*.E.

The affinity is even more evident in the examples of vermifugal roasting and fumigation in *MSI*.E. *MSI*.E.208 explicitly associates scabies with bugs which are expelled after the medicine-covered scabies are roasted. Scabies are treated by roasting in three more recipes (*MSI*.E.202, 204, 206), and other scabies recipes use well-known vermifugal drugs; for example, the feces of a ram and a rat (*MSI*.E.200, 211).[1] Correspondingly, fumigation is used to expel bugs in recipes for hemorrhoids, which also have a bug etiology. Hemorrhoids swarming with pinworms are fumigated by burning an unidentified drug in a pit while the patient kneels over it in *MSI*.E.149. The patient sits over a steaming jar of drugs boiled in urine in *MSI*.E.147 (the steam is so irritating to the throat that the recipe includes a formula for a soothing beverage to counteract it). Fumigation is one of the most potent demonifuges, and occurs frequently in the Shuihudi "Jie." In one entry the Yang Demon 陽 鬼, a reification of Yang, prevents the kitchen stove from cooking food; the remedy is to "burn pig feces inside the house, then it will stop" (*SHD*: 212). When the Pestilence Demon 癘 鬼 occupies a home, causing the occupants to suffer from itching, the remedy is to "burn fresh *tong* 桐 (paulownia) inside the house, then it will desist" (*SHD*: 216). These fumigations have parallels in received literature in *Zhouli* accounts of the exorcistic responsibilities of certain state officers.[2] Let me reiterate that fumigation and other forms of heat therapy in *MSI*.E belong to a medical tradition in which naturalistic theories were developing rapidly, while at the same time the therapies

[1]It is unlikely that the itch mite *Sarcoptes scabiei* was already observed in early Chinese medicine. There is probably some other basis for the observation of bugs in scabies.

[2]Harper (forthcoming) discusses the relation between magico-religious fumigation and fumigation in *MSI*.E.

applied to the body continued to be analogous to magico-religious activities.

Soaking in a hot bath of decocted *tao* 桃 (peach) leaves to treat itch (*MS*I.E.255), and soaking a wounded shin in a pot of water with pulverized drugs which is kept hot all day (*MS*I.E.199) are the two examples of balneotherapy—which I distinguish from the more numerous examples of washing the body with medicinal liquids. *Yun* "hot-pressing" occurs more frequently. The therapy takes its name from the instrument used to iron fabric. In *MS*I.E.19, hot-pressing the body with scorched salt wrapped in cloth expels the cold and wind which are the cause of "rigidity due to a wound." The hot-press expellent in *MS*I.E.25, used to treat rigidity in infants, is made of anthill loam and salt. There are two examples of hot-pressing hemorrhoids. In the first (*MS*I.E.146), oblong stones are burned in the fire, quenched in vinegar, and then used to hot-press the hemorrhoid.[1] The second is, strictly speaking, fumigation; the hemorrhoid is "hot-pressed" with the vapor of a rat boiled in urine (*MS*I.E.154). Equally unusual is the example of "hot-pressing" an abscess with *shanglao* 商牢 (pokeweed) soaked in vinegar (*MS*I.E.159)—perhaps the drug is understood to have "hot" properties.

Let me briefly mention several other forms of therapy in *MS*I.E. Urine retention is treated by roasting the affected area and having two people massage the patient's buttocks in *MS*I.E.104. *Yinshu*, "Exercises," includes a similar entry for urine retention in which the patient stands erect, puts his arms around a pillar, and pulls his buttocks while another person apparently grips his waist (the verb describing the other person's action is illegible in the text; *YSSW*: 84). Massage is of course related to the hygienic and therapeutic exercise tradition illustrated in *MS*II.C (as best as can be determined from its current state of preservation, *MS*II.C does not illustrate an exercise for urine retention). An anal fistula is surgically removed in a complicated procedure in *MS*I.E.153. Hemorrhoidal surgery

[1]Ma Jixing and Zhou Shirong (1978) broaden the definition of *bian* "lancing-stone" to include all stones used in therapy (they are used to massage in addition to hot-pressing). I find no written evidence that the term *bian* refers to stone medical instruments other than a lance and am not convinced by their argument.

also occurs in *MS*I.E.145-46. The first recipe seems to describe cupping the hemorrhoid before cutting it open.

As I stated at the outset, drugs alone or in combination with some of the therapies discussed above predominate in *MS*I.E. In addition to the emphasis on drug therapy I would note a corresponding lack of surgical procedures. The only reference to lancing is in the inguinal swelling recipe (*MS*I.E.135). None of the abscess recipes mention lancing, even though this is the classic application of the lancing-stone. The lack of surgical procedures does not mean that painful therapies are avoided. The cauterization described is hardly painless; and in one of the roasting therapy recipes (for a skin ailment) the patient is instructed to get drunk before beginning the therapy, which is stopped when "the heat is unbearable" (*MS*I.E.74).

MATERIA MEDICA

*MS*VI.A.9 includes the earliest drug descriptions attributed to a physician. Wen Zhi praises *jiu* 韭 (leek) as the "thousand-year herb" which concentrates the vapor of heaven and earth; and he declares it to be the "king of the hundred herbs." The leek calms skittishness, improves vision and hearing, and prevents illness. Liquor is the "vapor-essence of the five grains" which penetrates the vessels and permeates the body, thus it is the "medium for the hundred drugs." And when King Wei asks about eggs, Wen Zhi identifies the chicken as a "Yang creature." The context for Wen Zhi's observations is chiefly dietetic, but they are applicable to materia medica in general. In *MS*I.E as well as in the two macrobiotic hygiene recipe texts (*MS*III and *MS*IV), drugs are typically added to liquor and drunk. Various forms of liquor are the most frequently used substances in the recipe texts, both internally and externally; liquor, itself a drug, is the ideal medium for the other drugs. Bird eggs gathered in the second and third months of spring (when their potency is great) are used to make a skin medicine in *MS*I.E.74 (the medicine is applied before roasting the affected skin). "Spring-bird egg"—perhaps a dickeybird egg—is a tonic food in *MS*III.17; and is used as a male aphrodisiac in *MS*IV.4. Curiously, the leek does not occur in the recipe texts.

The three recipe texts and the section of recipes related to conception and childbirth in *MSV* are the main documentation of materia medica in the Mawangdui medical manuscripts.[1] Ma Jixing estimates the extant number of substances used in the manuscripts to be nearly four hundred, divided between plant, animal, mineral, and prepared substances (the last category covers condiments and food preparations as well as cloth, mats, and other manufactured goods).[2] It is convenient to refer to the inventory of substances as materia medica or as drugs, keeping in mind that foods (grain, fruit, meat, etc.) and other goods are also drugs; and that in addition to therapeutic or hygienic uses, the substances are used in a range of applications loosely related to medicine by virtue of their inclusion in the manuscripts. For example, a woman's menstrual cloth is an ingredient in a medicine taken internally to treat inguinal swelling in *MS*I.E.121; in *MS*III.85, a virgin's menstrual cloth is part of a magical technique to hasten the speed of travel. A similar catholicity is evident in the Shuanggudui *Wanwu*, whose significance for knowledge of early Chinese materia medica is discussed below.[3]

Information on the identity of the drugs or their properties is rarely included in the recipes. Two recipes in *MS*I.E and two in *MS*III are exceptions. *MS*I.E.95 concludes with a detailed discussion of the plant *dujin* 毒堇 (identity uncertain). We learn that "the stalks are red and the leaves have vertical cords," that the fruit has a "bitter taste," and that the fruit forms shortly before the summer solstice. A fresh supply of *dujin* must be gathered every year on the day of the summer solstice, dried in the dark (not in sunlight), and stored in a leather pouch. *MS*I.E.147 describes a plant named *qu* 蓲 (identity uncertain). The recipe first gives the name for the drug in Jing 荆 (i.e. Chu 楚); then it notes that "its leaves can be boiled and are sour; its stalks have thorns" (the Jing name for a second plant is also given). *MS*III.38 and 43, both aphrodisiacs, provide brief identifications for several ingredients (insects and plants); lacunae prevent clear understanding of the text.

[1]In addition, *MS*II.A names one drug; *MS*VI.A includes occasional references to drugs; and the recipes for philters in *MS*VII.A also provide evidence of drugs.

[2]Ma Jixing 1992: 123-26, 1073-98. Ma counts exactly 394; and he does not include some of the magical materials—like those used to exorcise ailments in *MS*I.E and to produce philters in *MS*VII.A—which brings the total to over four hundred.

[3]In the Index of Materia Medica I adopt a broad definition of materia medica as nearly everything that forms part of the treatment of ailments or the execution of techniques (cooking pots, dishes, and sundry utensils used to prepare drugs are not included); that is, if something seems to me to be playing an active role in a recipe—be it the *ge* 葛 (kudzu) used to make exorcistic arrows in *MS*I.E.132 or the *bai* 柏 (arbor-vitae) pestle used for exorcistic beating in *MS*I.E.118—I include it.

A recipe which gives the name for a drug in Jing implies that for the most part the drug names in the text are generally known and are not local names; Chu names were added to editions copied in places like Changsha. Like other elements of medicine, knowledge of materia medica was shared across the cultural and geographical regions of China in the third and second centuries B.C. We have no information on drug production or commerce for this period. Presumably the majority of the drugs named in the recipe texts were obtainable in Changsha, although one wonders how many could be gathered locally like *dujin*. Yoneda identifies three names of drugs used in *MS*I.E which had to have been imported from the north: *gancao* 甘 草 (licorice), *fangfeng* 防 風 (saposhnikovia), and *huangqi* 黄 耆 (astragalus; 1988: 52).[1] Several drugs are explicitly identified as imports: Rong salt in *MS*I.E.97 is salt from Rong 戎, the northwestern borderlands; *MS*III.69 uses a stone found in the vicinity of Song Mountain 嵩 山 (in present-day Henan); and the dark fungus in *MS*III.77 comes from Luo 雒 (the Luo River 洛 水 region, Henan).

Unschuld (1982b) and Yoneda (1988) address the problem of identifying the precise botanical, zoological, or mineralogical referents of drug names in *MS*I.E (the majority of drugs are plants and animals) as well as questions concerning the relation of drug knowledge in *MS*I.E to the *Shennong bencaojing* and later materia medica.[2] As Yoneda wisely cautions, the correlation between drug names and their referents in the natural world has hardly been constant. Already in medieval times, Tao Hongjing 陶 弘 景 (456-536) complained that physicians did not themselves know drugs and instead listened to the drug sellers in the market; and the sellers' knowledge was also faulty since they relied in turn on the drug gatherers (Yoneda 1988: 48-49; Unschuld 1986a: 38). Yoneda lists several factors influencing which plants, animals, or minerals went by which names in traditional materia medica: either identifications were imprecise and resulted in several natural referents for a single drug name; a substitute supplanted the chief referent of the drug name; or the same name was applied to different things in different regions. Yoneda adds that unchanging identity between a drug name and its natural referent from antiquity to the present is not common in materia medica (1988: 49-52). Despite the

[1] See the Index of Materia Medica for occurrences. *Fangfeng* also occurs in *MS*III.

[2] Other Mawangdui medical texts which utilize drugs were not available before publication of *MWD*, vol. 4. Detailed studies of all materia medica in the Mawangdui medical manuscripts have not yet been published.

twentieth century normalization of Chinese materia medica which includes scientific identifications, we should not become overconfident that we know the very plants, animals, and minerals named in the Mawangdui medical manuscripts. When the evidence is strong I provide a scientific identification using *ZY* as the standard reference. This does not mean, however, that I am equally confident of all of the identifications, many of which I still regard as tentative.

Unschuld utilizes a statistical model to estimate the correlation between *MS*I.E and later materia medica. Although my definition of materia medica is broader than Unschuld's, and my scientific identifications are not in complete agreement with his, Unschuld's conclusions bear repeating.[1] Based on a count of 224 drugs in *MS*I.E, Unschuld judges 27 to be unidentifiable, 109 to be identifiable with confidence, and another 47 to be identifiable with a fair degree of confidence. Thus, 156 out of 224 drugs (or roughly seventy percent) can be compared to later materia medica with relative confidence (1982b: 58). Comparing *MS*I.E to Tao Hongjing's *Bencaojing jizhu* 本草經集注 (the oldest extant recension of the *Shennong bencaojing*), Unschuld estimates that slightly more than half of the drugs in *MS*I.E can be correlated with drugs listed in the *Bencaojing jizhu* (1982b: 59). Even with generous margins of error for both figures, it is clear that *MS*I.E bears witness to an early tradition of materia medica which resulted several centuries later in the compilation of the *Shennong bencaojing*.[2]

The other recipe texts include some of the same drugs found in *MS*I.E along with additional drugs. I have not attempted to extend Unschuld's statistical analysis of *MS*I.E to all drugs in the Mawangdui medical manuscripts, but the relation with later materia medica is equally evident. Most importantly, the other recipe texts document hygienic drug use which is missing in *MS*I.E (it is wholly concerned with the use of drugs to treat ailments—ailments as understood in ontological pathology). To give two notable examples, *MS*III.2 details a recipe for a fermented beverage with *dianji* 顛棘 (asparagus), which is a well-known longevity drug in the Later Han *xian* cult; and *MS*III.71 provides the earliest record of mica

[1]Unschuld does not count as drugs substances which he judges to be carriers of the drugs (fats and various liquids), and does not include magical materials. It is well to remember that scientific identifications of drug names are subject to the caveats enumerated by Yoneda.

[2]Some drugs in *MS*I.E not listed in the *Bencaojing jizhu* are included in other, later materia medica. For further discussion of the *Shennong bencaojing* and Tao Hongjing's contribution to materia medica, see Unschuld 1986a: 17-43.

ingestion as part of macrobiotic dietetics. Thus, by the third century B.C. the therapeutic and hygienic uses of a variety of individual drugs were already determined. Moreover, the recipe texts sometimes call for as many as seven drugs in specified proportions, suggesting definite ideas about how drugs worked in combination.[1]

What kind of thinking or specific theories guided drug use? Unschuld estimates that among the *MSI*.E drugs with correlates in the *Shennong bencaojing*, about half show some degree of correspondence in terms of the ailments they treat; of course, the therapeutic indications for the other half are different (1982b: 59). Yet there is no evidence in the Mawangdui medical manuscripts of the *Shennong bencaojing*'s theoretical framework for materia medica.[2] The fact that *dujin* fruits are said to be "bitter" and *qu* leaves "sour" (*MSI*.E.95, 147) is not evidence of the formal classification of drugs by taste (sour, salty, sweet, bitter, acrid) for therapeutic purposes. Nor is Wen Zhi's classification of the chicken as Yang evidence of systematic Yin Yang classification. Vessel theory, either in connection with pathology or hygiene, also does not play an identifiable role in materia medica in the manuscripts. For that matter, we do not know how Chunyu Yi combined vessel theory diagnosis with drug therapy. In the medical case histories he refers to drug formulas by proper names and does not mention individual drugs or discuss principles of materia medica (Yamada 1985a: 100-107). Materia medica is insignificant in the *Huangdi neijing*, and drug theory in the *Shennong bencaojing* is not based on *Huangdi neijing* vessel theory pathology; in particular, the Yin Yang and Five Agent theories incorporated into vessel theory pathology do not figure in the *Shennong bencaojing* (Unschuld 1986a: 26-27).

The drug monographs in the *Shennong bencaojing* relate both hygienic and therapeutic information for individual drugs, which are additionally ranked in three grades and classified according to taste and warming or cooling properties. The ranking and classifications represent the application of theory to drugs already in use. Older drug knowledge was not discarded; it was simply incorporated into a new, more systematic materia medica. Theory is not needed to discover which substances in nature are medically effective; nor is theory a prerequisite for experimentation with

---

[1] *MSI*.E.157 describes a seven-drug compound used as an internal medicine for *ju* abscess; the proportions of the drugs vary depending on the location of the abscess.

[2] The classification of drugs and drug theory in the *Shennong bencaojing* are discussed in detail in Unschuld 1986a: 18-27.

combinations of drugs such as occur in the Mawangdui medical recipe texts. The recipe texts restore evidence of materia medica before the *Shennong bencaojing* systematization. While the recipe texts do not reveal an underlying theory, there are indications of ideas which informed early knowledge of materia medica.

I would note first of all the strong magico-religious component. Many of the substances used in the recipe texts had dual uses in medicine and in popular religion or occult practice; naturalistic explanations of their properties which emerged in Warring States medicine built on and did not invalidate their magical properties. The magical properties of drugs continue to be noted in the *Shennong bencaojing* and later materia medica, which identify certain drugs as demonifuges in addition to describing their properties according to naturalistic standards (Unschuld 1986a: 25-26). *Jiao* 椒 (zanthoxylum) is one of the important aromatics in early Chinese religion, used to both attract spirits and expel demons (Mizukami 1977: 521-50). Zanthoxylum is used nine times in the medical manuscripts—several times in combination with two other pungent aromatics which are used even more frequently, *jiang* 薑 (ginger) and *gui* 桂 (cinnamon).[1] Rationalization of the medicinal value of pungent substances was surely already accomplished in Warring States medicine, hence the frequency with which zanthoxylum, ginger, and cinnamon are used for therapeutic and hygienic purposes in the manuscripts. But their very prominence should be seen against the background of their prior and contemporary magico-religious uses.[2]

Magical properties are obviously foremost for the substances used in *MSI*.E. for exorcistic operations, including feces (*MSI*.E.233, 235) and peachwood (*MSI*.E.137, 276). The use of such substances in other contexts is not unrelated; their exorcistic efficacy is simply an assumed property. Feces have already been mentioned as a vermifugal, demonifugal drug associated with bug-related ailments in *MSI*.E. In *MSI*.E.71, dog

[1]For combinations of zanthoxylum, ginger, and cinnamon, see *MSI*.E.2, 157, 171; *MSIV*.5. There are more combinations of zanthoxylum with cinnamon, zanthoxylum with ginger, and ginger with cinnamon. Cinnamon—including *jungui* 菌桂 (curled cinnamon)—is used a total of twenty-three times; ginger a total of fifteen times.

[2]Mawangdui tomb 1 exemplifies the importance of aromatics in mortuary customs. The woman's corpse was holding in its hands silken pouches filled with zanthoxylum, cinnamon, and other aromatics. And all four storage areas in the burial chamber surrounding the coffins contained aromatics; notably six sacks in the storage area on the west side, five of which were filled with a mixture of zanthoxylum, cinnamon, ginger, and other aromatics (Hunan yixueyuan 1980: 261-66).

feces play an important role in treating "crazed seizure," evidently a demonically-inspired seizure. The feces are spread on an incision made along the back of the sufferer's head, which is then covered with a white chicken for three days. Afterwards the chicken is cooked and eaten by the sufferer. The therapy is like therapy in other recipes in which drugs are prepared and administered; yet it is barely one step removed from the overtness of an exorcistic ritual to drive the demon from the sufferer's body. The recipe represents a kind of sublimation of exorcistic behavior, which is replaced by the manipulation of drugs understood to be exorcistic. The exorcistic nature of consuming chicken flesh is best illustrated in *MSI*.E.274, which treats the demonic *gu* ailment by having the patient consume a medicine made from one black rooster and one snake. I suspect that the clay-wrapped baked chicken eaten to cure hemorrhoids in *MSI*.E.150 is also exorcistic, as is the dog medicine used to treat rigidity in *MSI*.E.22.[1]

Peachwood bows and figurines were a standard item in the Warring States magico-religious arsenal; their exorcistic properties were associated with the sun, Yang, and the east (see Section Five, "Varieties of Magic"). A bow is used exorcistically in *MSI*.E.137; a figurine in *MSI*.E.276. Perhaps the peach-leaf bath to treat itch in *MSI*.E.255 shares some of the same efficacy. The use of peach fruit (*MSIII*.23) and peach fuzz (*MSIII*.43; *MSIV*.3, 12) in aphrodisiacs may be due to their Yang potency, but magical associations are not absent. Eastward orientation alone is sufficient to render certain plants more efficacious, as in the case of the east-facing parts of *huai* 槐 (pagoda tree) used in *MSI*.E.264 to treat scabbing (*MSI*.E.265 uses an exorcistic incantation to treat the same ailment).

The variety of drugs and the elaborateness of their use indicate the other major aspect of ideas about materia medica in the Mawangdui medical manuscripts. Quite simply, within the community of physicians, knowledge of materia medica was organized; it was known that drug X was useful for application Y. Oral traditions—including those of drug gatherers and others—certainly played an important role in the diffusion of this knowledge, but I regard the Shuanggudui *Wanwu* as evidence that physicians compiled lists of drugs which noted their applications. Such written lists would have provided much of the therapeutic and hygienic information later incorporated into the *Shennong bencaojing*. Of course,

[1]Dog and chicken are well-known sacrificial animals used for exorcistic purposes. See *Fengsu tongyi*, 8.4a-b; and Bodde 1975: 317-25. The chicken is also Yang, another aspect of its exorcistic efficacy.

Wanwu is not exclusively a drug list. In addition to physicians, other specialists in natural philosophy and occult knowledge had reasons to record the uses of substances in nature. I estimate that slightly more than a hundred names of substances are extant on the fragmentary slips of *Wanwu*, of which at least one third can be identified with drugs named in the Mawangdui medical recipe texts (not all are used medicinally in *Wanwu*).

One drug, *wuhui* 烏喙 (monkshood), occurs four times in *Wanwu*, the most separate entries of any substance: monkshood "stops *jie* 節" (an ailment of uncertain identity);[1] "ingested for one hundred days monkshood improves a person's ability to run"; monkshood "makes horses run faster"; the last entry only preserves the name *wuhui* (Fuyang Han jian zhenglizu 1988: 36, 38, 39, 40). Notably, *wuhui* is the second most used drug in the Mawangdui medical recipe texts (excluding liquors, vinegars, and fats) with twenty-one occurrences.[2] In *MS*I.E its main use is external, for wounds (*MS*I.E.12-13), abscesses (*MS*I.E.162, 227), and scabies (*MS*I.E.209, 212, 215-16); it is used once internally for hemorrhoids (*MS*I.E.151). Its use in *MS*III is internal, chiefly in tonics and purgatives (*MS*III.60-61, 72, 74) as well as to increase one's speed when traveling by foot (*MS*III.77-80). The drug, an aconite, was one of the famous early Chinese poisons—a potion produced from it was used to coat arrowheads and other weapons (*MS*I.E.37-43 provide recipes for treating *wuhui* poisoning). All aconites are a source of aconitine, a narcotic alkaloid still in use as a sedative and pain killer (Heywood and Chant 1982: 11, 26). Appreciation of its toxic and narcotic properties in early Chinese medicine is well documented in both *Wanwu* and the Mawangdui medical manuscripts. *Wuhui* and other aconite drugs continued to be used internally as purgatives and stimulants in later materia medica, although they were no longer the poison of choice in recipes for rapid travel. The *Shennong bencaojing* assigns this use to *langdang* 莨菪 (henbane), which it states "makes a person walk vigorously, running in step with a galloping horse."[3]

I suspect that *yun* 雲 is an abbreviation of *yunmu* 雲母 (mica) in the *Wanwu* entry which states "to lighten the body use Yue Mountain *yun* 越

[1]The editorial committee reads it as *jie* 癤, but I remain skeptical because this word is not attested as a name for a kind of swelling before medieval times.

[2]Cinnamon and curled cinnamon combined occur twenty-three times.

[3]*GM*, 17.20; *ZY*: no. 0649, *Hyoscyamus niger* L. (cf. Unschuld 1986a: 22). The *Shennong bencaojing* also notes that eating too much henbane "makes a person run crazily."

山之雲" (Fuyang Han jian zhenglizu 1988: 38).[1] As noted above, mica is one of the drugs in a medicine which "makes a person longlived and not become aged" in *MS*III.71. *MS*III also includes a category of recipes to "lighten the body and increase strength," but all drug names are missing from the single extant recipe in *MS*III.45. Might not the original recipes have included mica? The conjectural nature of my argument notwithstanding, *Wanwu* and *MS*III can be seen to anticipate the *Shennong bencaojing* monograph on mica, which is placed in the upper grade along with the hygienic information that "when ingested for a long time (mica) lightens the body and extends one's years of life" (*GM*, 8.44).

Unschuld notes the emphasis on the hygienic uses of drugs in the *Shennong bencaojing*. He tabulates eighty-four upper-grade drugs which "lighten the body," thirty-nine which "extend years of life," thirty-one which "eliminate agedness," and another thirty-one which are also useful macrobiotic drugs (1986a: 24). Some drugs in the middle and lower grades are used hygienically, but most are primarily used therapeutically. Thus the chief purpose of ranking the drugs into three grades is to privilege those used in macrobiotic hygiene. At the time of the compilation of the *Shennong bencaojing* (roughly first century A.D.), the tradition of macrobiotic hygiene in medicine had already been influenced by teachings emanating from a kind of syncretistic Daoism and the *xian* cult, which introduced new ideas about the care of the body and immortality (see Section Four, "Intellectual Background"). It is likely that the privileging of macrobiotic drugs in the *Shennong bencaojing* derives from the cross-fertilization between medical hygiene and Daoist/*xian* macrobiotics at that time.[2] The Mawangdui medical manuscripts and *Wanwu* document the physicians' knowledge of materia medica in the third and second centuries B.C. Hygienic uses of drugs in the recipe texts are nearly as numerous as therapeutic uses; and the hygienic information anticipates the *Shennong bencaojing* ("lightens the body," "increases strength," etc.). This is significant evidence of the importance of macrobiotic drug use in the medicine taught by Warring States physicians before Daoist or *xian*-cult influences.[3]

---

[1]Minerals from Yue are noted in another entry which refers to working jade with Yue metal 越金 (Fuyang Han jian zhenglizu 1988: 38).

[2]It is interesting that the materia medica specialists responsible for the *Shennong bencaojing* embraced macrobiotic hygiene while the physician-authors of the *Huangdi neijing* distanced themselves from it.

[3]Unschuld characterizes the *Shennong bencaojing* as having a "Taoist orientation" (1986a: 24). I would argue that the intellectual affiliations of macrobiotic hygiene are complicated and are not

Much research remains to be done on the drugs in the Mawangdui medical manuscripts. In the Translation and in the Index of Materia Medica I attempt a judicious evaluation of the drug names. I generally refrain from comparing their uses (assuming that a drug can be identified with certainty) with uses recorded in later materia medica. I lack the medical and anthropological expertise for critical evaluation of drug use in specific therapeutic contexts, which is made all the more difficult when the evidence is in the form of newly excavated manuscripts. Perhaps this is the place to mention that the Mawangdui medical manuscripts usually do not identify which part of a plant is used as the drug. We may presume the root, but stalks, leaves, flowers, fruits, seeds, and pods of many plants are equally usable (later materia medica is clearer on this point). I trust that these kinds of questions will be addressed by scholars more qualified than myself, and that they will find the Translation an accurate basic guide.[1]

Let me conclude with a brief account of drug processing and of the varieties of medicines or hygienic preparations in the Mawangdui medical recipe texts.[2] The discussion of gathering and processing *dujin* in *MS*I.E.95 includes important details. We learn from it that the summer solstice—a significant day in magico-religious belief and the day the sun is at the peak of its Yang potency—was already an important day to gather certain plants by the third century B.C.; the earliest testimony of gathering plants on the summer solstice in received literature is sixth century A.D. The fifth month, the month of the summer solstice, is specified for the same reason in *MS*III.6-8 (other months and seasons for gathering drugs are occasionally indicated in the recipe texts). *Dujin* must be dried in the dark, not in the sun. The opposite instruction—to dry a plant in the sun or over heat—is given for other plants in other recipes. *Dujin* is one of several drugs stored in a leather pouch; pouches of silk and plain cloth are also used.

Most drugs are pounded with mortar and pestle. The most common term used is *ye* 冶, a word borrowed from metallurgy (where it means to

---

simply Daoist (whether one means the philosophy associated primarily with the *Zhuangzi* and *Laozi*, the syncretistic Daoism of the Former Han, or the nascent religious Daoism of the Later Han). Again, see Section Four.

[1]In addition to Unschuld 1982b and Yoneda 1988, Morimura 1981 and Murakami 1985 represent ambitious preliminary assessments of materia medica in *MS*I.E. Ma Jixing's survey of all Mawangdui materia medica is also a useful beginning (1992: 123-51, 1073-98).

[2]Ma Jixing's account is more detailed (1992: 128-51). Similar information in the *Shennong bencaojing* and Tao Hongjing's additional notes is translated by Unschuld (1986a: 18-39).

cast metal or perhaps to hammer metal). *Ye* denotes the fine pestling required to achieve a uniform powder before the introduction of sifting techniques (which were not common in medicine until after the Han). I adopt the translation "smith" for *ye* in order to preserve the metallurgical connotation.[1] Drugs are also chopped, minced, flaked, hammered, ground, and chewed.[2] Fresh or dried, some drugs are allowed to soak before further use, often in liquor or vinegar; sometimes it is the infusion which is used. When drugs are cooked, the chief methods are boiling, steaming, incinerating, scorching, and frying. Many drugs are incinerated before being pulverized. Boiling, which forms part of the preparation of many decoctions, is the most varied of the cooking methods. Besides simply boiling substances until they are done or boiling to produce a reduced concentrate, there are examples of "thrice boiling" at three degrees of heat: the substances are brought to a certain temperature, allowed to cool, and then cooked again for a total of three times. The lowest temperature is indicated by the verb *wen* 溫 (heat), the highest by *fei* 沸 (bubble). A third word written with the graph 沕 is unattested in received literature, but from the context it appears to represent a temperature in between the other two; I tentatively translate it as "scald."[3]

Therapeutic medicines which are to be drunk may be decoctions or infusions, but it is common to stir pulverized drugs into liquor, vinegar, or some other beverage. Hygienic drug use follows the same pattern. There are a few examples of forming the drugs into balls, which are either swallowed directly or are crushed and drunk in a beverage.[4] Macrobiotic beverages and food preparations are discussed in Section Four, "Techniques." The relation between therapy, pharmacy, and cuisine is evident in *MS*I.E recipes for baked chicken (*MS*I.E.150), a rich millet gruel (*MS*I.E.57), and a strained broth of chicken, rabbit, and grain

[1]See the first occurrence of *ye* in *MS*I.E.3 for details. I disagree with Ma Jixing, who interprets *ye* to mean grinding drugs (1992: 130).

[2]I assume that the many references to chopping, mincing, and flaking involve the use of knives, although it is not impossible that the terms might refer to pounding the drug to a certain degree of fineness as well. Drugs are chewed in the mouth in three recipes: *MS*I.E.197, *MS*III.74, *MS*IV.3. See Ma Jixing 1992: 130-31, for further discussion of pulverization vocabulary.

[3]The three words are discussed in the notes to *MS*I.E.102.

[4]Balls of a four-drug compound (including monkshood) are swallowed to treat hemorrhoids in *MS*I.E.151; in *MS*I.E.2, the balls are crushed and mixed into liquor. Macrobiotic balls are swallowed in *MS*III.16-17 and *MS*III.71 (where the main ingredient is mica); the balls swallowed in *MS*III.77 (also containing monkshood) speed travel.

(*MS*I.E.58).[1] Most ointments for external application are prepared either by frying the drugs in lard or by blending pulverized drugs with lard without cooking. Decoctions, infusions, and drugs in solution are also used externally. One innovative form of external application is used in *MS*III and *MS*IV exclusively for aphrodisiacs, usually applied to the region of the genitals. Cloth is repeatedly soaked in a drug liquid, allowed to dry, and soaked again until the liquid is gone. The drug-impregnated cloth is then rubbed on the body (*MS*III.23, 37-43; *MS*IV.3, 6, 7).[2]

[1]Note also the frequent use of grain throughout the recipes in *MS*I.E.

[2]In several recipes a mixture of drugs is spread on the cloth rather than the soaking method described. *Lingshu* 6, 2.5a, details a similar preparation (the cloth is soaked in an infusion of liquor, zanthoxylum, ginger, and cinnamon!), which is used to *yun* "hot-press" an ailment rather than as an aphrodisiac.

SECTION FOUR
MACROBIOTIC HYGIENE

The first text in the Zhangjiashan *Yinshu*, "Seasonal Regimen," opens with a hygienic maxim attributed to Ancestor Peng 彭祖, the paragon of longevity in late-fourth and third century B.C. received literature: "Spring, generate; summer, grow; fall, collect; winter, store—this is the way of Ancestor Peng" (*YSSW*: 82). The text continues with an amplification of the hygienic regimen appropriate to each season:

> Spring days. After rising in the morning, eliminate water,[1] scrub (the hands), rinse (the mouth), wash the teeth, and knock (the teeth);[2] unfasten the hair, stroll to the lower end of the hall to meet the purest of dew and to receive the essence of heaven,[3] and drink one cup of water—these are the means to increase accord. Enter the palace[4] from evening until greater midnight;[5] increasing it injures vapor.
>
> Summer days. Wash the hair frequently, bathe rarely; do not rise late; eat many greens. After rising in the morning and eliminating water, scrub and rinse with water, and clean the teeth; unfasten the hair, walk to the lower end of the hall, and after a while drink one cup of water. Enter the palace from evening until midnight; increasing it injures vapor.

---

[1] I.e. urinate.

[2] Later in *Yinshu* knocking the teeth when awaking is said to prevent tooth decay (*YSSW*: 85).

[3] Perhaps breath cultivation.

[4] "Enter the palace" translates *rugong* 入宫, which from the context denotes sexual intercourse. The term also occurs in the demonography "Jie" on the first Shuihudi hemerological manuscript, where I previously interpreted it to mean "married" (*SHD*: 213; Harper 1985: 496). *Rugong* is attested in received literature, but its proper denotation has not been recognized. An anecdote in *Hanfeizi*, 11.200, mentions ritual purification in which, "for half a year you must not enter the palace (*rugong*) nor drink liquor and eat meat." The phrase has been read as an injunction barring the ruler from entering his palace, but clearly it is sexual intercourse that is forbidden.

[5] "Greater half" 大半 and "lesser half" 少半 refer to two thirds and one third respectively (see *MSI*.E.90, 156). "Greater midnight" 夜大半 ought to be 1:00 A.M.; and "lesser midnight" 夜少半 11:00 P.M. (see below). Cf. Chen Mengjia 1965: 121, 126.

> Fall days. Bathe and wash the hair frequently. With drink and food, let hunger or satiation be whatever the body desires. Enter the palace however often the body finds it beneficial and comfortable—this is the way of benefit.
>
> Winter days. Bathe and wash the hair frequently. The hands should be cold, the feet warm, the face cold, the body warm.[1] One should rise from sleep late, and while recumbent must stretch out straight. Enter the palace from evening until lesser midnight; increasing it injures vapor.

Ancestor Peng's way of hygiene is directed to an elite, male audience; and it encompasses various activities that promote a healthy, enjoyable, and long life—personal cleanliness, cultivation of vapor (or "dew" and "essence"), diet, and sexual intercourse. In *MS*VI.A.6, Ancestor Peng teaches men to value the vapor associated with the penis, claiming that "longevity lies entirely with the penis." Daily exercise, breath cultivation, and diet serve to "secure" the penis and nurture its essential vitality. The final text in *Yinshu*, "Cultivation of the Body," provides teachings on the nature of health and illness. A distinction is made between the noble and the ignoble in society. The ailments of the noble are caused by imbalances of vapor; the "person of the way" 道者 prevents them from occurring by maintaining the proper balance of vapor with breathing techniques. Strenuous labor coupled with their ignorance (they do not even know about the breathing techniques!) make the ignoble prone to sickness and death (*YSSW*: 86). Similarly, "Care of the Body" in *Maishu* assumes that its hygienic teachings are intended for "those who ride in carriages and eat meat" (*MSSW*: 74).

The Mawangdui and Zhangjiashan macrobiotic hygiene texts provide a remarkably full record of a tradition of macrobiotic hygiene which by all appearances was taught to the elite by physicians in the third and second centuries B.C. Writing without knowledge of the Mawangdui and Zhangjiashan medical manuscripts, Graham speculates that the philosophies of Yang Zhu 楊朱 and Zhuangzi 莊子 borrowed physiological concepts

---

[1] Compare these statements to the ideal of cold head and warm feet in *MS*I.C. Perhaps exercise is understood as a way to maintain the proper temperatures.

from medicine in the fourth century B.C. based on circumstantial evidence, chiefly in the *Zhuangzi* (1989: 328). Graham seems to have in mind borrowing from basic medical ideas related to vapor and to Yin and Yang, not from a body of macrobiotic hygiene literature disseminated by physicians. Yet *MS*VI.A.9 presents the fourth century B.C. physician Wen Zhi teaching his "way" of macrobiotic hygiene to the founder of the Jixia Academy, King Wei of Qi. The cross-fertilization between Warring States philosophy and medicine was far more extensive than even Graham thinks.

INTELLECTUAL BACKGROUND

As the excavated macrobiotic hygiene texts make clear, the theory and practice of physical and spiritual cultivation were part of the medical knowledge that the elite acquired from physicians. We now know how philosophy came by the basic physiological ideas that underlie the philosophers' discussions of spiritual cultivation and meditation (none of the extant philosophical texts discuss physiological theory in any detail).[1] To be sure, medicine was hardly isolated from Warring States philosophical discourse and the philosophers contributed to medical thought, especially during the third century B.C. when the nature of the body and spirit became a prominent philosophical issue. At the same time, there is esoteric knowledge in the Mawangdui and Zhangjiashan macrobiotic hygiene texts that has no counterpart in Warring States, Qin, and Han philosophical literature; nothing comparable exists before the cultivation literature of religious Daoism of roughly the third century A.D. and after (see "Techniques" below).

Physiological ideas are the basis for the conception of the sage in the *Guanzi*, "Neiye," as the man who trains his heart to cultivate vapor (*qi* 氣), essence (*jing* 精), and spirit (*shen* 神)—these being the basic elements of human physiology. Meditation in the "Neiye" is this heart/mind training, which produces "perfect virtue" (*cheng de* 成 德) and consequently wisdom (*Guanzi* 49, 16.269). I concur with Graham that the "Neiye" is the oldest Chinese meditation text, probably composed in the late fourth century B.C. and associated with the Jixia Academy (1989: 100). The "Neiye" alternates between discussion of the mystical transformation

---

[1]Roth notes the absence of physiological theory in the philosophical literature, but like Graham is not aware of the excavated macrobiotic hygiene texts (1991: 602–603).

wrought by the heart and concerns of a more hygienic nature. For example, the discussion of the "way of eating" 食之道 is reminiscent of passages in the Mawangdui and Zhangjiashan macrobiotic hygiene texts (*Guanzi* 49, 16.272; see "Philosophy and Macrobiotic Hygiene" below). As Graham notes, the "Neiye" is not a Daoist text. "Way" 道 has both cosmological and moral dimensions; and the goal of meditative cultivation is to perfect human potential (1989: 105). I would add that its hygienic concerns indicate an affinity with the hygienic teachings of contemporary physicians like Wen Zhi.

A focus on the spirit and meditative cultivation of the heart/mind is evident in the *Zhuangzi*, which at the same time distances its more mystical understanding of cultivation from commonplace hygiene. "Xiaoyao yu" 逍遙遊—probably also late fourth century B.C.—pointedly belittles the ordinary folk who admire Ancestor Peng's longevity and try to emulate him (*Zhuangzi* 1, 7). The same essay later describes a "spirit-being" 神人 who "does not eat the five grains, but sucks wind and drinks dew." His body rendered light by this diet, he "mounts clouds and vapor, driving flying dragons, and journeys beyond the four seas" (*Zhuangzi* 1, 15). The spirit-being's dietetics and breath cultivation have counterparts in macrobiotic hygiene; *MS*II.A relates the technique of "eliminating grain" and "eating vapor." Cosmic flight as the result of long cultivation is described near the end of *MS*VI.A.4; perhaps the *xian* 仙 cult with its ideas about transcendence has influenced both the *Zhuangzi* and *MS*VI.A.4. However, I do not read the *Zhuangzi*'s ideal of the spirit-being as condonation of macrobiotic hygiene or nascent *xian* ideas, nor does it necessarily allude to the *Zhuangzi*'s own program of cultivation. The spirit-being is fashioned to serve as yet another image of perfect freedom which stands in contrast to human endeavors (like the Peng bird which opens "Xiaoyao yu"). The *Zhuangzi* is concerned with the cultivation of the spirit in connection with matters beyond bodily well-being, long life, and immortality; it does not share the goals of medical macrobiotic hygiene or the *xian* cult. A program of cultivation is detectable in many *Laozi* passages, which appear to encode specific teachings in verse and metaphor. The precise intent of these passages hinges on what the original frame of reference may have been. Similar use of verse and metaphor to encode techniques in the Mawangdui macrobiotic hygiene texts bear out the physio-spiritual interpretation of *Laozi* passages in Han commentaries like the "Heshang gong" 河上公 and "Xianger" 想爾 (see "Techniques" below). However, cultivation in the *Laozi* is fused to a political plan in which longevity and immortality are not the central goals.[1]

The Mawangdui and Zhangjiashan macrobiotic hygiene texts describe a kind of baseline macrobiotic hygiene for the elite that focuses on care of the body, not on the more philosophical and mystical programs of the "Neiye," *Zhuangzi*, or *Laozi*. In addition, the texts' goal of long life is not identical to the *xian*-cult goal of immortality and transcendence. The formation of the *xian* cult in the third and second centuries B.C. remains unclear. Eremitism, shamanic religion, and ideas about flight to spirit paradises each played a role, as did new ideas about a drug of deathlessness and alchemical elixirs which began to circulate in the third century B.C. Most importantly, the physiological theories on which macrobiotic hygiene was founded also furnished the rationale for immortality—to go from the belief that macrobiotic hygiene can lengthen life to the belief that an individual can create an imperishable body is in many respects a logical progression of ideas (all that is necessary is the assumption that humans can achieve perfection). The promise of immortality seems to have been instrumental in establishing the reputation of the *xian* cult as a superior tradition of macrobiotic hygiene.[2] Rather than adopt Ancestor Peng, the early *xian* cult attributed its macrobiotic traditions to a new pair of legendary adepts, Chisongzi 赤松子 and Wangzi Qiao 王子喬. Their longevity is briefly noted in several third-century B.C. sources; second-century B.C. sources are more numerous and detailed, including references

---

[1]The scholarly convention is to treat the complex of ideas associated with both macrobiotic hygiene and the belief in *xian* as aspects of a belief system loosely called Daoist. However, Graham notes that in the whole of the *Zhuangzi* (which contains a variety of material down to the second century B.C.) there are only two passages concerning the pursuit of immortality; that is, even the later authors whose writings are incorporated in the received text of the *Zhuangzi* were not preoccupied with the theme of immortality (1981: 176). The *Laozi* is an equally unlikely point of origin for ideas about longevity and immortality. The Mawangdui and Zhangjiashan macrobiotic hygiene texts are evidence enough that macrobiotic hygiene did not originate in so-called Daoist philosophy. The case of the *Huainanzi* is more complicated; most of its chapters appear to represent a syncretistic Daoism which crystallized in the second century B.C. Like the *Zhuangzi*, the *Huainanzi* focuses primarily on the more rarefied cultivation of the spirit, yet its rationale of spiritual cultivation incorporates elements from medical and *xian* ideas (see below). This syncretistic Daoism clearly influenced second-century B.C. thought, but it is still difficult to gauge its influence on ideas about longevity and immortality. In short, efforts to understand the development of ideas concerning macrobiotic hygiene and the *xian* cult are not well served by a too easy use of the label Daoist.

[2]The basic elements of the *xian* cult are well summarized in Kaltenmark 1953: 8-26; and Needham 1954-, vol. 5, part 2: 93-126. Qin and Han recipe gentlemen played a major role in the spread of the *xian* cult.

to immortality and cosmic flight.[1] The word *xian* does not occur in the Mawangdui and Zhangjiashan macrobiotic hygiene texts; the only mention of ideas related to immortality and other possibly *xian* beliefs is the brief passage in *MS*VI.A.4 (discussed in "Body and Spirit" below). Given the prominence of the *xian* cult by the end of the third century B.C., we could expect to find signs of its influence in the excavated texts; what is surprising is how slight the influence is.[2]

By the time Li fils practiced the techniques of macrobiotic hygiene described in his manuscripts, the situation regarding physical and spiritual cultivation must have been complex. First, the Daoist authors of the probably second-century B.C. "Keyi" 刻 意 in the *Zhuangzi* criticize people who strive to match Ancestor Peng's longevity by practicing breath cultivation ("spitting out the old and taking in the new" 吐 故 納 新) and exercises ("guiding and pulling" 道 引; *Zhuangzi* 15, 237); a criticism which is seconded in a parallel passage in *Huainanzi*, 7.105. In the words of the *Huainanzi*, the "realized man" 真 人 focuses on the condition of the spirit; his spiritual communion with the ultimate does not depend on exertion to "nurture the form" 養 形 because he knows that physical decay is inevitable. Thus he is not distracted by the popular hygienic regimens. I expect that the criticism did little to dissuade the elite from practicing the techniques described in the Mawangdui and Zhangjiashan macrobiotic hygiene texts.

Then we have the syncretistic Daoism reflected in the *Huainanzi*, which has a definite program of cultivation—an amalgam of Daoist, *xian*, and medical ideas.[3] Finally, there were people who declared themselves followers of Wangzi Qiao or Chisongzi. According to the *Shiji*, Zhang

---

[1]A speech in *Zhanguoce*, 5.13a, alludes to the "longevity of Qiao and Song." *Huainanzi*, 11.178, enumerates the macrobiotic techniques of Wang Qiao and Chisongzi, which culminate in leaving behind the mortal form and taking flight. The *Chuci* poem "Yuanyu" 遠 遊 is a kind of *xian*-cult credo; Wangzi and Chisong are named along with others who became *xian* (*Chuci*, 5.2b, 4b; cf. Hawkes 1985: 199-200).

[2]Sakade notes the more medical orientation of macrobiotic hygiene in the Mawangdui texts; Sakade distinguishes between this type of hygiene, which he associates with the figure of Ancestor Peng, and the beliefs and practices of the *xian* cult (1985: 426-29). It has been argued that Ancestor Peng's interlocutor in *MS*VI.A.6, Wangzi Qiaofu 王 子 巧 父, is none other than Wangzi Qiao; I think the identification is doubtful (in any case, nothing in the content of the passage bespeaks *xian* ideas). Parallels between the technique of breath cultivation in *MS*II.A and *Chuci*, "Yuanyu," also raise the possibility of *xian*-cult influence, but it is possible that the technique was shared by both traditions.

[3]Roth gives a thorough account of physiological and spiritual cultivation in the *Huainanzi* (1991: 628-48).

Liang 張良 (d. 187 B.C.) wished to "abandon affairs among men to wander with Chisongzi," which led him to study "avoidance of grain" (*bigu* 辟穀), "guiding and pulling," and "body lightening" (*Shiji*, 55.12b). All three were also part of what I shall call standard second-century B.C. hygiene and are attested in the Mawangdui macrobiotic hygiene texts (see *MS*II.A on "elimination of grain," *MS*II.C on "guiding and pulling," and *MS*III.45 for a tonic to "lighten the body"). I do not doubt Chisongzi's reputation among enthusiasts, but I wonder how different from standard hygiene the practices were. I also wonder whether everyone who professed admiration for the legendary *xian* adepts actually participated in the *xian* cult or whether it was the convention to glamorize any form of macrobiotic hygiene with a *xian* pedigree.[1]

I assume that the hygienic practices in Li fils' manuscripts were customary rather than exceptional among people of his class; and that the "way of Ancestor Peng" in *Yinshu* was a standard guide to healthful living. If a distinctive *xian* macrobiotic hygiene literature was already circulating, I can only conclude that we have not recovered it in the manuscripts excavated to date. Yet there are signs of a trend to associate macrobiotic hygiene with *xian* ideas by the first century B.C. The changing perception of hygiene is formalized in the rubric adopted for the subcategories of medical literature in the *Hanshu* bibliographic treatise: sexual cultivation literature is placed in a separate category, even though sexual cultivation is one of the branches of macrobiotic hygiene; the rest of the macrobiotic hygiene literature is in a category entitled "Shenxian" 神僊 (Spirit transcendence; *Hanshu*, 30.82a). The summary appended to the category states that "Shenxian" literature, "provides the means to secure the real nature of life and to explore what lies beyond it," making *xian*-style "exploration of the beyond" part of the definition of macrobiotic hygiene. The summary also strikes a note of warning to practitioners of macrobiotic hygiene: "Yet because some people devote themselves solely to this endeavor, grandiose, deceptive, weird, and obtuse texts proliferate all the more—this is not how the sage kings instructed. Confucius said,

[1]The *Shiji* account of Zhang Liang represents his "grain avoidance" dietetics as a kind of self-imposed starvation which Zhang abandoned at the behest of Dowager Lü 呂太后. Before assuming that all such dietetic practices were regarded as ascetic extremism—which is not the impression one gets from *MS*II.A—we should consider Sima Qian's motive for portraying macrobiotic hygiene as he does (for the historian the issue is whether an official should quit government service for selfish reasons).

'To seek the occult and engage in weird practices in order to leave a mark for later ages—this I will not do.'"

The accusation could have been leveled (and was) at all *fang*-literature, which lay outside "canonical art" in Han intellectual and social orthodoxy (see Section Two, "Recipes, Techniques, Calculations, Arts"). Orthodox censure of both macrobiotic hygiene and the *xian* cult focused on the issue of selfishness. Even the *Huainanzi* gives voice to the orthodox complaint in a passage which states that for devotion to macrobiotic hygiene Chisongzi and Wangzi Qiao "can be said to have nurtured life, but cannot be said to have been filial sons" (*Huainanzi*, 20.354). Horiike surveys the attitudes of Han intellectuals towards macrobiotic hygiene and *xian* ideas; unsurprisingly, expressions of skepticism and disapproval outnumber approval (1988: 298-311).

The physician-authors of the *Huangdi neijing* acknowledge that according to physiological theory a person will not become ill so long as he maintains the natural harmony of the organism. This is the subject of *Suwen* 2, which concludes with the dictum: "The sage does not treat those who are already ailing, he treats those who do not yet ail; he does not treat what is already chaotic, he treats what is not yet in chaos" (*Suwen* 2, 1.9b). The kind of preventive medicine implied in this statement is of course the individual practice of hygiene. Yet, vessel theory in the *Huangdi neijing* is vessel theory pathology; and the physician uses vessel theory to diagnose illness, which he treats with the nine needles of acupuncture. The *Huangdi neijing* physician does not necessarily condemn macrobiotic hygiene. *Suwen* 2 opens with a discussion of harmonizing the body with the seasons which is clearly related to the "way of Ancestor Peng" in the *Yinshu* (*Suwen* 2, 1.6a-7b). There is the same correlation of spring/generate, summer/grow, fall/collect, and winter/store; and there are recommendations about times for rising and going to bed. But the real point of *Suwen* 2 is to demonstrate the correlation between the microcosmic body and macrocosmic processes across the seasons. Where the *Yinshu* details a specific hygienic regimen, *Suwen* 2 substitutes general principles. *Lingshu* 55 increases the distance between vessel theory pathology and macrobiotic hygiene by quoting the dictum on "treating those who do not yet ail" in a new context. The ideal no longer concerns working to keep patients healthy, but rather concerns the physician's skill in diagnosing the entire course of a patient's illness. The superior physician "treats *what* does not yet ail," meaning that his acupuncture therapy is applied not to the morbid condition which is already manifest in the organism ("what is already ailing")—it is too late for that—but to the next stage of the illness which he can expect to treat. Preventive hygiene has disappeared.[1]

In the midst of *xian*-cult enthusiasm, Daoist critique, syncretistic-Daoist approval, orthodox disapproval, and neglect by the medical establishment represented in the *Huangdi neijing*, I think a medical tradition of macrobiotic hygiene—a kind of standard hygiene—remained a part of everyday elite life. The *Lunheng* attests to its continued vitality in the first century A.D. Wang Chong states that he himself wrote a "book on nurturing life" in sixteen fascicles which treated of "nurturing vapor and self-preservation," "ingesting drugs and pulling and guiding," and other subjects in hopes of extending his own life (*Lunheng*, "Ziji," 30.592). The book is lost, but Wang Chong's sympathy for macrobiotic hygiene comes out at various points in the *Lunheng*, even as he savages what he regards as the unfounded belief in immortality and transcendents (*xian*). According to Wang, "swallowing drugs and nurturing life can make a person free of ailments; they cannot increase his longevity to become a transcendent" (*Lunheng*, "Daoxu," 7.148). And again, "there has tended to be proof of ingesting drugs to lighten the body and increase vapor, but (the idea) that it extends your years so that you transcend (*du* 度) the world—of this the world has no verification" (*Lunheng*, "Daoxu," 7.157).

A distinction between the medical tradition of macrobiotic hygiene and the newer *xian*-cult hygiene is not an issue in the Mawangdui and Zhangjiashan macrobiotic hygiene texts; it became an issue for Wang Chong because by the first century A.D. macrobiotic hygiene was so closely associated with *xian* ideas in the popular mind. In subsequent centuries, religious Daoism developed its own macrobiotic theory and practice out of the legacy of Han medical and *xian* ideas, while at the same time more popular hygienic traditions coexisted with and borrowed from religious Daoism. The Mawangdui and Zhangjiashan texts invite comparison to later popular and religious Daoist hygienic literature—a large-scale undertaking which I do not attempt here except for the occasional illustration. The following discussion focuses on the characteristics

[1]In vessel theory pathology individual ailments are manifestations of a physiological dysfunction whose location within the organism continues to shift, producing new manifestations until the physician intervenes. Unschuld discusses both passages and the elaboration on the *Lingshu* meaning in the *Nanjing* (1986b: 633-34).

of early macrobiotic hygiene, of which the excavated texts are our first significant evidence.

BODY AND SPIRIT

The *Guanzi*, "Neiye," provides the best testimony of the fourth century B.C. formulation of physiological theories which fused the physical and spiritual components of the human organism, and which made vapor the source of each. The "Neiye" opens with the declaration that *jing* 精 (essence) is the source of life (*Guanzi* 49, 16.268). Then in a series of statements spread across its rhymed stanzas the text identifies the heart as the "abode of essence" 精舍, defines essence as the "essence of vapor" 氣之精者, and links essence with the indwelling *shen* 神 (spirit)—which like essence comes to rest in the body so long as the body is cared for properly (*Guanzi* 49, 16.270). In later usage *jing* and *qi*, either singly or in compound form, are ubiquitous terms for the vital stuff which lies at the base of human existence. In the fourth century B.C., the physiological denotation of *jing* was new. Like *shen*, the original meaning of *jing* was related to religious conceptions. Things that were pure and refined were considered "essence," be they the offerings presented to the external spirits or the potency of the spirits themselves.

Shibata (1984) discusses the religious background of essence and spirit, and their naturalization in the physiological theory of the "Neiye." In religion, external spirits were believed to descend to human beings; or humans might draw them down with the power of *de* 德 (virtue; another philosophical concept with religious origins). The "Neiye" transfers this religious transaction to the physiological plane, and equates essence with vapor. Having opened with the statement on essence as life, the text shifts to a discussion of "human vapor" 民氣, and identifies the role of virtue: "This vapor cannot be stopped with strength, yet it can be made to rest with virtue" (*Guanzi* 49, 16.269). The chief innovation in the "Neiye" is the equation of essence and vapor, which unites essence and spirit (with their old religious connotations) with vapor. Moreover, every human being possesses an indwelling spirit which is particular to the body in which it resides yet is similar in nature to the external spirits. Virtue serves to explain the mechanism by which vapor, essence, and spirit are drawn to the body and stored inside.

The "Neiye" mentions the combination of blood and vapor in passing (*Guanzi* 49, 16.271), but the focus throughout the essay is on the triad of vapor, essence, and spirit, which must be stored and concentrated inside the body in order to create a wellspring of vitality. If virtue is the philosophical explanation of how the three are cultivated, it is clear that at the very least the "Neiye" assumes the practice of breath cultivation. The same focus is evident in the Mawangdui macrobiotic hygiene texts. The breath cultivation technique in *MS*VI.A.1 is entitled "the way of the Heavenly Teacher to eat spirit vapor." References elsewhere in *MS*VI.A to "essence and spirit," "essence and vapor," and other combinations are frequent, as are references to wellsprings inside the body. The techniques of cultivation are breathing, sex, exercise, and diet; several paths to one goal. As already noted, the "Neiye" has a philosophical plan that goes beyond macrobiotic hygiene. One need not claim a fourth-century B.C. date for the Mawangdui and Zhangjiashan texts to argue that they restore examples of medical ideas that were part of the intellectual context within which "Neiye" physiological theory was formulated.

The physio-spiritual fusion in the Mawangdui macrobiotic hygiene texts is expressed most clearly in the term *shenming* 神 明 (spirit illumination), used in *MS*VI.A-B and *MS*VII.B. The term already occurs with a physiological denotation in the "Neiye" where it means something like the divine spark of intelligence (*Guanzi* 49, 16.270). *Shenming* originated in religion, referring to the external spirits or to the magical efficacy possessed by spirits or permeating sacred objects. The religious meanings continued to be used by Warring States philosophers alongside newer meanings referring to numinous powers in nature and to human intelligence.[1] On the one hand, the idea of spirit illumination gave specificity to the mental faculties of the heart and the indwelling spirit, further rationalizing the conception of the human organism. Yet the ambiguity of the term admitted the possibility of a natural sympathy between man and external spirits. This sympathy is expressed in the "Neiye" in a passage which states that when meditative concentration fails to "penetrate" (*tong* 通), "demons and spirits will penetrate it"; followed by the explanation, "this is not due to the strength of the demons and spirits, but to the supremacy of essence and vapor" (*Guanzi* 49, 16.271). The idea that cultivation of essence and vapor leads to contact with external spirits recurs in the *Huainanzi*, in praise for the person who "makes Yin and Yang his model": "His virtue forms a triad with heaven and earth, his illumination

[1]The best account of the early history of the term *shenming*, including complete text references, is Knoblock 1988: 252-55.

is a mate for the sun and moon, his *essence joins with demons and spirits*" (*Huainanzi*, 8.120).[1]

The breath cultivation technique in *MS*VI.A.1 is also called the "doubly marvelous recipe to penetrate spirit illumination." The remaining occurrences of spirit illumination are closely associated with sexual cultivation. Cultivating essence by thrusting his penis in the vagina without ejaculating culminates in "penetrating spirit illumination" in *MS*VI.A.3, which has parallels in *MS*VI.B.2 and *MS*VII.B.3. Female orgasm in *MS*VI.B.8 brings sexual cultivation to a successful conclusion, described as follows: "Essence and spirit enter and are deposited, then engendering spirit illumination." The direct references to sexual cultivation in *MS*VI.A.3 and *MS*VII.B.3 are preceded by more general statements regarding accumulating essence—in the words of *MS*VII.B.3, "to cultivate the body the task lies in accumulating essence." And both refer to an internal space called the "jade enclosure" (a physiological metaphor of uncertain identity) where spirit illumination accumulates. Again, *MS*VII.B.3 provides the more explicit statement:

> The matter of spirit illumination lies in what is enclosed. Vigilently control the jade closure, and spirit illumination will arrive.

Spirit illumination in the Mawangdui macrobiotic hygiene texts is obviously related to spirit illumination in the "Neiye" and other Warring States philosophical texts. But whereas the philosophical texts use ideas of spirit and spirit illumination to speculate on the nature of mental faculties, in macrobiotic hygiene spirit illumination is a kind of mana which those who practice cultivation can concentrate in their body. I suspect that the macrobiotic concept of spirit illumination is older than the philosophical one, and that it retains a deeper awareness of the human organism as a sacred vessel. This awareness may explain some of the physiological metaphors in descriptions of techniques which are attested with a religious meaning in received literature, but not with a physiological meaning. As

---

[1]One of the effects of theorizing about vapor, essence, and spirit was to add another dimension to the understanding of the spirit world; manifestations of demons, spirits, and other things in nature were explained as functions of vapor and essence which could influence the human world. In medicine, the *Huangdi neijing* denies the validity of such ideas. Its theories of vapor, essence, and spirit deal purely with the relation between the indwelling spiritual and mental elements of the individual and the physiological substrate; the external spirit world is not relevant to the functioning of the human organism. This viewpoint was not universal. See Harper 1990: 224-25; and Ishida 1981.

in later religious Daoist cultivation, the language for the body projects a vision of its divinity (see "Techniques" below).[1]

Hun 魂 (ethereal-spirit) and *po* 魄 (earthly-spirit) appear twice, in *MS*VI.A.4 and *MS*VI.A.10. The references are conventional; the view of human life as the fusion of ethereal-spirit and earthly-spirit is theoretically insignificant in the Mawangdui and Zhangjiashan macrobiotic hygiene texts. Yin and Yang are prominent. When Yao 堯 asks Shun 舜 how to cultivate life in *MS*VI.A.5, Shun replies, "investigate Yin and Yang." In *MS*VI.A.1, the Heavenly Teacher teaches the Yellow Thearch that, "when you examine heaven's nature, Yin and Yang are the rulers," then exhorts the Yellow Thearch to "eat Yin and secure Yang; attain spirit illumination." A rhymed breath-cultivation technique follows in the text, headed by the phrase "the way to eat Yin" (this is the same technique which at the end of *MS*VI.A.1 is called the "doubly marvelous recipe to penetrate spirit illumination" and the "way of the Heavenly Teacher to eat spirit vapor"). Many passages in the Mawangdui and Zhangjiashan macrobiotic hygiene texts refer to cultivating vapor, essence, spirit, and the like without specific reference to Yin and Yang. But, whenever human life as a Yin Yang construct is at issue, the texts are unanimous in identifying Yin (or Yin vapor, Yin essence, etc.) as the primary element of life that must be cultivated.

Yinshu, "Cultivation of the Body," provides the most theoretical statement on the subject:

> The reason why people are prone to collapse and suffer early degeneration of Yin is because they are unable to regulate their vapor. Those who can regulate their vapor well and solidify Yin will then benefit their body. (*YSSW*: 86.)

Yin is associated with the body in general and with the genitals in particular (referred to as the Yin); at times the two referents are indistinguishable. Loss of Yin causes irreparable damage: "If there is a calamity for that life, it is invariably because Yin essence leaks out; and the hundred vessels are clogged and derelict" (*MS*VI.A.4). For those who fail to follow a regular program of cultivation, "at the age of forty, Yin vapor has halved itself" (*MS*VII.B.4). And impotency portends physical collapse. In *MS*VI.A.5, Yao asks Shun, "why is it that the Yin is born together with a man and

[1]This concept of spirit illumination is not the concept of the *Huangdi neijing*, which is closer to the philosophical idea of mental faculties (see Ishida 1981: 31).

yet departs ahead of the body?" Shun replies that the Yin (the penis) is too often neglected, even shunned, except in times of unbridled lust. Shun instructs Yao to "cherish it and delight in it; instruct and counsel it; and give it drink and food"; that is, all hygienic activity should focus on nurturing the Yin. Ancestor Peng offers the same advice when he declares, "let penetrating breathing be together with the penis; let drinking and eating be together with the penis" (*MS*VI.A.6). In short, cultivation of Yin encompasses sexual cultivation, breath cultivation, exercise, and dietetics (see "Techniques" below). There is no Yang counterpart to the emphasis on Yin cultivation in the texts.[1]

The texts assume that vapor and essence are inside the vessels, which are sometimes referred to generically as the "hundred vessels." During intercourse, one of the stages the man achieves while thrusting his penis without ejaculating is referred to as "the hundred vessels pass clear through" in *MS*VI.A.3; parallels in *MS*VI.B.2 and *MS*VII.B.3 refer to the same stage as "the waterway passes through." The meaning is that vapor and essence now move freely in the vessels; the idea of the vessels as a waterway reinforces the analogy between the body's vessels and water channels in the earth (see Section Three, "Physiology"). Conversely, when vapor is blocked, "the hundred vessels produce illness" (*MS*VI.A.6).

Except for the heart, none of the usual internal organs are mentioned by name. There are, however, references to the "five depots" (*wu zang* 五臟) and "six cavities" (*liu fu* 六腑). We can probably assume that the depots are the heart, kidney, liver, lung, and spleen. The cavities probably include gall bladder, stomach, large intestine, small intestine, and bladder; it is improbable that the sixth is the *Huangdi neijing*'s "triple burner" (*san jiao* 三焦; see *MS*VI.A.4). The five depots and six cavities are not explicitly linked to the vessels in the Mawangdui and Zhangjiashan macrobiotic hygiene texts, but they are places where vapor and essence are stored (see *MS*VI.A.1, 4, 10). More important as places for storage than the five depots or six cavities are places particular to macrobiotic hygiene: jade closure (*MS*VI.A.3, *MS*VII.B.3), jade wellspring (*MS*VI.A.3, *MS*VII.B.3), womb (*MS*VI.A.7-8; see "Techniques" below), progenitive

[1]Perhaps aphrodisiacs to stiffen the penis and tonics to increase strength in *MSS*III-IV are understood to bolster the Yang element, but Yang is never mentioned. There is one passage in the *Yinshu* which equates illness with imbalances of Yin and Yang vapor, manifested in the emotions of anger and joy respectively. Breathing techniques are used to remedy the excess of each vapor and restore somatic harmony (*YSSW*: 86).

gate (*MS*VI.B.1), central cavity (*MS*VI.B.7), central bourne (*MS*VI.B.8), blood gate (*MS*VII.B.13). Some of the places seem to have a closer association with one form of cultivation than another (progenitive gate and blood gate are evidently synonyms for the place where essence is stored following successful sexual cultivation), and some of the names are attested in later received literature. But we still know too little about early macrobiotic hygiene to be able to specify the exact location and function of the storage places named. A similar caution applies to many unattested physiological terms (some of which are discussed in "Techniques" below).

The conclusion to *MS*VI.A.4 warrants separate discussion because it is the only passage in the Mawangdui and Zhangjiashan macrobiotic hygiene texts that reflects the likely influence of *xian* or syncretistic-Daoist ideas about immortality. The regular perspective in the texts is on the care of the body and on longevity. The conclusion to *MS*VI.A.4 begins with the unexceptional statement that "longevity is born of growth and accumulation." Then it moves in a new direction, declaring that "the person who is capable of it invariably becomes a spirit"; and that such a person achieves *xingjie* 形解. *Xingjie* is attested in the *Shiji* in connection with the *xian* cult and recipe gentlemen during the reign of the First Qin Thearch. *Xingjie* is thought to be synonymous with the term *shijie* 尸解, first attested in the first century A.D. *Shijie* was understood to be the moment of *xian* transformation, and became an important religious Daoist concept. Having fashioned the immortal body within the shell of the mortal body, the *xian* adept's immortal body emerged from the mortal body, which it sloughed off. In this context *shijie* seems to mean "release from the corpse." I am uncertain whether the concept of a second body—the immortal body—which sloughs off the mortal body was already the understanding of *xingjie* in the third and second centuries B.C. *Xingjie* is plausibly interpreted as "release *of* the form," meaning that cultivation renders the one body a person is born with imperishable and it is released from mortal constraints to live as the spirits. To me this is the more likely meaning in *MS*VI.A.4. But I am uncertain of the connection between *xingjie* in the Mawangdui text and in the *xian* cult; and I am not entirely certain that the term originated in the *xian* cult rather than in macrobiotic hygiene.[1]

---

[1]See the notes to *MS*VI.A.4 for text citations. Resurrection is also part of the background to *shijie*, and is examined in Harper 1994.

Following a description of cosmic flight which is reminiscent of the spirit-being in *Zhuangzi*, "Xiaoyao yu," and of *xian* flight, *MS*VI.A.4 rationalizes immortality based on Yin and Yang:

> Wuchengzhao 巫成柖 (identity uncertain) was born together with Yin and Yang. Yin and Yang do not die, and Wuchengzhao is coequal with them. The gentleman who possesses the way is also like this.

The "way" described here is in keeping with passages in the *Huainanzi* which argue that death does not come to someone who is above life and death, someone who renders himself identical to the ultimate source of change which itself is eternally unchanging:

> What gives life to living things has never died; the things that it gives life to are what die. The transformer of things has never transformed; the things that it transforms are what transform. (*Huainanzi*, 7.105.)

The promise of immortality is given in *MS*VI.A.4; and one suspects the influence of literature more focused on that goal. Immortality is not the unifying theme of the Mawangdui and Zhangjiashan macrobiotic hygiene texts.

TECHNIQUES

The true focus of the Mawangdui and Zhangjiashan macrobiotic hygiene texts is on techniques. Unlike the "Neiye," which is a theoretical exposition on the physiology of the sage, the excavated texts are meant to teach how to do it—whether it be breath cultivation, exercise, sexual cultivation, or dietetics. Prior to their discovery, the only ancient example of a macrobiotic technique was a rhymed inscription on a dodecagonal block of jade bearing the title *xing qi* 行氣 (To circulate vapor). The artifact is thought to be late Warring States (perhaps late fourth or early third century B.C.). The technique is presented in nine trisyllabic phrases which describe the stages of breath cultivation from first swallowing the vapor to completion; four explanatory phrases conclude the text:[1]

[1]Rubbings of the twelve faces were published over fifty years ago. The artifact has been referred to as either a jade hilt or a set of jade plaques. The artifact itself was lost and only recently resurfaced; it is indeed a dodecagonal block not twelve plaques. According to Chen Banghuai (1982) the jade is not a hilt and its original function remains uncertain. The inscription has been studied by a

> Swallow, then it travels; traveling, it extends; extending, it descends; descending, it stabilizes; stabilizing, it solidifies; solidifying, it sprouts; sprouting, it grows; growing, it returns; returning, it is heaven. Heaven—its root is above; earth—its root is below. Follow the pattern and live; go against it and die.

The verbs that identify the stages of cultivation are not obscure words (travel, extend, descend, etc.), but neither is it obvious exactly how the technique is executed. Like the "Neiye" and the *Laozi*, the text is an example of verse meant for recitation by initiates who would have received fuller knowledge of its meaning either orally or in ancillary texts. The verse itself is the verbal distillation of the technique, each verb an icon of the act of circulating vapor.[1]

The jade-inscription verse does, nevertheless, describe initial downward movement of vapor, followed by transformation and return upwards—the pattern of circulation recommended in *MS*I.C. The verse has a counterpart in a longer, more esoteric verse on breath cultivation in *MS*VI.A.1, and in another esoteric verse on sexual cultivation in *MS*VI.B.1, as well as in numerous shorter technique records (often rhymed) in *MS*II.A, *MS*III, *MS*VI.A-B, *MS*VII.B, and the Zhangjiashan *Yinshu*. This trove of techniques is complemented by exact recipes for everyday tonics and aphrodisiacs in *MS*III and *MS*IV, and illustrations of exercises in *MS*II.C. Esoterica mix easily in the texts with common knowledge in a way that is characteristic of other *fang*-literature. With the "Neiye" or the single, contextless jade-inscription technique, one is inclined to think of Warring States cultivation theory and practice as an arcane matter with few actual practitioners. The Mawangdui and Zhangjiashan macrobiotic hygiene texts paint a rather different picture of the popularity of macrobiotic hygiene among the elite in the third and second centuries B.C. The techniques and recipes need not all have been practiced daily by everyone. But it is clear that macrobiotic hygiene literature was available, and that it represented the ideal which the elite emulated.

There is considerable overlap between the four main branches of macrobiotic hygiene: breath cultivation, exercise (and massage), sexual cultivation, and dietetics (which I define broadly to include aphrodisiacs and

---

number of scholars. My tentative translation is based on Chen Banghuai's transcription. Cf. Li Ling 1993: 320-23.

[1] For discussion of didactic verse in Warring States philosophy, see Harper 1987b: 560-64.

the like). The four were indivisible elements of a single enterprise. Breath cultivation sometimes occurs simultaneously with sexual intercourse; or a combination of breath cultivation with exercise may be a counterpart to sexual cultivation. The following discussion aims to give a summary of both the shared and distinctive features.

Let me begin with esoterica, using the verse in *MS*VI.A.1 as my example.[1] Encoding a technique in esoteric verse is a well-known feature of religious Daoist cultivation and meditation, beginning with the ca. third century A.D. *Huangting jing* 黃庭經 (Scripture of the Yellow Court). The scripture uses a secret, metaphorical language to describe the inner regions of the body and the spirits who dwell there. Embedded within the text of the *Huangting jing* are instructions for performing the practices essential to achieving the Daoist goal of corporeal perfection and spiritual transcendence, including sexual cultivation. Learning the physio-spiritual denotations of the metaphors was part of initiation into the secrets of the religion; current interpretation of the scripture relies on several extant medieval commentaries.[2] Metaphorical language in certain *Laozi* passages has also been interpreted to refer to physiological and meditative cultivation, although the passages do not describe actual techniques to be performed. The Later Han "Heshang gong" and "Xianger" commentaries provide the earliest evidence of this reading of the *Laozi*.[3] In *MS*VI.A.1, *MS*VI.B.1, and other shorter technique passages in the excavated texts we have the oldest examples of recording cultivation techniques in esoteric verse. Ideas about secrecy and initiation must have been an important part of the social and intellectual background. At the same time, the metaphors made the body a more cosmic and spiritual site. Lacking a contemporary commentary, the metaphorical language is difficult to decipher. But occasionally the denotations are clear and their symbolic significance is evident.

Here is the core of the breath cultivation verse in *MS*VI.A.1:

---

[1]The verse in *MS*VI.B.1 is analyzed in Harper 1987b.

[2]I refer to the so-called "outer" scripture (*Huangting waijing jing* 黃庭外景經), not the later "inner" scripture (*Huangting neijing jing* 黃庭內景經) which was probably composed within the Shangqing 上清 sect of Daoism in the fourth to sixth centuries (see Schipper 1975: 1-11). Maspero's translation of passages related to breath cultivation and sexual cultivation in the *Huangting jing* is classic (1981: 491-94, 524-28).

[3]Needham translates the "Heshang gong" commentary for several such *Laozi* passages (1954-, vol. 5, part 5: 130-35).

> Still your spirit wind, make fast your two racks, triply pound, and let nothing escape. The spirit wind then is born; the five tones then are matched.
>
> Suck it in not more than five times, bring it to the mouth, and still it with the heart—this being what the four assistants prize. The dark winepot then arrives.
>
> Drink it not more than five times; the mouth invariably finds the taste sweet. Bring it to the five depots. The form then is extremely relaxed.
>
> Make it spread to your flesh and skin, and reach to those hair tips. The hair vessels then are permeated. The Yin water then arrives, drenching that Yang blaze. Firm, sturdy, and undying; drink and food enter the body as guests.

A rough synopsis (see *MS*VI.A.1 for fuller explanation): external vapor is inhaled, the two racks (the ribcage?) compress it to produce the spirit wind (an internal vapor?); the spirit wind is brought to the mouth where it is transformed into the dark winepot (saliva); the dark winepot is swallowed, stored in the five depots, and then circulated outward to the skin; an internal transformation produces Yin water, which tempers the Yang blaze inside the body; the body itself is now tempered and benefits from the drink and food introduced into it.

The only metaphor attested in third and second century B.C. sources is "dark winepot" (*xuanzun* 玄 尊), which is attested in a religious not a physiological meaning. Dark winepot is the name for holy water used to worship the *shenming*—in religion, the glowing manifestation of the external spirits. The water was obtained from a Yin mirror-pan set beneath the moon; the condensation in the pan was regarded as Yin fluid from the moon. In the context of *MS*VI.A.1, dark winepot certainly denotes saliva. The technique provides the earliest evidence of saliva ingestion, which was a regular practice in religious Daoism. The technique seems to understand a parallel between the holy water used in religion and saliva; the holy water given to the *shenming* to drink becomes the ingested saliva which produces Yin water—a numinous internally generated fluid. Yang blaze evidently designates an alchemical zone in the abdominal region (anticipating later alchemical metaphors for the body, particularly in religious Daoism). Tempering it with Yin water prepares the body for realizing the full benefit of whatever drink and food are consumed; that is, the technique concerns dietetics as well.

Breath cultivation, exercise, sexual cultivation, and dietetics share the goal of continually replenishing and refining the body's supply of vapor and essence. The following statement in *MS*VI.A.4 is representative:

> The essence of cultivating vapor is to exit from death and enter into life. With zest and gusto, let the taste suckle. To fill the form with this is called "concentrating essence." To cultivate vapor there is a norm; the task lies in accumulating essence. When essence reaches fullness, it invariably drains; and when essence is lost, it must be replenished.

The activity of storing accumulated vapor and essence somewhere and the activity of circulating it throughout the body are equally important; one or both of the activities occur in many techniques (breath cultivation in *MS*VI.A.1 above includes both). *MS*VI.A.4 provides a statement related to breath cultivation:

> It must be made to reach to the extremities[1] so that essence is generated and not deficient. . . . He who is skilled at cultivating vapor lets the old vapor disperse at night and the new vapor gather at dawn, thereby penetrating the nine apertures[2] and filling the six cavities.

Tonics contribute to vapor production, as evidenced by the medicine in *MS*III.61 which "increases the vapor, and also makes a person's face lustrous"; and the liquor in *MS*IV.25 which ensures that the interior of the body "has an abundance of essence-fluid."

"Eating vapor" 食氣 is the usual expression for breath cultivation. The most common verb for inhaling vapor is *xi* 噏 (suck). I identify the term "dual-entry doorway" in *MS*VI.A.4 as the nostrils, providing the only direct reference to inhaling external vapor through the nose: "During the ingress, gauge that dual-entry doorway as if storing it in a deep pool." The nose is the port of entry for external vapor in the "Heshang gong" commentary to the *Laozi* and in religious Daoist breath cultivation. There are three verbs for exhaling through the mouth: *hu* 呼, *xu* 呴, and *chui* 吹. *Hu* is both the usual word for "exhale" and one of the three manners of exhalation in breath cultivation technique. *Xu* and *chui* are more techni-

[1] I.e. the four limbs.

[2] Mouth, eyes, nostrils, ears, genitals, anus.

cal. Based on their usage in *Yinshu*, *xu* is associated with heat and Yang, *chui* with dampness and Yin. In later breath cultivation *xu* exhalation is performed with a round open mouth, *chui* exhalation with lips spread flat (see *MS*II.A for text citations). Exhalation technique is discussed in *MS*II.A:

> Those who eat vapor practice *xu* exhalation and *chui* exhalation when they first go to bed and first arise. Whenever doing *xu* exhalation, in mid-breath change to *chui* exhalation.

The passage continues with details on the timing of the exhalation routine and the number of repetitions during each performance (which is based on the age of the practitioner).

*MS*II.A also details a seasonal routine for breath cultivation. The text identifies six types of vapor in the external atmosphere which the practitioner mixes with his breath in different combinations according to the season. A two-vapor mixture is inhaled in spring, summer, and fall; in winter, four of the six vapors are mixed and eaten. Dusk and dawn are the times of day when cultivation is allowed (*MS*VI.A.4 specifies dawn, daytime, dusk, and midnight as appropriate times). In addition, there are five harmful atmospheric vapors (one each in spring, summer, and winter; two in fall) which must be dispersed by the practitioner before breath cultivation can begin (four of the five are named in the parallel in *MS*VI.A.4). Damage to the silk has destroyed most of the final section of *MS*II.A. However, some of the fragments concern the characteristics of the vapors (atmospheric conditions which produce them, color, appearance, etc.). The knowledge of atmospheric vapors required to practice the technique is similar to the knowledge of the astrological specialists who interpreted the portents signified by similar kinds of atmospheric conditions. The technique is evidence of the specificity applied to the classification of atmospheric vapors for the purpose of "eating vapor."

*MS*II.A several times contrasts "those who eat vapor" with "those who eat grain," expressed in cosmological terms near the end of the text:

> Those who eat grain eat what is square; those who eat vapor eat what is round. Round is heaven; square is earth.

The contrast is not made elsewhere in the Mawangdui and Zhangjiashan macrobiotic hygiene texts; "eating vapor" is simply the term for breath cultivation and the regular consumption of drink and food is assumed. The contrast in *MS*II.A is part of the rationale for the technique of "eliminating grain" which opens the text (and which only occurs in *MS*II.A). Grain is, of course, the basis of the normal human diet, but is also associated with decay. This explains the *Huainanzi* statement that, "those who eat vapor achieve spirit illumination and are long-lived; those who eat grain have quick minds and are short-lived" (*Huainanzi*, 4.60; a final phrase adds that, "those who do not eat do not die and are spirits"). The grain-elimination technique in *MS*II.A involves daily consumption of the drug *shiwei* 石 韋 (pyrrosia) in specified amounts over the course of a lunar cycle, which is obviously coupled with "eating vapor" as described later in the text. According to the text, *xu* exhalation and *chui* exhalation are used to counter some of the physical effects of grain elimination (heavy head, light feet, itchy body); the drug must have also ameliorated symptoms that accompanied grain elimination.

Han sources tend to associate grain elimination with the *xian* cult, whose adepts eschewed human food in favor of macrobiotic drugs and the pure diet of the spirits. Wang Chong dismissed the idea as simply misguided starvation (*Lunheng*, "Daoxu," 7.156). In religious Daoism, grain elimination was additionally related to purging the corpse-worms inside the body—a necessary first step towards undertaking a Daoist program of cultivation (Maspero 1981: 333-35). I remain uncertain of the nature and purpose (or purposes) of grain elimination in *MS*II.A. The text does not seem to be influenced by *xian* ideas of immortality, nor is a belief in corpse-worms evident. No drug besides pyrrosia is mentioned. Yet the dietetics recommended to King Zhao of Qin 秦 昭 王 (r. 306-251 B.C.) in *MS*VI.A.10 could be understood to be a grain-elimination regimen in which food is replaced by macrobiotic drugs like *song* 松 (pine) and *bai* 柏 (arbor-vitae):

> You must face the sun and moon and suck in the rays of their essence; eat *song* (pine) and *bai* (arbor-vitae); and drink running beasts' wellspring blossom.

In both *MS*II.A and *MS*VI.A.10 it is not clear whether the macrobiotic diet cum breath cultivation is to be practiced in perpetuity (as in religious Daoism) or periodically (in *MS*II.A the expectation may be to complete just one mensual cycle). Short-term practice might have served as a method of fasting with therapeutic benefits. Still, the contrast between vapor-eaters (who partake of heaven) and grain-eaters (who partake of earth) suggests a macrobiotic asceticism in which the former are more privileged (dietetics is discussed further below).

The drawing captioned "bear ramble" in *MS*II.C.41 is one of the *daoyin* 導引 (guiding and pulling) exercises named in the *Zhuangzi* criticism of macrobiotic hygiene (*Zhuangzi* 15, 237). There is no doubt that the forty-four drawings in *MS*II.C represent the early *daoyin* exercise tradition. The drawings are skillful, yet few of the captions remain and the original exercises are often difficult to reconstruct from the static poses of the figures. The descriptions of exercises in *Yinshu*, "Exercises," are more informative. "Exercises" includes both single exercises and combinations of exercises in more complicated routines to achieve a specific purpose, often to treat an ailment. Although both the *Yinshu* and *MS*II.C refer only to *yin* "pull," which probably has the sense of "physical exercise" in the compound *daoyin*, breathing is an integral part of many routines in "Exercises."[1] Some single exercises have animal names or are related to Yin and Yang: extending the lower leg and curling the toes thirty times is the "measuring worm";[2] extending both feet out straight thirty times is "pulling the Yang muscles" (*YSSW*: 82); putting one foot forward, kneeling, raising one arm, and bending back is the "tiger pull"; clasping the hands with palms facing out, raising them, and bending down as low as possible—a basic toe-touch—is "pulling Yin"; clasping the hands with palms in and lifting them as high as possible is "pulling Yang" (*YSSW*: 83). "Exercises" concludes with a list of exercises that identifies what part of the body or physiological function they benefit. It is clear from the list that basic calisthenics was very much a part of the early *daoyin* tradition.

The *Yinshu* is a rich source; its documentation of exercise as a branch of macrobiotic hygiene far exceeds anything in the Mawangdui macrobiotic hygiene texts. A full study of the manuscript and its contribution to knowledge of early *daoyin* cannot be undertaken here. I propose to examine just two exercise routines described in "Exercises." Their significance lies in their focus on Yin cultivation, and in their relation to several techniques in the Mawangdui macrobiotic hygiene texts that combine exercise with breath cultivation. Moreover, the Mawangdui techniques

[1]Sakade (1980) examines the meaning of the term *daoyin* beginning with Warring States occurrences. As a compound, *daoyin* often seems to refer to exercise combined with breathing, but there are examples where *daoyin* is exclusively exercise and others where it refers to breath cultivation. The *MS*II.C drawings illustrate different mouth positions which must represent the specific manner of breathing performed along with the exercise.

[2]Measuring worm is also the name of a sexual position in *MS*VI.B.3.

overlap with sexual techniques as a way of cultivating Yin and shed light on aspects of early sexual cultivation technique. The first *Yinshu* exercise is called "increasing Yin vapor":

> Increasing Yin vapor. Sit in the regular position with thighs straddled. Do not feel remorse for food. Press the left hand on the ground. Grasp cooked grain in the right hand and suspend it over the mouth. Then inhale the vapor of the cooked grain, doing it to the utmost. Then eat it. Let both thighs press down, bend the waist, and extend the lesser abdomen forward, using force to do it to the utmost. Do not drink or swallow. Repeat again, stopping after the third time. (*YSSW*: 84.)

This exercise routine, which combines dietetics (ingestion of the vapor of grain and the grain itself) with exercise and breath cultivation (clearly the Yin vapor is circulated internally), is a variation on another exercise called "pulling Yin" (not the toe-touch which is also called "pulling Yin"):

> Pulling Yin. Sit squarely and spread both thighs. Place the left hand on the ground and reach up with the right hand. Bend the waist, extend the lesser abdomen forward, and use force to pull the buttocks. (*YSSW*: 84.)

The additional instruction to pull the buttocks suggests that anal constriction is used to propel the vapor being forcefully compressed in the lesser abdomen. The technique is similar to several passages in *MS*VI.A and *MS*VII.B which refer explicitly to anal constriction. *MS*VII.B.7 describes "eight benefits," most of which arise from sexual cultivation. The first two, however, are techniques which do not involve intercourse:

> To rise at dawn, sit upright, straighten the spine, open the buttocks, suck in the anus, and press it down is "cultivating vapor." When drinking and eating, to relax the buttocks, straighten the spine, suck in the anus, and let the vapor pass through is "bringing the fluid."[1]

The benefits from intercourse begin with the third technique; and the fourth once again concerns anal constriction: "While having intercourse,

[1]"Sucking in the anus" refers to constriction, not to introducing vapor into the body via an open anus. Similarly, "letting the vapor pass through" refers to transmitting vapor internally (the anus is not the port of entry). The sense of "pressing down" is discussed in connection with sexual cultivation below.

to relax the spine, suck in the anus, and press it down is 'gathering vapor.' " The specific role of anal constriction in sexual cultivation is discussed below. A parallel to *MS*VII.B.7 occurs in *MS*VI.A.7, where it is called the "way for coitus with Yin (sexual intercourse) and eating spirit vapor."[1] Moreover, Yin is also understood as the Yin, the male genitals:

> First, relax the limbs, straighten the spine, and flex the buttocks; second, spread the thighs, move the Yin, and contract the anus; third draw the eyelashes together, do not listen, and suck in the vapor to fill the womb;[2] fourth, contain the five tastes and drink that wellspring blossom; fifth, the mass of essence all ascends, suck in the great illumination.

The second stage adds the instruction to "move the Yin" which suggests penile action during intercourse, but other aspects of the technique indicate a second, non-coital application similar to *MS*VII.B.7 and to the two *Yinshu* exercises.[3] Of course, the dual technique is also evidence of the simultaneous practice of sexual cultivation and breath cultivation.[4]

There is an ambiguous reference to "pulling Yin" in *MS*VI.A.8:

> To awaken from sleep and pull Yin, this is called "refining the muscles." To first stretch and then curl, this is called "refining the bones."

More in the nature of a wake-up routine, "pulling Yin" is certainly not a sexual cultivation technique (besides, morning is not the recommended time for men to practice sexual cultivation).[5] Is it the dawn exercise called "cultivating vapor" in *MS*VII.B.7, which then corresponds to the *Yinshu* technique of "pulling Yin"? Or is it something as simple as the toe-touch also called "pulling Yin" in the *Yinshu*? I remain uncertain. Still, the direct

---

[1]The sexual cultivation technique in *MS*VI.A.3 is called "coitus with Yin and cultivating spirit vapor." The sense of "eating spirit vapor" may be purposefully ambiguous in *MS*VI.A.7 (recall that the breath cultivation technique in *MS*VI.A.1 is "eating spirit vapor," "eating Yin," and "penetrating spirit illumination").

[2]"Womb" represents my identification of the graph 脇. The term is discussed under sexual cultivation below.

[3]I have already noted above ("Body and Spirit") that cultivation of Yin is also cultivation of the genitals, which must be included in all cultivation activity (as taught by Shun in *MS*VI.A.5 and by Ancestor Peng in *MS*VI.A.6).

[4]*MS*VI.A.10 and *MS*VII.B.13 also combine sexual cultivation with breath cultivation.

[5]See the statements on proper times for sexual intercourse in the *Yinshu*, "Seasonal Regimen," quoted above; and *MS*VI.B.1, *MS*VII.B.13. *MS*VI.A.6 also describes a morning routine of self-massage and breath cultivation.

references to anal constriction in *MS*VI.A.7 and *MS*VII.B.7 are important evidence of a broader use of anal constriction in early macrobiotic hygiene beyond its role in male sexual cultivation.[1]

Sexual intercourse is denoted by the following terms in the Mawangdui macrobiotic hygiene texts: "coitus with Yin" (*jie* Yin 接 陰), "conjoin vapor" (*heqi* 合 氣), "conjoin Yin and Yang" (*he* Yin Yang 合 陰 陽), "conjoin male and female" (*he nan nü* 合 男 女), "conjoin forms" (*jiexing* 接 形), and "approach the inner (chamber)" (*jin nei* 近 内).[2] Sexual relations are, of course, complicated by the matter of lust. The problem is addressed in *MS*VII.B.9:

> When a person is born there are two things that do not need to be learned: the first is to breathe and the second is to eat. Except for these two, there is nothing that is not the result of learning and habit. Thus, what assists life is eating; what injures life is lust. Therefore, the sage when conjoining male and female invariably possesses a model.

The summary appended to the sexual cultivation category of medical literature in the *Hanshu* bibliographic treatise is in the same vein (*Hanshu*, 30.81a).

The literature recorded in the bibliographic treatise includes books like the *Rong Cheng Yindao* 容 成 陰 道 (Rong Cheng's way of Yin), the *Yao Shun Yindao* 堯 舜 陰 道 (Way of Yin of Yao and Shun), and the *Huangdi sanwang yang Yang fang* 黃 帝 三 王 養 陽 方 (Recipes of the Yellow Thearch and the Three Kings for nurturing Yang). All of the books are lost. Rong Cheng, Yao, Shun, and the Yellow Thearch are associated with macrobiotic hygiene and sexual cultivation teachings in *MS*VI.A. Presumably the books in the bibliographic treatise were also composed in dialogue form, but with far more detail—similar to the style of the *Huangdi neijing*. The oldest sex manuals in received literature are preserved in extensive quotations in chapter twenty-eight of the tenth century *Ishinpô* 醫 心 方, compiled by the Japanese physician Tanba Yasuyori 丹

---

[1]Wile discusses anal constriction in later macrobiotic hygiene, in particular in sexual cultivation (1992: 59). See also, Li Ling 1993: 345.

[2]For "conjoin vapor" see *MS*III.89 and *MS*VI.A.3; for "conjoin Yin and Yang," *MS*VI.B.1; for "conjoin male and female," *MS*VII.B.9; for "conjoin forms," *MS*VI.B.1 and *MS*VII.B.13; for "approach the inner (chamber)," *MS*III.34. "Coitus with Yin" is used mostly in *MS*VI.A. In addition, *MSS*III-IV use *yong* 用 and *wei* 爲 idiomatically in the sense of "engage in intercourse, have intercourse" (see *MS*III.23, 39).

波康賴 from medieval Chinese sources. The *Sunü jing* 素女經 (Scripture of the Immaculate Maid) and *Xuannü jing* 玄女經 (Scripture of the Dark Maid), which may be as old as third century A.D., are composed as dialogues in which the Immaculate Maid and the Dark Maid teach the Yellow Thearch the principles of sexual cultivation. Ancestor Peng also offers occasional teachings.[1]

The medieval sex manuals provide theoretical background for sexual cultivation, but their chief objective is to translate the erotic subtleties of intercourse into a technique which, like other cultivation techniques, guides a man towards success. Each aspect and every stage of intercourse are analyzed, including: foreplay, sexual positions, signs of female arousal, the art of using the penis, and the culminating moment when the man successfully achieves his goal. And the analysis takes a numerical form: there are "five signs" to watch for in the woman as intercourse gets underway, "ten movements" to be made by the penis as it thrusts, "nine manners" in which to thrust it, etc. The same kind of analysis of sexual intercourse is detailed in *MS*VI.B and *MS*VII.B, minus the dialogue manner of presentation; both are realizations of the sage's "model for conjoining male and female."[2] The parallels between *MS*VI.B, *MS*VII.B, and the medieval sex manuals show the Mawangdui texts to be the textual antecedents to the later literature.[3] Previously, a lack of evidence led to speculation that the sexual cultivation technique of the later sex manuals was a Han development (Schipper 1969: 14). We now know that both the technique and the literature came into being as part of Warring States macrobiotic hygiene.

The goal in sexual cultivation is to generate vapor and essence, which the man absorbs and stores inside his body. The description of female orgasm in *MS*VI.B.8 and the statement concerning "nurturing the woman's

---

[1]Evidence of Han sexual cultivation literature is examined by Gulik, who traces the Immaculate Maid and Dark Maid to Later Han times (1961: 70-79); Gulik also discusses the medieval sex manuals in the *Ishinpô* (1961: 121-60). Wile (1992) provides a fine translation of the *Ishinpô* sex manuals along with a general study of traditional Chinese sexology. See also, Harper 1987b; Li and McMahon 1992; and Li Ling 1993: 356-402.

[2]There is a brief dialogue between the Yellow Spirit (the Yellow Thearch by another name) and the Left Spirit in *MS*VII.B.1. For the "five signs," "ten movements," and "nine manners" and their counterparts in the Mawangdui texts, see *MS*VI.B.1, 2, 4.

[3]Passages on sexual cultivation in *MS*III.88-89 and in *MS*VI.A seem to borrow selectively from fuller accounts of sexual cultivation technique like *MS*VI.B and *MS*VII.B. *MS*III.89 is notable for casting the ladies at Yu's court as sex instructresses, anticipating the role of the Immaculate Maid and Dark Maid in the later sex manuals.

essence with my essence" in *MS*VI.B.7 suggest that the woman may also benefit from intercourse, but the technique is designed for the man's benefit. The attention paid to the woman is a necessary part of realizing a true "conjoining of Yin and Yang"—the man must be certain that his mate reaches sexual climax. *MS*VII.B.20 includes one of several statements on the male flaw of haste in intercourse:

> If when having intercourse he is unsuccessful, the blame can be placed entirely on haste. The essential task in the pleasures of play is to be slow and prolonged. If only he can be slow and prolonged, the woman then is greatly pleased. She treats him with the closeness she feels for her brothers, and loves him like her father and mother.

In the later sex manuals male sexual cultivation takes several forms. The man might absorb the sexually generated essence and withdraw from the woman without reaching orgasm. Needham adopts the term *coitus conservatus* for this technique. Alternatively, the man might reach climax but prevent ejaculation and retain the essence inside his body. Needham calls this *coitus thesauratus*. Needham associates *coitus thesauratus* with a method of applying hand pressure to a spot between the anus and the scrotum, which prevents ejaculation by blocking the urethra and redirects the essence internally. He further equates *coitus thesauratus* with the form of sexual cultivation called *huanjing bunao* 還精補腦 (returning the essence to replenish the brain). Needham notes that while the Chinese maintain that the essence passes up the spine to the brain, physiologically the ejaculate—*jing* now become semen—passes to the bladder. In sexual cultivation without male orgasm, the man's *jing* remains an internal essence similar in nature to *jing* in breath cultivation; with male orgasm, *jing* also becomes fluid semen. Whether what passes up the spine to the brain is *jing* become semen or is the vaporous form of sexually generated *jing* is variously understood in the sex manuals (1954-, vol. 5, part 5: 197-99).

Based on careful review of the medieval sex manuals, Wile objects to Needham's definitions on several grounds. First, causing *jing* to ascend by means of "returning the essence" is not exclusively associated with Needham's *coitus thesauratus* in the sex manuals; non-orgasmic *coitus conservatus* also results in "returning the essence." Thus male orgasm is not the defining characteristic of "returning the essence to replenish the brain" as Needham proposes in his definition of *coitus thesauratus*. And the matter of the ejaculate—the *jing* become semen—is less central to cultivation theory. The predominant view in the sex manuals is that whether or not male orgasm occurs, what ascends is vaporous *jing*. Furthermore, anal constriction is a common method for "returning the essence," with or without orgasm. Blocking the urethra with hand pressure is used only with orgasm. Wile prefers the term "retrograde ejaculation" for sexual cultivation in which male orgasm occurs (1992: 59).

In the Mawangdui macrobiotic hygiene texts *jing* appears to consistently name something inside the body similar in nature to vapor; there are no examples of *jing* denoting semen. In fact, no word for semen occurs. Semen is implicit in several passages in *MS*III. An aphrodisiac recipe in *MS*III.5 states that "if (the semen) is already spent, splash (the penis) with cold water," which is intended to cause detumescence. *MS*III.63-64 are recipes for "if a man experiences scantness when engaging in intercourse and (the semen) is clear." But none of the passages on sexual cultivation use *jing* or any other term to denote semen as distinct from vapor and essence. There were surely ideas about semen and *jing* which are simply not elucidated by the Mawangdui macrobiotic hygiene texts. However, I suspect that the conception of *jing* in connection with other forms of cultivation influenced the conception of *jing* in sexual cultivation, not vice versa. I am inclined to think that Wile's understanding of *jing* in the later sex manuals applies to the Mawangdui texts as well. Thus, rather than adopt Needham's "retention of semen" as a general term for male sexual cultivation (1954-, vol. 5, part 5: 30), I prefer "essence retention."

Whether essence retention in the Mawangdui macrobiotic hygiene texts includes both non-orgasmic cultivation (*coitus conservatus*) and orgasmic cultivation (*coitus thesauratus*, retrograde ejaculation) is not certain. The passages on thrusting the penis uniformly describe the benefits of repeated thrusting without ejaculating; none describe male orgasm, ejaculation, or retrograde ejaculation (*MS*VI.A.3, *MS*VI.B.2, *MS*VII.B.3). Passages which describe the culmination of intercourse and what actions the man takes are ambiguous. Let me cite two of the more ambiguous lines first:

> Enter the dark gate (the vagina); ride the coital muscle; suck the essence and spirit upward. (*MS*VI.B.1.)

> Conjoin forms after sunset; and send the vapor to the progenitive gate. (*MS*VI.B.1.)

The section on "cultivation of the eight benefits" in *MS*VII.B.7 refers explicitly to anal constriction in connection with sexual cultivation:

> While having intercourse, to relax the spine, suck in the anus, and press it down is "gathering vapor." While having intercourse, to not hurry and not be hasty, and to exit and enter with harmonious control is "harmonizing the fluid." When getting out of bed, to have the other person make it erect and let it subside when angered is "accumulating vapor." When nearly finished, to not let the inner spine move, to suck in the vapor and press it down, and to still the body while waiting for it is "awaiting fullness." To wash it after finishing and let go of it after becoming angered is "securing against upset."

This is from the same section quoted above which opens with the morning exercise: "To rise at dawn, sit upright, straighten the spine, open the buttocks, suck in the anus, and press it down is 'cultivating vapor.' " In both the exercise and in intercourse, the "it" in the phrase "press it down" 抑下之 refers to the vapor which is compressed by means of anal constriction; there is no evidence of hand pressure as in the one form of retrograde ejaculation. At the culmination of intercourse ("when nearly finished . . ."), the man once again "sucks in the vapor and presses it down" using anal constriction. Because anal constriction is used to influence the vapor at several stages during intercourse, anal constriction alone is not proof of orgasmic retrograde ejaculation in *MS*VII.B.7; but neither is the occurrence of orgasm positively disproven. The text is simply not clear on the question of orgasm.

The same ambiguity applies to *MS*VI.A.7 (quoted above), where the instruction to "contract the anus" occurs at the second stage of a five-stage technique, followed in the third stage by the instruction to "suck in the vapor to fill the womb." The technique culminates in the fifth stage when "the mass of essence all ascends, suck in the great illumination." "Womb" translates *liu/*ljəgw* 腳, which I read as a phonetic loan for *bao/*prəgw* 胞 (womb, uterus) and understand as a womb-like organ where men as well as women store vapor and essence (see *MS*VI.A.7 for details). Other scholars conjecture that the graph should be read as *nao* 腦 (brain), and conclude that the passage is the earliest documentation of "returning the essence to replenish the brain." The conjecture is disproved by the passage itself. "Returning the essence to replenish the brain" culminates sexual cultivation. Assuming that the *MS*VI.A.7 technique concerns sexual cultivation (recall that breath cultivation is also probable), filling the *liu* takes place at the midpoint of the technique; culmination occurs in the fifth stage when "the mass of essence all ascends." In short, the internal place which is filled in the third stage of the technique is not the brain.

However, "sucking the essence and spirit upwards" (*MS*VI.B.1) and "sucking in the great illumination" (*MS*VI.A.7) are evidence of an early idea of "returning the essence," of using sexual cultivation technique to reverse the flow of essence as sexual climax nears and the imminence of ejaculation threatens. *MS*VII.B.3 expresses the concern nicely:

> Conjoin in a sitting position; tailbone, buttocks, nose, and mouth each participate at the proper time. Passing by fleetingly and coming momentarily, the culminant essence is about to be lost. How can I stay it?

Whether orgasm is part of male sexual cultivation in *MS*VI.B and *MS*VII.B or not, the texts do teach the technique of "staying the culminant essence."

*MS*III and *MS*IV devote considerable space to aphrodisiac recipes for both men and women. The use of aphrodisiacs to arouse desire, increase strength, and stimulate the genitals was evidently quite acceptable in sexual cultivation. Wasps are the basic ingredient in *MS*III.12–13. Snails are used in many recipes, as in *MS*III.14:

> Pingling Lü's way of pleasure. Dry in the dark snails (removed) from the shell and smith. If you want twenty, use seven pinches; if you want ten, use three pinches—and one cup of liquor.

The frequency of intercourse and the number of different partners are not discussed in *MS*VI.B and *MS*VII.B. *MS*III.14 is one of several recipes with numbers attached to the dosage ("if you want twenty, use seven pinches"). The numbers probably represent anticipated sexual conquests; the dosage gives a man the strength to finish. The recipe for dried dog-meat prepared with snails in *MS*III.75 is clearer: "Eat one *cun* of the dried-meat slices to overcome one person, and ten *cun* to overcome ten people" (the recipe is intended to fortify a man for encounters with opponents, which is basically the same as encounters with sexual partners).

Turning to dietetics, the tonic drugs, beverages, and foods in *MS*III and *MS*IV supplement the usual diet; nothing in the recipes suggests the kind of ascetic dietetics represented by grain elimination. The recipe for drinking raw eggs in liquor (*MS*III.15) stipulates that the eggs are consumed before the morning meal; taking tonics after meals is more frequent (for example, *MS*III.60-62). Several recipes describe foods that are simply meals in themselves. A dish of boiled *dianji* 顛 棘 (asparagus), chicken parts, and dog parts in *MS*III.34 is "eaten at the late afternoon meal, in whatever amount you wish." Its purpose is to "facilitate approaching the inner (chamber)"; that is, to prepare for sexual intercourse in the evening. *MS*III.50 gives a recipe for boiled beef, concluding with the statement that "you may eat whatever amount of meat you wish" (it fortifies the body).

The *MS*III recipes are grouped under headings, a number of which directly describe their hygienic purpose. Some of the headings, selected from the list in *MS*III.92, are: non-erection due to agedness, cultivation, to lighten the body and increase strength, to purge the inside and increase vapor, to cultivate strength, mash-liquor to benefit the inside. These represent the kinds of properties associated with certain drugs in the *Shennong bencaojing* (see Section Three, "Materia Medica") as well as in the Shuanggudui *Wanwu*, which includes entries like: to firm the body, to double strength, to lighten the body, to increase vapor (Fuyang Han jian zhenglizu 1988: 36, 38, 39). Some of the drugs with macrobiotic properties in the *Shennong bencaojing* figure in the *xian*-cult dietetics of the Han period. The *Liexian zhuan* often records the drugs consumed by famous *xian* adepts, including: *songshi* 松實 (pine fruit), *songzhi* 松脂 (pine rosin), *yunmu* 雲母 (mica), and *gui* 桂 (cinnamon; Kaltenmark 1953: 53, 59, 81-82). In the *xian* cult, these drugs were claimed to replace food in a grain-elimination regimen. The recommendation to "eat *song* (pine) and *bai* (arbor-vitae); and drink running beasts' wellspring blossom" in *MS*VI.A.10 suggests a similar ideal (see above). *MS*III and *MS*IV document the normal use of the drugs in the medical tradition of macrobiotic hygiene.

Two examples will suffice. In *MS*III.71, equal amounts of pulverized mica and pine rosin are combined with whole-wheat flakes and made into balls (the heading under which the recipe comes is missing in the body of the text as well as in the list in *MS*III.92). The recipe details the regimen for swallowing the balls. Beginning with one ball, for the first decade the person swallows an additional ball each day until on the tenth day he swallows ten. For the second decade he gradually decreases the number of balls until on the tenth day he swallows just one. Over successive decades the result is to "make a person longlived and not become aged." The mica-rosin-wheat balls do not replace meals; the mixture of horseflesh and drugs in *MS*III.70 also "increases longevity," and is to be eaten in a dosage of "a three-fingered pinch after the meal." *MS*III.74 is the best preserved of the fermentation recipes in *MS*III and *MS*IV.[1] Received sources indicate that *lao* 醪 (mash-liquor) is a liquor produced by adding a mash of freshly cooked grain to already fermented liquor for a second fermentation (see *MS*III.10). The mash-liquor in *MS*III.74 is a sophisticated and potent cordial worthy of Wen Zhi's praise for liquor (*MS*VI.A.9), and representative of the tradition of medicinal liquors among early physicians.[2] *Wuhui* 烏喙 (monkshood) is one of the drugs added during the fermentation process (see Section Three, "Materia Medica"). The finished cordial is a valued daily tonic:

> Drink one cup at the late afternoon meal. After drinking, rub any places on the body that itch. When ingested for one hundred days, it makes the eyes bright and ears perceptive; the extremities all become strong.

Wen Zhi says of liquor:

> Liquor is the vapor-essence of the five grains. When it enters the inside it disperses and flows; when it enters the internal network (of vessels) it penetrates and circulates.

Each afternoon to drink a cordial and massage the body as the liquory spirits circulate is nice macrobiotic work.

PHILOSOPHY AND MACROBIOTIC HYGIENE

The Mawangdui and Zhangjiashan texts restore the first examples of medical literature on macrobiotic hygiene of the third and second centuries B.C. Their significance for the study of Warring States thought is certain. We can no longer investigate knowledge of the human organism in

---

[1]These recipes are significant for the history of fermentation; the earliest received fermentation recipes are in the sixth century *Qimin yaoshu* 齊民要術.

[2]This tradition is reflected in the word *yi* 醫 (physician). *SW*, 14B.40a, explains the lower part of the graph, which represents "liquor," in terms of the centrality of liquor to medical treatment.

philosophy without considering the interaction between philosophers and physicians. Physicians had the ear of the elite, who also collected their books—books which taught of the body and its care. And their hygienic ideas and techniques were put to use as the elite daily observed dietary recommendations and engaged in various forms of cultivation. Medical ideas and techniques belonged to a pool of knowledge of nature from which the philosophers drew in formulating their ideas about human existence. Philosophers might reject ideas—as did the author or authors of the *Zhuangzi* essay "Keyi" in criticizing the practice of breath cultivation and exercise—and they might tacitly incorporate ideas into their philosophical program.

My purpose here is not to examine standpoints on macrobiotic hygiene among Warring States philosophers, nor to prove that one or another philosopher's ideas were borrowed from the medical tradition of macrobiotic hygiene. To the extent that medical knowledge was a common intellectual property, a philosopher was simply formulating his ideas within the intellectual framework of his time. Some ideas were ubiquitous by the third century B.C. Everyone was talking and writing about *shenming* "spirit illumination," although its exact significance was understood differently in different contexts. Other ideas were better known in connection with a particular philosopher or philosophical book—or, as we now know, a particular physician or medical book. We are accustomed to examining Warring States philosophical literature for signs of cross-influences. We acknowledge that Mencius' idea of vapor owes something to the *Guanzi*, "Neiye," and that the *Laozi* is behind the mystical strain of thought in the political theory of the *Hanfeizi* (Graham 1989: 126-27, 285-92). Because it was lost, medical literature has not been considered as a source of ideas paralleling philosophical literature.

Yet it is evident from the Mawangdui and Zhangjiashan macrobiotic hygiene texts that certain ideas were probably more widely known in medical literature than in philosophical literature. I suspect, for example, that the readership for texts like *MSVI.A* was greater than for the *Guanzi*, "Neiye." Moreover, there is evidence in the excavated texts of hygienic maxims which probably arose in a medical context but which have only been known to us through quotation in philosophical literature. Similarly, theoretical discussions of hygiene in philosophical literature sometimes incorporate phrases which I suspect are culled from accounts of macrobiotic techniques in medical literature. In a text like *MSVI.A*, such phrases fit in a sequence which corresponds to stages of the actual technique. The same phrases in the philosophical literature are like shorthand allusions which assume that the reader already knows of the original technique. The Mawangdui and Zhangjiashan macrobiotic hygiene texts give us the techniques.

I identify several passages from the excavated texts below to illustrate ways in which philosophy may have drawn upon medicine. Again, my purpose is not to review philosophy, nor is it to make claims about textual borrowing. I simply wish to introduce a body of medical literature which, circulating concurrently with philosophical literature, played a role in the formation of ideas about physical and spiritual cultivation. Knowing what the physicians were teaching—which I would argue reflects the elite consensus—we gain a new perspective on the philosophers.

The Zhangjiashan *Maishu*, "Six Constituents" (see Section Three, "Physiology") concludes with a warning against obesity:

> Thus, if the gentleman becomes fat and loses the standard measure, this is called "muscle and bone do not succeed in their responsibilities." His vapor then becomes abundant; his blood then becomes uncontrolled. Blood and vapor putrefy and rot; the hundred joints all collapse. They clog the twenty extremities and turn back, racing to the heart. If this is not treated in advance, one will hear the sound of weeping. (*MSSW*: 74.)

Maishu, "Care of the Body," precedes "Six Constituents" with a maxim and positive advice:

> Now, the reason why flowing water does not become putrid and the doorway pivot is not devoured by bugs is because they move. By moving, you fill the four limbs and empty the five depots. When the five depots are empty, the jade body will benefit.

The discussion of the "way of eating" in the *Guanzi*, "Neiye," warns against either overeating or undereating, observing that, "when overstuffed, injury results and the form does not store things; when undernourished, the bones wither and the blood cakes." Thus: "*When hunger and satiation lose the standard measure*, devise a strategy for it. When oversated, *move rapidly*" (*Guanzi* 49, 16.272). I expect that such advice was common in medical literature. The key to health is to prevent stagnation of blood and vapor, lest they putrefy—a teaching which "Care of the Body" presents figuratively. In received literature the *locus classicus* for the "flowing water" analogy is the *Lüshi chunqiu* essay "Jinshu" 盡數 (Fulfill the calculation):[1]

> The reason why flowing water does not become putrid and the doorway pivot is not devoured by bugs is because they move. The form and vapor are also thus. If the form does not move, the essence does not flow. If the essence does not flow, the vapor clogs. (*Lüshi chunqiu*, 3.26.)

The passage continues with a list of specific ailments caused by vapor clogging in various parts of the body.

"Jinshu" is one of two essays in the third chapter of the *Lüshi chunqiu* which treat of care of the body; it is followed by "Xianji" 先己 (Put oneself first). The first and second chapters of the *Lüshi chunqiu* are thought to contain four essays which represent the self-preservation philosophy associated with the figure of Yang Zhu: "Bensheng" 本生 (Life as the root), "Zhongji" 重己 (Emphasize self), "Guisheng" 貴生 (Prize life), and "Qingyu" 情欲 (Essential nature and desire; Graham 1989: 55). The titles of the chapter three essays (Fulfill the calculation, Put oneself first) appear thematically related to the Yangist essays. However, their emphasis on macrobiotic hygiene sets them apart from Yangist philosophical issues. In my judgment "Jinshu" reads like an adaptation of a medical text; "Xianji" opens with a passage straight from the medical tradition, and then moves on to other topics.

Let me be specific. "Jinshu" opens with Yin and Yang as the models for cultivating life (as does *MS*VI.A.1), next discusses the importance of cultivating essence, and then presents the "flowing water" analogy—probably a well-known hygienic maxim in medicine (as we can see from the *Maishu*, "Care of the Body"). Dietary advice follows the list of ailments, culminating with a statement on the "way of eating":

> Be neither hungry nor sated—this is called the "treasure of the five depots." The mouth invariably finds the taste sweet. Blend the essence, right the figure, and fortify it with spirit vapor. The hundred joints rejoice and all advance to receive the vapor. Invariably drink in small swallows. Be square and erect, do not be hunched. (*Lüshi chunqiu*, 3.26.)

[1]The title refers to fulfilling one's allotted years of life.

I note a marked similarity between this passage and the breath cultivation technique in *MS*VI.A.1, which is a technique for "eating spirit vapor" (see "Techniques" above). The "Jinshu" passage appears to paraphrase a related technique. Do not "blending essence, righting the figure, and fortifying it with spirit vapor" parallel stages of the *MS*VI.A.1 technique, as the practitioner first produces the spirit wind and then the dark winepot (saliva)? And after swallowing the dark winepot five times, "the mouth invariably finds the taste sweet." Is this not the sense of the same statement in "Jinshu"? "Drinking in small swallows" may refer to swallowing in breath cultivation. "The hundred joints advancing to receive the vapor" alludes to the circulation of the vapor (or saliva) after ingestion. Of course, "Jinshu" may still refer to eating and drinking. But eating and drinking are combined with cultivation activity in the Mawangdui and Zhangjiashan macrobiotic hygiene texts. I have no doubt that a late-third or second century B.C. reader of "Jinshu" knew of the cultivation technique underlying the passage, a full account of which was to be found in texts like *MS*VI.A.

The medical passage in "Xianji" is an exchange between King Tang of the Shang 商湯王 and his minister Yi Yin 伊尹 on how to become the supreme ruler.[1] Yi Yin advises King Tang that the first order of business is to *zhi* 治 (order, cultivate) his body, for self-cultivation is the key to ordering the world. The idea was ubiquitous by the third century B.C.[2] Yi Yin recommends a plan:

> Utilize the new, discard the old, and the skin's webbed pattern is permeated. Essence-vapor is daily renewed; evil vapor is entirely eliminated. (*Lüshi chunqiu*, 3.27.)

Rong Cheng's "way to suck in vapor" in *MS*VI.A.4 clarifies Yi Yin's intent:

> It must be made to reach to the extremities, so that essence is generated and not deficient. Above and below are all essence; cold and warm are tranquilly generated. Breathing must be deep and long, so that the new vapor is easy to hold. The old vapor is that of agedness, the new vapor that of longevity. He

[1] Yi Yin is a legendary medical and culinary expert. The *Lüshi chunqiu* essay "Benwei" 本味 (Taste as the root) has Yi Yin teaching King Tang that cuisine is the key to becoming a true Son of Heaven (*Lüshi chunqiu*, 14.140). For Yi Yin in medicine, see Harper 1982: 44-46.

[2] *MS*VI.A.8 introduces the idea in the form of advice to Yu 禹, whose body is ravaged by his labors to control the flood: "As a rule, the mainstay for ordering government must begin from the body."

> who is skilled at cultivating vapor lets the old vapor disperse at night and the new vapor gather at dawn, thereby penetrating the nine apertures and filling the six cavities.

Yi Yin's recommendation and Rong Cheng's technique concern the practice of breath cultivation—"spit out the old and take in the new"—criticized in *Zhuangzi*, "Keyi" (*Zhuangzi* 15, 237).

What we learn from the Mawangdui and Zhangjiashan texts is that the elite regarded macrobiotic hygiene as normal. Medical advice on the care of the body provided a common base of belief and practice. The philosophers addressed their ideas about the body and about heart/mind cultivation to a clientele already versed in the basics.

SECTION FIVE
MAGIC

*MS*I.E.120 offers the following recipe for the treatment of inguinal swelling:

> On the sixteenth day of the month when the moon first begins to deteriorate, perform the Pace of Yu thrice. Say: "Moon is matched against sun" and "Sun is matched against moon"—three times each. "Father is perverse, Mother is strong. Like other people they bore Sons, and only bore inguinal swelling bulges. Perverseness desist. Grasp the hammering stone and strike your Mother." Immediately, exorcistically beat and hammer the person twice seven times with an iron mallet. Do it at sunrise, and have the person with inguinal swelling face east.

In a magical operation which on one level might be construed as the conquest of Mother moon by Father sun, the time (sunrise of the day after full moon), the eastward orientation, the ritual acts, and the incantation all work in concert to overwhelm the demonic Mother blamed for giving birth to the ailment. A similar combination of magical elements is applied to a different end in *MS*III.87:

> If while traveling you wish to have your feet not hurt, face south, perform the Pace of Yu thrice, and say: "Whatever the water, no disaster; whatever the way, no withering. Give me [2]." When finished, take chimney soot [5] and insert it inside the shoe.

The Pace of Yu (Yu *bu* 禹 步) and other magical devices are discussed below ("Varieties of Magic"). The point to be made now is that the Mawangdui medical manuscripts are perfect illustrations of the blending of natural philosophy and occult thought, and of the everyday uses of magic among the elite. Related magical material in the Shuihudi and Fangmatan hemerological manuscripts provides further proof that the Mawangdui medical manuscripts are not exceptional. Whatever the sources—religion, folklore, occult specialists—by the third century B.C. this material circulated in manuscript within the several geographical and cultural regions of the ancient Chinese world.

Any attempt to discuss magic encounters formidable problems of definition. Without minimizing the importance of theory and definitions, I propose to take a primarily descriptive approach with the Mawangdui medical manuscripts.[1] One does not need a definition in order to recognize that the two recipes just cited are relevant to the investigation of magic in early China. Indeed, it is only with this kind of evidence that we will come to know more about the subject of early Chinese magic.

A few basic observations are necessary. I assume the relation between religion and magic in Chinese antiquity; were it not stylistically cumbersome I would consistently use the compound forms "magic and religion" and "magico-religious." Magic, whether from the perspective of ancient text sources or of modern investigation, concerned human actions undertaken in the belief that spirits and divine powers were present in nature. Having encountered particular circumstances, humans tapped the divine presence with voice, gesture, and select materials; likewise religion. Qualifications can be proposed, but it is difficult to justify the discreteness of religion except on relativistic grounds. When such grounds are expressed in an ancient text they are an invaluable record of how an individual or a group (religious or political) judged the action in question; they do not define the action absolutely. Astrology, divination, and other occult systems of knowledge arose in the same spiritual environment. I treat them as specialized systems alongside religion and magic. Astrology and divination blended with Warring States naturalistic theories—astrologers and diviners were among the formulators of correlative cosmology. The bond between Warring States natural philosophy and occult thought as represented by astrology and divination was one reason (but not the only reason) for the easy accommodation of magico-religious viewpoints. Knowledge of demons and deities, incantations, rituals, and sundry magico-religious devices became part of the occult knowledge dispersed in *fang*-literature like the Mawangdui medical manuscripts and the hemerological manuscripts from Shuihudi and Fangmatan.

There is further discussion of these matters in "Magical Recipes" below. In studying a subject that has received scant attention in sinology, I

[1] I take for granted the obsolescence of earlier theories which attempt to relate magic developmentally to either the history of religion or of science (with the implicit understanding that religion and science are more evolved civilizational forms); nor is magic simply degenerate religion. The issues arising from the question "what is magic?" in the Greco-Roman context are ably set forth by Phillips (1991).

am indebted to scholars investigating Greco-Roman occult thought and magic (see Section Two, "Recipes, Techniques, Calculations, Arts"). Their investigations reveal complex patterns of intellectual and spiritual syncretism in which magic plays an important role.[1] The evidence of magic in the Mawangdui medical manuscripts is significant for ancient magic studies as well as for the history of early Chinese medicine.

MAGICAL RECIPES

I identify fifty-six entries in *MS*I.E, *MS*III, *MS*IV, and *MS*VII.A as magical. All are recipes that detail magical techniques. The thirty-nine magical recipes in *MS*I.E involve incantations, ritual acts,[2] or both: *MS*I.E.9, 27, 34, 48-49, 56, 59-60, 65-70, 93, 107, 114, 118-20, 124-26, 128, 131-32, 134, 137-38, 178, 225, 229, 233-35, 265, 273, 276-77. With one exception (*MS*I.E.9) the recipes are exorcistic. *MS*III includes a group of five magical recipes related to travel (protection when stopping overnight, increasing speed, and easing foot pain): *MS*III.83-87. The six magical recipes in *MS*IV all concern ways to avoid the attack of the venomous creature named *yu* 蜮: *MS*IV.28-29, 32-35. *MS*VII.A.1 describes a charm and six applications (among them, to stop a dog's barking and an infant's crying). *MS*VII.A.2 is an agonistic charm intended to magically defeat an adversary. *MS*VII.A.3-6 are recipes for philters, which when administered serve to seduce or in one instance to separate. They form a set with the preceding charms and share with the charms a similar coercive effect (one of the applications of the charm in *MS*VII.A.1 is for seduction).

The fifty-six magical recipes are not the only evidence of magic in the Mawangdui medical manuscripts. Except for the philters in *MS*VII.A I have omitted other recipes in which the use of drugs is demonstrably magical. For example, *MS*IV.30-31 prescribe chewing *suan* 蒜 (garlic), *lan* 蘭 (eupatorium), or *lingji* 菱芰 (water chestnut) every morning to avoid the *yu*'s attack; the effect of the drugs is surely apotropaic. In *MS*I.E.271-

---

[1]For medicine, I would mention Scarborough's masterly study of Greek pharmacology and magico-religious assumptions (1991). Lloyd's investigations of the formation of scientific ideas (especially medical ideas) within a broad context of natural philosophy and occult thought give new direction to the history of ancient science (1979).

[2]I use "ritual act" as a broad term for gestures ranging from the most simple to elaborate rituals. Thus "using the hem-band from a robe to bind the thumb of the left hand once" in *MS*I.E.114 is a ritual act, as is "scratching twice seven times with the middle finger" in *MS*I.E.131. I also use the term "magical device," which overlaps with "ritual act" but refers additionally to strategies like timing and orientation or the use of certain materials.

75, the ailment category *gu* 蠱 is a demonic ailment, like the category "child sprite" which follows in *MSI*.E.276-77 (both magical recipes). Why not identify all of the recipes for *gu* as magical, not just *MSI*.E.273 which uses talisman water? I have already noted in Section Three ("Materia Medica") the exorcistic nature of the rooster and snake medicine in *MSI*.E.274. And why not include other recipes for ailments whose names suggest demonic possession, in particular the exorcistic dog feces cure for "crazed seizure" in *MSI*.E.71 (see Section Three, "Materia Medica")?[1]

I restrict my identification of magical recipes to the fifty-six for several reasons. First of all, I wish to focus attention on the two things that for someone like Li fils were unambiguously magical: incantations and ritual acts. At a time when naturalistic explanations were forming the foundation for a rationalized understanding of the medical properties of drugs and of the effects of other therapies on illness, to chant an incantation or perform a ritual act was to align oneself with divine powers. Notably, stipulations regarding time in the magical recipes mostly relate to the positions of the sun and moon (as in *MSI*.E.120). Only three magical recipes specify days in the sexagenary cycle based on hemerological ideas (*MSI*.E.107, 124, 126; see "Varieties of Magic" below). Because the evidence is so slight, the Mawangdui medical manuscripts do not require that we deal with the issue of whether hemerology and other occult knowledge ought to be called magic.[2] The medical manuscripts themselves imply that incantations and ritual acts were the essence of magic.

Even though I call *gu* a demonic ailment, I am wary of using the ailment name as the basis for identifying all *gu* recipes as magical. I prefer to allow the possibility that any ailment might have been perceived at several levels (after all, the physician-authors of the *Huangdi neijing* reject demonic causation). Perhaps a naturalistic understanding of *gu* lies behind the two recipes which have the patient drink a medicine made from a woman's menstrual cloth (*MSI*.E.272, 275). A dual view combining naturalistic causation and demonic causation is even more likely for crazed seizure. Moreover, most of the ailment categories with magical recipes randomly

[1]Yamada's identification of magical recipes in *MSI*.E is more inclusive, counting forty-nine magical recipes to my thirty-nine (1985b: 256).

[2]The techniques for determining a child's fortune and for burying the afterbirth in *MSV*.1-2 are based on astrological, calendrical, and hemerological ideas. Magic does not seem like the best description of them.

intersperse them with non-magical recipes (twelve inguinal swelling recipes are magical, twelve are not). The same caveat applies to drugs, whose multiple uses were surely viewed multiply. To cure *gu*, drink the ash of a woman's menstrual cloth (*MS*I.E.272); to speed travel, tie a virgin's menstrual cloth around the waist after first tossing it at a whirling wind (*MS*III.85); soak a menstrual cloth and spread the liquid on a burn (*MS*I.E.184); use the same liquid to boil meat, and consume both meat and liquid to treat inguinal swelling (*MS*I.E.121). Ailments and drugs considered individually lead us into a middle ground where magical and naturalistic conceptions overlap.

The philters in *MS*VII.A.3-6 are, of course, drugs. They obviously belong together with the charms as examples of coercive magic. Just as obviously, magical ideas inform the use of drugs and therapies elsewhere in the Mawangdui medical manuscripts. The virtue of focusing primarily on incantations and ritual acts as the identifying sign of magic is that we are identifying clear-cut types of magical behavior from the perspective of those who performed the techniques. From the fifty-six magical recipes we learn something of the magico-religious side of their personality.

One of the surprises about the magical recipes is the knowledge that the Warring States, Qin, and Han elite were far more involved in a variety of magico-religious activities than we previously knew. Before recent archaeological discoveries, the conventional wisdom was that their religious beliefs and practices chiefly concerned family ancestral cults and ritual observances associated with state and family. If there was a popular religion, it was presumed to have been part of regional *wu* 巫 (shaman) cults. The mechanisms of interaction with the spirit world (incantation, exorcism, and the like) were, so far as was recorded in received sources, in the hands of shamans and religious officiants, whose activities were paralleled by the astrologers and diviners. Other than that, general superstition was widespread but was not a defining characteristic of elite religious life.[1]

[1]I follow Hawkes in rendering *wu* as "shaman" in view of the importance of spirit mediumism as the chief *wu* specialty (1985: 42-51). *Wu* ideas are thought to lie behind the Shang concept of divine kingship (the classic statement of the thesis is Chen Mengjia 1936). The exact identity of the shamans in Shang and Zhou society is far from clear. Warring States legends trace the origins of medicine, divination, and other skills to them. However, in Warring States society shamans underwent a decline in status. With the intellectual transformations of the Warring States period, physicians (*yi* 醫) participated in the text-based traditions of the other specialists in natural philosophy and occult knowledge. As I argue below, it is important to distinguish the continuing religious role of the shamans from the activities of these specialists. The connotations of the word *wu* also

Seidel's investigation of Later Han religious life based on archaeological evidence changes this picture of popular religion during the time when religious Daoism was born. Demonstrating that first and second century A.D. popular religion revolved around notions of administrative procedures and judgments issued to individuals by a bureaucratic spirit world, Seidel observes that this religion—which was practiced at all levels of society—"is definitely not the mediumistic folk religion we assume to have preceded Taoism" (1987: 46). Basic religious ideas in the early Daoist communities were clearly derived from popular religion. Similar evidence of Warring States popular religion is now emerging in the archaeological record. Shamans were an important part of the religious scene (the core of Seidel's "mediumistic folk religion"), but the elite themselves were already engaged in transactions with a highly organized spirit world. The most intriguing find is a Fangmatan text recounting the resurrection of a man named Dan 丹 in 297 B.C. Written as a first person account, the text describes how Dan was released from the underworld because of a petition submitted by his former employer to the Scribe of the Director of the Life-mandate 司命史 (Li Xueqin 1990; Harper 1994; Harper 1995).

While the Fangmatan text attests to the bureaucratizing of the spirit world and to ideas about death in Warring States popular religion, the Mawangdui magical recipes (together with the Shuihudi and Fangmatan hemerological manuscripts) show the elite in another light utilizing incantations and ritual acts for everyday, personal needs. Some of the magic is simple folklore; for example, treating warts by rubbing them against something onto which the warts are magically transferred (*MS*I.E.65–70). But there are many examples of incantations and rituals like *MS*I.E.120 and *MS*III.87. The few references in received literature of the period only occur in the context of the performances of shamans and religious officiants. The magical recipes indicate that it was usual for the elite to perform comparable magico-religious techniques on their own.

The archaeological record is supplementing the received picture of Warring States elite society as religiously cool with a picture of religious

---

changed. By Han times *wu* was applied to what in English could be called "witchcraft"; and what was perceived as witchcraft was not simply the activities of shamans.

Mair (1990) argues that *wu*/**mjag* is a loan from Old Persian *magus*, and speculates on archaic contacts between China and the Near East, including migration of foreign magi to China. Mair's ideas are provocative, but I remain skeptical. In any case, they pertain to religion and magic prior to the Warring States transformations that concern me here.

engagement.[1] And apart from religious life, magico-religious traditions were one element in the syncretistic mixing of ideas in natural philosophy and occult thought. Describing the whole of this complex phenomenon and determining precisely where within it the Mawangdui magical recipes fit is infeasible. Let me attempt to isolate a few distinctive features. By the third century B.C. popular religion as we now understand it emphasized individual magico-religious practices. Practices once left to shamans and religious officiants were in general use, and probably spawned a boom in magic which greatly enriched folkloristic practices. Concurrently, natural philosophy and occult thought were reshaping intellectual and spiritual conceptions. Rather than isolating a world of strictly natural phenomena from a world inhabited by spirits and demons, the two worlds were merged in varying composites fashioned by the specialists and recorded in *fang*-literature. Books which treated magic as one among a number of techniques in the broad fields of natural philosophy and occult thought made magic all the more appealing.

The *Hanshu* bibliographic treatise classifies books on demonology, exorcism, and incantation together with divination literature in the subcategory "Zazhan" 雜占 (Assorted divination) of the "Shushu" 數術 division. Titles include: *Rengui jingwu liuchu bianguai* 人鬼精物六畜變怪 (Human and demonic spectral entities and the mutant prodigies of the six domestic animals), *Zhi buxiang he guiwu* 執不祥劾鬼物 (Seizing the unpropitious and subjugating demonic entities), *Qingdao zhifu* 請禱致福 (Favor-granting prayers to bring good fortune; *Hanshu*, 30.75a–76a). The demonography "Jie" in the first Shuihudi hemerological manuscript exemplifies occult literature on "spectral entities" and "mutant prodigies." "Jie" contains seventy entries which identify the causes of uncanny phenomena in everyday life, most attributed to demons, and provide remedies. Here is one of several entries dealing with domestic animals: "When people or birds and beasts as well as the six domestic animals continually go into a person's home—these are spirits from above who are fond of

[1] Graham sums up received opinion when he contrasts what he regards as the folk-religious beliefs of the Mohists (a reflection of their lower social origins) with the general tendency in Warring States thought: "The tendency throughout the classical age is to ignore the spirits of the dead and of the mountains and rivers after paying them their customary respects, and to regard Heaven as an impersonal power responsible for everything outside human control, including the undeserved misfortune to which you resign yourself as your destiny" (1989: 47). The archaeological record (in particular the manuscripts under discussion) suggests that the elite tendency deduced from received literature is less general than has been supposed.

those below and enjoy entering." The remedy is to have virgin boys and girls beat drums, ring bells, and screech (*SHD*: 213; Harper 1985: 496). The Mawangdui magical recipes furnish the best examples of incantations and exorcistic rituals to "seize the unpropitious and subjugate demonic entities." Prayers to counteract the demonic evil of nightmares in both Shuihudi hemerological manuscripts exemplify the genre of "favor-granting prayers" (*SHD*: 210, 247; Harper 1987a: 270-71).

Part of the rationale behind the naturalistic/demonic composites in occult thought is expressed in the word *jing* 精, which I translate both as "essence" and as "specter, spectral." In its origin *jing* was understood to be the "stuff of spirits," which the *Guanzi*, "Neiye," links to *qi* "vapor" (see Section Four, "Body and Spirit"). In later use *jing* continued to signify spectral qualities associated with the transmutability of things. With time the concentration of *jing* in certain things became "spectral" and the thing became a "specter," as evidenced by the *SW* definition of *mei* 魅 (a kind of goblin) as "the *jing* of an aged entity" (*SW*, 9A.41a). Spectral manifestations of vapor itself are documented in "Jie" entries which blame uncanny phenomena on vapor. Vapor makes it possible for a demon to impinge on a person, either because vapor is the medium of transfer or because vapor is the stuff of demons just as it is the stuff of things that exist in the natural world.[1] Theories of vapor as well as Yin Yang and Five Agent theories served to reanimate the world of spirits and demons in a more complex religious viewpoint.[2]

In the Mawangdui magical recipes and "Jie" we have the magic recommended to the elite by occult specialists ranging from recipe gentlemen to physicians. Much of it surely circulated orally in an environment that included shamans. However, the committing of magic to writing and the transmission of magical literature within *fang*-literature set this magic apart from oral tradition and connected it to occult thought as a field of knowledge. Shamans also contributed to the dispersion of magico-religious practices among the elite (the fame of Yue 越 shamans and Thearch Wu's 武帝 patronage of them in the second century B.C. is dis-

[1]Cloud vapor which enters the home covertly is remedied by building a fire (*SHD*: 215); the vapor of "Bug-misfortune" (*yang* 恙) causes a person's hair to stand on end (*SHD*: 214; Harper 1990: 227); the vapor of the "Whirling Wind" (*piaofeng* 飄風) causes animals to speak to people (*SHD*: 212; Harper 1985: 495). Several entries also reify Yin and Yang as demons (*SHD*: 212, 214). On this point and for further discussion of the bivalence of *qi* and *jing*, see Harper 1990: 224-25.

[2]Yin Yang and Five Agent cycles provided a new *modus operandi* for spirits and demons. See the preceding note for reification of Yin and Yang.

cussed in "Recipes of Yue" below). But their activities belonged more to the sphere of religion than to occult thought. Shamans were both admired and feared for their commerce with spirit powers. And the arbiters of socio-intellectual orthodoxy held their cults in low regard as a source of social unrest.[1] Although all manner of occult practice was potentially suspect, shamanic activities were the most suspect, no doubt because shamans as a group were outside the elite mainstream and were predominately female. Whether perpetrated by shamans or not, Han terms for witchcraft or black magic tend to utilize the word *wu* (see below).

The Mawangdui magical recipes provide techniques that like the other recipes are expected to work. The magical recipe for infant convulsions (*MS*I.E.27) concludes with word "excellent," one of several terms used in *MS*I.E to indicate that certain recipes are known for their efficacy. Similarly, "Jie" concludes most entries with phrases like "it will stop," "it will desist," "it will not come," "it will leave," "it will die of terror." The idea is that the magical remedy "will work." We find in both texts a kind of everyman's magic, a magic that addresses the exigencies of everyday life. This continued to be the focus of medieval popular magic as we know it from works like the fourth century *Baopuzi* and from Dunhuang 敦煌 manuscripts of the Tang period like the *Baize tu* 白澤圖 (Diagrams of White Marsh). Text parallels between these works and the newly excavated manuscripts testify to the durability of magical literature from its Warring States origins into the medieval period.[2]

The Mawangdui magical recipes do not treat of unusual feats of magic for which recipe gentlemen and their occult brethren as well as shamans were famed: conjuring up the dead, magic flight, invisibility, and various acts of magical transformation (assuming multiple forms, changing the forms of other things, and the like).[3] The elite appreciated the difference between the kind of magic that they practiced ordinarily and the more powerful magic of those rare individuals who had a true calling. Yet their

---

[1]The *Shiji* account of the Warring States official Ximen Bao 西門豹 is paradigmatic. As the newly installed magistrate in a Yellow River district, Ximen is credited with eliminating the annual bride sacrifice made to the river god by tossing the head shamanka and her cohorts into the river in place of the local virgin required by the cult (*Shiji*, 126.12b).

[2]A version of the nightmare prayer in the Shuihudi hemerological manuscripts occurs in the Dunhuang *Baize tu*, which is a medieval demonographic counterpart to "Jie" (Harper 1985; Harper 1988). The incantation text shared between *MS*III.83 and the *Baopuzi* is discussed in "Varieties of Magic" below.

[3]See Ngo 1976: 160, 195-202.

own involvement in magico-religious activity was not insignificant. Conditions favored a flourishing occult culture with the elite as active participants.

The approbation of magic evidenced in the excavated manuscripts helps to put the disapprobation of received sources in perspective; despite its problematic nature, everyone did it. Sima Tan 司馬談 (d. 110 B.C.) approves of the art of Yin Yang—by which he means cosmological and calendrical knowledge—for the order it brings to seasonal cycles, but he reproves it for "the multitude of prohibitions and avoidances, which cripple the people and increase their fears"; that is, he accuses the Yin Yang specialists of abetting superstition (*Shiji*, 130.3b). The summary of the Yin Yang specialists in the *Hanshu* bibliographic treatise is even more explicit: "When (the Yin Yang art) is practiced in a crippling way, it becomes snarled in interdictions and prohibitions, and mired in specious calculations. It abandons the business of humankind and relies on demons and spirits" (*Hanshu*, 30.40a). Both criticisms are directed at popular hemerological books like those discovered at Shuihudi and Fangmatan (Harper 1985: 462-70). The *Hanshu* objection does not concern ideas—that belief in demons and spirits is in principle wrong—but concerns the social consequences of the ideas. From the standpoint of the Han socio-intellectual orthodoxy expressed in the *Hanshu*, if ideas encouraged undesirable behavior they had to be regulated. What was the basis for distinguishing between desirable and undesirable behavior? In Han times, one standard was established by *jingshu* 經術 (canonical art; see Section Two, "Recipes, Techniques, Calculations, Arts").

To be sure, anything perceived to be potentially damaging to the person and the authority of the Han thearch and to accepted social norms was suspect, including the Warring States philosophical books which a first century B.C. court official branded as inimical to "canonical art" (*Hanshu*, 80.8a). By engaging in religious practices other than approved state observances and in any form of occult practice one risked running afoul of the government, even though the practices themselves were customary and were not specifically outlawed. The fact that magic had been performed was not so important as the circumstances of its performance. For example, in the late first century B.C. Xifu Gong 息夫躬, dismissed from court for his involvement in political intrigues, was harassed by robbers at home and was taught a magical technique to keep them away:

> He fashioned a ladle from a mulberry branch that faced southeast and drew the seven stars of the Northern Dipper on it. At night Gong unfastened his hair, stood in the central courtyard, and faced the Northern Dipper. He gripped the ladle and waved it while chanting the incantation against robbers. (*Hanshu*, 45.18a.)

The astrological and magical significance of the Northern Dipper (the Big Dipper) in Warring States, Qin, and Han times is well documented (Harper 1978-79; Kalinowski 1983). The description of Xifu's magical exploitation of the constellation to subdue robbers is comparable to techniques in the Mawangdui magical recipes. However, someone reported Xifu Gong to the authorities claiming that Xifu harbored hatred for his ruler; moreover, that Xifu was examining astrological signs to discover his ruler's fortune and was chanting "shaman curses" (*wu zhuju* 巫 祝 詛). Xifu was promptly arrested and died in jail. Perhaps his intent was sinister. The Mawangdui magical recipes indicate that the magical performance itself was not out of the ordinary. Might not Li fils have found himself in similar difficulty if his performance of one of the magical recipes were to have been viewed in the wrong light by a hostile party?

Ill-purposed magic or witchcraft—that is, magic perceived by others as witchcraft—is commonly denoted by compounds using *wu* in Han sources. *Wu*, the majority of them female shamankas, were known to aid people in achieving whatever goal they desired. The *Hanshu* account of Liu Xu 劉 胥 (d. 54 B.C.), one of Thearch Wu's sons, must represent a common pattern. When Liu Xu did not succeed his father, he employed the shamanka Li Ruxu 李 女 須 to curse Thearch Zhao 昭 帝 (r. 87-74 B.C.). Ruxu first entered a shamanic trance. When she announced that Thearch Wu occupied her body, everyone present bowed while the deceased ruler declared, "I command that Xu become Son of Heaven" (*Hanshu*, 63.15a-b). Delighted, Liu Xu sent the shamanka to offer prayers to the spirits that he be granted a favor—the demise of Thearch Zhao and his own succession. Shortly thereafter, Thearch Zhao died. Although Liu Xu failed to succeed to the throne, he remained convinced of Ruxu's shamanic powers and continued to employ her to perform her "shaman curses" on other occasions (the same curses Xifu Gong was accused of performing).

Such activities contributed to a generalized notion of black magic or witchcraft as the work of women. Accounts of Thearch Wu's reign provide notable examples. In 130 B.C. it came to light that Dowager Chen 陳皇后 had been practicing the "women's way of seduction" (*furen meidao* 婦人媚道) in her efforts to secure her uncertain position (*Hanshu*, 97A.11a; Twitchett and Loewe 1986: 174). Shortly thereafter the lady's daughter and others were arrested for attempting to aid her by practicing "shaman *gu* (*wugu* 巫蠱), sacrificial worship, and curses." Her daughter was beheaded. The lady was demoted in a decree that opened with the words, "the Dowager has failed to observe propriety and is deluded by shaman curses." Yet another more serious *wugu* scandal occurred in the last years of Thearch Wu's reign (Loewe 1974: 37-90; Twitchett and Loewe 1986: 177-78).

The association of *gu* with demonic evil and with female seduction was already made in the Warring States (see *MS*I.E.271). The compound *wugu* reflects the perception that women's magic was inherently dangerous (especially for men). As in all accusations of witchcraft, the deed and its name are defined by the accusers. I am particularly struck by the accusation that Dowager Chen practiced a "women's way of seduction," implying witchcraft. Did her "way of seduction" perhaps include the use of philters like those in *MS*VII.A which ensure that "seduction will occur" (*MS*VII.A.4) or that the object of desire "will be obtained" (*MS*VII.A.5)? Was the use of philters by men to seduce women perceived differently from their use by women? As in the case of Xifu Gong, I suspect that some of the activities were not in themselves exceptional; it was simply riskier for women to engage in them.

VARIETIES OF MAGIC

In the Han mind the south was where magico-religious traditions were strongest. Chu 楚 and Yue 越 shamans were the most powerful; inhabitants of Chu and Yue were most given to worship of spirits and demons; the southern genius for magic was attributed to the sultry environment itself. The contents of the Mawangdui magical recipes reflect in part southern magico-religious traditions. The prominence of spitting and spouting when chanting incantations in the magical recipes suggests the southern breath magic called "recipes of Yue" (Yue *fang* 越方) in Han sources. Breath magic is discussed below under incantation. My thesis regarding the Mawangdui magical recipes and the recipes of Yue is presented separately in "Recipes of Yue." Other aspects of the magical recipes clearly belong to beliefs and practices that were already common to magic in the north and south during the third century B.C. Parallels in the Shuihudi and Fangmatan hemerological manuscripts provide the proof, the Pace of Yu being the best single piece of evidence. There is evidence as well of deities in the Later Han popular religion reconstructed by Seidel (1987). In short, the Mawangdui magical recipes bear witness to widespread magico-religious traditions in the third to second centuries B.C.

Consequently, although the context is most often the treatment of specific ailments (the thirty-nine recipes in *MSI*.E and the eight in *MSIV*), the contents of the Mawangdui magical recipes are not exclusive to medicine. Li fils would have understood the magical recipes as the medical application of magico-religious techniques; we can use the same recipes to reconstruct magic and religion.[1] My survey of the Mawangdui magical recipes is brief, more a list of salient details than an exegesis. I begin with incantation, followed by ritual acts and other magical devices. There is a slight amount of corroborative evidence in received literature. For the most part, the magical recipes themselves are our first records of the wording of incantations and of all the directions needed to actually work magic. The Shuihudi and Fangmatan hemerological manuscripts corroborate and supplement the Mawangdui magical recipes. I refer to the hemerological manuscripts on occasion, but I leave thorough treatment of them for another time.

The majority of incantations in the magical recipes are indicated as direct speech with the verb *yue* 曰 (say), the standard verb for any kind of direct speech. Next in frequency is *zhu* 祝 (chant the incantation; the right side of the graph signifies a mouth atop a human figure, the left side signifies the presence of the spirits). The texts of several incantations are simply prefaced by words for spitting and spouting, indicating breath magic (see below); and there are two examples of a word denoting "curse" (see *MSI*.E.124). Mostly rhymed and occasionally punctuated by magical utterances, the Mawangdui incantations represent the third to second century B.C. manifestation of a long tradition of magical communication with the spirits.[2]

---

[1]Of course, the belief that illness was demonically inspired made faith-healing a key element of shaman cults and popular religion.

[2]Harper summarizes some of the material relevant to the history of incantation in early Chinese religion, for which the Shang bone and shell inscriptions provide the earliest documentation (1982: 69-79). As early as the Shang, the act of speaking to the spirits in incantation was complemented by written communication with them. Evidence of oral and written communication is discussed in Harper 1985: 472-74. It is worth noting that most Shang vocabulary for speaking and writing was

A feature shared by all of the incantations is their intelligibleness. Nonsense and phrases from other languages are not used.[1] The purpose of the incantations is to deliver a particular kind of message, and most of them state their information in straightforward fashion. The magical recipe to stop bleeding in *MS*I.E.9 includes the simplest, most direct incantation: "Man, staunch! Woman, vinegar!" The incantation conjures the presence of a man to stop the flow of blood and a woman to cleanse the wound with vinegar. An incantation may also take the form of a wish, as in the *MS*III.87 recipe to prevent foot pain quoted at the beginning of this section ("Whatever the water, no disaster; whatever the way, no withering.").

The majority of the incantations occur in *MS*I.E and are exorcistic curses. The curses typically threaten the demonic agent blamed for causing the ailment with mutilation and death if it does not leave the patient's body. The graphic quality of the phrases is illustrated by the following portion of the incantation in *MS*I.E.229: "With a *zuo* 柞 (oak) rod I stab you; with tiger claws I gouge and grab you; with a knife I butcher you; with *wei* 葦 (reeds) I sever you. . . . If you do not depart, it will be bitter." Oak, tiger claws, and reeds are all exorcistic materials used in ritual acts; the use of the first person pronoun indicates that the very person chanting the incantation intends to punish the agent (the "you"). Usually the incantations request spirit assistance in dealing with the demonic agent; and an exorcistic act follows the chanting of the incantation, like flagellation (with an iron mallet in *MS*I.E.120 quoted above) or spitting (see below).

This scenario for exorcism mirrors the one complete account of a Han state-sponsored exorcism in received literature, the Great Exorcism (*da nuo* 大儺) performed at New Year's and recorded in the *Hou Hanshu* treatise on ritual.[2] The Great Exorcism clears away the pestilential evil of the old and dying year, inaugurating a new purified cycle of time. It is

originally related to spirit communication in religion; application to human communication was secondary. I suspect that the fundamentally sacred nature of speech itself continued to inform ideas about the magic of speech in Warring States, Qin, and Han times. Vocabulary for different types of incantations and written documents is attested in ritual books like the *Zhouli*, along with the hierarchy of officiants charged with executing them (Harper 1982: 71). The influence of incantation on the writing of poetry is studied in Harper 1987a.

[1]Chinese incantations were enriched by Indic speech and pseudo-Indic speech following the introduction of Buddhism. The use of foreign speech meshed with religious Daoist ideas about celestial speech and script known only to initiates (Bokenkamp 1983: 462–65).

[2]Bodde studies the account and reviews earlier scholarship on it (1975: 75–138).

performed by the chief exorcist leading a troupe of youths and palace officiants. The curse comes at the climax of the ceremony when twelve spirit beasts—played by twelve costumed officiants—are commanded to each devour one of twelve evils (some illnesses, some demons) of the old year. Having conjured their assistance, the curse continues:

> These twelve spirits are all charged to pursue the evil and baleful. May they scorch your carcass! May they rip apart your skeleton! May they strip away your flesh! May they tear out your lungs and guts! If you do not depart quickly, whoever remains will become food.

Brandishing torches, the exorcistic party passes through the palace, finally delivering the torches to horsemen outside the south gate who dispose of them (and the evil they contain) in the river (*Hou Hanshu*, "Zhi" 志, 5.10b; Bodde 1975: 81-82).

The *MSI*.E incantations are the chief source for the names of spirits and demons, who are either invoked to assist or are the objects of the exorcism (similar to the Great Exorcism). The religious viewpoint reflected in the incantations is animistic. The ontological view of ailments as entities fuses with the belief that each entity has its spirit—which is one reason for alternation between treating ailments medically and treating them with exorcism. The scorpion spirit is cursed in *MSI*.E.48-49; the lizard spirit in *MSI*.E.56, 59-60; in *MSI*.E.65 the person with warts plays the role of the wart spirit who is exorcised by being forced to name himself. Some of the spirits who assist are personifications of elements of nature. The incantation in *MSI*.E.49 calls upon a spirit Father and Mother to trap the scorpion:

> Father dwells in Shu. Mother is the Wind Bird who punishes. Do not dare flee up or down. The Wind Bird bores your heart.

Father, Mother, and Son groupings are sometimes associated with spirit powers in the environment (as above); and are sometimes part of the demonic etiology of an ailment (as in *MSI*.E.120, in which the incantation commands the inguinal swelling Sons to attack the Mother who bore them).

There is evidence of a more formal pantheon. The magical recipes for the rash caused by lacquer include incantations which accuse the Lacquer King 漆 王 of failing to perform the tasks assigned to him by the Thearch of Heaven 天帝 (*MSI*.E.233-35). The incantation in *MSI*.E.124 calls upon the Spirit of Heaven 天神 and Spirit Maids 神女 to expel the fox blamed for inguinal swelling. The Yellow Spirit 黃神 is summoned in *MSI*.E.178 (a burn) and *MSI*.E.265 (scabbing). The fox's demonic reputation in China is well known; *MSI*.E.124 and 128 are now the earliest attestation of fox possession. Thearch of Heaven, Spirit of Heaven, and Yellow Spirit all refer to the same supreme deity in Han popular religion (Seidel 1987: 28-30). Spirit Maids are divine agents associated with hemerology (*MSI*.E.124 is to be performed on a specific day in the sexagenary cycle; see below); they figure prominently in religious Daoism. The bureaucratic aspect of human relations with this pantheon is reflected in two incantations that mimic the formula used by officials to address their superiors: "I dare to declare." The announcement of an abscess in *MSI*.E.229 is made to Tai Mountain (the sacred peak of the east, in present-day Shandong, whose presiding deity was one of the arbiters of human fate): "I dare to declare to the Tai Mountain Barrow." A similar address is made to the East Lord and Bright Star 東君明星 (perhaps the astral deity Taiyi 太一) when securing a campsite in *MSIII*.84.

Let me turn to breath magic. The evidence is of two kinds: magical utterances and acts of spitting and spouting. The two are not unconnected. Like spitting and spouting, utterances concentrate the vapor which is the breath as it is ejected from the mouth. A vocabulary of utterances used by shamans and religious officiants can be traced to the Shang bone and shell inscriptions. Shirakawa demonstrates that *yi* 殹—both a phonetic and signific in 醫 "physician"—belongs to a family of Shang words for exorcistic weapons, the sounds of exorcistic beating, and exorcistic utterances (1976, vol. 2: 232-33). The etymology of the word *yi* "physician" as the "shaman who heals with exorcistic techniques" proposed by Shirakawa is convincing.[1] Warring States ideas about vapor, breath, and saliva added to the magico-religious conception of magical utterances.

MSI.E includes five magical utterances, each one occurring just once and always at the beginning of the incantation (I list them with Old Chinese reconstruction as they appear in the translation): **tsjar* 嗟 (*MSI*.E.56); **gwjag* 吁 (*MSI*.E.128); **sjit *sjit, *khwət *khwət* 胒胒詘詘 (*MSI*.E.178); **kəgw* 罿 (*MSI*.E.229); **tsjəm *tsjəm, *hjəkw *hjəkw* 浸浸

[1]For further speculation on the early vocabulary of magical utterances, see Harper 1982: 76-79.

熇熇 (*MSI*.E.265). ⋆*Gwjag* ⋆*tsjar* is attested as a compound utterance in several *Shijing* 詩經 poems in which the utterance is part of the magic of conjuring spirit beasts (see *MSI*.E.56). A variant of the first of the two four-syllable utterances is attested in the *Zuozhuan* 左傳 as a monitory prophecy; the graphs in *MSI*.E.178 may additionally mean "swarm, submit." ⋆*Kəgw* represents the sound of a cry that reaches into the spirit world. The utterance forms part of the *Yili* 儀禮 ritual of summoning back the soul of a person recently deceased; and it is used to summon assistance in exorcising nightmare demons in the two Shuihudi hemerological manuscripts. In *MSI*.E.229 the cry reaches the Tai Mountain Barrow. One occurrence each hardly constitutes heavy usage, but the fact that the utterances occur indicates that the Mawangdui incantations utilize widely shared conventions of incantation.

The examples of spitting (*tuo* 唾) and spouting (*pen* 噴) I judge to be more characteristic of a southern style of breath magic. Let me inventory the occurrences. In *MSI*.E.27 spitting precedes the incantation; the incantation first invokes a "spouter" to "spout ferociously" and continues with a typical curse of the demonic agent who is expelled by the spirit spouter (surely the act of invoking the spouter involves spouting action by the person chanting). The incantation in *MSI*.E.48 is preceded by spitting and spouting; in *MSI*.E.59 by spouting and blowing; in *MSI*.E.93 by spouting and snorting thrice. The incantation in *MSI*.E.118 again invokes a spouter to expel the demonic agent, as does the incantation in *MSI*.E.277. In *MSI*.E.178 the person spits thrice after the incantation; *MSI*.E.229 says simply to spit after the incantation. Spitting precedes the incantation in *MSI*.E.233, and the first word of the incantation is "spout" as the utterance ⋆*pən*; ⋆*pən* is again the initial utterance in the incantation in *MSI*.E.235. Spitting follows the incantation in *MSI*.E.234, seven times for men and twice seven times for women. In *MSI*.E.48, 178, 229, and 234 the recipes instruct the person to spit on the ailments; that is, to spit on the demonic agent who is localized in the affected part of the body.

As a universal human custom spitting does not require elaborate explanation. The Chinese custom of spitting at demons is already well documented in post-Han sources (Liu Zhiwan 1974: 338-48; Harper 1982: 92-93). From the standpoint of the demons, the fact that they dislike being spat at is now on record for the third century B.C. in the Fangmatan resurrection account. The account concludes with a list of graveyard rules, including the following: "Let those who offer sacrifices at tombs not dare to spit. If they spit, the ghosts depart and flee in fright" (Harper 1994:14). Surely spitting and spouting were employed exorcistically in the north and south in the third century B.C. and earlier. My argument for a southern style of breath magic involving spitting and spouting is based on two forms of evidence: first, Wang Chong's 王充 rationalization of incantation in the *Lunheng* 論衡, which uses vapor theory to explain what others would have understood to be breath magic; and second, accounts in the *Lunheng* and elsewhere of the potent breath of the inhabitants of Chu and Yue, and of the techniques of the recipes of Yue. The Han tradition of the recipes of Yue probably grew out of the blending of magic and occult thought in the south during the Warring States. Originally a southern tradition, the recipes of Yue gained wider fame during the Han. I submit that the examples of spitting and spouting in the Mawangdui magical recipes are the breath magic of the recipes of Yue.

The southern tradition of breath magic is treated in "Recipes of Yue" below. Wang Chong's statements on why incantations work are necessary background information. Wang Chong's purpose is to demystify incantation by showing that it is a natural phenomenon involving vapor, Yin and Yang, and the Five Agents. His arguments shed light on probable ways in which Warring States naturalistic theories bolstered the magico-religious understanding of incantation and breath magic. Even in the first century A.D. I suspect that Wang Chong's rationalization served to justify the elite's belief in the magical efficacy of incantation.

Wang Chong's basic premise is that all phenomena can be explained as manifestations of vapor. What people take to be demons are momentary agglomerations of Yang vapor, which is volatile, fiery, and red. Yang vapor burns like fire and can harm people, but the harm of seeing a demon—that is, of encountering a mass of Yang vapor—is no different than the harm of being poisoned by certain substances, which Wang Chong explains as being burned by the Yang vapor concentrated in them. Wang Chong further equates speech and fire, citing as his authority the canonical "Hongfan" 洪範 (Great plan) treatise of the *Shangshu* 尚書, which Graham dates to the fifth century B.C. (1989: 326). The "Hongfan" lists of symbolic correlations name Fire as the second of the Five Agents and Speech as the second of the Five Human Functions.[1] The *Lunheng* essay

[1]These matters are discussed in two essays: *Lunheng*, "Dinggui," 22.453-54; and "Yandu," 23.459. As explained by Graham, the lists of correlations in the "Hongfan" predate the concept of a five-fold cycle in later Five Agent theory (1989: 340-56)

"Yandu" 言毒 (Explanation of poison) appeals both to the "Hongfan" and to folk belief:

> There is a folk saying, "A multitude of mouths melts metal." The mouth is Fire. Among the Five Agents the second is Fire; among the Five Human Functions the second is Speech. Speech is matched with Fire, hence the saying that it "melts metal." (*Lunheng*, "Yandu," 23.459.)

Wang Chong's argument weaves together his own ideas about Yang vapor, the "Hongfan" correlation of Fire and Speech, and folk belief. His argument continues with an explanation of why the folk saying must be grounded in Five Agent theory (according to which Fire conquers Metal), but this is part of his rationalization. The folk saying itself simply indicates a popular belief that breath works like fire, which probably reflects magico-religious ideas about the properties of fire prior to Five Agent theory (see Section Three, "Therapy"). Having provided a theoretically satisfying explanation, Wang Chong has no difficulty affirming that the incantations chanted by shamans are efficacious because shamans are naturally endowed with greater concentrations of Yang vapor. Moveover, the speech of the inhabitants of the south (which is a Yang region) is naturally more potent:

> In the lands of Grand Yang the people are frenzied. When a person is frenzied his mouth and tongue become poisonous. Thus the people of Chu and Yue are frenzied and febrile. When they speak with another person and the saliva from their mouth strikes the person, then his vessels swell up and form sores. In the extremely hot lands of the Southern Commandery, when the inhabitants chant an incantation at a tree the tree dies, and when they spit at a bird the bird drops down. The reason why Shaman Xian was able to use incantations to alleviate the people's sicknesses and cure the people's misfortunes is because he was born in Jiangnan and possessed burning vapor. Now as for poison, it is the vapor of Yang. Thus when it strikes a person it is like fire scorching the person. (*Lunheng*, "Yandu," 23.457.)

Wang Chong rationalizes the effects of speech and incantation as natural phenomena. Others would have understood the words spoken in incantation to be oral fire, whose power was increased by the use of utterances, spitting, and spouting. Breath magic partook of the magic of fire.

The incantation in *MS*III.83 is a notable example of travel magic. The recipe is used "when traveling and stopping overnight," evidently when camping in the open. Both the incantation and the ritual acts which accompany it secure the campsite by creating a magically protected space. This kind of magic is well documented in the fourth century A.D. *Baopuzi* 抱朴子 as part of the essential knowledge for anyone who would go into the wilds in search of spirits and the magical substances which confer immortality, and who must beware of tigers, wolves, and demonic machinations. *MS*III does not explain why a traveler would find it necessary to camp; I presume that lodges even along better known routes were not plentiful in the third and second centuries B.C. No doubt the hazards of the road were similar to those experienced by the *Baopuzi* traveler. Remarkably, there is a parallel version of the incantation in the *Baopuzi*, which includes the same phrases "the Yang side of Tai Mountain" and "walls and ramparts that are not intact, seal with the metal bar." In *MS*III.83, following the incantation the traveler performs the Pace of Yu and draws a circle on the ground saying, "With a stick of fresh *jing* 荆 (vitex) two *cun* long I draw a circle around the inside." In the *Baopuzi* the traveler draws a square on the ground with a knife, and the knife is laid on the square at an astrologically significant position. The phrase "seal with the metal bar" suggests that in earlier versions of the technique a knife was also used, but has been replaced by a magical stick of vitex in *MS*III.83. The parallel techniques may be due to oral transmission, but I think it probable that we are witnessing continuity in the transmission of *fang*-literature.

Discussion of ritual acts and magical devices must begin with the Pace of Yu 禹步. Prior to the evidence in the Mawangdui magical recipes and the Shuihudi and Fangmatan hemerological manuscripts, the earliest occurrence of the term was in the *Shizi* 尸子, in a description of the physical deformities suffered by Yu (the hero of the Chinese flood myth and legendary founder of the Xia ruling house) as a consequence of his labor to control the flood:

> His hands did not have nails and his shins had no hair. He was afflicted with hemiplegia. One foot would not step past the other foot, which the people called the Pace of Yu. (*Shizi*, 1.16b.)

Granet (1925) adduces *Shizi* and other passages in pre-Han philosophical literature that describe Yu's physical deformities (treated by the philosophers as an example of the ruler sacrificing himself for his people) as evidence of an underlying religious conception in which such traits constituted the mark of the shaman. Granet proceeds to hypothesize that the Pace of Yu, which was a trademark of religious Daoism during the centuries after the Han, originated in shamanistic traditions of early popular religion; and that key elements of religious Daoism were derived from this earlier popular religion. There is, of course, other evidence in the excavated manuscripts of the relation between ancient popular religion and religious Daoism. But the eight occurrences of the Pace of Yu in the Mawangdui magical recipes (*MS*I.E.60, 67, 118, 120, 128, 225, 276; *MS*III.83) are the most striking proof, and confirm Granet's inspired hypothesis.[1]

I believe Granet is correct. However, the exact nature of its shamanic origin is not clarified in the manuscript evidence, in which the Pace of Yu is already part of the occult tradition transmitted in *fang*-literature.[2] In *MS*I.E performing the Pace of Yu magically subdues; it always occurs at the beginning of a magical operation, either before or simultaneously with the incantation. *MS*III.83, the first Shuihudi hemerological manuscript (*SHD*: 223), and the first Fangmatan hemerological manuscript (Qinjian zhengli xiaozu 1989: 5) all employ the Pace of Yu in magical techniques related to travel. The incantation accompanying the Pace of Yu in the Shuihudi technique declares the traveler's wish: "Let so-and-so travel and not suffer odium; he first acts as Yu to clear the road." The Pace of Yu clears away the hazards of the road, replicating Yu's taming of water, earth, spirits, and demons during his legendary travels. The legend of Yu's caldrons (magical talismans emblazoned with the images of the spirits and demons) and the talismanic *Shanhaijing* (the prototypical demonography which enumerates the habitats and marvelous inhabitants of the earth) belong to the same Warring States occult tradition which made the Pace

---

[1]When I first examined a transcription of *MS*I.E in 1977 the occurrence of the Pace of Yu immediately reminded me of Granet's hypothesis, launching my research on the Mawangdui medical manuscripts.

[2]Granet traces the Pace of Yu to the ancient royal cult in which the shaman-king controlled the world by virtue of his contact with the spirits. The pace represents the themes of initiatory sickness and ecstatic trance which are universal in shamanism. Evidence in Shang bone and shell inscriptions suggests that the Shang king was the chief shaman and experienced shamanic sickness as part of his kingship (Harper 1982: 99-100). The *Fayan* notes a Han "shaman pace" (*wubu* 巫步) attributed to Yu: "In the past the chief of the Yao clan (i.e. Yu) controlled the water and earth and the shaman pace makes much of Yu" (*Fayan*, "Chongli," 10.28; the word *wu* in *wubu* probably connotes popular magico-religious tradition, not just the shaman cults).

of Yu a popular magico-ritual step (Harper 1985: 479; Harper forthcoming; Kudô 1990: 44-57).

The regular instruction to perform the pace thrice in the manuscripts suggests that the early Pace of Yu was similar to the technique described in *Baopuzi*, 17.78, which is the earliest extant account of how to execute it. Beginning with the right foot in front and the left foot behind, the performer steps ahead with the left foot and then again with the right foot, finally bringing the left foot even with the right foot—which concludes the first pace. The second pace continues by stepping ahead with the right foot, followed by the left foot, finally bringing the right foot even with the left foot. The third pace repeats the first pace.[1]

The inguinal swelling recipes in *MSI*.E are notable for descriptions of exorcistic rituals and for references to ritual acts attested in received literature. Several provide precise stage directions, as in the *MSI*.E.125 sunrise ritual: the patient faces east beneath the roof gutter; the designated officiant grasps a rammer and faces west opposite the patient; after chanting the first incantation (which blames the ailment on Father, Mother, and Sons), the officiant hits the patient twice seven times; finally, in a second incantation the officiant commands the patient to rise and inguinal swelling to desist. Archery is described in *MSI*.E.132 and 137; the latter recipe uses a peach-branch bow, which is well attested in received descriptions of formal exorcistic rituals (see *MSI*.E.132). Exorcistic archery with peachwood bow and jujube arrows (the material for arrows specified in received literature) also occurs in the Shuihudi "Jie" (*SHD*: 212; Harper 1985: 492-93). There are three occurrences of a rare, technical term for "exorcistic beating" (*si* 敀; see *MSI*.E.118). Creating a magical, protected space by drawing on the ground in *MSIII*.83 has an exorcistic counterpart in *MSI*.E.134. The patient kneels beneath a wall facing east and inserts his testicles and penis into a gourd. Then twice seven pegs made of oak are poked into the ground around him, creating a magical demon-trap. A similar technique using peach stakes to exorcise nightmare demons is described in "Jie" (*SHD*: 214).

The two recipes to exorcise the child sprite warrant mention, *MSI*.E.276 for the use of peachwood figurines fastened above the door-

[1]Andersen (1989-90) surveys the Pace of Yu in religious Daoism, where it is identified with the cosmo-ritual practice of *bugang* 步綱 (walking the guideline). I do not agree with Andersen's assumption that the Pace of Yu in the excavated manuscripts is already a cosmo-ritual walk as in religious Daoism.

way. The custom is associated with New Year's observances in received literature. The bundles of peachwood figurines placed in the coffin in Mawangdui tomb 1 (see *MSI*.E.276) and the "Jie" recommendation to hit demons with a peachwood figurine (*SHD*: 215) attest to their wider use. *MSI*.E.277 describes an exorcistic procession. A cart made from a winnowing basket mounted on gourds is harnessed to a black pig and led through the patient's home. The accompanying incantation declares that the Shamanka Mistress is searching for the child sprite, and that it will be cast into the water (recall that the Great Exorcism concludes with casting the torches into the river).

Synchronization of incantations, ritual acts, and magical devices into a whole operation must be examined for each magical recipe, which I will not do here. Nor will I inventory the magical recipes for everything that is magically significant. However, I would like to indicate representative magical devices employed in the recipes. Let me begin with the idea of magical transfer. Water, gourds, gourds filled with water, clods, brooms, and various plants are all used to trap and contain demonic pathogens, which are then discarded. The water is often a preparation called "silted water" (see *MSI*.E.27). In *MSI*.E.60 (a lizard bite), the designated officiant carries a gourd holding one cup of silted water in his left hand, faces north towards the patient to perform the Pace of Yu, chants incantations, and has the patient drink one half cup of the water in the gourd. The recipe concludes with the instruction, "cover the gourd flask and discard it." A gourd is placed over the man's genitals during the exorcism in two inguinal swelling recipes (*MSI*.E.134, 137). Clods, brooms, and plants are most common in the recipes for warts (*MSI*.E.65–70). And after brushing the warts with a broom in *MSI*.E.66 the broom is discarded in an abandoned well.

Specifically demonifugal materials include peach and arbor-vitae wood. Both have well-known associations with the sun, Yang, and the east (*MSI*.E.118, 137, 276) which are usually cited in explanations of why these two kinds of wood are magical. Certainly the magical exploitation of the sun and the east in the inguinal swelling recipes (*MSI*.E.118–20, 125–26, 132, 134, 137) overlaps with the use of peach and arbor-vitae; and the peachwood figurines in *MSI*.E.276 are made from a branch cut from the east side of the tree. Whether the woods are magical because of the sun and the east is another question. In discussing peachwood Bodde makes a useful distinction between the ancient belief that the wood *is* magical and attempts to explain *why* it is magical (1975: 128-34). Bodde cites the Han legend of the peach tree in the eastern sea which is a demon barrier. As demons pass through the barrier from the northeast, two spirit guards seize the evil ones and feed them to tigers. While the legend served in Han times to explain the tradition of the peachwood figurines (they are the two spirit guards), we still cannot say why the tree in the eastern sea is a peach and why peachwood is magical. The logic to why some materials are believed to be magical and others not remains unexplained (and there may not be an explanation).[1]

The demonifugal use of feces to expel the lacquer demon in *MS*I.E.233 and 235 is supplemented in "Jie" by fumigation with feces (see Section Three, "Therapy"), throwing balls of dog feces at demons (*SHD*: 213; Harper 1985: 495), and bathing in dog feces to exorcise a demon (*SHD*: 215; Harper forthcoming). There are notable examples of prophylactic clothing to protect the wearer from the *yu* in *MS*IV.32-34, especially the red and black silk garments trimmed with horsehair in *MS*IV.33. Similar attire is worn by the chief exorcist in the Great Exorcism and is used to dress the body of the deceased in the *Yili*.[2]

Timing and orientation have been in evidence throughout this section. Sunrise and east are preferred for exorcising inguinal swelling; night and north are preferred for warts.[3] *MS*I.E.120 schedules the exorcism of inguinal swelling to coincide with the waning moon in order to weaken the influence of the "Mother who is strong." The last day of the month, the point of juncture between one lunar cycle and the next, is usual for warts (except for *MS*I.E.69 which schedules the exorcism on the first day of the month). The symbolism is reasonably clear. North is the realm of water and is where noxious things are imprisoned (the dead, demons, and the like). The act of "brushing the warts to the north" (*MS*I.E.66) on the last day of the month is a lesser version of the Great Exorcism at New Year's.

---

[1]Not wanting to belabor the point, let me just note that it would be incautious to assume that solar associations can be used as the primary criterion for classifying various materials as magical. Yin Yang and Five Agent correlations also influenced people's perceptions, yet why something is magical cannot be explained by reference to correlative cosmology. Faraone's observations on attempts to explain why Greco-Roman binding spells were inscribed on lead are instructive (1991: 7).

[2]There are standard correlations between red and fire, Yang, heaven, and life; between black and water, Yin, earth, and death. I will not try to explain how these correlations are related to warding off the *yu*'s attack with red and black clothing.

[3]Actually, only *MS*I.E.67 specifies that the technique be performed after dark. The preference for the last day of the month may imply the night of the last day.

East has its own exorcistic associations (including the peach tree legend); and the rising sun expels darkness and evil. In the third and second centuries B.C. Yin Yang classifications of spatial orientations and temporal cycles would have added to the rationale underlying the magical operations. It is worth noting, however, that none of the magical recipes refer to Yin and Yang or to the Five Agents.

Two inguinal swelling recipes (*MS*I.E.124, 126) and one urine retention recipe (*MS*I.E.107) are scheduled for specific days in the sexagenary cycle. The three days must be hemerologically significant, but I cannot explain their selection. Both days in the inguinal swelling recipes are in the *xin* 辛 decade, and both incantations open with a declaration of cyclical day designation. The *MS*I.E.123 incantation then exhorts Spirit Maids to "according to sequence hear the spirit pronouncement." The sequence must be the sequence of the sexagenary cycle, thus the Spirit Maids are the hemerological spirits associated with days. The day in *MS*I.E.126 serves as the occasion for the patient to get rid of the ailment by changing his name to Yu, the flood hero.

The significant numbers in the magical recipes are three, seven, and twice seven (fourteen). Seven is odd and thus Yang; twice seven is Yin. In *MS*I.E.67 a man rubs his warts with seven clods, a woman with twice seven; in *MS*I.E.234 a man spits on the lacquer rash seven times, a woman twice seven times. The two examples are interesting, but gender is not a consideration in other occurrences. Moreover, all three numbers are used regularly in non-magical recipes (as well as in later medical recipe literature). Their use is important in the magical recipes, but is not a definitive sign of magic.

I conclude with an example of associative magic in *MS*VII.A.6 involving words, materials, and objectives. The philter recipe is short:

> Put the person's left eyebrow in liquor and drink it. You invariably obtain the person.

The word for eyebrow in *MS*VII.A.6 is *mei* 眉 (written 麋 in the recipe). Eyebrows figure in the etymology of the word for seduction, *mei* 媚. In *MS*VII.A.6, the object of desire's left eyebrow compels her or him to submit to the magic of your seduction.

RECIPES OF YUE

A scattering of received sources from the Han to the early twentieth century indicates the existence of a southern tradition of breath magic, called Yue *fang* 越方 (recipes of Yue) in Han times. According to the *Baopuzi*, the technique "consists of augmenting the vapor (of the breath) and that is all" (*Baopuzi*, 5.24). Down the centuries, southern "vapor charms" (*qijin* 氣禁) were associated with various legendary practitioners and were known by several names. And southern breath magic mingled with Daoist and popular occult traditions. The examples of spitting and spouting in *MSI*.E are now the earliest documentation of this southern breath magic; several magical recipes are remarkably similar to much later received accounts. To show how breath magic in *MSI*.E is related to the recipes of Yue I must first examine received documentation concerning the latter. Even without the new manuscript evidence, the history of the recipes of Yue demonstrates the durability of a distinctive tradition of magic which has been handed down in the region of the Yangzi River since Han times. With the discovery of *MSI*.E we can verify its transmission in third century B.C. *fang*-literature.

The term Yue *fang* first occurs in the *Hou Hanshu* account of two occult specialists: Xu Deng 徐登 and Zhao Bing 趙炳. Xu Deng was from Min 閩 (a region identified with Yue culture and peoples in Han times, situated in present-day Fujian); he "excelled in performing shaman arts (*wushu* 巫術)." Zhao Bing was from Dongyang 東陽 (in the old Yue heartland, present-day Zhejiang) and "was able to perform the recipes of Yue" (*Hou Hanshu*, 82B.9a; Ngo 1976: 127-28). The men, who lived during the Later Han, met at the Ji River 溪水 (Zhejiang):

> It was a time of war and chaos, and sickness was rampant. After meeting on the banks of the Ji River at Wushang the two men made a compact to use their arts to cure ailments. They said to one another, "Now that we share a mutual determination, let us each test our ability." Deng then charmed (*jin* 禁) the Ji River causing its water to not flow. Bing followed that by charming a dead tree, which immediately sprouted buds.

The account continues with details of their sometimes miraculous activities, noting that "solely by practicing these charms (the ailments) they treated were always eliminated." Xu Deng's and Zhao Bing's abilities are reminiscent of the southern incantation skills described by Wang Chong (see "Varieties of Magic"). I suspect that Wang Chong had knowledge of the recipes of Yue when he composed his argument concerning the south, Yang vapor, and human breath.

Xu Deng and Zhao Bing were Later Han inheritors of magico-religious traditions that were already highly regarded in the second century B.C. The *Huainanzi* relates that "people of Jing 荆 (i.e. Chu 楚) worship demons, people of Yue are habitual demon-worshippers" (*Huainanzi*, 18.306). Han references to Jing/Chu designate a broad geographical and cultural sphere in the central and eastern regions of the Yangzi, tending to overlap with Yue and Wu 吳 in the southeast. In addition, the deep south which stretched from Min to Southern Yue 南越 (including present-day Fujian and Guangdong, and extending into Vietnam) was known as the land of various groups of Yue people. Thus references to Yue apply both to the southeast Yangzi region and the deep south.[1] Yue magic and religion were officially sponsored by Thearch Wu around 110 B.C. when the Yue shamanka Yongzhi 勇之 convinced Thearch Wu that Yue magic was not only spiritually potent, but was also the key to longevity (the reason for Thearch Wu's active patronage of recipe gentlemen). Thearch Wu ordered Yue shamans to establish cult sites for Yue *zhu* 越祝 (Yue incantation) at Chang'an; Yue-style worship and divination with chicken bones are said to have become popular as a result (*Shiji*, 28.33b; *Hanshu*,25B.1a-b).[2] Thearch Wu's faith in Yue shamans and their magic was reconfirmed in 104 B.C. when the Arbor-vitae Beam Terrace 柏梁臺 burned. Thearch Wu followed Yongzhi's counsel regarding the Yue custom of averting the danger of fire by replacing a burned structure with an even larger one; and he built the grandest of his palace complexes, the Establishing Brilliance Palace 建章宮 (*Hanshu*, 25B.4b).

Zhang Heng 張衡 (78-139) makes a stock allusion to "Yue shamans putting forth recipes" 越巫陳方 in the "Xijing fu" 西京賦 account of the building of the Establishing Brilliance Palace (*Wenxuan*, 2.6a). A later passage on a man known as Yellow Sire 黄公 from Donghai 東海

[1]For a summary of the political geography of the south in Former Han times, see Twitchett and Loewe 1986: 451-57. The Kingdom of Southern Yue was independent of Han rule until its defeat by Thearch Wu in 111 B.C.

[2]Thearch Wu's conquest of Southern Yue in 111 B.C. was the prelude to his sponsorship of Yue magic and religion. The Yue cult sites are mentioned again in *Hanshu*, 28A-1.30a, and were known for their exorcisms (see *MSI*.E.124).

(present-day Shandong) is more suggestive of the occult tradition represented by the recipes of Yue during the Han:

> Donghai's Yellow Sire, he of the red knife and Yue incantations.
>
> He hoped to subdue the white tiger, and in the end could not be rescued. (*Wenxuan*, 2.16a-b.)

According to the Li Shan 李善 commentary (seventh century): "In Donghai there was a man who was able with a red knife and the Pace of Yu to use the incantation method of the Yue people to subdue tigers, and who was called Yellow Sire." Various post-Han sources give anecdotal accounts of Yellow Sire, explaining how in old age his powers weakened and how he was eaten by a tiger when his magic failed to work.

The Yellow Sire's technique of Yue incantation surely represents the same magical tradition as Zhao Bing's recipes of Yue. Moreover, while the existence of cult sites for Yue incantation at Chang'an is significant evidence of the dispersal of Yue magic, the man who went by the alias Yellow Sire and hailed from present-day Shandong was not a Yue shaman but was an occult specialist like Xu Deng and Zhao Bing. Called either recipes of Yue or Yue incantation, by the first century A.D. Yue magic was being transmitted orally and in writing among occult specialists. The magical recipes in *MSI*.E reflect the knowledge of Yue-style incantation in *fang*-literature collected by the elite several centuries earlier.

The terms "recipes of Yue" and "Yue incantation" became obsolete after Han times. However, the *Baopuzi* proves that southern breath magic continued to be transmitted:

> In Wu and Yue there is a method for charm spells (*jinzhou* 禁呪)[1] that produces very clear results. It consists of augmenting the vapor (of the breath) and that is all. Those who know it can enter into the midst of a great pestilence and share the bed with a sick person without themselves being infected. Again, in a group of several tens of travelers, all can be made to lose their fear. This demonstrates that vapor can exorcise heavenly calamity. It may happen that evil goblins and mountain specters invade the home, throwing tiles and stones at people or setting fire to the roof. At times they manifest

[1] *Zhou* 呪 (spell) is interchangeable with *zhu* 祝 (incantation).

> their forms as they go and come; at times only the sound of their speech is heard. If someone skilled at charms charms them with vapor, they all cease immediately. This demonstrates that vapor can charm demons and spirits. When entering mountains and forests where the land abounds in streams and poisonous snakes, none who venture there will not be attacked and injured. If someone skilled at charms charms them with vapor, they can be repelled for over a distance of several tens of square *li*; and none of his companions will suffer harm. Moreover, he can charm tigers and leopards as well as snakes and wasps, causing them all to lie prostrate and be unable to rise. If he charms a metal wound with vapor the blood stops flowing the moment it wells up. Moreover, he can reattach bones and reconnect muscles. If he charms a bare blade with vapor he can stamp on it without injury, and stab without having it penetrate. If a person is struck by a snake or viper and charms it with vapor, it is immediately cured. In recent times Zuo Ci 左 慈, Zhao Ming 趙 明,[1] and others have used vapor to charm water, making the water flow in the opposite direction for one or two *zhang*. Or again, lit a fire on a thatch roof; cooked food and eaten it; and the thatch roof was not singed.[2] Or again, nailed a large nail into a pillar seven or eight *cun* and blown on it with the vapor (of the breath); and the nail popped out as if shot from a bow. (*Baopuzi*, 5.24.)

The enumeration of southern breath magic concludes with several more examples of vapor charms.

The mention of charming tigers and leopards brings to mind Yellow Sire and his Yue incantations which failed to subdue the white tiger; Zhao Bing's well-known expertise in the recipes of Yue is referred to directly. The everyday aspect of vapor charms is evident in the passage on demonic nuisances in the home. The Shuihudi "Jie" provides remedies for the same kinds of hazards. I expect that the techniques of spitting and spouting in the *MSI*.E magical recipes were also used to rid the home of demons (note especially the exorcistic procession through the home to capture the child sprite in *MSI*.E.277, and the incantation which summons a "spouter"). Vapor charms to stop bleeding and to cure snake bites

---

[1] I.e. Zhao Bing.

[2] This feat is attributed to Zhao Bing in the *Hou Hanshu* account.

have counterparts in *MSI*.E.9 (even though recipe does not include spouting and spitting)[1] and in several recipes for bites by poisonous creatures (*MSI*.E.48, 59). In short, there is good evidence to link the fourth century A.D. southern breath magic in the *Baopuzi* not only with the recipes of Yue and Yue incantation, but also with the techniques of spouting and spitting in *MSI*.E.

After the *Baopuzi* description of Wu and Yue vapor charms, I have found only two likely references to the transmission of southern breath magic prior to the seventeenth century. The Li Xian 李 賢 (seventh century) commentary to the *Hou Hanshu* account of Xu Deng and Zhao Bing notes that, "it is said that in Jiangnan the charm method of Lord Zhao to cure sickness is still being transmitted" (*Hou Hanshu*, 82B.9b). And Xue Bozong 薛 伯 宗, a fifth century southerner, knew the art of vapor charms:

> Gongsun Tai suffered from (an abscess) on his back. Bozong sealed it with the vapor (of his breath) and transferred it, lodging it on the willow in front of the studio. (*Nanshi*, 32.18a.)

Xie Zhaozhe 謝 肇 淛 (1567-1624), from a prominent Fujian family, picks up the thread of the tradition in the *Wuzazu* 五 雜 俎. His discussion of vapor charms follows that of shamans in Jiangnan and Min:

> In antiquity those skilled at vapor charms could extract a spearhead from bone and transfer an abscess to a tree in the courtyard.[2] As for being able to drive dragons and bind goblins, such things were all the easier to do! This is, to be sure, the genuine talisman spell-casting (*fuzhou* 符 呪) and not an illusory art. The various kinds of talisman spell-casting are all to be found in the Daoist Canon (*Daozang* 道 藏). One must simply undergo a process of refinement and training (to practice them). At present there are certain wandering monks who singe their eyebrows, set fire to their fingers, and go for up to thirty-five days without starving. They are not genuine possessors of the way. They are also able to perform vapor charms, but the spuriousness of their practices needs no discussion. (*Wuzazu*, 6.32b.)

[1] It is tempting to speculate that the missing penultimate word in *MSI*.E.9 might be "spit," making the sentence read, "Draw five lines on the ground and [spit] on it."
[2] Alluding to Xue Bozong's feat.

Extracting spearheads, transferring abscesses, and binding goblins are activities consistent with the Wu and Yue vapor charms discussed in the *Baopuzi*. By placing the entry after the entries on Jiangnan and Min shamans, Xie Zhaozhe appears to have a regional tradition in mind. However, he is quite definite in attributing the genuine art to talisman spell-casting in the scriptures of the Daoist Canon. The local "wandering monks"—no doubt popular occultists—practice a false art.

Xie Zhaozhe's evaluation suggests one answer to why the record of the recipes of Yue vanished in medieval times. Quite simply, the popular use of charms, spells, and talismans was subsumed by religious Daoism. The use of magic in Daoism and the record of it in the Daoist Canon came to represent the genuine source in the minds of the elite and of popular occultists who would have tended to identify their practices with the prestige of Daoism.[1] Moreover, breath magic in the later occult tradition was regarded as an extension of breath cultivation; the ability to perform incantations and spells was one of the fruits of cultivating vapor (the refining and training referred to in the *Wuzazu*). Already in the *Baopuzi* the purpose of discussing Wu and Yue vapor charms was not to describe a notable southern tradition of breath magic for its own sake; the passage follows a discussion of macrobiotic hygiene which advocates ingesting drugs, circulating vapor, and sexual cultivation. The purpose of the passage on Wu and Yue vapor charms is to illustrate the importance and utility of vapor cultivation with examples of vapor's magical potency (hence the refrain of "this demonstrates that vapor can exorcise heavenly calamity" and "this demonstrates that vapor can charm demons and spirits").

Ideas about vapor must have already influenced the Warring States conception of the power of incantation and breath magic. However, in the third century B.C. the acts of spitting and spouting in *MSI*.E were likely to have still been regarded as magical acts in themselves, not yet assimilated with vapor theory. Southern breath magic was grounded in magico-religious tradition, not in naturalistic or occult theories concerning vapor. The *Lunheng* offers the first explanation of breath magic based on vapor theory (see "Varieties of Magic"). In the *Baopuzi* we have the first references to the idea that breath magic is "augmenting vapor" and "charming with vapor," and the oldest statement linking breath magic to hygiene

[1] I of course do not fault the received record for failing to provide the kind of information that interests me; writing about regional magico-religious customs would have been of minor interest to most Chinese authors.

(religious Daoism also assumes the connection). The new rationale of breath magic would have tended to diminish the significance of a regional tradition of breath magic, for now the regional tradition was one example among others of phenomena associated with vapor and its cultivation. Along with the rise of religious Daoism, changes in the perception of breath magic also affected the old southern breath magic called recipes of Yue. Nevertheless, neither Daoism nor changed perceptions stifled its continued transmission.

Writing in the first quarter of the twentieth century, Chai E 柴萼 argues that the current name for the Han recipes of Yue is Chenzhou *fu* 辰州符 (Chen District talismans; Chen District is present-day Yuanling 沅陵, several hundred kilometers west of Changsha):

> The *Hou Hanshu*, "Account of Recipes and Arts," states that Zhao Bing was skilled at the recipes of Yue. I note: The former Chen District in Hunan is the ancient region of Southern Yue.[1] Thus it is also called Chen District talismans. In the *Nanshi*, Xue Bozong was skilled at transferring abscesses. When Gongsun Tai suffered from (an abscess) on his back, Bozong transferred it for him onto a tree. Something like one *dou* of yellow-red liquid came out (from the tree) and the tree withered because of it. Thus one already sees the transfer of illness by means of *zhuyou* 祝由 (incantations for removal) in the Northern and Southern Dynasties. (*Fantianlu conglu*, 33.28a.)

Whereas Xie Zhaozhe attributes breath magic to sources in the Daoist Canon, Chai E argues that an old southern tradition of breath magic lies behind the Chen District talismans. Chai E deserves credit for being the first scholar to identify the recipes of Yue with the Chen District talismans. His reason for making the identification requires explanation.

---

[1]Chai E's claim that Chen District belonged to Southern Yue is plausible, however his geographical argument to prove the identity of the recipes of Yue and the Chen District talismans is not entirely convincing. In the second century B.C. the kingdom of Southern Yue extended northwards from its center in present-day Guangdong to a frontier with Changsha and the ancient Chu region. Riegel (1976) discusses the border between Changsha and Southern Yue based on maps discovered in Mawangdui tomb 3. As for the recipes of Yue, Zhao Bing was from Dongyang in the old Yue heartland (present-day Zhejiang). While the name Chen District talismans as well as the occurrence of spitting and spouting in *MSI*.E are significant evidence of the distribution of this southern breath magic in the region of present-day Hunan, the later appearance of the name Chen District talismans is not likely to have been because Chen District was geographically part of ancient Southern Yue.

Like other Qing writers, Chai E understood medicine to contain thirteen divisions of which the thirteenth is the division of magical medicine, called *zhuyou ke* 祝由科 (division of incantations for removal). The *locus classicus* of *zhuyou* is in the *Suwen*.[1] The classification of medicine into thirteen divisions is first attested in the fourteenth century in the *Chuogenglu* 輟耕錄, which attributes the classification to the twelfth century Song medical compendium *Shengji zonglu* 聖濟總錄 (*Chuogenglu*, 15.227; the classification does not appear in extant editions of the *Shengji zonglu*). Chai E and other writers discuss magical medicine under the heading *zhuyou ke*, and their examples mostly date to the Song and later. By linking the recipes of Yue, the Chen district talismans, and Xue Bozong's magical removal of the abscess in his entry on *zhuyou ke*, Chai E breaks new ground with his claim that "the transfer of illness by means of *zhuyou*" can be traced to the Northern and Southern Dynasties (i.e. third to sixth centuries A.D.). Chai E's purpose is to clarify the history of the *zhuyou ke*. He cites magical traditions besides the Chen District talismans in the entry; other writers cite still other magical traditions in their entries on *zhuyou ke*.[2]

The virtue of the idea of the *zhuyou ke* is that regional traditions of magic became the focus of attention; magical medicine was not treated as just an adjunct of religious Daoism. One must bear in mind, however, that the Qing writers did not pursue research on the Chen District talismans or other magical traditions beyond noting their significance for the history of the *zhuyou ke*; nor did they cast themselves in the role of ethnographers. My thesis regarding southern breath magic is supported chiefly by several accounts of specialists in the Chen District talismans and occultists from Yuanling (who presumably practice the Chen District talismans) in sources like the *Qingbai leichao* 清稗類鈔. Evidence that might provide us with a better picture of the Chen District talismans in more recent times is lacking, although I suspect that written materials exist and that oral traditions are still alive in Hunan and elsewhere.[3] I do not

---

[1]The Yellow Thearch asks why drugs and other therapies are necessary in the present age whereas he has heard that in antiquity "incantations for removal" were sufficient to cure ailments. Qi Bo replies that people of old enjoyed a simpler life and that as a result evil did lodge in their bodies; incantations sufficed to remove an ailment (*Suwen* 13, 4.2b).

[2]The *zhuyou ke* is also discussed in *Qingbai leichao*, vol. 30: 102; *Kechuang xianhua xuji*, 1.4b; and *Jianhu guangji*, 1.3a.

[3]In a study of the interpretation of talismans Chen Xiangchun (1942) refers to a book entitled *Chenzhou zhenben lingyan fuzhou quanshu* 辰州真本靈驗符咒全書 (Complete book of

doubt that there have been changes in the tradition of magic whose most recent name is Chen District talismans; and that the Chen District talismans incorporate much Daoist magic (especially the use of talismans). At the same time, comparison of the *MSI*.E recipes which make use of spitting and spouting (see the list in "Varieties of Magic" above) with the *Qingbai leichao* accounts indicates to me that we are dealing with the same core tradition of breath magic, which has been transmitted in the region of Hunan and elsewhere in the south since at least the third century B.C.

The plausibility of my thesis is best illustrated by one *Qingbai leichao* account, which has a counterpart in *MSI*.E.27. The specialist in the Chen District talismans was an anonymous salt official from Hangzhou 杭州 (Zhejiang):

> There was a local man who had a sore on his back. A physician diagnosed it for him and it did not get better. The oozing and rotting became increasingly severe and the mouth of the wound was already about three *cun* across. Then he went to the gate of the salt official and sought a diagnosis from him. He examined it closely and said, "Sir, your coming is already ten days delayed. Nevertheless I must remove it for you. Just ten days will be needed, then it will be cured." Thereupon he hooked his finger and drew a talisman. At the same time he applied an ointment. Further, he got a cup of pure water for (the patient) to carry home and place on the stove as an offering. He instructed him saying, "Tomorrow morning when you come again for diagnosis, bring along the water. I will cure (the sore) for you." The next morning the man arrived bearing the cup of water. Then he had him sit with his back facing east. Once again he hooked his finger and drew a talisman. He sucked up the water in the cup and spouted (*pen* 噴) it. Then he pinched the wound with three fingers, hurled (his hand) towards the wall, and there seemed to be a sound.[1] Continuing, he covered (the wound) with an ointment and the mouth of the wound subsequently closed.

---

divinely verified talisman-spells in the genuine edition of Chen District), published in 1922. I have not been able to examine the book. The talismans cited by Chen are Daoist in nature, but it is possible that other parts of the book contain material related to the breath magic of the Chen District talismans tradition. I delivered a paper on the magical recipes in *MSI*.E, the recipes of Yue, and the Chen District talismans at the International Symposium on Mawangdui Han Tombs in Changsha in August 1992 (Xia De'an 1994). I did not acquire new evidence while in Hunan.

[1]The demonic pathogen hitting the wall is the source of the noise.

> After that, he took a talisman and pasted it on, saying, "You are better now." As for the man at this point, his ailment was as if vanished. (*Qingbai leichao*, vol. 30: 154.)

The magical operation in *MSI*.E.27 could easily be taken for yet another of the salt official's Chen District talisman cures. The ailment is infant convulsions and may be related to a tetanus infection. The treatment focuses on drawing the demonic pathogen out from the opening of a wound, like the removal of the cause of the festering sore above. Let me quote the relevant part of the recipe:

> Take vegetation from the upturned slope of the roof. Incinerate it using kindling and [1] it in a ladle. Make silted water that is roiled thrice and fill a cup with it. Then spit on the ladle and chant this incantation over it: "Spouter, spout ferociously. On high be like the sweeper star. Down below be like congealed blood. You will be seized left of the gate. You will be cut apart right of the gate. Should you not desist, you will be quartered and exposed in the marketplace." Then stroke with the ladle in a circle around the spot where the infant convulsions are, and rinse it in the cup of water. Watch it. When there is blood like a fly wing, discard it by the wall. Take fresh water. Once again spit on the liquid in the ladle[1] and stroke with it as before. There should be no trembling. Repeat it over and over again. When the trembling has ceased, stop. Excellent.

The salt official drew talismans, spouted consecrated water on the sore and extracted the demonic pathogen from the sore with his fingers, hurling it at the wall. The related sequence of actions in *MSI*.E.27 is as follows: the designated officiant spits on the ladle filled with roof vegetation ash (perhaps the ash has solar, exorcistic properties) and chants an incantation over it; the incantation commands a spouter to spout and exorcise the demonic agent, who is directly threatened with execution; with the power of the spouter transferred to the ladle, the ladle is then used to stroke the spot where the ailment is located (probably a wound); the demonic agent is caught by the ladle; once caught, the agent becomes manifest as blood in the shape of a fly wing in the rinsing water; and the rinsing water is discarded by the wall. The sequence of actions is repeated

---

[1]See *MSI*.E.27 for comments on the meaning of this phrase.

until the demonic pathogen is entirely removed, as indicated by cessation of trembling.

The salt official also drew talismans with his finger and chanted spells to remove a writing brush lodged inside a man's throat—the counterpart to vapor charms for removing nails from pillars which the *Baopuzi* associates with occult specialists like Zhao Bing (*Qingbai leichao*, vol. 30: 154).[1] A skeptic may object that there is simply not enough evidence to prove that the Chen District talismans, the recipes of Yue, and *MSI*.E belong to a continuous tradition of breath magic. I admit that my argument is conjectural and that we will probably never have better evidence. However, I think the similarity between *MSI*.E.27 and the salt official's use of the Chen District talismans coupled with historical references to southern traditions of incantation, to the recipes of Yue, and to southern vapor charms satisfy the burden of proof; it is up to the skeptic to prove me wrong.

[1]According to the account, the brush slowly emerged from the patient's throat as the salt official chanted.

TRANSLATION

INTRODUCTION

The Translation is based on the photographic reproduction and transcription of the Mawangdui medical manuscripts in *MWD*, vol. 4. *MWD*, vol. 4, assigns column (C) or slip (S) numbers to all of the manuscripts (the numbers appear both in the transcription and the photographic reproduction, excepting *MS*II and *MS*V). I provide column or slip numbers for each entry in the texts in parentheses at the beginning of the entry. Citations to *MWD*, vol. 4, "Transcription," are to the appropriate columns or slips in the transcription portion of *MWD*, vol. 4.

Because *MWD*, vol. 4, does not take account of the editions of *MS*I.B, *MS*I.C, and *MS*I.D in the Zhangjiashan *Maishu*, I have made a new transcription of the three texts in Appendix 1. I explain my transcription method there, but I would like to note here that I do not attempt to produce a collated edition of the texts in question. Rather, I have used the more complete *Maishu* editions to fill lacunae in the *MS*I editions (*MWD*, vol. 4, "Transcription," resorts to filling many of the lacunae in *MS*I.B based on text parallels in *Lingshu* 10). I trust that the transcription in Appendix 1 is a fairer representation of the texts.

In order to explain my translation conventions, I must briefly review the *MWD*, vol. 4, transcription conventions (set forth in the "Fanli" 凡例 at the front of the volume). I am grateful to Professor Li Xueqin, who performed the final editing of the "Transcription," for clarifications. The "Transcription" uses modern *kaishu* 楷書 graphs, changing some graphs to conform with current convention (歙 is written 飲, 衠 becomes 衝, etc.). Modern punctuation is used throughout (which at times I judge to be incorrect). Of three text markers in the original manuscripts, the dot • is retained in the "Transcription" (it is used most often before new entries or to distinguish one passage from another within a single entry in the texts). Two other markers are excised in the "Transcription": a double-bar sign = placed at the bottom right of a graph meaning that the graph is repeated ("Transcription" writes the graph twice); and a hook-like sign ㇄ that is used occasionally to punctuate words or phrases within a line of text.

Lacunae in the texts are either graphs that are judged to be illegible or places where the material of the manuscripts (silk, bamboo, wood) is actually destroyed. When lacunae occur and it is possible to estimate the number of missing graphs, each missing graph is marked in the "Transcription" with a box; if the number is indeterminable, a box with a slash through it is used. Missing graphs in lacunae are sometimes restored based on parallels within the text, with other Mawangdui medical texts, or with received literature. These emendations are indicated by placing heavy brackets around the graph(s). The "Transcription" does not identify the basis for the emendation in each instance, but Li Xueqin informs me that emendations based on received literature affect only *MS*I.B, *MS*II.B (another edition of *MS*I.B), *MS*III.91, and *MS*V.3. In addition, if a graph is barely legible in the text and the transcription necessarily tentative, the graph is placed in the same heavy brackets. Finally, the heavy brackets are also used to emend the text when the "Transcription" judges that a graph has been erroneously omitted by the scribe; these emendations are always identified in the "Transcription" notes. When the "Transcription" judges that the scribe miswrote a graph, the graph deemed correct is placed in caret-shaped brackets < > after the graph in question.

Most of the graphs are readily identifiable. Quite often they are written without the signific (or "radical") usually used in received literature, but there is little difficulty in reading the intended word. The "Transcription" places the fuller graph in parentheses after the graph as written in the text. Sometimes the graph as written in the text is attested for the appropriate word and meaning in received literature, but it is a rare usage or is a loan graph. To facilitate reading, the "Transcription" again uses parentheses to indicate a more usual graph for the word in question; the same is true of variant graphs and simple cases of unattested graphs. When identification of a graph is problematic the "Transcription" notes often propose a solution, but the proposed graph is not introduced parenthetically into the text.

My translation is complete but for *MS*II.B. Although it differs in small details from *MS*I.B (see Appendix 1), I have decided to let the latter edition represent the text (a major reason for my decision is the number of lacunae in both editions and my judgment that

MSI.B is more similar to the *Maishu* edition, leaving me less certain of emending *MSII.B*). I do not rely on the punctuation in the "Transcription" and usually do not comment when my own punctuation differs. As a rule I accept the "Transcription," minus any of the material placed in heavy brackets, caret-shaped brackets, and parentheses. Between forty and fifty graphs have been mistranscribed in the "Transcription." Some are obvious printing errors, some involve fine points of transcription. Qiu Xigui (1992) is responsible for identifying most of the incorrect graph transcriptions; I discovered some during the course of my research. The revisions are noted in the Translation and are also listed in Appendix 2. In several instances the correct transcription of a graph remains difficult to determine (I am grateful to Li Xueqin for re-examining the photographic reproduction and giving me his considered opinion).

I accept most of the "Transcription" emendations (graphs placed in heavy brackets and caret-shaped brackets). When I accept them, I simply translate without comment. When I do not, I note my reasons. Words placed in brackets [ ] in the Translation indicate either that my acceptance of the "Transcription" emendation is tentative or that I am introducing an emendation of my own. Again, I note my reasons. Lacunae are indicated in the Translation with brackets as well, the enclosed arabic numeral representing the estimated number of missing graphs; [?] means that the number is indeterminable. Whenever lacunae leave me perplexed as to the meaning of the graphs before or after, I indicate these graphs with braces { } enclosing the number of graphs involved. I use parentheses sparingly as needed to fill out the meaning; and also to provide common English names for the drugs which are given in romanization.

The parenthetical graphs in the "Transcription" lie at the heart of text explication. It would be a dry exercise to note every instance when my reading of a graph differs from the parenthetical graph-gloss given in the "Transcription"; and I do not do so. My reading and interpretation of difficult graphs are discussed in the Translation notes, including of course the unattested and other problematic graphs discussed in the "Transcription" notes.

Reconstructions of Old Chinese are based on Li Fang-kuei's system as represented in Schuessler 1987 (I have removed tone markers used by Li and Schuessler). At times I have had to improvise, usually a matter of using the phonetic of a graph in the manuscripts as the basis for determining the reconstruction; and I bear the responsibility for any errors committed. Mostly the reconstructions serve to test the probability of phonetic loan graphs and to identify rhyming words in the incantations in *MS*I.E.

Materia medica presents special difficulties. Traditional Chinese drug names are not like modern botanical, zoological, and chemomineralogical nomenclature. Whether we can know exactly which plant, animal, or mineral is denoted by the name is frequently open to doubt. The situation is all the more uncertain for materia medica in the Mawangdui medical manuscripts. Items like cultivated grains, domesticated animals, foods and food products, common minerals (soils, salt, mercury, etc.), and manufactured articles are simply translated. Where appropriate, a technical identification is provided in the Index of Materia Medica, using *ZY* as the standard reference. Most other plant, animal, and mineral names are romanized. If I am sufficiently confident of its identity, a common English name is placed in parentheses in the Translation (often I adopt the expedient of using the genus of the item in question). The scientific name is provided in the Index of Materia Medica, based on *ZY*. Many of these identifications should, of course, still be regarded with suspicion, but the possible continuities in traditional knowledge of materia medica leading up to the compilation of works like *ZY* outweigh my skepticism. Other names are left in romanization. If there is room for speculation, likely identifications are discussed in the Translation notes.

Facsimiles of portions of *MS*I.A (Fig. 1), *MS*III (Fig. 13), and *MS*VI.A (Fig. 17) are the work of Mr. Xu Datong. They are based on the photographic reproduction in *MWD*, vol. 4, which while discernible—especially with bright light and magnifying glass—loses considerable clarity when reproduced itself. The facsimiles both illustrate the manuscripts and exemplify several types of script and calligraphic styles. Fig. 13 was also chosen to illustrate the *MS*III.91 drawing of the female genitals. In addition, Mr. Xu has made facsimiles of eleven of the *MS*II.C exercise drawings (Figs. 2-12). The photographic reproduction of *MS*II.C in *MWD*, vol. 4, was supplemented by color photographs in Fu and Chen 1992: 148-50; and in Mawangdui Han mu boshu zhengli xiaozu 1979. The original is severely damaged; of the forty-four drawings we chose eleven that lend themselves to accurate replication (captions are also copied when they are legible in the photographs). A reconstruction of *MS*II.C in Mawangdui Han mu boshu zhengli xiaozu 1979 provides renderings of all forty-four drawings, even the most fragmentary, and should be regarded as conjectural in many details. My parenthetical description of the *MS*II.C drawings in the Translation is based on photographic reproductions, not on this reconstruction.

MSI.A

ZUBI SHIYI MAI JIUJING

足臂十一脈灸經

CAUTERIZATION CANON OF THE ELEVEN VESSELS OF THE FOOT AND FOREARM

MSI.A.1 (CC1-4)

Foot[1]

Foot Great Yang vessel.[2] It emerges[3] in the hollow by the outer malleolus.[4] Ascending, it penetrates the calf and emerges at the po-

---

[1]*Zu* 足 (foot) is written in a raised position about one centimeter above the main text in C1. It serves as the heading for *MSI*.A.1-6. Each of the six foot vessels occurs symmetrically on the left and right side, for a total of twelve vessels.

[2]𧖴 represents the word *mai* "vessel," which is consistently written with this graph throughout *MSI*.A. It is composed of three parts: 血 (blood); 水 (water); and 目 (eye). According to *MWD*, vol. 4, "Transcription," n. 2, the graph is composed of a variant form of 衇 (the graph for *mai* attested in *SW*, 11B.6b) with the addition of 目. The "Transcription" also notes that the graph occurs on Warring States seals, and thus may be a Warring States seal script graph for the word *mai*. Two other graphs are used to write *mai* on *MSI*. *MSI*.B consistently writes 眽 (still using 目); and *MSI*.E.1 writes 脈 (attested in *SW*, 11B.6b). The reason for writing the graph with *mu/*mjəkw* 目 is not clear (it is definitely not a phonetic for *mai/*mrik*).

[3]The verb *chu* 出 occurs many times in *MSI*.A-B when describing the path of the vessels. All occurrences are uniformly translated "emerge," in the sense of "rise forth." According to *SW*, 6B.2b, *chu* means "advance" and the graph depicts a plant rising. Like English "emerge," *chu* includes the sense that something becomes apparent, that it "rises into notice." When *chu* is used at the beginning of a vessel description, as in the present case, it designates the point from where the vessel arises (see *MSI*.B.1 and *MSI*.B.4 for examples of other words used to denote a vessel's point of origin). Ma Jixing argues that occurrences of *chu* at subsequent points in a vessel description mean simply "ascend" or "reach" (1992: 176, n. 11). I suspect that the sense of "rise into notice" is applicable, and that *chu* means not only that the path of the vessel reaches a particular point on the body, but also that the presence of the vessel is detectable at that point.

[4]*Huai* 踝 denotes the bony prominence on either side of the ankle (see *SW*, 2B.24a); i.e. the malleolus. For the most part the use of "outer" and "inner" as well as "upper" and "lower" to designate positions on the body in *MSI*.A-B is readily comprehensible. However, in some contexts the use of *nei* 内 is ambiguous, since it also means "in" or "inside" in addition to designating an "inner" surface in contrast to an "outer" surface on the exterior of the body.

ples.[1] A branch goes to the lower *xun*.[2] The direct path penetrates the [1] and presses laterally on the spine.[3] It [2] and ascends to the head.[4] A branch at the lower part of the center of the forehead goes to the ear. The direct path penetrates the inner canthus of the eye and goes to the nose.

The ailments: ailing from the loss of function in the little toe;[5] calf pain; cramping in the poples; buttock pain;[6] the occurrence of hemorrhoids;[7] waist pain; pain pressing laterally on the spine; [1] pain; nape pain; hand pain;[8] coldness in the center of the forehead; the occurrence of deafness; eye pain; stuffy nose and bloody nose;[9]

---

[1]胳 in *MWD*, vol. 4, "Transcription," should be transcribed as 郤, which represents the word *xi*, written 郄 in *Suwen* 41, 11.7a. According to the Wang Bing commentary, *xi* denotes the place at the center of the back of the knee where there is a fold in the skin; roughly the center of the poples.

[2] 脾 is not attested in received literature; the reading *xun* is conjectural, based on reading 旬 as the phonetic. Wei and Hu argue that the graph may be a phonetic loan for *tun* 臀 (buttock; 1992, vol. 1: 2, n. 6). Phonological evidence does not support a loan between *xun*/**sgwjin* and *tun*/**dən*; hence I do not accept the proposed loan usage. It is worth noting that Li Fang-kuei's reconstruction of a velar in the Old Chinese initial of *xun* departs from Karlgren (1957), who reconstructs a dental affricate. Ma Jixing argues that the graph is a phonetic loan for *shen*/**sthjin* 胂, attested at *SW*, 4B.23b, as a term for the flesh that presses laterally on both sides of the spine (1992: 177, n. 14). Thus the "lower *xun*" would designate a point at the lower end of the spine. Ma's proposed loan usage is arguable and I am not firmly convinced. For the time being I leave the graph unidentified.

[3]"Press laterally" translates *jia* 夾. The meaning is that the left and right foot Great Yang vessels pass along either side of the spine. All other occurrences of *jia* in describing the path of the vessels have the same meaning; e.g. *MSI*.A.3, "press laterally on the lesser abdomen" and "press laterally on the mouth."

[4]I follow Ma Jixing in reading 豆 as *tou* 頭 (head), and not as a word for the nape as suggested in *MWD*, vol. 4, "Transcription" (1992: 177, n. 20).

[5]"Loss of function" translates *fei* 癈. See *Lingshu* 10, 3.8b, for an example of the medical sense of *fei* in connection with the vessels: "When (the vessel) is full then the joints grow slack and the elbow has loss of function (*fei*)." The sense of *fei* includes numbness as well as physical impairment.

[6] 脽 (read *shui*) in *MWD*, vol. 4, "Transcription," should be transcribed as 雎, which is attested in *SW*, 8A.71b, as a variant graph for *tun* "buttock." *Shui* also denotes "buttock," and is glossed with *tun* in *SW*, 4B.25b.

[7]On hemorrhoids (*zhi* 痔) see *MSI*.E.142.

[8]Because the hand does not lie on the path of the foot Great Yang vessel, Ma Jixing proposes reading *shou* 手 as the homophonous 首 "head" (1992: 181, n. 12). While there is reason for suspicion about the graph written in the text, the evidence is insufficient and I do not accept Ma's reading.

[9]尪 in *MWD*, vol. 4, "Transcription," should be transcribed as 尳. The graph represents the word *qiu*, written 鼽 in *SW*, 4A.17a, and defined as "ailing from coldness affecting the nose so that it is blocked." *SW*, 5A.51a, defines *niu* 衄 as "blood coming out from the nose."

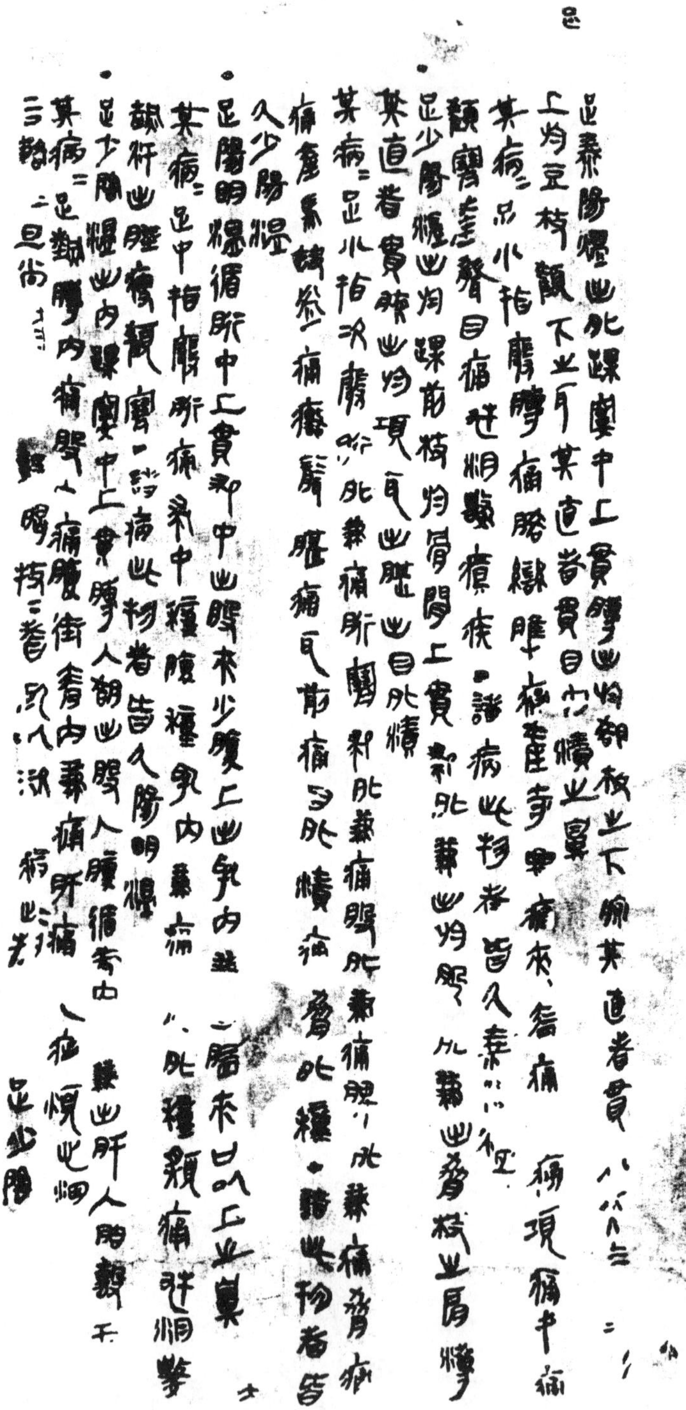

Fig. 1 Facsimile of *MS*I.A.1-4

continual seizure sickness.[1] In all cases of ailing from these things, cauterize the Great Yang vessel.

MSI.A.2 (CC5-9)

Foot Minor Yang vessel. It emerges in front of the malleolus.[2] A branch is situated in the bone.[3] (The direct path) ascends[4] and penetrates the outer edge of the knee.[5] It emerges at the outer edge of the thigh and emerges at the side. A branch goes to the shoulderblade. The direct path penetrates the underarm, emerges at the nape and at the ear, emerges at the *zhen*,[6] and emerges at the outer canthus of the eye.

The ailments: ailing from the loss of function in the (toe) next to the little toe;[7] pain in the outer edge of the shin; coldness in the shin; pain in the outer edge of the knee; pain in the outer edge of the thigh; pain in the outer edge of the ham;[8] pain in the side; [1] pain; the occurrence of *ma*;[9] pain in the broken basin;[10] neck

---

[1]"Seizure" translates *dian* 癲 (see *MSI*.E.71).

[2]The outer malleolus must be understood here.

[3]Ma Jixing suggests that the bone is the malleolus (1992: 184, n. 4), but the shinbone is also plausible. Ma also cites evidence for understanding *jian* 間 in the sense of "in, inside."

[4]Usually *MSI*.A explicitly distinguishes a branch path from the main path of the vessel with the phrase 其直者 "the direct path." I have added the phrase parenthetically for clarity.

[5]*MSI*.A-B regularly use *lian* 廉 (edge) to add specificity to the identification of points on the exterior of the body.

[6]䐶 is not attested in early sources. It is attested later as a variant graph for *nan* 腩, which refers to a form of cooked meat (Morohashi 1957-60, vol. 9: nos. 29692-29693). The reading *zhen*/**tjəm* is based on the phonetic 甚. *MWD*, vol. 4, "Transcription," reads the graph as a phonetic loan for *zhen*/**tjəm* 枕 (headrest), and interprets it as a reference to the occipital bone based on *Suwen* 60, 16.4a. The argument is plausible. Equally plausible is the argument cited in *KGS*, vol. 1: 90, n. 29, that the graph is a phonetic loan for *zhun*/**tjən* 肫, defined as "cheekbone" in *SW*, 4B.20b. The difference of consonant **-n* in place of **-m* does not invalidate a phonetic loan. Luo and Zhou cite evidence which suggests that several groups of words with consonant **-m* already changed to **-n* in some Former Han dialects (1958: 53). Hence 䐶 may have already been read **tjən* in the dialect reflected in *MSI*.

[7]I.e. the fourth toe. The phrase in the original text consists of three graphs 小指次, literally "(the one) next to the little toe." *MWD*, vol. 4, "Transcription," emends the text by adding a fourth graph 指 "toe" to the end of this phrase, arguing that it was omitted due to scribal error. I judge the text to be acceptable as written.

[8]"Ham" translates *bi* 髀, defined as "outer part of the thigh" in *SW*, 4B.15a. My translation derives from the use of *bi* to gloss *tun* "buttock" in *SW*, 8A.71b, which indicates that the "outer thigh" denotes the buttock and back part of the thigh; i.e. the ham.

[9]*MWD*, vol. 4, "Transcription," n. 4, and Ma Jixing (1992: 188, n. 7) both identify *ma* 馬 as an abbreviation of *madao jiaying* 馬刀俠癭, which is attested in *Lingshu* 10, 3.6a (in the description of the foot Minor Yang vessel), as the name for lumps (probably scrofula) that appear by the underarm (*madao*) and the neck (*jiaying*). *Ma* also occurs as an ailment name

lumps;[1] deafness; pain in the *zhen*; pain in the front of the ear; pain in the outer canthus of the eye; swelling in the outer part of the side. In all cases of (ailing from) these things,[2] cauterize the Minor Yang vessel.

MSI.A.3 (CC10-12)

Foot Yang Brilliance vessel. It follows along in the shin. Ascending, it penetrates the knee, emerges at the thigh, and presses laterally on the lesser abdomen.[3] Ascending, it emerges at the inner edge of the breast and emerges at the throat. It presses laterally on the mouth and, ascending, goes to the nose.

The ailments: ailing from the loss of function in the middle toe; shin pain; swelling in the knee; swelling in the abdomen; pain in the inner edge of the breast; swelling in the outer part of the [1]; cheekbone pain; stuffy nose[4] and bloody nose; continual hotness with sweating; loss of flesh at the *cuo*;[5] coldness in the center of the

---

in the Zhangjiashan *Maishu*, "Ailment List": "When it is located below the underarm—it is *ma*" (*MSSW*: 72). Although *ma* and *madao* are both said to occur in the underarm region, I remain skeptical of the identity between the two ailment names. The ailment name *madao* was probably derived from the resemblance of the lump to a type of mussel known as *madao*. I question whether *ma* in *MSI*.A.2 and in "Ailment List" can be an abbreviation of the proper name of the mussel. Another possible explanation is to identify *ma* with *ma* 瘍, which occurs in *MSI*.E.280-82. From the descriptions there, the ailment is characterized by the formation of pustules on the face which burst.

[10]"Broken basin" (*quepen* 缺盆) denotes the clavicle (see *Shiji*, 105.20a, and commentary).

[1]*Lou* 瘻 is defined as "swellings on the neck" in *SW*, 7B.29a—most likely scrofula. *Maishu*, "Ailment List," also specifies that *lou* is an ailment located on the neck (*MSSW*: 72). Ma Jixing cites evidence for identifying *lou* as a kind of abscess and argues that *lou* in *MSI*.A.2 refers more generally to this condition rather than specifically to lumps on the neck (1992: 188, n. 10). Ma's identification of *lou* is in part related to the fact that if *lou* denotes "neck lumps" it overlaps with the same kind of scrofulous ailment that Ma has already identified with the ailment name *ma* above.

[2]*MWD*, vol. 4, "Transcription," emends the text by adding 病 on the presumption that the final sentence in each vessel description in *MSI*.A should begin 諸 病 此 物 者, as in *MSI*.A.1. I judge the phrase as written to be scribal abbreviation and would not emend the text (adding words parenthetically for clarity).

[3]According to *Shiming*, 3.61, *shaofu* 少 腹 (lesser abdomen) is the name for the part of the abdomen that lies below the navel. Medical literature also refers to this region as the "small (小) abdomen."

[4]㾓 in *MWD*, vol. 4, "Transcription," should be transcribed as 鼽 (see *MSI*.A.1).

[5]From the context here and in two later occurrences in *MSI*.A.6, *cuo* 脞 is the name of a part of the body. The graph is attested in pre-Han literature meaning "small" or "chopped" (Morohashi 1957-60, vol. 9: no. 29508). *MWD*, vol. 4, "Transcription," n. 4, argues that in all three occurrences the graph is a scribal error for *bi* 髀. The earliest attestation of *bi* is in medieval sources where it designates the upper thigh region. I am skeptical that a scribe would commit the same error thrice; and I suspect that the graph as

forehead. In all cases of ailing from these things, cauterize the Yang Brilliance vessel.

MSI.A.4 (CC13-15)

Foot Minor Yin vessel. It emerges in the hollow by the inner malleolus. Ascending, it penetrates the calf and enters the poples.[1] It emerges at the thigh, enters the abdomen, and follows along the inner [1] edge of the spine. It emerges at the liver,[2] enters the upper side,[3] and is attached to the tongue [1].

The ailments: ailing from hotness in the foot; pain in the calf;[4] pain in the thigh; pain in the abdomen crossroads[5] and the inner

---

written is a phonetic loan for an anatomical term. Zhou and Xiao (1988: 9, n. 13) cite an argument that *cuo/*tshuar* is a loan for *zui/*tshuəd* 朘 , which is attested as a word for the penis (see *MSI*.E.134). In *MSI*.A.6 the path of the foot Ceasing Yin vessel terminates at the *cuo*; and according to *Lingshu* 10, 3.6b, the foot Ceasing Yin vessel passes by the genitals on the way to the lesser abdomen, stomach and liver. Thus the argument is plausible. My own proposal is to identify *cuo/*tshuar* with *duo/*duar* 脩. The latter graph occurs several times in *MSI*.E; although it is also unattested, it probably denotes the navel (see *MSI*.E.88). This speculation receives added support from *Maishu*, "Ailment List," where there is the following description of a type of *jia* 瘕 (conglomeration): "When on the inside it constricts the *duo* (navel?), so that there is no passage from above to below—it is feces conglomeration" (*MSSW*: 72). Assuming that *cuo* refers to the navel in *MSI*.A.3, there remains the problem of explaining what it means to have a "loss of flesh at the navel." Perhaps it refers to an ailment similar to the one described in "Ailment List" when the *duo* becomes "constricted." An analogous condition is described in *Lingshu* 29, 6.la: "When above the navel (*ji* 臍) the skin is hot and it is hot inside the intestines, then (the feces) expelled are yellow like gruel; when below the navel the skin is cold and it is cold inside the stomach, then the abdomen becomes bloated." Further speculation in the absence of more certain evidence seems unwise.

[1]郤 in *MWD*, vol. 4, "Transcription," should be transcribed as 郄 (see *MSI*.A.1).

[2]The reference to the liver is intended to describe the path that the vessel takes and is not related to the correlation between internal organs and vessels as described in *Lingshu* 10. According to *Lingshu* 10, 3.4b, the foot Minor Yin vessel is associated with the kidney. *KGS*, vol. 1: 93, n. 43, argues that the reference to the liver should not be interpreted as meaning the internal organ itself, but rather a location on the surface of the body corresponding to the internal position of the liver. The argument is plausible since *MSI*.A-B generally specify external points on the body or points near the surface when describing the path of a vessel; further, they treat the vessels as a set of separate paths in the body that are neither interconnected nor connected to the internal organs.

[3]According to *SW*, 4B.24b, *qu* 胠 specifies the region of the side below the underarm, hence the translation "upper side."

[4]Ma Jixing argues that *nei* 内 in this phrase means the "inner surface" of the calf, not "in" the calf; and Ma adopts the same interpretation of *nei* at various points below (1992: 194, n. 2). I agree that in the descriptions of the vessel paths, which locate a vessel mainly by reference to external points, *nei* occurring by itself refers to the "inner surface"; e.g. *MSI*.A.6 ("the inner part of the thigh") and *MSI*.A.7 ("the inner part of the upper arm"). However, in the ailment lists I suspect that *nei* alone simply means "in."

edge of the spine; liver pain; heart pain; feverishness of the heart;[1] throat [4];[2] tongue splitting;[3] [1] exhaustion;[4] rising [vapor];[5] [2]; being continually parched;[6] coughing accompanied by muteness and a craving to sleep. (In all cases of)[7] ailing from these things, cauterize the foot Minor Yin vessel.

*MS*I.A.5 (CC16-18)

Foot Great Yin[8] vessel. It emerges at the inner edge of the big toe alongside the bone and emerges at the upper edge of the inner

---

[5]The term *fujie* 腹街 (abdomen crossroads) is not attested in received literature. Ma Jixing (1992: 194, n. 4) associates the term with *qijie* 氣街 (vapor crossroads), which has two meanings in medical literature. It is used to name four regions of the body where vapor collects in the process of being transported, one of which is the abdomen (see *Lingshu* 52, 8.7b). And it is the name of an acupuncture point on the groin (see *Lingshu* 10, 3.2a). In either meaning, the concept of *qijie* relies on medical theories that are absent from *MS*I.A-B. In my judgment the term cannot be used to interpret *fujie* in *MS*I.A.4.

[1]"Feverishness of the heart" translates *fanxin* 煩心, an ailment name that also occurs as *xinfan* (see *MS*I.A.7). In *MS*I.A.6, *MS*I.B.7, and *MS*I.B.8, *fanxin* is associated with incurable, fatal conditions in the vessels. Although *fanxin* occurs many times in the *Huangdi neijing*, I am not convinced that its meaning there is the same (see Ma Jixing 1992: 250, n. 2, for one definition). It should also be noted that there was an older concept of *fanxin* that did not rely on vessel theory. *Fan* itself refers to a burning, feverish pain that disturbs a person's mental and physical composure (Yu Yan 1972: 172). *Hanfeizi* 34, 13.247, uses *fanxin* to describe a condition of unbearable pain. And the Shuanggudui *Wanwu* includes a fragment concerning a drug that "stops *fanxin*" (Fuyang Han jian zhenglizu 1988: 36).

[2]I follow Ma Jixing in reading 洇 as *yan* 咽 (throat; 1992: 195, n. 9). *MS*I.B.9 includes throat-related ailments in the description of the foot Minor Yin vessel. The ailments following the lacuna contain more textual problems which may be resolved by referring to the text of *MS*I.B.9.

[3]I follow Ma Jixing in reading *lu/*glag* 輅 as a phonetic loan for *ce/*thrak* 坼 (1992: 195, n. 10). While the phonological evidence is arguable, the parallel in *MS*I.B.9 which reads *shece* 舌坼 (tongue splitting) is convincing.

[4]I follow Ma Jixing in reading *dan/*tan* 旦 as a phonetic loan for homophonic 癉 based on the parallel in *MS*I.B.9 (1992: 195, n. 11). *SW*, 7B.33b, glosses *dan* as an "exhaustion ailment." For discussion of *dan* as a type of exhaustion associated with hotness, see Yu Yan 1972: 144. Ma Jixing interprets the ailment differently (see *MS*I.B.9).

[5]I follow Ma Jixing in filling the lacuna with 氣 based on the parallel in *MS*I.B.9 (1992: 195, n. 12). The ailment concerns the contrary movement of vapor in the vessels (see *MS*I.B.1).

[6]*MWD*, vol. 4, "Transcription," reads 腸 as *he* 喝 (hoarse). I agree with Qiu Xigui that the graph should be read as *ke* 渴 (parched, thirsty; 1992: 529).

[7]*MWD*, vol. 4, "Transcription," emends the text by adding 諸. The emendation is unnecessary.

[8]陽 in *MWD*, vol. 4, "Transcription," is a printing error for 陰.

malleolus. It follows along[1] the inner edge of the shin, [1] the inner edge of the knee, and emerges at the inner edge of the thigh.

The ailments: ailing from the loss of function in the big toe; pain in the inner edge of the shin; pain in the thigh; abdomen pain; bloated abdomen; *fu* [1];[2] no craving to eat; a tendency to belch; heart [1];[3] a tendency for *zhou*.[4] In all cases of ailing from these things, cauterize the foot Great Yin vessel.

MSI.A.6 (CC19-24)

Foot Ceasing Yin vessel. It follows along in the big toe and, ascending, emerges at the inner edge of the shin. Eight *cun* up, it intersects the Great Yin vessel.[5] It [1] the inner part of the thigh and, ascending, enters in the *cuo*.[6]

The ailments: ailing from loss of flesh at the *cuo*; frequent urination; a craving to drink; swelling in the back of the foot; affliction with numbness.[7] In all cases of ailing from these things, cauterize the Ceasing Yin vessel.

In all cases of having these five ailments and in addition suffering feverishness of the heart, death occurs. When ailments of the three

---

[1]循 in *MWD*, vol. 4, "Transcription," should be transcribed as 揗; the meaning, however, is the same as other occurrences of *xun* 循 (follow along).

[2]Wei and Hu argue that *fu* 復 should be read as 腹 "abdomen" (1992, vol. 1: 10, n. 3). Even though the two previous occurrences of the word for "abdomen" are written with the usual graph, the reading is plausible.

[3]The ailment must be either "feverishness of the heart" or "heart pain."

[4]*MWD*, vol. 4, "Transcription," n. 1, suggests reading *zhou* 肘 as *zhou* 疛. The latter is glossed in *SW*, 7B.29a, as "ailment of the heart and abdomen." *Maishu*, "Ailment List," describes *zhou*, written with the graph 肘, as a type of "vapor conglomeration" (*qijia* 氣瘕): "As for *zhou*, when it arises from the spine and chest causing the abdomen to become bloated, and it is eased slightly when vapor (i.e. breath) is obtained—it is vapor conglomeration" (*MSSW*: 72). The reference to "obtaining vapor" suggests that the ailment is accompanied by shortness of breath.

[5]Based on the description of the foot Ceasing Yin vessel in *MSI*.B.8, the lower point of reference for the upward measurement of eight *cun* must be the inner malleolus.

[6]See *MSI*.A.3 on *cuo* and my conjecture that it refers to the navel. In *MSI*.B.8 the path of the foot Ceasing Yin vessel is said to pass from the lesser abdomen (located below the navel) upwards to the canthi. Although the identification of *cuo* remains speculative, reference to the navel in *MSI*.A.6 would be a logical counterpart to the lesser abdomen in *MSI*.B.8.

[7]"Numbness" translates *bi* 痹. *Maishu*, "Ailment List," describes *bi* as follows: "When it is located on the body, and (the person) is in a stunned state so when he is [1] he has no feeling—it is *bi*" (*MSSW*: 72). For further discussion of the association of *bi* with numbness, see Yu Yan 1972: 229-32.

Yin (vessels) create disorder,[1] death occurs within ten days. If when pressing a vessel it is like three men triply pounding,[2] death occurs within three days. When the vessels are severed for the time it takes to eat,[3] death occurs within three days. When there is feverishness of the heart and in addition bloating of the abdomen, death occurs. When unable to sleep and in addition suffering feverishness of the heart, death occurs. When muck and leaking slop continually come out, death occurs.[4] When ailments of the three Yin (vessels) are mixed with ailments of the Yang (vessels), it can be treated. As for ailments of the Yang (vessels), when the back seems to be streaming with hot water,[5] death occurs. In the case of Yang (vessel) ailments where bones are broken and muscles severed, yet there are not Yin (vessel) ailments, death does not occur.[6]

MSI.A.7 (CC25-26)

Forearm[7]

---

[1]I.e. the foot Minor Yin, Great Yin, and Ceasing Yin vessels.

[2]The phrase likens the abnormal, erratic pulse in a vessel to the pounding action of pestle in mortar when three people pound simultaneously. The phrase "like triply pounding" also occurs in *Suwen* 20, 6.10b, to describe an abnormal pulse.

[3]To say that the vessels are severed means that the pulse in the vessels ceases. The term *shiqing* 食頃 in Han texts refers to the amount of time required to consume a meal, not to simply swallow a mouthful of food. I do not know how many minutes a meal was supposed to last, and depending on the context the exact duration of *shiqing* seems to range from a few moments to a rather longer stretch of time. A passage in *Suwen* 63, 18.2a-3a, describes the length of time following acupuncture therapy before the patient recovers using four terms to indicate relative time: *li* 立 (immediately); *youqing* 有 頃 (some time); *shiqing*; and *xing shili qing* 行 十 里 頃 (the time it takes to travel ten *li*). By implication, "the time it takes to eat" is longer than "immediately" and "some time."

[4]"Muck and leaking slop" translates *tangxie* 溏 泄, referring to diarrhea-like conditions. *Tang* is glossed as "muck" in *Guangya*, 5A.5b. I translate the two words as two ailment names because of *Maishu*, "Ailment List," which describes two ailments, one *tangjia* 溏 瘕 (muck conglomeration) and the other *xie*: "When it is located in the intestines, is painful, nothing transforms, and slop leaks out (*xie*; here the word describes a symptom)—it is muck conglomeration"; "When immediately after eating (the food) is discharged—it is leaking slop" (*MSSW*: 72). It is also possible that *tangxie* is a single ailment name in *MSI*.A.6, since the compound occurs in *Suwen* 69, 20.3b; and in *Suwen* 74, 22.6b.

[5]I.e. a hot sweat.

[6]The Yang vessels are associated with heaven and external things, hence the association of external injuries with the Yang vessels. This idea is stated explicitly in *MSI*.D. However, in *MSI*.D broken bones and severed muscles are regarded as fatal in connection with Yang vessel ailments.

[7]*Bi* 臂 (forearm) is written in a raised position about one centimeter above the main text in C25. It serves as the heading for *MSI*.A.7-11. *Bi* can also refer to the entire arm. I adopt the narrower meaning because the vessel descriptions in *MSI*.A-B regularly use *bi* to spec-

Forearm Great Yin vessel. It follows along the upper edge of the muscle[1] and runs along the inner part of the upper arm.[2] It emerges at the inner edge of the underarm and goes to the heart.

The ailments: heart pain; feverishness of the heart with belching. In all cases of ailing from these things, cauterize the forearm Great Yin vessel.

MSI.A.8 (CC27–28)

Forearm Minor Yin vessel. It follows along the lower edge of the muscle[3] and emerges at the lower edge on the inner part of the upper arm. It emerges at the underarm and runs to the side.

The ailments: pain in the side. In all cases of ailing from (these)[4] things, cauterize the forearm Minor Yin vessel.

MSI.A.9 (CC29–30)

Forearm Great Yang vessel. It emerges at the little finger and follows along the lower edge of the bone.[5] It emerges at the lower edge of the upper arm, emerges at the outer edge of the shoulder, and emerges at the nape. It [3] outer canthus of the eye.

The ailments: pain in the outer edge of the forearm. In all cases of ailing from these things, cauterize the forearm Great Yang vessel.

MSI.A.10 (CC31–32)

Forearm Minor Yang vessel. It emerges at the middle finger, follows along the lower edge of the upper bone of the forearm,[6] and runs to the ear.

The ailments: the occurrence of deafness; [1] pain. In all cases of ailing from these things, cauterize the forearm Minor Yang vessel.

---

ify the forearm and another word for the upper arm. Each of the five forearm vessels occurs symmetrically on the left and right side, for a total of ten vessels.

[1]The muscle is the muscle of the forearm, and the reference to the upper edge is to the radius (or thumb) side of the forearm (see Ma Jixing 1992: 208, n. 2; and *KGS*, vol. 1: 97, n. 68).

[2]"Upper arm" translates *ru* 臑, which usually denotes the forequarter of an animal in Han sources (*SW*, 4B.24b). *Lingshu* 10, 3.1a, attests to medical usage denoting the arm from the elbow to the shoulder. *Zou* 湊 is well attested in received literature in the sense of *zou* 走 (run; see Ma Jixing 1992: 208, n. 3).

[3]The lower edge of the muscle is on the ulna (or little finger) side of the forearm (see Ma Jixing 1992: 210, n. 2; *KGS*, vol. 1: 97, n. 68).

[4]*MWD*, vol. 4, "Transcription," emends the text by adding the graph 此. The emendation is unnecessary.

[5]The bone must be the ulna.

[6]I.e. the lower edge of the radius.

MSI.A.11 (CC33-34)

Forearm Yang Brilliance vessel. It emerges in the middle finger, follows along the upper edge of the bone,[1] and emerges at the [2] of the upper arm. Ascending,[2] it runs to the *zhen*[3] and goes to the mouth.

The ailments: ailing from tooth pain; [4]. In all cases of ailing from these things, cauterize the forearm Yang Brilliance vessel.

In the above, the foot vessels are six; the hand vessels are five.

---

[1]I.e. the upper edge of the radius.
[2]*MWD*, vol. 4, "Transcription," places a comma after 上, connecting it to the preceding sentence. In this instance *shang* clearly has the meaning "ascend," and should be read as translated.
[3]See *MSI.A.2*.

MSI.B

YIN YANG SHIYI MAI JIUJING, JIABEN

陰陽十一脈灸經甲本

CAUTERIZATION CANON OF THE ELEVEN YIN AND YANG VESSELS, ED. A

MSI.B.1 (CC35-38)

Great Yang vessel. It is attached to the heel, in the outer malleolus. It emerges in the poples. Ascending, it bores the buttock, emerges in the hip joint,[1] and presses laterally on the spine. It emerges at the nape, ascends the corner of the head,[2] descends the center of the forehead, presses laterally on the bridge of the nose, and is attached to the inner edge of the eye.

When this (vessel) is moved, one ails from:[3] dashed head;[4] the eye is as if being torn; the nape is as if being axed; chest pain; the waist

---

[1]According to Wang Bing's commentary to *Suwen* 58, 15.7b, *yan* 厭—literally, "press down"—designates the space between the hip joint and the head of the femur. By analogy, the femur is likened to the pestle pressing on the hip-joint mortar.

[2]The term *toujiao* 頭角 (corner of the head) is not attested in received literature. *MWD*, vol. 4, "Transcription," n. 6, associates it with *ejiao* 額角, which is attested in *Lingshu* 13, 4.1b, where it refers to the boundary formed by the hairline along the side of the forehead.

[3]This phrase and the companion phrase "the ailments that it produces are" (see below) introduce separate lists of ailments for each vessel in *MSI*.B. Additionally, a count for the number of ailments in the second list is recorded at the end of each vessel description. A similar form of listing ailments occurs in *Lingshu* 10. Ma Jixing cites five different explanations of the two lists found in traditional medical commentaries, all of which assume that the two lists have a basis in etiological and nosological classification (1992: 221, n. 1). However, the explanations are based on a level of medical theory not yet in evidence in the Mawangdui medical manuscripts. My interpretation of the first ailment list in *MSI*.B is that *dong* 動 (move) connotes vascular disturbance arising from a contrary movement of vapor in the vessels, a condition also known as *jue* 厥 (reversal). Significantly, it is stated below that the ailments in the first list in *MSI*.B.1 "constitute heel reversal (*jue*)"; and five other vessel descriptions also attribute the ailments in the first list to "reversal" stemming from a part of the body with which the vessel is associated (*MSI*.B.2, which speaks of "Yang reversal," is an exception). *Shiming*, 8.255, gives a basic definition of *jue* which reflects ideas prior to the elaboration of *jue* in the *Huangdi neijing*: "*Jue* is when contrary vapor rises from below in a reverse direction and goes upward to enter the heart and side" (cf. Yu Yan 1972: 233). The idea that vapor (especially vapor entering the body through

is as if being snapped; the ham cannot rotate;[1] the upper side is as if knotted; the calf is as if being ripped. These constitute heel reversal.[2] For these (ailments), the Great Yang vessel controls the treatment.

The ailments that it produces are: head pain; ear deafness; nape pain; strain in the *qian*;[3] cold and hot syndrome;[4] back pain; waist

---

respiration or eating) should move downward, and that a reversal of that pattern causes illness is the central point of *MSI*.C (although the word *jue* does not occur in *MSI*.C). The first paragraph in *MSI*.C explains that maintaining warm feet and a cool head ensures that vapor, which moves in the direction of warmth, will move downward. This was evidently a fundamental teaching in early hygiene.

But if the first ailment list is to be associated with vascular disturbance, what is the essential difference between it and the second list which enumerates ailments that are "produced by the vessel," especially when many of the ailments are forms of pain occurring in both lists? I agree with Liao Yuqun (1989: 21) that the two lists are not based on specific etiological or nosological theories. However, I disagree with Liao when he argues that the first list belongs to the older, core text; and that the second list arose as a form of commentary expanding on the core text. For Liao, the notion of canonical text and appended commentary explains the fact that *Lingshu* 10 expands on the second list (often more than doubling the number of ailments) while leaving the first list relatively intact. I would attribute the existence of two lists to two kinds of concerns in early medicine. The first list may reflect a concept of the relation between the vessels and illness that arose in the context of early hygiene as documented in *Maishu* and *Yinshu* (Prolegomena, Section Three, "Physiology"). The prominence of *jue* "reversal" in the first list might also be explained as the influence of hygiene, since the idea of *jue* reflects early hygienic theory of how vapor should move in the vessels. In contrast, the second list appears to focus on medical diagnosis and treatment as practiced by physicians. I suspect that the reason for counting the number of ailments in the second list in *MSI*.B and for the expansion of the second list in *Lingshu* 10 is because it was in this category that vessels were associated with ailments for diagnostic purposes. It is also noteworthy that most ailments with technical names occur in the second list (the exception is *MSI*.B.8, which includes inguinal swelling and *shan* in the first list); and that references to medical prognosis and treatment form part of the second list in *MSI*.B.7-9. Thus, it is the second list that is comparable to the list of ailments in *MSI*.A, whose diagnostic/therapeutic nature is evident in the conclusion to each vessel description which states that the vessel in question is to be cauterized whenever one of the ailments occurs.

[4]Ma Jixing suggests that "dashed" (*chong* 冲) refers to vapor moving counter to the proper direction of flow and "dashing" against the head; i.e. that "dashed head" is a "reversal" ailment (1992: 222, n. 2).

[1]No doubt due to pain in the thigh and hip joint.

[2]*Maishu* writes *zhong* 踵 (heel). The graph in the corresponding position in the text of *MSI*.B.1 is fragmentary. Undoubtedly because the *Lingshu* 10, 3.4a, parallel writes *huai* 踝 (malleolus), *MWD*, vol. 4, "Transcription," writes the latter graph. On re-examination, the graph should be written 踵.

[3]*Qian/*dzjiəm* 潛 clearly represents an anatomical name, but I am unable to identify it. Ma Jixing argues that it is a phonetic loan for *zhen/*tjəm* 枕 (headrest), referring to the occipital bone (1992: 224, n. 3; cf. *MSI*.A.2). The parallel in *MSII*.B writes *er* 耳 (ear) in place of *qian*. As noted by Ma Jixing, *er* undoubtedly resulted from miswriting the graph 潛 as *er* 潛, which was then altered to 耳.

pain; buttock pain; hemorrhoids; pain in the upper side;[1] calf pain; numbness in the little toe—making twelve ailments.

*MS*I.B.2 (CC39–42)

Minor Yang vessel. It is attached to the front edge of the outer malleolus. Ascending, it emerges at the outer part of the fish-thigh[2] and emerges at the side. Ascending, it emerges at the front of the ear.

When this (vessel) is moved, one ails from: pain in the heart and side; inability to turn from side to side; when severe, lacking fat;[3] the foot turning outward. These constitute Yang reversal.[4] For these (ailments), the Minor Yang vessel controls the treatment.

The ailments that it produces are: [3] pain; nape pain; side pain; cold and hot syndrome; sweating; pain in all the joints; pain in the edge of the ham; pain in the fish-thigh; pain in the outer edge of the knee; shaking from coldness; numbness in the middle toe—making twelve ailments.

*MS*I.B.3 (CC43–47)

Yang Brilliance vessel. It is attached to the outer edge of the shinbone and ascends following along the shin. It bores the kneecap and emerges at the edge of the fish-thigh. Ascending, it bores the breast, bores the cheek, emerges at the outer edge of the eye, and circles the center of the forehead.

---

[4]*SW*, 7B.31a, defines *nue* 瘧 as "the ailment when cold (chill) and hot (fever) stop and start." According to *Maishu*, "Ailment List": "When the body is cold and hot, is parched, and the four limbs are painful—it is *nue*" (*MSSW*: 72). The name *nue* is also applied to malarial disease in early sources (Yu Yan 1972: 235).

[1]*Maishu* writes *qu* 胠 (upper side; n.b., 胘 in the *MSSW* transcription is a printing error). The graph in the corresponding position in the text of *MS*I.B.1 is fragmentary and is written *xi* 郤 (poples) in *MWD*, vol. 4, "Transcription." On re-examination, and also based on comparison with one occurrence of *qu* in C46 and one of *xi* in C62, the graph in *MS*I.B.l should be written 胠.

[2]The term *yugu* 魚股(fish-thigh) is not attested in received literature. However, there is evidence of anatomical names that liken parts of the body to the shape of a fish. For example, *Suwen* 41, 11.8a, refers to the calf as the "fish belly" (*yufu* 魚腹). *MWD*, vol. 4, "Transcription," n. 1, suggests that "fish-thigh" refers to the quadriceps of the thigh.

[3]The wording of the parallel at *Lingshu* 10, 3.6a, indicates that the lack of fat refers to the body's loss of moisture and fat. Perhaps the fat is literally cooked out of the body by the heat of "Yang reversal" in the vessel.

[4]The other "reversals" in *MS*I.B are named according to a part of the body associated with the vessel in question. Yang Shangshan's commentary to *Taisu*, 8.83, associates Yang reversal with morbific heat.

When this (vessel) is moved, one ails from: shivers and ailing from coldness; fondness for stretching;[1] continual yawning; blackness in the center of the forehead;[2] ailing from swelling; when severe,[3] detestation for people and fire; when hearing the sound of wood, panicked alarm;[4] panicky heart; the desire to close doors and windows and dwell in isolation; when the ailment is severe, the desire to mount high and sing, and to cast off clothing and run. These constitute shin reversal. For these (ailments), the Yang Brilliance vessel controls the treatment.

The ailments that it produces are: pain in the center of the forehead; stuffy nose; neck pain;[5] breast pain; calf pain;[6] pain in the heart and the upper side; swelling in the outer part of the abdomen; intestinal pain; knee rigidity;[7] numbness in the back of the foot—making ten ailments.

*MS*I.B.4 (CC48-49)

Shoulder vessel.[8] It arises behind the ear, descends the shoulder, and emerges at the inner edge of the elbow.[9] It emerges at [3],[10] and mounts the back of the hand.

---

[1]It is evident from the *Maishu* text and from *MS*II.B that the word in the text of *MS*I.B.3 should be *shen* 伸 (stretch) and not *long* 龍 (dragon). *MWD*, vol. 4, "Transcription," n. 5, argues that the original graph was probably 申, and speculates on how the graph 龍 came to be written in the text.

[2]Yang Shangshan's commentary to *Taisu*, 8.74, explains the blackness as the presence of Yin vapor.

[3]I follow Yang Shangshan's gloss of *zhi* 至 as "severe" in the commentary to *Taisu*, 8.74. Ma Jixing interprets *zhi* to mean "when (an ailment) arises" (1992: 234, n. 7).

[4]Yang Shangshan's commentary to *Taisu*, 8.74, explains the antipathy for fire and wood in terms of Five Agent theory. Since there is no evidence of Five Agent theory in *MS*I.B, these antipathies have some other basis.

[5]The text writes *ling* 領 (neck). According to *MWD*, vol. 4, "Transcription," this is a scribal error for *han* 頜 (jaw). The apparent reason for emending *ling* is the occurrence of *ling* in *MS*I.B.4, where the parallel in *Lingshu* 10, 3.3b, writes *han*. However, *MS*I.B, *MS*II.B, and *Maishu* consistently write *ling*. Given that the meaning "neck" fits in each context, I do not accept the proposed emendation.

[6]For identification of *qi* 胻 as a name for the calf, see *Guangya*, 6B.9b. In *MS*I.B.3 there is a lacuna in the text extending from "neck" above to "heart" below. The five graphs added from *Maishu* easily fit the space left by the lacuna.

[7]"Rigidity" translates *tiao* 跳, which according to *SW*, 2B.28a, refers to stiffness in the leg joints that causes stumbling.

[8]The shoulder vessel corresponds to the forearm Great Yang vessel in *MS*I.A.

[9]*Maishu* writes *zhou* 肘 (elbow). The graph in the corresponding position in the text of *MS*I.B.4 is fragmentary and is written *ru* 臑 (upper arm) in *MWD*, vol. 4, "Transcription." On re-examination, and comparing the graph to one occurrence of *zhou* in C52, the graph in *MS*I.B.4 should be written 肘. Similarly, the graph following *zhou* is illegible and I

When this (vessel) is moved, one ails from: swelling and pain in the neck; inability to look back; the shoulder is as if being torn; the upper arm is as if being snapped. For these (ailments), the shoulder vessel controls the treatment.

The ailments that it produces are: neck pain; throat numbness; shoulder pain; pain in the outer part of the elbow—making four ailments.

MSI.B.5 (CC50-51)

Ear vessel.[1] It arises at the back of the hand and emerges at the outer part of the forearm between the two bones, at the lower edge of the upper bone.[2] It emerges at the elbow and enters the ear.

When this (vessel) is moved, one ails from: ear deafness with blurring; swelling in the throat. For these (ailments), the ear vessel controls the treatment.

The ailments that it produces are: pain in the outer canthus of the eye; cheek pain; ear deafness—making three ailments.

MSI.B.6 (CC52-53)

Tooth vessel.[3] It arises at the index finger and thumb, emerges at the upper edge of the forearm, enters the elbow, and mounts the upper arm. It bores the cheek, enters the teeth, and presses laterally on the nose.

When this (vessel) is moved, one ails from: tooth pain; cheekbone swelling.[4] For these (ailments), the tooth vessel controls the treatment.

---

follow the *Maishu* text which writes *nei* 内 (inner). The text of *MSII*.B.4 appears to be different since it writes *wai* 外 (outer; the graph is fragmentary and there is a lacuna above it).

[10]At this point the *Maishu* text writes four graphs 臂外捥上 "the outer part of the forearm by the wrist." There is not space for four graphs in the lacuna in *MSI*.B.4 (C48); and at the same time, I am unable to determine a plausible abbreviation of the four graphs in *Maishu*. Two possibilities occur to me. Perhaps the restored silk of *MSI* as shown in the plate is inaccurate and the lacuna in C48 is larger than it appears to be; or perhaps the fourth graph was omitted from the text due to scribal error and must be added to the three graphs that fit the lacuna. I am unable to prove either possibility, and it is equally likely that the text of *MSI*.B.4 is simply different.

[1]The ear vessel corresponds to the forearm Minor Yang vessel in *MSI*.A.

[2]The upper bone is the radius.

[3]The tooth vessel corresponds to the forearm Yang Brilliance vessel in *MSI*.A.

[4]*Zhuo* 䪼 refers to the cheekbone (*SW*, 9A.10b), and to the space above the cheekbone and below the eye.

The ailments that it produces are: tooth pain; cheekbone swelling; yellowing of the eye; dry mouth; upper arm pain—making five ailments.

*MS*I.B.7 (CC54-57)

Great Yin vessel. This is the stomach vessel.[1] It goes alongside the stomach,[2] emerges at the lower edge of the Yin part of the fish-thigh[3] and at the upper edge of the calf, and emerges at the upper edge of the inner malleolus.

When this (vessel) is moved, one ails from: (vapor) ascending [1] and racing to the heart;[4] bloated abdomen; a tendency to belch; wanting to vomit after eating—when able to defecate and pass vapor[5] there is welcome relief. For these (ailments), the Great Yin vessel controls the treatment.

The ailments that it produces are: feverishness of the heart by itself—death occurs; heart pain and bloated abdomen—death occurs; inability to eat, inability to sleep, and strained yawning—when the three are combined, death occurs; muck and leaking slop—death occurs; water and blockage—when combined, death occurs[6]—making ten ailments.

---

[1]The identification of the foot Great Yin vessel with the stomach is unrelated to the correlation between vessels and organs in *Lingshu* 10.

[2]"Go alongside" translates *pi* 披, which represents my reading of *bi* 彼 in the original text. For attestation of *pi* in the sense of "go alongside," see *Shiji*, 1.4b and 1.28a. *MWD*, vol. 4, "Transcription," n. 2, reads 彼 as *bei* 被, glossed as "cover over." The phrase in *MS*I.B.7 begins the description of the path of the vessel, and the meaning "cover the stomach" does not fit the context well. In addition, *Lingshu* 10, 3.6b, describes the foot Ceasing Yin vessel as "pressing laterally on the stomach," which lends support to reading the phrase in *MS*I.B.7 as translated.

[3]Yin and Yang are used to refer to positions on the exterior of the body, corresponding to inner and outer respectively.

[4]The ailment name is composed of four graphs 上 [1] 走 心, with one graph missing in the lacuna at the bottom of C54. Perhaps the lacuna is *dang* 當, which appears in the corresponding position in *MS*II.B. The *Maishu* text writes 上 走 心. I concur with *MWD*, vol. 4, "Transcription," n. 4, that the ailment is a reversal ailment where vapor harms the heart by moving in a contrary direction.

[5]I.e. intestinal gas.

[6]Both "blockage" (*bi* 閉) and "water" (*shui* 水) are included in *Maishu*, "Ailment List," the former referring to not being able to urinate and the latter to abdominal bloating: "When it is located at the forbidden spot (i.e. the genitals) and one is unable to urinate—it is blockage"; "When the abdomen is full while the body, face, feet, and legs all diminish—it is water" (*MSSW*: 72). For discussion of the two ailments in later medical literature, see Ma Jixing 1992: 250, n. 8.

MSI.B.8 (CC58-61)

Ceasing Yin vessel. It is attached to the clump of hair on the big toe. It mounts the upper edge of the back of the foot, one *cun* away from the inner malleolus. It rises five *cun* above the malleolus and emerges behind the Great Yin (vessel).[1] Ascending, it emerges at the inner edge of the fish-thigh, encounters the lesser abdomen, and presses laterally[2] on the canthi.

When this (vessel) is moved, one ails from: in men, inguinal swelling[3] and *shan*;[4] in women, swelling in the lesser abdomen; waist pain; inability to raise the head skyward; when severe, the throat is dry; facial blemish. For these (ailments), the Ceasing Yin vessel controls the treatment.

The ailments that it produces are: internal hotness; urine retention;[5] inguinal swelling; *pian*; *shan*[6]—making five ailments. If in

---

[1]The phrase "emerges behind the Great Yin (vessel)" is lost in the lacuna at the bottom of C58, and there is also a lacuna in the corresponding position in *Maishu*. Although there is only space for five graphs at the bottom of C58, I fill the lacuna with the six graph phrase from *MSII*.B since either one of the two grammatical particles in this phrase (於, 之) can be omitted without affecting the meaning.

[2]*Maishu* writes *jia* 夾 (press laterally). *MWD*, vol. 4, "Transcription," writes *da* 大 in the corresponding position in *MSI*.B.8. On re-examination, and comparing it to *jia* 夾 in C62, the graph in *MSI*.B.8 should be written 夾.

[3]For *tui* 癩 (inguinal swelling), see *MSI*.E.118.

[4]*Shan* 疝 is applied to several morbid conditions characterized by pain and swelling in the region of the heart and abdomen, and sometimes is treated synonymously with *tui*. Various meanings of *shan* are discussed in Ma Jixing 1992: 253, n. 2; and Yu Yan 1972: 218-20, 225.

[5]For *long* 癃 (urine retention), see *MSI*.E.88.

[6]The last two ailment names pose a problem that is not easily resolved. They can be plausibly read as a single ailment name, *pianshan* 偏 疝 (see below); but if they are read thus, there are only four ailments instead of the five stated in the text. Of course, the number five is only extant in *Maishu* (there are lacunae in *MSI*.B.8 and *MSII*.B in the corresponding position), and we might feel justified in emending the text to read "four" on the presumption that *Maishu* is in error. This solution seems unacceptable because of *MSI*.A.6 which lists five ailments for the foot Ceasing Yin vessel and also describes the fatal prognosis when these ailments occur together with feverishness of the heart, providing a clear parallel to *MSI*.B.8. To be sure, the ailments listed are not identical, but the number five undoubtedly has a significance of its own. Ma Jixing resolves the problem by reading *pianshan* together and speculating that the fifth ailment name has been omitted in *MSI*.B.8 as well as in the corresponding position in *MSII*.B and *Maishu* (1992: 255). My approach to the problem is to read the text as written and to treat *pian* and *shan* as two ailments. *Shan* already appears in the first ailment list above. *Pian* is attested in *Xunzi* 5, 3.47, referring to hemiplegia, usually written *pianku* 偏 枯 (withering on one side). *Lingshu* 23, 5.4b, describes *pianku* as follows: "The body is useless on one side and is painful. Speech is not altered and the will is not disordered."

addition to these five ailments there is feverishness of the heart, death occurs—there is no treating it. If there are Yang vessels with ailments at the same time, it can be treated.

MSI.B.9 (CC62-66)

Minor Yin vessel. It is attached to the outer edge of the inner malleolus, bores the calf, and emerges at the center of the poples. Ascending, it bores the inner edge of the spine, is attached to the kidney,[1] and presses laterally on the tongue.

When this (vessel) is moved, one ails from: hoarse panting; when rising from a sitting position the eyes become clouded as if sightless; the heart is as if suspended; ailing from hunger; insufficiency of vapor;[2] a tendency to become angry; panicky heart with the fear that one is about to be seized by someone; no desire to eat; the face is moldy black[3] like the color of lampblack; when coughing, there is blood. These constitute bone reversal. For these (ailments) the Minor Yin vessel controls the treatment.[4]

Despite my skepticism of reading *pianshan* as a single ailment in *MSI*.B.8, the alternative merits careful consideration since the usage is attested in the *Huangdi neijing*; however, the first graph of the name has been altered in the received text. In the second ailment list of the foot Ceasing Yin vessel in *Lingshu* 10, 3.6b, the ailment *hushan* 狐疝 (fox *shan*) occurs. Akahori argues that the *Lingshu hu* 狐 is a corruption of *MSI*.B.8 *pian* 偏 (1989: 21). The Yang Shangshan commentary in *Taisu*, 8.84, explains the ailment as follows: "The fox cannot urinate at night and is first able to do it at dawn. The human ailment resembles the fox. The list (in the description of the foot Ceasing Yin vessel) reads *hushan*; and there are editions that write *tuishan* 㿗疝. It refers to the ailment *piantui* 偏㿗." The name *hushan* also occurs in *Lingshu* 47, 7.9a; 49, 8.4b; and in *Suwen* 64, 18.7a. And in medical literature after the *Huangdi neijing*, "fox *shan*" continues to be described as a distinctive type of *shan* ailment associated with inguinal hernias (Yu Yan 1972: 228-29). Yang Shangshan's commentary is significant because it documents the name *piantui* "inguinal swelling on one side" when identifying "fox *shan*." Evidently even after *hu* "fox" replaced *pian* "on one side" in the name of the ailment—and the fox was introduced into its etiology—the identification of the ailment as a form of asymmetrical "inguinal swelling" was still understood.

[1]The kidney happens to be the organ correlated with the foot Minor Yin vessel in *Lingshu* 10. While reference to the kidney in *MSI*.B.9 may have some bearing on the later vessel-organ correlations, it cannot be interpreted as evidence of such correlations in *MSI*.B.

[2]The ailment may refer to a general shortage of vapor in the body and its vessels as well as to shortness of breath. *Taisu*, 8.79, connects this ailment to the next one, which is fear rather than anger: "When there is insufficiency of vapor, there is a tendency to become frightened." According to the Yang Shangshan commentary, the "insufficiency" is of the vapor in the foot Minor Yin vessel.

[3]"Moldy black" translates *yan* 黬, defined in *SW*, 10A.59a, as the "deep black of (molded) fruit."

[4]*Zhi* 治 (treatment) is not written in the text and should be regarded as a case of scribal omission.

The ailments that it produces are: hotness in the mouth; tongue splitting; throat dryness; rising vapor;[1] choking; pain in the throat; exhaustion;[2] a craving to sleep; coughing; mutism—making ten ailments. When cauterizing the Minor Yin vessel, eat raw meat heartily, leave the belt loose and the hair unbound, and walk with a large stick wearing heavy shoes. The moment the cauterization is finished the ailment will desist.

MSI.B.10 (CC67-69)

Forearm Great Yin vessel. It is situated in the palm of the hand and emerges at the inner Yin part (of the forearm)[3] between the two bones, at the lower edge of the upper bone above the muscle.[4] It emerges at the inner Yin part of the arm[5] and enters the heart.

When this (vessel) is moved, one ails from: heart pain with throbbing;[6] pain in the broken basin;[7] when severe, one is shaking with both hands clasped.[8] These constitute forearm reversal. For these (ailments) the forearm Great Yin vessel controls the treatment.

---

[1]I.e. a "reversal" of the movement of vapor in the vessels.

[2]"Exhaustion" translates *dan* 癉 (see *MSI*.A.4). The second ailment list in *Lingshu* 10, 3.4b, has the ailment *huangdan* 黃疸 (yellow *dan*; i.e. jaundice) instead. Ma Jixing argues that because received medical literature generally associates the foot Minor Yin vessel with jaundice the ailment in *MSI*.B.9 should be understood as jaundice rather than as exhaustion (1992: 264, n. 7). In received literature the use of *dan* 癉 and homophonous *dan* 疸 is confused (see *SW*, 7B.33b, and Duan Yucai commentary), so Ma's interpretation is plausible.

[3]The forearm must be understood here (the word for forearm is written in *Maishu*). Inner and Yin are synonymous, both referring to the inner surface of the forearm.

[4]The upper bone is the radius.

[5]*Bi* 臂, which in all other occurrences in *MSI*.A-B refers to the forearm, is suspect. Although *bi* can refer to the arm in general, which is how I have translated it here, it is likely that *bi* is an error for *ru* 臑 (upper arm). There is a lacuna in the corresponding position in *Maishu*, while *MSII*.B also writes *bi*. The best evidence for scribal error is the description of the path of the forearm Minor Yin vessel in *MSI*.B.11 which is similar to *MSI*.B.10, and which specifies the upper arm at this point.

[6]*Pangpang* 滂滂 is a descriptive compound that suggests the quality of surging water (*Guangya*, 6A.10b). The corresponding position in *MSII*.B uses the same compound, but in *Maishu* the compound is *pengpeng* 彭彭. *SW*, 5A.34a, glosses *peng* as the "sound of drumming."

[7]I.e. the clavicle.

[8]Even clasping one's hands cannot suppress the excruciating pain.

The ailments that it produces are: chest pain; pain in stomach sack;[1] heart pain;[2] pain in the four extremities; conglomeration[3]—making five ailments.

*MS*I.B.11 (CC70-71)

Forearm Minor Yin vessel. It arises in between the two bones of the forearm and goes along the upper edge of the lower bone below the muscle.[4] It emerges at the inner Yin of the upper arm and enters the heart.[5]

When this (vessel) is moved, one ails from: heart pain; parched throat with the desire to drink. These constitute forearm reversal. For these (ailments) the forearm Minor Yin vessel controls the treatment.

The ailments that it produces are: side pain—making one ailment.

[1]瘱 is not attested in received literature (the same graph appears in the corresponding position in *MS*II.B). I follow *MWD*, vol. 4, "Transcription," in reading the graph as *wan* 脘, for which the variant graph 腕 also occurs. *Wan* refers to the stomach in its capacity as the receptacle for food (see *Suwen* 33, 9.10b, which attributes the inability to get food to go down to blockage in the "stomach sack"). *Maishu* writes *qi* 脊 (calf). While the inclusion of "pain in the four extremities" just below in the second ailment list increases the plausibility of *qi*, I suspect that *wan* is the better reading.

[2]I follow the emendation in *MWD*, vol. 4, "Transcription," which adds *xintong* 心痛 (heart pain) to the text. The ailment is included in *Maishu* and *MS*II.B. It is a clear case of scribal omission since the text only names four ailments and yet gives a final count of five ailments.

[3]"Conglomeration" translates *jia* 瘕. *Jia* refers to a variety of growths or internal blockages that occur primarily in the abdomen and intestines (Yu Yan 1972: 129). *Maishu*, "Ailment List," gives the names of the following types: male conglomeration (intestinal), blood conglomeration (intestinal), vapor conglomeration (abdominal), fat conglomeration (abdominal), feces conglomeration, and muck conglomeration (*MSSW*: 72).

[4]The lower bone is the ulna.

[5]Both *Maishu* and *MS*II.B conclude the description of the vessel path with the phrase 入心中 "enters the heart." In *MS*I.B.11 there is a lacuna at the bottom of C70 that begins where this phrase should be and extends into the beginning of the next paragraph. I differ with *MWD*, vol. 4, "Transcription," which omits this phrase and adds only the subsequent five graphs to fill the lacuna. According to my calculations there is sufficient space to add all eight graphs as written in the corresponding positions in *Maishu* and *MS*II.B.

*MS*I.C

MAIFA

脈法

MODEL OF THE VESSELS

*MS*I.C (CC72-83)

May the model of the vessels be clearly taught to those below.[1] The vessels are also something the sage prizes. As for vapor, it goes to the lower part (of the body) and harms the upper part;[2] it follows warmth and departs from coolness. The sage has a cold head and warm feet.[3] To treat ailments, take away the surplus and increase

---

[1]This sentence is not included in *Maishu*. The term *maifa* 脈 法 (model of the vessels) refers to the physiological theory of the vessels and its medical application as well as to a genre of medical literature. Both meanings occur in the *Shiji* account of Chunyu Yi. Beginning with the first of Chunyu Yi's medical case histories, at *Shiji*, 105.9b, Chunyu Yi regularly quotes from a *Model of the Vessels* to provide theoretical support for his diagnoses. And at *Shiji*, 105.21b, Chunyu Yi refers to the "model of the vessels" as the invention of ancient sages for the purpose of elucidating the structure of the body and classifying the ailments that affect it. See also, *Suwen* 4, 1.15b, which concludes a discussion of the effects of the seasons on the body and its ailments with the statement, "this is the model of the vessels for the average person"; and *Suwen* 67, 19.9b, which quotes from a work entitled *Model of the Vessels* to demonstrate an argument.

[2]"Goes to the lower part" translates *dao xia* 到 下. The corresponding position in *Maishu* writes *li xia* 利 下 (benefits the lower part). Since "benefit" is the standard antonym of "harm," it is tempting to emend *dao* in *MS*I.C. I hesitate to make the emendation for several reasons. *Dao* is grammatically acceptable and to reject it solely because it does not form the standard antonym pair is incautious. In addition, *dao* does express the contrast between where the vapor should go and the harm it causes if it ascends instead. Given other instances where *Maishu* adds rhetorical words and rewords difficult phrases, it is possible that an earlier *dao* was altered to *li*.

[3]This observation on the physiology of the sage concludes the brief paean to the theory of the vessels, and *MS*I.C next shifts to a discussion of how to apply vessel theory to treating ailments. The image of the sage, whose warm feet ensure that vapor is drawn downward, is related to Warring States ideas about macrobiotic hygiene. Similar ideas occur in the Warring States jade inscription on circulating vapor, in which downward movement is the key (see Prolegomena, Section Four, "Techniques"). The sage's warm feet also call to mind the passage in *Zhuangzi* 6, 103, which speaks of the "perfected man of antiquity" who "breathes with the heels." Both the warm feet theory of *MS*I.C and the *Zhuangzi*'s "heel-breathing" have their origins in forms of breath cultivation designed to circulate vapor by generating warmth in the lower limbs.

what is insufficient.[1] When vapor ascends and does not descend, discern which vessel has excess and cauterize it at the ring.[2] If the ailment is severe, go up two *cun* above the ring and perform an additional cauterization.[3] If vapor emerges, lance the vessels at the poples and elbow with a lancing-stone.[4]

The idea of a cold head to balance the warm feet in *MSI.*C differs from *Huangdi neijing* passages that refer to the face as able to withstand coldness because it is the place where all Yang vessels meet. See Ma Jixing 1992: 281, for relevant citations; and Unschuld 1986b: 446, for a translation of the *Nanjing* passage concerning the face (Ma's interpretation of *MSI.*C based on the *Huangdi neijing* misses the significance of the idealized physiology of the sage described in *MSI.*C).

[1]The principle of treating ailments by restoring equilibrium in the vessels is standard in the *Huangdi neijing*. For example, *Suwen* 60, 16.la, states that, "to regulate the Yin and Yang, replenish when there is insufficiency and drain when there is surplus." The same principle also existed in ancient macrobiotic hygiene as attested in the *Maishu*, "Care of the Body," passage which states that, "when the vessels are brimful, drain them; when empty, fill them; when still, stay in attendance on them" (*MSSW*: 74).

[2]*Suwen* 80, 24.5b, discusses "having surplus" and "vapor ascending and not descending" as aspects of the morbid condition of *jue* 厥 (reversal). In my judgment, the condition described in *MSI.*C is comparable to the reversal ailments of *MSI.*B (see *MSI.*B.1). The part concerning cauterization is more problematic—especially the interpretation of the word *huan* 環, which I translate as "ring." The grammar of the phrase "cauterize it at the ring" 當環而灸之 is parallel to the phrase below, "lance the vessels at the poples and elbow with a lancing-stone" 郄與肘之脈而砭之; and I am convinced that the best explanation of the two occurrences of *huan* in *MSI.*C is to treat the word as a noun for a part of the anatomy. Ma Jixing cites the acupuncture point named *huangu* 環谷 located in the navel and suggests that *huan* in *MSI.*C refers to the navel region (1980: 23). My own speculation is that *huan* "ring" refers to the waist (*yao* 要). A related term in *MSVI.*B.1, *zhouhuan* 周環 (encircling ring), I also identify as the waist. Although this usage is unattested in received literature, the idea of the waist as the central ring around the body is well documented. *SW*, 3A.39b, glosses *yao* "waist" as the "middle of the body," and explains the graph as a depiction of a person clasping both hands around the waist. The *Huangdi neijing* acknowledges the importance of the waist for vessel theory by including a special vessel that rings the waist even with the navel called the *daimai* 帶脈 (belt vessel). Its nature and function differ from the twelve Yin and Yang vessels of the hands and feet (cf. Unschuld 1986b: 322), yet *Suwen* 44, 12.10a, states that the Yin and Yang vessels "belong to the belt vessel" 屬於帶脈. The idea in *MSI.*C is to correct the ascending vapor in the vessels by cauterizing a central point on the body that might induce the vapor to re-descend (since vapor "follows warmth"). Even though one is supposed to determine which vessel "has excess," I doubt that cauterization was performed at discrete places around the waist corresponding to the path of each vessel (impossible in any case for the hand vessels). The treatment appears to be relatively simple and unrelated to the vessel theory and therapy found in the *Huangdi neijing*. Ma Jixing (1992: 282–83) rejects his earlier identification of *huan* as an anatomical term in favor of a more theoretically elaborate interpretation of *MSI.*C. His new understanding of *huan* is grammatically implausible, and I am skeptical of his general interpretation.

[3]Presumably when the reversal ailment is severe, a single cauterization at the waist is insufficient to induce the vapor to descend and a second cauterization must be performed

The use of the lancing-stone to open vessels must conform to the plan. When an abscess or swelling has pus, gauge its size and then lance it. When lancing there are four harms.[1] When the pus is deep and lancing is shallow, it is called "not reaching"—the first harm. When the pus is shallow and the lancing is deep, it is called "exceeding"—the second harm. When the pus is large and the lancing-stone is small, it is called "seeping"; when seeping occurs, the pollution is not eliminated—the third harm.[2] When the pus is

---

higher on the body than the first. I interpret *yang* 陽 in the sense of "rise, go up," not as a reference to Yang.

[4]For the phrase 氣 出 "if vapor emerges," the corresponding position in *Maishu* writes 氣 一 上 一 下 "if vapor now ascends and now descends." I suspect that the latter version is a paraphrase of the former. The grammatical use of *yi* 一 in the sense of "either/or" or "now/now" when referring to an unstable physiological condition is attested in *Suwen* 62, 17.4a: "Blood and vapor leave their abodes, *now full and now empty*. Blood bonds to Yin and vapor bonds to Yang, thus causing panicky wildness." For "vapor to emerge" or "vapor to now ascend and now descend" appears to designate the most severe form of the reversal ailment, one where treatment with cauterization is inadequate. Perhaps the ailment is similar to the ailment suffered by the Prince of Guo 虢 太 子 as described in *Shiji*, 105.3b-6a. According to the account, the palace experts believe that he has died of "violent reversal" (*baojue* 暴 蹷): "The Prince was ailing from blood and vapor being untimely so that they crossed one another and could not be drained. When it violently erupted to the outside, this caused internal harm. The essence and spirit were unable to stop the evil vapor so that the evil vapor accumulated and could not be drained. Therefore Yang was slack while Yin was tense. Thus he experienced violent reversal and died." While Bian Que's diagnosis is that the Prince's ailment is "corpse reversal" (*shijue* 尸 蹷) and that the patient is still alive, his description of the ailment continues to focus on disorder among the vessels: "The Yang vessels plummet downward and the Yin vessels fight upward. The converging vapor is blocked and does not pass through." It is plausible to interpret "vapor emerging" in *MSI*.C as related to the "violent eruption which caused internal harm" in the *Shiji* account, the idea being that a morbid condition (perhaps vapor that ascends and descends) makes it impossible for vapor to flow normally and that even cauterization does not prevent it from erupting. Under these circumstances *MSI*.C introduces the use of the lancing-stone (*bian* 砭, more often written 砭) to cut open vessels at the poples and elbow and allow the vapor to drain.

SW, 9B.32a, defines *bian* as a verb meaning "lance an ailment with a stone"; and the word is used both as a verb and a noun in *MSI*.C. *MSI*.C and the single occurrence of *bian* in *MSI*.E.135 confirm pre-Han and Han sources that describe the use of sharpened stones to drain pus from abscesses and to relieve pressure in swellings. The significance of the lancing-stone in *MSI*.C in connection with the transition from cauterization to acupuncture is discussed in the Prolegomena, Section Three, "Therapy."

[1]See the Prolegomena, Section Three, "Therapy," for discussion of a *Lingshu* parallel to this account of draining pus with the lancing-stone, which speaks instead of acupuncture needles.

[2]"Seeping" translates *lan* 濫, which is listed among words meaning *zi* 漬 (soak) in *Guangya*, 2B.7a. The third and fourth harms concern the choice of a lancing-stone, which depends on the amount of pus to be drained: large lancing-stones for large amounts of pus and small

small and the lancing-stone is large, it is called "overflow"; when overflow occurs, good flesh is injured—the fourth harm. When pus is abundant and deep, the top is black and large. When pus is slight and deep, the top is black and small. When pus is abundant and shallow, the top is white and large. When pus is slight and shallow, the top is white and small. It is imperative to investigate this. When there is pus, cauterization cannot be used.[1]

The way to examine the vessels. Place the left [hand five *cun* up from the malleolus] and press on it.[2] Place the right hand at the malleolus and palpate it.[3] If other vessels are full and this one alone

---

lancing-stones for small amounts. If the lancing-stone is too small for the amount of pus, the undrained pus "seeps" and the abscess continues to fester.

[1]Due to the fragmentary condition of the silk, *MWD*, vol. 4, "Transcription," errs in identifying a single column in this part of the text as two columns (CC79-80). *Maishu* permits correction of the error ("Transcription," n. 4 states that CC79-80 may be a single column). The error is corrected in my transcription. In *MWD*, vol. 4, "Transcription," C81 should be renumbered C80 and so forth to the end of the numbering sequence with C88 in *MSI*.D, which should be renumbered C87.

[2]The bracketed words represent lacunae in both *MSI*.C and *Maishu* that have been filled in accordance with the emendation proposed by Ma Jixing, who adds the graphs 手 上 去 踝 五 寸 from a parallel passage in *Taisu*, 14.185 (1992: 292, n. 2). Textual parallels also occur in *Suwen* 20, 6.11a; and *Zhenjiu jiayi jing*, 4.27a. The lacuna in *MSI*.C has sufficient space for the six graphs. *MWD*, vol. 4, "Transcription," and the new transcription of *MSI*.C appended to *MSSW*: 74, do not include this emendation; but both transcribe two graphs 走 而 at the end of the lacuna, which conflict with the proposed emendation. On re-examination, I find that 而 is in fact the top of 案 (*an* "press") below. As for 走, I am unable to discern the graph written in the text.

[3]"Palpate" translates *tan* 撢, glossed with *tan* 探 in *SW*, 12A.44b. While the primary meaning of both words is "search out," they are also used to refer to grasping something and feeling it with the hand (*Erya*, 2.10b, and commentary). The parallels in *Taisu*, *Suwen*, and *Zhenjiu jiayi jing* all write *dan* 彈 (strike), meaning that the right hand should strike the malleolus with a tapping motion. Ma Jixing argues convincingly that *tan* "palpate" is the best reading (1992: 108).

MSI.C and the parallels in received medical literature present a paradigm of vessel diagnosis, but none specify which vessel is being diagnosed. According to the Yang Shangshan commentary in *Taisu*, 14.185, the vessel is the foot Great Yin vessel because it emerges at the upper part of the inner malleolus and then intersects the foot Ceasing Yin vessel eight *cun* above the malleolus. The diagnostic technique as described in the *Taisu* text and explained by Yang Shangshan entails tapping the vessel at the malleolus with the right hand while the left hand feels for a response up above. It is likely that *MSI*.C also understands the foot Great Yin vessel as the one being diagnosed. According to *MSI*.B.7, the path of the foot Great Yin vessel descends from the stomach and ends at the "upper edge of the inner malleolus"; and in *MSI*.B.8, the foot Ceasing Yin vessel "rises five *cun* above the malleolus and emerges behind the Great Yin vessel." Thus in *MSI*.C, the left hand is pressing precisely at the intersection of the Great Yin and Ceasing Yin vessels while the right hand is probably palpating the Great Yin vessel at the malleolus. The similarity be-is empty, it controls the ailment. If other vessels flow evenly[1] and this one alone is blocked,[2] it controls the ailment. If other vessels are still and this one alone is moved, it controls the ailment. Now, the vessels that have constant movement are the Minor Yin of the shin and the Great Yin and Minor Yin of the forearm. These (vessels) normally have movement;[3] and when it is rapid, ailments occur. These provide the basis for deciding when there is excess in the vessels. For the remainder, carefully discern the excess in the corresponding vessel.[4] The vessel connections[5]—let it be written and

---

tween *MSI*.C and received medical literature ends here. In the sentences below, *MSI*.C judges the condition of the vessel by comparing the vessel being diagnosed—called "this one" (*ci* 此)—to "other vessels" (*tuo mai* 它 脈), whereas received medical literature looks at the response within the vessel being diagnosed. Ma Jixing interprets *mai* in the sense of the "pulse" in the vessel and argues that *tuo mai* refers to the "other pulse," meaning the pulse where the right hand is positioned, while "this one" refers to the pulse where the left hand is positioned (1992: 295, nn. 1-2). Thus he argues that the diagnostic technique is basically similar to the received medical literature. Even if one accepts the identification of *mai* as the pulse (which is unlikely here, and occurs nowhere else in the Mawangdui medical manuscripts), the grammar of *tuo mai* and *ci* requires considerable forcing to produce Ma's interpretation. I think it best to simply acknowledge that the diagnostic technique described in *MSI*.C is different.

1 "Flow evenly" translates *gu/*kwət* 汩, glossed in *SW*, 11A-2.43a as "well-ordered water." The corresponding position in *Maishu* writes *gu/*kwət* 滑 (smooth).

2 "Blocked" translates *shuai/*sljət* 率, glossed in *SW*, 13A.40b as a "bird-catching net" (the graph is explained as a depiction of a net on a pole). This meaning is not attested outside of the *SW*, and my speculation that it may have the extended meaning of "block" is tentative (most occurrences of *shuai* borrow the graph to represent a word meaning "lead" or "follow"). *Shuai/*sljət* contrasts with *gu* "smooth" in *Maishu* (the first word is missing in *MSI*.C). The *SW* includes two words that both are glossed as "not smooth," i.e., "rough, blocked": *SW*, 2A.40b, *se/*srjəp* 歰; and *SW*, 11A-2.11b, *se/*srjək* 濇. Although they are phonetically distinct, the two words were used interchangeably in Han texts as antonyms of *gu* "smooth." Perhaps *shuai/*sljət* represents a third previously unattested antonym of *gu*.

3 The blood pulse is responsible for the idea that certain vessels "normally have movement."

4 *MSI*.C leaves many matters unexplained. Assuming that the technique for diagnosing the foot Great Yin vessel has been described above, details concerning where and how to diagnose the other foot vessels are missing; and nothing is said about diagnosing the hand vessels. After this sentence *Maishu* has a different conclusion which does not include the final sentences of *MSI*.C: "The method for treating ailments. Discern which (vessel) erupted first and treat it. When several vessels erupt in ailments together, pick the one that is most severe and treat it first."

5 "Connection" translates *xuan/*gwian* 縣, glossed in *SW*, 9A.17b, as *xi* 繫 (attach, connect). The term "vessel connections" probably designates the set of vessels "attached" to the body along paths described in *MSI*.A-B. I reject *MWD*, vol. 4., "Transcription," which reads 縣 as a phonetic loan for *xuan/*gwin* 玄 (darkness, subtlety). The phonological evidence is arguable, and the meaning "subtlety of the vessels" has nothing to recommend it.

thoroughly studied. Pupils, be devoted and respectful. Study [4] {4} [6] words, it is imperative to investigate them.

MSI.D

YIN YANG MAI SIHOU

陰陽脈死候

DEATH SIGNS OF THE YIN AND YANG VESSELS

MSI.D (CC84-87)

All three Yang (vessels) are the vapor of heaven. Among their ailments, only the cases where bones are broken and skin is ripped are the sole occasion when death occurs.[1] All three Yin (vessels) are the vapor of earth, and are the vessels of death. When ailments of the Yin (vessels) create disorder, death occurs within ten days.[2] The three Yin (vessels) putrefy the depots and rot the intestines, and they control killing.[3]

[2] the five forms of death.[4] When the lips turn outward and the groove beneath the nose is full,[5] flesh has died first. When the gums become level and the teeth long,[6] bone has died first. When the face is black and the eyes—fixed with fear[7]—gaze obliquely, vapor has

[1]Compare the statement in *MSI*.A.6 on the Yang vessels.

[2]Compare the statement in *MSI*.A.6 on the Yin vessels.

[3]The sentence identifies the Yin vessels as the source of decay in the body. Reference to the depots (liver, heart, spleen, lung, kidney) and intestines (large and small) is metonymy for the body and does not imply any theoretical correspondence between the Yin vessels and these organs. In *Maishu* this sentence occurs ahead of the previous sentence ("When ailments of the Yin. . . .").

[4]*Maishu* has a different opening sentence: "Whenever discerning the signs of death." *Lingshu* 10, 3.7a-b, lists fatal signs for five Yin vessels (the hand Ceasing Yin vessel is not included) using language that is sometimes similar to *MSI*.D. For example, when "the vapor is severed in the foot Great Yin (vessel)," one of the signs is that "the lips turn outward"; and the conclusion is that "flesh has died first." The contents of *MSI*.D reflect older physiological ideas which were later subsumed within *Huangdi neijing* vessel theory (see Prolegomena, Section Three, "Physiology").

[5]I translate *ren* 人 as "groove beneath the nose" on the basis of *Lingshu* 10, 3.7a, which has the compound *renzhong* 人 中 (human middle). The compound denotes the nasolabial groove (see Ma Jixing 1992: 308, n. 4).

[6]I.e. the gums recede, exposing the teeth.

[7]I follow *MWD*, vol. 4, "Transcription," in reading 環 (i.e. *huan* "ring") as *qiong* 睘 (also written 瞏), glossed in *SW*, 4A.5b, as "eyes gazing startledly."

died first. When floss-like strands of sweat emerge that stick and do not flow, blood has died first.[1] When the tongue binds and the testicles curl up,[2] muscle has died first. When all five occur, he will not live.[3]

---

[1] *Maishu* reverses the third and fourth signs, making the third a sign of blood dying first and the fourth a sign of vapor dying first.

[2] "Bind" translates *jun* 稛, glossed in *SW*, 7A.48a, as "bind with a cord." The graph is written 捆 in *MSI*.D, and is miswritten as 掐 in *MWD*, vol. 4, "Transcription," which reads the latter graph as *xian* 陷 (drop down). *Lingshu* 10, 3.7b, uses the phrase "the tongue curls up and the testicles contract" to describe "muscle dying first." In *MSI*.D, "bind" refers to the stiffening of the tongue as it contracts, and it is the testicles that "curl up. "

[3] *Maishu* has a different conclusion: "In all, the signs are five. When one signs appears, act first to keep the person alive."

MSI.E

WUSHIER BINGFANG

五十二病方

RECIPES FOR FIFTY-TWO AILMENTS

MSI.E.1[1]

Various Wounds (*MSI*.E.2–18)
Rigidity Due to a Wound (*MSI*.E.19–24)
Infant-cord Rigidity (*MSI*.E.25)
Infant Ailing from Spasms (*MSI*.E.26)
Infant Convulsions (*MSI*.E.27)
Mad Dog Bites a Person (*MSI*.E.28–30)
Dog Bites a Person (*MSI*.E.31–33)
Nest (*MSI*.E.34–35)
Xixia (*MSI*.E.36)
Wuhui (Monkshood) Poisoning (*MSI*.E.37–43)
Scorpion (*MSI*.E.44–49)
Leeches Bite (*MSI*.E.50–51)
Lizard (*MSI*.E.52–63)
Warts (*MSI*.E.64–70)
Seizure Sickness (*MSI*.E.71–72)
Baichu (*MSI*.E.73–75)
Dadai (*MSI*.E.76–77)
Ming (*MSI*.E.78)
Quan (*MSI*.E.79)
[1] *zhe* (*MSI*.E.80–83)
Yun (*MSI*.E.84–85)

---

[1]The names of the fifty-two ailment categories that form the main contents of *MSI*.E are listed in four registers. Throughout *MSI*.E these names (or slight variations) appear as headings written just above the first column of the first recipe in a given ailment category. When there is more than one recipe in an ailment category, subsequent recipes are usually headed by *yi* 一 (another).

To Make a Person Ailing from the Horse not Have Spasms (*MSI*.E.86)
To Make a Person Ailing from the [1] not Have Spasms[1]
To Make a Person Ailing from the Sheep not Have Spasms
To Make a Person Ailing from the Snake not Have Spasms
Various Eating Ailments
Various [1] Ailments
Urine Retention Ailment (*MSI*.E.88-114)
When Urine Has [1] Sediment (*MSI*.E.115)
Lard Urine (*MSI*.E.116)
Swollen Scrotum (*MSI*.E.117)
Intestine Inguinal Swelling (*MSI*.E.118-41)
Vessel Hemorrhoid (*MSI*.E.142)
Male Hemorrhoid (*MSI*.E.143-46)
Female Hemorrhoid (*MSI*.E.147-54)
Anus Itchiness (*MSI*.E.155-56)
Ju Abscess Ailment (*MSI*.E.157-73)
[2] (*MSI*.E.174-75)
[1] Burns (*MSI*.E.176-93)
Shin Burns (*MSI*.E.194-97)
Shin Wounds (*MSI*.E.198-99)
Scabies (*MSI*.E.200-223)
Snake Bite (*MSI*.E.224)
Abscess (*MSI*.E.225-32)
Lacquer (*MSI*.E.233-39)
Chewing by Bugs (*MSI*.E.240-48)
Dry Itch (*MSI*.E.249-56)
Old Scabbing (*MSI*.E.257-70)
Gu (*MSI*.E.271-75)
Child Sprite (*MSI*.E.276-77)
Removing a Person's Horse Warts (*MSI*.E.278-79)
Treating Facial Pustules (*MSI*.E.280-82)
Altogether Fifty-two

MSI.E.2 (CC1-2)

Various Wounds[2]

---

[1]The recipes for this ailment category as well as for the next four ailment categories are missing in the text.

[2] lard[1] and *gancao* (licorice), two portions of each; *gui* (cinnamon), *jiang* (ginger), *jiao* (zanthoxylum),[2] [22]. Crush one ball in a cup of liquor and drink it.[3] Drink once daily. {1} [1] {1} [?].

MSI.E.3 (CC3-4)

Another. [4] *qu*,[4] made to be the size of small beans.[5] Then combine with one *dou* of *chida* (adzuki beans) and [1]. Again smith[6] [11] {1} [3]. Drink the liquid, entirely consuming the dregs along with the liquid. Eat it as you wish. It relieves pain {1} [?].

---

[2]Judging from *MSI*.E.6, 12, 17, and 18—which all refer specifically to "blade wounds" or "metal wounds"—this category is mainly concerned with stab wounds and accidental cuts. The usual term for such wounds in Han and post-Han medical nomenclature is *jin chuang* 金 創 (metal injuries). A recipe manual for treating "metal injuries" is listed in the *Hanshu* bibliographic treatise (*Hanshu*, 30.80a); and the Wuwei recipes include "metal injuries" (*WWYJ*: 2b-3a, 8a-b).

[1]*Gao* 膏 (lard) and *zhi* 脂 (suet) are the two standard terms in the Mawangdui medical manuscripts for animal fat. Li Zhongwen (1980) examines the use of both words in *MSI*.E and concludes that their meaning corresponds to the definition in *SW*, 4B.36b. *Gao* is the soft fat from animals without horns, principally the pig (i.e. lard); *zhi* is the hard fat from horned animals, principally oxen and sheep (i.e. suet).

[2]*Jiao* 椒 refers to several species in the genus *Zanthoxylum*. *MSI*.E occasionally specifies Shu *jiao* 蜀 椒, which is the drug name listed in *BC*.

[3]The standard practice in *MSI*.E is to form medicine balls which are crushed before using; *MSI.E*.151 provides the only example of swallowing the balls directly. Balls are also swallowed in *MS*III.71.

[4]*Qu/*gjug* 朐 is glossed in *SW*, 4B.33b, as "strips of dried meat." I doubt the graph has this meaning in *MSI*.E.3 and suspect that it is a loan for a herbal drug name. One possibility is *ju/*kjug* 蒟. *Ju* is glossed in *SW*, 1B.31b, as "a fruit"; and is also mentioned as the chief ingredient of a spicy sauce produced in Shu 蜀 in *Shiji*, 116.2b. Hui-lin Li presents evidence for identifying *ju* as the word for black pepper (*Piper nigrum*) in Former Han times (1979: 46-53).

[5]*Da* 荅 (small bean) is the adzuki bean, also called *xiaodou* 小 豆 and *chi xiaodou* 赤 小 豆 (see *chida*). In *MSI*.E.3, "small bean" is used as a relative measure of size in drug preparation. A similar usage occurs in the Wuwei recipes, which mention making medicine balls "the size of *chidou* 赤 豆" (*WWYJ*: 3b). The use of the adzuki bean as a metrological standard in early medicine is confirmed by Tao Hongjing, who explains that references in old medical recipes to a measurement "like a small bean" are to the *chi xiaodou* of his day, and that the measurement is equivalent to three large hemp seeds (*GM*, 1.38).

[6]*Ye* 冶 is used regularly in *MSI*.E to denote the fine pounding of a drug. My literal translation "smith" is based on Akahori (1985), who argues that *ye*—which means to cast metal according to *SW*, 11B.8b—also had the sense of hammering metal; and was then extended to the pestling of drugs. As noted by Akahori, sifting techniques were not common in medicine until after the Han period. Before that time, long pestling was necessary to reduce a drug to a uniform powder; and *ye* "smith" was borrowed from metallurgy to denote the pounding process. *Ye* appears frequently in the Wuwei recipes, but it is rare in later medical literature (and when it does occur in received literature it is regularly miswritten as *zhi* 治). Evidently the word *ye* became obsolete once sifting simplified the process of pulverizing drugs.

*MS*I.E.4 (CC5-7)

Another. Smith *ji*[1] [2] soak using pure liquor,[2] and shape into wafers. Bake in a pottery kettle, using charcoal [13] soak [1]. Bake as [before].[3] Then smith. Put a three-fingered pinch into a half cup of warmed liquor.[4] [15] ones, smith one hundred times; for large [1] ones, (smith) eighty times; and for small ones, (smith) forty times. Smith until fine.[5]

*MS*I.E.5 (CC8-9)

Another. Incinerate the feathers of a white chicken and scalp hair.[6] Smith each in equal amounts. Smith eight times that amount of hundred-grass-residue ash[7] and [6]. [Crush][8] one ball in one cup of warmed liquor and drink it.

*MS*I.E.6 (C10)

Another. For a blade wound, incinerate sheep feces and spread (the feces) on it.

---

[1]It is probable that 齊 should be read as *ji* 薺 (see *MS*I.E.18).

[2]*Chunjiu* 淳 酒 (pure liquor) is undiluted liquor (see the definition of *chun* 醇 in *SW*, 14B.35a).

[3]The repetition of the words "soak" and "bake" following the thirteen-graph lacuna above suggests that there is a second drug prepared in the same fashion as the first. Filling the lacuna here with "before" is based on the repeated use of the phrase *ru qian* 如 前 (as before) in *MS*I.E.

[4]*SW*, 12A.32b, glosses *cuo* 撮 (pinch) as "four spatulas" and as "a three-fingered pinch"; i.e. the amount of medicine that can be picked up using the thumb, index, and middle fingers. Measurement by spatulas is not mentioned in the Mawangdui medical manuscripts, and measuring drugs was undoubtedly still performed with the fingers. *MS*I.E.18 provides a more precise indication of the measurement when it specifies using "one three-fingered pinch reaching to the knuckles." The three-fingered pinch also occurs in *Suwen* 46, 13.2b; and in the Wuwei recipes (*WWYJ*: 3a, 8b).

[5]Despite the lacuna, it is evident that the conclusion of *MS*I.E.4 discusses the technique of pestling relative to the size of the drug being powdered. Determining the fineness of a drug by counting the number of times it is pounded was probably a standard procedure in early medicine, although this is the only place in the Mawangdui medical manuscripts that specifies a pounding count.

[6]In materia medica *fa* 髮 refers to hair clipped from the scalp as distinct from loose hair that collects in brushes and combs (*GM*, 52.81). Loose hair is specified in *MS*I.E.205.

[7]*Baicao mo* 百 草 末 (hundred grass residue) is not attested in received literature. *MWD*, vol. 4, "Transcription," n. 3, suggests that it may be similar to *baicao shuang* 百 草 霜 (hundred grass frost), which is the name for the soot that collects in the stove flue in later medical literature (*GM*, 7.87). Wei and Hu argue that *ba/*priat* 八 is not the number eight, but rather is a phonetic loan for *ba/*briat* 炦, glossed in *SW*, 10A.44a, as "fire vapor" (1992, vol. 1: 48, n. 3). *Ba* is unattested outside of the *SW*, but the reading *bahui* 炦 灰 (fire-vapor ash) is plausible; in which case the translation would be, "Smith hundred-grass-residue fire-vapor ash."

[8]Filling the lacuna here with "crush" (*hui* 毀), based on *MS*I.E.2.

MSI.E.7 (C11)

Another. To stop blood from coming out, incinerate scalp hair and press it on the wound.

MSI.E.8 (C12)

Another. To cause the wounded person not to feel pain and not to have blood coming out, take an old cattail mat {1} [3] incinerate [4] the wound.[1]

MSI.E.9 (C13)

Another. When blood is coming out of the wounded person, chant this incantation: "Man, staunch! Woman, vinegar!"[2] Draw five lines on the ground and [1] it.[3]

MSI.E.10 (C14)

Another. To cause the wound to not form a scar, take pig lard and [1] *yan*.[4] Smith together and spread (the salve) on it.

MSI.E.11 (C15)

Another. Spread a man's slime on it.[5] Every time, a scar does not form.

---

[1]The ashes of the cattail mat are probably pressed on the wound, like the scalp hair in *MSI*.E.7.

[2]"Vinegar" translates *dai* 胾, glossed in *SW*, 14B.41a, as "vinegar beverage." *Dai* was a common beverage in Han times, made by allowing rice-preparation water to ferment (see Hayashi 1975: 69). Elsewhere in *MSI*.E rice-cleaning water is used as a bathing solution. In the incantation, I interpret "vinegar" as a verb meaning "apply vinegar to the wound." The incantation conjures a man to stop the bleeding and a woman to apply the vinegar.

[3]The act of drawing five lines on the ground creates a magical diagram. *MSIII*.83 describes a magical technique to protect a traveler from harm at night that includes drawing a circle on the ground. A similar procedure is described in the first Shuihudi hemerological manuscript, which gives instructions for a ritual to be performed before departing on a journey. The last part of the ritual entails drawing five lines on the ground, picking up soil from the center of the lines, and carrying it in the bosom (*SHD*: 223). The exact manner of executing the five-line diagram remains unclear. Perhaps it is a kind of magic square composed of five lines. Kudô examines the Mawangdui and Shuihudi manuscript evidence in the light of later religious Daoist practices; he speculates that the five lines may be related to a Daoist cross-hatch design consisting of four vertical lines and five horizontal lines (1990: 50–57). I would prefer better evidence. In *MSI*.E.9 the five-line diagram is intended to create a magical space that protects the wounded person from further harm.

[4]The drug name [1] *yan* 衍 is unidentified.

[5]"Slime" translates *ji* 洎, which has two attested meanings: "pour water into a vessel" (*SW*, 11A-2.30b); and "juice from meat" (*Zuozhuan*, Xiang 28, 38.13b). Both meanings occur in *MSI*.E. Although the meaning is unattested, *MWD*, vol. 4, "Transcription," n. 1, argues that *ji* refers to semen in *MSI*.E.11, citing as support later medical literature that records the use of semen to prevent scars. Qiu Xigui argues that 洎 should be read as *yi* 洟 (snot) in *MSI*.E.11, citing as evidence the Mawangdui *Yijing* manuscript in which the text for the hexagram Cui 卒 writes 洎 instead of 洟 in the received text (1992: 530; the Mawangdui

MSI.E.12 (C16)

Another. For a metal wound, use lard, *wuhui* (monkshood), and [2] {2} [1] fry.[1] Apply (the salve) to it.

MSI.E.13 (CC17-18)

Another. For a wound, use one handful of *xuduan* (teazel), two long sticks[2] of *du* [1],[3] two sticks of *huangqin* (skullcap), [1] sticks of *gancao* (licorice), two [1] of autumn *wuhui* (monkshood),[4] and two saucers of [4].[5] Then fry together [1] cooked. Wring it in a cloth to obtain the liquid.[6] Use old hemp-wadding[7] [2]. Spread (the salve) on it.

MSI.E.14 (CC19-20)

Another. For [1], smith *huangqin* (skullcap) and [5] pig lard [2] it. Then wring it in a cloth [8]. Swab[8] (the salve) on it.

---

graph could be analyzed literally as "fluid that comes from the nose"). Ma Jixing accepts the identification with semen and rejects snot, in part because he questions why *MSI*.E.11 should distinguish between a man's snot and a woman's (1992: 339-40). I am inclined to agree that in *MSI*.E.11 *ji* refers to a substance like semen or snot (both viscous fluids, one from the nose and the other from the penis). Rather than pass judgment on the relative probability of semen or snot, I use "slime" in the sense of a viscous body fluid.

[1]*Jian* 煎 (fry) means to cook something until the liquid is cooked away. Fat may or may not be used for frying.

[2]According to *SW*, 6A.23b, *ting* 梃 is a measure word for stick-like objects. The scribe failed to write the complete graph in this occurrence in *MSI*.E.13, for there is merely an oblique stroke ＼ in the text. The subsequent two occurrences are written 梃 and 廷 respectively.

[3]*Du* [1] 獨 also occurs in *MSI*.E.138; unfortunately the second graph is again missing. The drug may be the herb *duhuo* 獨活, listed in *BC* and recommended for "metal injuries" (*GM*, 13.49). *ZY*: no. 3510, lists seven plants identified with this drug name.

[4]Reference to autumn probably specifies when the drug is to be gathered.

[5]Probably two saucers of lard are added.

[6]*Bu* 布 refers to cloth woven from hemp or kudzu fibers (*SW*, 7B.54a, and Duan Yucai commentary). The practice of squeezing a lard-based medicine through cloth is explained by Tao Hongjing, who recommends using the dregs separately (*GM*, 1.40). In *MSI*.E.13 the "liquid" is probably liquid fat being squeezed through a cloth to separate out the fried debris of the drugs. Other recipes in *MSI*.E describe the preparation of lard salves that are not strained before use.

[7]*SW*, 13A.38a equates *yun* 縕 with *fu* 紼, which is glossed as "matted hemp fiber." The main uses of hemp-wadding were as padding for clothing, as tinder for starting fires, and for twine.

[8]*Wei/*mjəd* 浘 is attested as a variant graph for *mei/*məd* 浼 (*Shijing*, Mao 43, 2C.9a, and commentaries). *Mei* is glossed with *wu* 污 in *SW*, 11A-2.40a; and the third of three glosses for *wu* in *SW*, 11A-2.29a, is *tu* 涂 (daub). Like *tu*, which occurs frequently in *MSI*.E, *wei* must mean "daub, swab."

MSI.E.15 (C21)

Another. For an old wound, mince[1] *xing* (apricot) pit kernels. Beat in rancid lard[2] and seal the wound. The bugs then come out. Previously tested.[3]

MSI.E.16 (C22)

Another. Put *xiaoshi* (niter)[4] in hot water and wash the abscess with it.[5]

MSI.E.17 (CC23-24)

Another. Recipe to cause a metal wound not to be painful. Take a *fenshu* (mole),[6] and dry and smith it. Take a *zhiyu*,[7] and incinerate and smith it. [2] *xinyi* (magnolia bud) and *gancao* (licorice), each in the same amount as the *fenshu* (mole). Combine them all, stirring. Take one three-fingered pinch, put it in one cup of warmed liquor,

---

[1]"Mince" translates *ji* 齏, which refers to the fine mincing of ingredients for relishes (*SW*, 7B.3b, and Duan Yucai commentary; the *SW* records several graphs used to write the word, and several variants also occur in *MSI*.E). It is likely that "mincing" could also be accomplished with a mortar and pestle.

[2]"Rancid" translates *zhi* 膱. The Zheng Xuan commentary in *Zhouli*, 42.9b, explains *zhi* as "grease that is rancid and spoiled." The same word is written 殖 in *SW*, 4B.13a, and glossed as "grease that is old and rancid." *MSI*.E often calls for rancid lard in preparing salves because it is more viscous than fresh lard. I read text 弁 as *pan* 拚, which *SW*, 12A.42b, glosses as "clapping the hands." *KGS*, vol. 1: 148, n. 64, argues that in *MSI*.E *pan* refers to a kneading action with the hands necessitated by the stiffness of the ingredients (other occurrences of *pan* in *MSI*.E also involve rancid lard or thick substances). I suspect that *pan* may also refer to beating something with a stick, hence the translation "beat in."

[3]*Changshi* 嘗試 (previously tested) is one of several terms used in *MSI*.E to praise the effectiveness of a recipe. Wang Chong alludes to the term in the *Lunheng* in his criticism of those who exploited the demand for secret recipes (see Prolegomena, Section Two, "Readership and Transmission").

[4]Needham examines the evidence concerning various soluble salts in early China, and concludes that the name *xiaoshi* 消石 (solvent mineral) was applied to niter (1954-, vol. 5, part 4: 179-94).

[5]"Abscess" translates *yong* 癰, which is also the name of the ailment category beginning in *MSI*.E.225. In *MSI*.E.16-17 *yong* probably refers to a wound that becomes abscessed. *Yong* occurs in the Shuihudi text *Fengzhen shi* meaning "wound" (*SHD*: 162, n. 8). Thus it is possible that *yong* in *MSI*.E.16-17 refers to a wound, not an abscessed wound. It is also possible that *yong* in this context refers to ulceration.

[6]*SW*, 10A.37a, identifies *fen* 鼢 as *yanshu* 偃鼠, the latter being the name listed in *BL* (*GM*, 51.67).

[7]*Zhi*/★*drjad* 彘 means "pig." *MWD*, vol. 4, "Transcription," n. 2, proposes reading it as a phonetic loan for *ti*/★*diəd* 鮧. *Tiyu* 鮧魚 is the name of a fish listed in *BL* (*GM*, 44.114); identified in *ZY*: no. 5359, as *Parasilurus asotus* (L.). Although the phonological evidence supports the proposed loan, I hesitate to make a conclusive identification. *Zhiyu* might also mean "pig fish" and represent a name that is not recorded in received literature.

and drink it. If this does not work, increase the medicine a bit.[1] Stop when it is no longer abscessed. Excellent.[2]

*MS*I.E.18 (CC25-29)

Another. To cause a metal wound not to be painful. Take one portion of the thoroughly dried fruits of *ji* (capsella), scorched until blackened and smithed; and two portions of *zhu* (atractylodes) root,[3] peeled and smithed. Blend the two substances together. Take one three-fingered pinch reaching to the knuckles and put the medicine into one brimming-full cup[4] of pure liquor. Stir and drink. For those who do not (usually drink), use one half cup of liquor. Having drunk it, after some time there is no pain. If pain occurs again, drink the medicine following the same procedure.[5] If there is no pain, do not drink the medicine. (Take) the medicine before eating or after eating as you wish.[6] While treating the ailment, do not eat fish, pork, horseflesh, turtles, snakes, odorous foods,[7] and *mazhu* greens.[8] Do not approach the inner (chamber).[9] When the ailment

---

[1]For the use of *cai* 財 (also written 裁 and 才) to mean "a few, a bit," see *Hou Hanshu*, 17.6a, and commentary. In other contexts in *MS*I.E *cai* has the sense of "a sufficient amount."

[2]*Ling* 令 (excellent) is another term of praise for a recipe that occurs frequently in *MS*I.E.

[3]In *BC* only *zhu* 朮 is listed. Tao Hongjing (*GM*, 12B.4) distinguishes between *baizhu* 白朮 (*Atractylodes macrocephala*) and *chizhu* 赤朮 (i.e. *cangzhu* 蒼朮; *Atractylodes lancea* and other spp.).

[4]I interpret *zhong bei* 衷杯 to mean a "brimming cup." For the use of *zhong*, written 衷 or 中, in the sense of a full measure, see *Hanshu*, 8.18a, and the Yan Shigu commentary.

[5]The expression *ru shu* 如數 occurs six more times in *MS*I.E (with slight variations depending on the context): *MS*I.E.20 (C36), 75 (C131), 94 (C160), 142 (C238), 146 (C247), and fragment 1 (*MWD*, vol. 4: 76). *Shu* means literally "a calculation." Considered in isolation, *shu* in *MS*I.E.18 might seem to mean "amount" (making the translation read, "drink the medicine using the same amounts"). However, judging from all seven occurrences, *shu* refers to the steps involved in executing a particular operation, hence my translation "following the same procedure."

[6]Instructions concerning whether to take medicine before or after eating a meal occur a number of times in *MS*I.E; and *MS*III contains similar instructions for tonics. I believe the meaning of the expressions *xian shi* 先食 (before eating) and *hou shi* 後食 (after eating) is as translated. Curiously, the Wang Bing commentary in *Suwen* 46, 13.2b, explains the expression *hou fan* 後飯 to mean, "make the meal come after and the medicine come before"—exactly the opposite of my translation. However, the Yang Shangshan commentary to the parallel passage in *Taisu*, 30.450, corresponds to my interpretation.

[7]*Xun* 葷 refers to strong-smelling, sharply-flavored vegetables like onions and garlic (see *SW*, 1B.7b).

[8]The term *mazhu* 麻洙 is also used in the Wuwei recipes (*WWYJ*: 6a). It clearly denotes a food preparation that was known in the cuisine of the Former and Later Han periods, yet there is no mention of it in received literature.

desists, (you may do things) as before. While treating the ailment, there are no temporal (restrictions).[1] Smith enough medicine to treat the ailment. After smithing the medicine, store it in a silk pouch. When smithing the *zhu* (atractylodes), let it dry by putting it in the sun or by some other means,[2] then smith. Excellent.

MSI.E.19 (CC30–33)

Rigidity Due to a Wound[3]

Rigidity occurs when there is a wound, wind enters the wound, and then the body becomes straight and cannot bend. To treat it, scorch salt until it turns yellow. Wrap one *dou* of it in a cloth. Quench it in pure liquor, dipping it in and then immediately taking it out. Cover it with an apron,[4] and hot-press the head with it.[5] If it is too hot, lift it off and lower it when all right. {1} [1] {1} and once again hot-press. When the hot-press becomes cold, once again scorch salt and use it to hot-press. Continue hot-pressing without

---

[9]I.e. entry to the bedroom for sexual intercourse is forbidden. For *jin nei* 近 内 (approach the inner chamber) as a term for sexual intercourse, see *MSIII*.34.

[1]*MSI*.E gives few examples of what constitute temporal restrictions, the statement that there are none being the usual formula. There is one calendrical prohibition in *MSI*.E.69, and it is probable that the restrictions derive from hemerological and astrological symbolism.

[2]Other methods of drying drugs besides in the sun are leaving them in a dark place or drying them over a fire.

[3]In *SW*, 7B.33a, *jing* 痙 (rigidity) is glossed simply as "acute stiffness." The etiology of *jing* "rigidity" in *MSI*.E is consistently linked to the prior existence of a wound, which permits wind to enter the body—and it is the wind that causes *jing* to occur. The third ailment category (*MSI*.E.25) is a kind of *jing* that affects infants, apparently occurring when the removal of the umbilical cord permits the pathogen to enter; and the fifth ailment category (*MSI*.E.27) is similar in that the treatment focuses on drawing the pathogen out of the opening of a wound. In the discussion of "rigidity" brought on by "metal injuries" in *Chaoshi zhubing yuanhoulun*, 36.12a, wind is also the pathogen. It is difficult to judge what modern ailments might correspond to *jing*, although tetanus is one likely choice (Yu Yan 1972: 142).

[4]The *fu* 巿 (apron) was a regular article of clothing in male and female dress (Hayashi 1976: 16–17).

[5]"Hot-press" translates *yun* 熨, glossed in *SW*, 10A.46b, as "pressing down from above" and "what one smooths silk with." Several specimens of the *yundou* 熨 斗 (iron) of Han date have been discovered (Sun Ji 1991: 346). They have shallow flat-bottomed pans to hold hot coals and are attached to long handles. As a form of medical therapy, *yun* is attested in *Hanfeizi* 21, 7.118, where Bian Que recommends "hot-pressing" when an ailment first lodges on the surface of the body and has not penetrated deeply inside (see also *Shiji*, 105.6b). *MSI*.E provides the earliest descriptions of the methods of hot-pressing; and the frequency of hot-pressing in *MSI*.E suggests that it was a common form of therapy in the third and second centuries B.C. A variety of materials are used, from the salt in *MSI*.E.19 to hot stones in *MSI*.E.146 (see Prolegomena, Section Three, "Therapy").

interruption. With the first hot-pressing, cold and sweat come out. After a great amount of sweat has come out, and (the body) can bend and straighten, stop. While hot-pressing as well as for four days after hot-pressing, [2] clothing, and do not let (the body) be exposed to wind. After four days (the body) feels good again. Hot-press before eating or after eating as you wish. There are no prohibitions and no temporal (restrictions). Excellent.

*MS*I.E.20 (CC34-36)

Another. For rigidity due to a wound, boil *li* (plum) fruit in a sufficient amount of water. Let it bubble rapidly and then remove (the liquid). Sieve (the fruit) to obtain the liquid.[1] When cooled to lukewarm, give it to the ailing person to drink. When drinking, take [2] as the measure.[2] If the ailment is severe and (the ailing person) cannot drink, open his mouth forcibly and pour it in for him. If at the time there is no *li* (plum) fruit, [6] boil, and drink the liquid following the same procedure as for the fruit.[3] There are no prohibitions. Previously tested. Excellent.

*MS*I.E.21 (CC37-40)

Another. For various wounds when wind enters the wound, which becomes abscessed and painful. Treat it using wadded hemp to make {1} [3] the wound. Soak [5] pig lard {2} [3] {1} continually [1] pour the lard downward without interruption, thereby expelling the cold vapor. [4] {1} [5] and spread it on the opening of the wound. Cover with a napkin [1] {3} [20] {1} [5]. Spread the medicine on (the wound) before eating or after eating as you wish. There are no prohibitions and no temporal (restrictions). [1] *yu* (arsenopyrite)[4] {1} [3] {1} [1].

---

[1]I.e. the fruit is placed in a sieve and strained separately to obtain the liquid still in it. This is the only recipe where *shu* 抒 (remove) and *jun* 浚 (sieve) occur together. Other recipes either say to "sieve (a boiled decoction) to obtain the liquid" (thereby removing the solid matter) or say to "remove the liquid" (apparently without straining it through a sieve). In just one instance, *MS*I.E.117 says to "sieve to remove the liquid" when it is the solid matter that is wanted for the recipe.

[2]*MS*I.E.99 contains the phrase "take a large amount as the measure," which is syntactically the same as the fragmentary phrase here.

[3]Missing in the lacuna is the drug to be substituted for plum fruit when the latter is unavailable. According to the recipe, the preparation and consumption of the substutite drug follow the procedure already described for plum fruit.

[4]Obviously arsenopyrite is used in preparing a medicine earlier in the recipe. The occurrence of the word at the end of the recipe is part of an added comment on the drug and its use in medicine.

MSI.E.22 (CC41-42)

Another. For rigidity due to a wound, chop finely one dog and allow it to rot with one half *dou* of malt.[1] Do not remove its feet. Place both in a [1][2] and soak at the bottom[3] of a well. [3] and take it out. Dry in the dark for one hundred days. Then if someone has rigidity, smith, blend one three-fingered pinch into one cup of warmed liquor, and drink it.

MSI.E.23 (C43)

Another. For rigidity due to a wound. Take one handful of *xie* (scallions)[4] and boil in one half *dou* of pure liquor until it bubbles. Drink it, and immediately sit with warm clothing pressed around all four sides. When sweat comes out and reaches the feet, then [1].

MSI.E.24 (C44)

Another. Smith *huangqin* (skullcap) and *gancao* (licorice), half and half. Then fry it in a sufficient amount of pig lard. Fry it until it bubbles, then wring it in a cloth to remove the liquid. [1] spread [1].[5]

MSI.E.25 (CC45-47)

Infant-cord Rigidity[6]

---

[1] *Nie* 糵 (malt) is sprouted grain used for fermentation (*SW*, 7A.60b). "Allow to rot" is a tentative translation of *beng* 澌, which is not attested in received literature until well after the Han period; and not in a meaning appropriate to *MSI*.E.22. Perhaps it is related to the primary graph *beng* 崩, glossed in *SW*, 9B.8a, as "destruction of a mountain" and also used in the sense of "ruin, spoil." I suspect that in *MSI*.E.22 *beng* refers to the degenerative effect of the malt on the chopped dog.

[2] Evidently the "rotting" process involves packing the chopped dog together with the malt in a vessel.

[3] 鐖 occurs again in *MSI*.E.31 where the context also suggests the meaning is "bottom"; and the same meaning is indicated for *duan* 斷 in *MSI*.E.155. The meaning "bottom" for *duan* is not attested in received literature.

[4] *ZY*: no. 5545, lists *Allium chinense* G. Don and *A. macrostemon* Bge. as the two main plants for the onions identified by the name *xie* 薤. However, as with English "scallion," *xie* has been applied to several other small onions.

[5] Probably the liquid obtained after wringing the lard medicine is spread on the affected part of the body.

[6] *MWD*, vol. 4, "Transcription," n. 1, argues that the ailment is a female ailment that occurs in women after childbirth, and then offers the alternative explanation that it is an infant ailment. The fourth and fifth ailment categories (*MSI*.E.26-27) are both related infant ailments, a good indication that *MSI*.E.25 is also an infant ailment and not a post-partum female ailment. *Yinger suo* 嬰兒索 (infant cord) is not attested in received literature, but there is no difficulty identifying it as a term for the umbilical cord. *MSI*.E.27 treats of the ailment *chi* 瘛 (convulsions) in infants. *SW*, 7B.35a, glosses *chi* as "the ailment *chizong* 瘛瘲 in infants." Yu Yan hypothesizes that *chi* refers specifically to infections like

Cord rigidity occurs if at the time of birth (the infant) remains on damp ground for a long time. The flesh by the bones stiffens and the mouth locks;[1] the muscles cramp and are hard to straighten. Take anthill loam[2] and smith it. [2], two portions; and salt, one portion. Combine them, stirring, and steam. Use it to hot-press all round the areas of stiffened flesh and cramped muscles. Starting from the head gradually [1] the hands and feet and no more. When the hot-press becomes cold [2] and steam it again. When the hot-press dries out, make a new one. Excellent.

MSI.E.26 (CC48-50)

Recipe for Infant Ailing from Spasms[3]

Take three nodules of *leishi* (bamboo truffle) and smith. Blend fried pig lard into it. For a small infant use one half *dou* of water, and for a large one use one *dou*. Divide the blended mixture into three parts. Place one part in the water, stir, and bathe the infant with it. When bathing, begin at the top of the head and proceed downward over the entire body, without letting the four limbs get wet. Bathe once a day for three days.[4] It desists after three days. Af-

---

tetanus that often occur when the newborn infant's umbilical cord is cut (1972: 115). Although the umbilical cord is not mentioned in *MSI*.E.27, there is reference to "stroking around the spot where the infant convulsions are"—perhaps a wound where the umbilical cord was cut. *MSI*.E.25 does not mention the cutting of the umbilical cord as a factor contributing to the occurrence of the ailment, but the umbilical cord or navel might still have been regarded as the point of entry for the pathogen.

[1]"Lock" translates *kou* 釦, which means literally "metal plating around the mouth of a vessel" (*SW*, 14A.8a).

[2]*Feng* 封 could have several meanings, but the meaning "anthill" is attested in *Fangyan*, 10.6a, as a Chu dialect word, which is probably the correct meaning of *feng* in *MSI*.E.25. The friable soil from anthills is included in *GM*, 7.77.

[3]*Xian* 癇 (spasms) refers to an ailment characterized by spasmodic fits. According to *Chaoshi zhubing yuanhoulun*, 45.7a, *xian* is the name for the ailment when it occurs in children younger than ten, and the same ailment is called *dian* 癲 when it occurs in someone older. It is unlikely that the twinned identity and age-based differentiation apply to *xian* and *dian* in *MSI*.E. Besides this recipe for Infant Ailing from Spasms, *MSI*.E.86 is the only extant recipe in *MSI*.E of what was originally a sequence of four categories of *xian* ailments; and age is apparently not a factor. *Maishu*, "Ailment List," also makes no mention of age when it identifies *xian*: "When (the body) snaps in a reverse direction, it is *xian*" (*MSSW*: 72). Although the ailment is not described, *MSI*.E.71-72 treat of *dian* as a separate ailment category. *Dian* was associated with mental derangement in Han times, and perhaps included epileptic seizure (see *MSI*.E.71).

[4]*MWD*, vol. 4, "Transcription," n. 4, argues that *san* 三 (three) is excrescent, making the line read, "bathe once a day." I suspect that the original wording is an elliptical way of saying that for a duration of three days the infant should be bathed once each day.

ter bathing always discard the water immediately in the privy. When spasms occur the body is hot and continually trembles. The neck and spine are rigid and the abdomen is enlarged. [1] spasms are many and various. Using this medicine, they all desist.

MSI.E.27 (CC51-55)

Infant Convulsions[1]

When infant convulsions occur, the eyes are fixed in a sidelong gaze.[2] The sides are painful, the breath is quick and shrill, and the feces remain green without transforming. Take vegetation from the upturned-slope of the roof.[3] Incinerate it using kindling[4] and [1] it in a ladle. Make silted water that is roiled thrice and fill a cup with it.[5] Then spit on the ladle and chant this incantation over it:

---

[1]See *MSI.E.25* for the association of *chi* 瘛 (convulsions) with tetanus. The exorcistic removal of the pathogen in *MSI.E.27* focuses on a wound from which blood is magically expelled. Although the umbilical cord is not mentioned, cutting the umbilical cord is a likely cause for a wound on a newborn infant. Among the symptoms described in *MSI.E.27* are pain in the sides and shortness of breath. "Inability to breath" is also one of the signs of *chi* in *Maishu*, "Ailment List" (*MSSW*: 72); and *Yinshu* specifies the sides as the location of *chi* when describing an exercise routine to alleviate it (*YSSW*: 85; it is highly unlikely that *chi* in the *Yinshu* passage has any connection with tetanus).

[2]*Jie/*krig* 繲, which I translate as "fixed," was previously a *hapax legomenon* in *Zhuangzi* 4, 82. Commentaries gloss the word as "wash clothes." However, the textual variant *xian* 繲 (thread) occurs in some *Zhuangzi* editions. This variant must also reflect the correct meaning of *jie*, which I interpret as "thread-work, sewing" in the *Zhuangzi* passage (complementing the reference to "wielding the needle" immediately preceding in the *Zhuangzi*). *Jie/*krig* is undoubtedly cognate with *xi/*kig* 係 (bind) and other words meaning to fasten with a cord. Ma Jixing interprets *mu jie* 目 繲 as equivalent to *mu xi* 目 系, a term for an attachment at the back of the eye attested in *Lingshu* 10, 3.6b (1992: 375, n. 2). I doubt that this technical denotation applies to *MSI.E.27*. 睮, which I read as *xie*, is not attested in received literature. Either it is a specialized word for oblique gazing, or perhaps a fusion of two graphs written by the scribe as one (目 and 邪).

[3]*Rong* 榮 is an architectural term that refers to the upturned edges of the roof by the eaves—also known as *wuyi* 屋 翼 (roof wing; *SW*, 6A.18b, and Duan Yucai commentary). "Vegetation from the upturned-slope of the roof" is probably the various plants that can still be seen today sprouting from the roof tiles of Chinese buildings. The use of roof vegetation in *MSI.E.27* must have symbolic significance related to the solar potency of something that grows on the roof, which makes roof vegetation an appropriate exorcistic material.

[4]Ma Jixing argues that *xin* 薪 forms a compound with *cai* 蔡 (vegetation) in the previous sentence, meaning "vegetation and grassy material" (1992: 377, n. 12). However, *MSI.E.244* and *MSI.E.271* exhibit similar grammar in which *xin* "kindling" refers to the kindling used to incinerate the drug.

[5]"Silted water" translates *yanji* 湮 汲, which means literally "make freshly-drawn water silty." It is used often in *MSI.E. MWD*, vol. 4, "Transcription," n. 4, identifies *yanji* with *dijiang* 地 漿 (earth juice), which is listed in *BL* (*GM*, 5.51). Tao Hongjing describes the method for preparing it as follows: "Dig a pit three *chi* deep in ground where there is

"Spouter, spout ferociously.[1] On high be like the sweeper star.[2] Down below be like congealed blood.[3] You[4] will be seized left of the gate. You will be cut apart right of the gate. Should you not desist, you will be quartered and exposed in the marketplace." Then stroke with the ladle in a circle around the spot where the infant convulsions are, and rinse it in the cup of water. Watch it. When there is blood like a fly wing, discard it by the wall. Take fresh water. Once again spit on the liquid in the ladle[5] and stroke with it as before. There should be no trembling.[6] Repeat it over and over again. When the trembling has ceased, stop. Excellent.

MSI.E.28 (C56)

Mad Dog Bites a Person

---

yellow earth. Pour freshly drawn water into it and stir until turbid. After a little while, take the clear part and use it." The term *san hun* 三 渾 (roiled thrice) in *MSI*.E.27 must mean that the water is stirred together with the dirt and allowed to clarify thrice before use.

[1] A purely exorcistic act of spouting through the mouth or nostrils (the word is *pen/*pən* 噴) often precedes the chanting of an incantation in *MSI*.E; and sometimes the first utterance in the incantation is the word for "spout" (in which case I adopt the reconstructed sound of the word to reflect its value as an exorcistic utterance). The person chanting the incantation in *MSI*.E.27 is undoubtedly spouting while uttering the words "Spouter, spout ferociously." The distinctive element in *MSI*.E.27 is that the person summons a "spouter"—a spirit—to assist in the expulsion of the demonic agent responsible for the ailment.

[2] I.e. a comet.

[3] *SW*, 5A.50b, glosses *pei* 衃 as "congealed blood." The compound *pei xie* 衃 血 is used to describe the bloody blob of an aborted fetus in the Shuihudi *Fengzhen shi* (*SHD*: 161; cf. Hulsewé 1985: 205). The word is cognate with *pei* 肧, glossed in *SW*, 4B.20a, as "first month of a pregnancy"; i.e. the stage when the fetus is still an amorphous blob. In *MSI*.E.27 it appears that the "spouter" is ordered to enter the infant's body and assume the form of "congealed blood" to expel the demonic agent.

[4] "You" represents a direct address to the demonic agent who is threatened with death.

[5] "Liquid in the ladle" renders the grammar of the text and agrees with the earlier instruction to spit on the ladle (and not on the cup of silted water); yet why would the ashed vegetation in the ladle would be referred to as a "liquid"? Another possible interpretation is that the person spits on both the ladle and the cup of water, referred to here as the "liquid."

[6] "Trembling" translates *zheng* 徵. The graph is often used for *zheng* 征, which occurs in compounds for extreme fright; e.g. *zhengying* 征 營 (trembling and shaking), a conventional expression used by court officials in addressing the monarch (see *Hou Hanshu*, 60B.16a: "Your servant trembles and shakes with alarm and terror"). *Fangyan*, 10.5b, identifies *zhengzhong* 征 伀 as another expression for terrified trembling used in the region of the Yangzi and Xiang Rivers (i.e. around Changsha). Ma Jixing interprets *zheng* to mean "a sign of being cured"; and the phrase to mean "if there are no signs" (1992: 379, n. 34). However, the second occurrence of *zheng* in the phrase *zheng jin* 徵 盡 below leads Ma into the forced interpretation, "when the signs of cure are completed."

Take two *hengshi*[1] and grind them against each other. Take the bits which are ground to the consistency of gruel and spread them on the dog bite. It will desist.

MSI.E.29 (CC57-59)

Another. When a mad dog bites a person, thoroughly clean[2] silted water. Pour it into a cup, the amount equivalent to the second serving of beverage.[3] Take a three-fingered pinch of stove residue ash[4] and [2] in the water. Give it to the ailing person to drink. After drinking, have him vigorously shake both hands, like [2] {2} [1] {1} [9] the person bitten by the mad dog [3] spread nothing on it.

MSI.E.30 (C60)

Another. When a mad dog wounds a person, smith *yu* (arsenopyrite) and *tuomo*.[5] Drink it in one half cup of gruel vinegar.[6] Women use the same medicine. {1} [?].

MSI.E.31 (CC61-62)

Wound Caused by a Dog Biting a Person

Take two *sheng* of earthworm excrement[7] along with an equal amount of dirt deposited at the bottom of the water jar kept by the

---

[1]*MWD*, vol. 4, "Transcription," n. 2, identifies *hengshi* 恒石 with *changshi* 長石, which is listed in *BC* (*GM*, 9.75). The identification is plausible, but uncertain. *ZY*: no. 0915, identifies *changshi* as anhydrite.

[2]*SW*, 11A-2.37a, glosses *sao* 澡 as "wash the hands." In *MSI*.E.29 *sao* refers to "cleaning" the silted water, probably to make it more suitable for drinking. *KGS*, vol. 1: 164, n. 173, reads *sao* as *lao* 撈, in the sense of "pick out floating debris." *MWD*, vol. 4, "Transcription," reads *sao* as *cao* 操, which Ma Jixing interprets to mean "manage, prepare" (1992: 381, n. 3). I reject the latter reading; the first reading is more plausible in that it still relates to cleaning the silted water.

[3]A "second serving of beverage" clearly represents a form of measure (perhaps related to rules governing the serving of drink at rituals and banquets), but there is no record of it in received literature.

[4]"Stove residue ash" is one of several terms used in the Mawangdui medical manuscripts for ash removed from the stove. *MWD*, vol. 4, "Transcription," n. 4, identifies "stove residue ash" with *fulong gan* 伏龍肝, which Tao Hongjing identifies as the yellow soil that accumulates inside the stove (*GM*, 7.8l).

[5]*MWD*, vol. 4, "Transcription," n. 1, identifies *tuomo* 橐莫 with *tuowu* 橐吾, which is undoubtedly correct. *BC* gives *tuowu* as an alternate name for *kuandong* 款冬 (*GM*, 16.102), identified in *ZY*: no. 4782, as *Tussilago farfara* L. However, the Wuwei recipes indicate that in Han times *tuowu* and *kuandong* were two distinct plants. Akahori demonstrates that *tuowu* was the name for *T. farfara*, while the early identity of *kuandong* is not known (1978: 104, nn. 191-92).

[6]*Xi* 醯 is a rich vinegar made from rice gruel fermented in liquor (*SW*, 5A.48a).

[7]Earthworm excrement is the fine soil produced by earthworms. Tao Hongjing discusses this substance in his commentary to the entry on earthworms (*GM*, 42.40), and observes that it was a regular ingredient in the lute used to seal alchemical vessels.

well. Scorch them together and take fine gruel vinegar [4] it. Shape roughly into balls and hot-press the wound with them. When the dog fur is completely removed, spread (the medicine balls) on the wound and it desists.

*MS*I.E.32 (C63)

Another. Boil stalks.[1] Wash it with the liquid. During winter days, boil the root.

*MS*I.E.33 (CC64-65)

Another. Recipe to make a dog bite not be painful and to make it easy to cure. Have the person who was bitten lie down and have someone else pour a sufficient amount of liquor over the wound. After pouring, [1] {1} it. Previously tested. There are no prohibitions.

*MS*I.E.34 (C66)

Nest[2]

Watch for lightning in heaven; then rub both hands together, face the lightning, and chant this incantation: "Eastern Quarter Sovereign, Western Quarter [4] preside over the dark. Darken this person's stars."[3] Do it twice seven times and [1].

---

[1]*MWD*, vol. 4, "Transcription," n. 1, notes that the name of the plant whose stalks are used must have been omitted by the scribe. Ma Jixing argues that *jing* 莖 (stalk) should be read as *jing* 葝, which is the name of a kind of wild onion (1992: 385, n. 1). The instruction below to boil the root in winter leads me to doubt Ma's interpretation.

[2]The ailment name *chao* 巢 (nest) is not attested in received literature. *Chao* occurs again in *MS*I.E.152-53 below designating an anal fistula. The ailment denoted by *chao* in *MS*I.E.34-35 is uncertain. It is probably a condition affecting the skin and flesh. *MWD*, vol. 4, "Transcription," n. 1, speculates that *chao/*dzragw* might represent a phonetic loan for *sao/*tshagw* 臊, and that the ailment is "body odor." Continuing with this speculation, it is suggested that *xing* 星 (star) in the incantation should be read as *xing* 腥, interpreted as "stench." I agree with the reading of the word *xing* in the incantation, but not the meaning "stench." *SW*, 4B.36a-b, distinguishes between the *xing* written 胜, which means "stench of dog fat"; and written 腥, which means "small hard growths produced in the flesh of pigs when they are fed while the stars are out." The Duan Yucai commentary notes several passages in the *Liji* that apply this word to hard, inedible lumps in pork. I would argue that in *MS*I.E.34 *xing* represents a pun which links the ailment to the influence of stars on the body. It seems likely that a transfer of stellar essence was believed to produce small growths in the flesh, and that these growths had the appearance of a "nest." Thus I reject the identification of the ailment as body odor in favor of some kind of growth, perhaps including polyps. It is because of the astral etiology that *MS*I.E.34 exploits a flash of lightning and an incantation ordering spirits to "darken the stars/growths."

[3]Spirits from the east and west who "preside over the dark" may be deities of the sun and moon. The incanted request to "darken the stars" refers both to the stars that have caused

MSI.E.35 (C67)

Another. Take choice[1] beef, *wuhui* (monkshood), and *gui* (cinnamon). Smith in equal amounts and blend. [1] fumigate, thereby [1] the ailment.[2]

MSI.E.36 (CC68–70)

Xixia[3]

Take a three-*cun* long piece of *huangqin* (skullcap) and thirty *helu* the size of [2] beans, skins removed;[4] and smith them together. [7]. Pestle, and boil until it bubbles. Squeeze to remove the dregs.[5] Then using the liquid [2] chill[6] the *xixia*. When finished, use suet [7] the smithed medicine and spread (the medicine) on it. If you are going to spread (the medicine) on it again, chill and spread as before. When finished, the *xixia* vanishes.

MSI.E.37 (C71)

Wuhui (Monkshood) Poisoning[7]

---

the growths and the growths themselves. The rhyming words in the incantation are *ming/*ming* 冥 (dark) and *xing/*sing* 星 (star).

[1]"Choice" translates *niu* 朒, glossed in *SW*, 14B.28b as "edible meat" (i.e. a choice cut of meat for fine eating).

[2]Apparently the blend of beef, *wuhui*, and *gui* is burned as a fumigant to treat the ailment.

[3]The name *xixia* 夕 下 is not attested in received literature. It appears to be another skin or flesh ailment. Reading the name literally, it might refer to "darkening" or "dark blotches" on the skin. *MWD*, vol. 4, "Transcription," n. 1, notes that *xi/*rjiak* might be a phonetic loan for *yi/*rak* 腋 (underarm), in which case it would be an ailment that affects the underarm region—perhaps a scrofular condition.

[4]*Helu* 合 盧 is an unidentified herbal drug. The quantity thirty, the size indication, and the instruction to remove the skins suggest that the drug is a fruit or seed.

[5]There are two different drug preparations used to treat *xixia*. The first is a salve of *huangqin* and *helu*—apparently mixed with suet and spread on the affected area (see below). In addition, there is a decoction whose ingredients are missing in the seven-graph lacuna above. This decoction is strained and applied to the affected area before the salve. *Jin* 搢, translated as "squeeze," is not attested in received literature. *MWD*, vol. 4, "Transcription," n. 3, reads the word as *jin* 晉, glossed as "restrain, press" in the Zheng Xuan commentary in *Zhouli*, 32.10b (the passage concerns horsemanship). My guess is that with the addition of "water," the word means to press the liquid out of something. The instruction to "squeeze to remove the dregs" suggests the technique of straining a decoction through cloth as described by Tao Hongjing: "Use a new cloth. Two men wring it using a piece of wood that is one *chi* long" (*GM*, 1.39).

[6]"Chill" is a literal translation of *qi/*tshiəd* 淒. *MWD*, vol. 4, "Transcription," n. 4, proposes reading it as a phonetic loan for *kai/*krəd* 揩 (rub), which is phonologically inadmissible—and besides, it is unlikely that a decoction would be "rubbed" on the body. Perhaps *qi* refers to cooling the *xixia* by bathing it with the decoction (and the unknown ingredients of the decoction also may have had cooling properties).

[7]*Wuhui* is an aconite and was a well-known poison in early China. Presumably incidents of poisoning could have been accidental or purposeful. *MSI*.E.42 describes applying medicine

Roast [2]. Drink the urine of a young boy or fresh *jichi*,[1] and then with water drink [?].

*MS*I.E.38 (C72)

Another. Flake *shaoyao* (peony). With one half cup of [1] take a large three-fingered pinch and drink it.

*MS*I.E.39 (C73)

Another. Take a one-*chi* long piece of *qi* (lycium) root the thickness of a finger. Peel it. Pound it in a wooden mortar. Boil in liquor [?].

*MS*I.E.40 (C74)

Another. Using [1] liquid, swallow soybeans[2] or *ku*.[3] It desists.

*MS*I.E.41 (C75)

Another. Boil iron and drink it.

*MS*I.E.42 (C76)

Another. When there is an occurrence of a person being poisoned, take *miwu* (lovage) root or [1] *ji*,[4] one [9]. Spread (the medicine) on the wound.[5]

*MS*I.E.43 (C77)

Another. Dig up the ground to a depth of [1] *chi*, and then boil one jar of water [11] one cup.

*MS*I.E.44 (C78)

Scorpion

[7] {3} *xie* (scallion) [?].

---

to a wound, providing the earliest evidence of the practice of coating weapons—especially arrow tips—with the poison (called *shewang* 射罔 by Tao Hongjing; *GM*, 17.46).

[1]*Jichi* 齊赤 is an unidentified drug name. For several guesses, see Ma Jixing 1992: 392, nn. 5-6; and *KGS*, vol. 1: 169, n. 203.

[2]*Shu* 菽 sometimes serves as a general term for bean plants, but regularly denotes *dadou* 大豆 (soybean; *Guangya*, 10A.34b). In *MS*I.E, *shu* consistently refers to the soybean.

[3]*Ku* 苦 is a herbal drug of uncertain identity. I favor identifying it with *kucai* 苦菜, listed in *BC* (*GM*, 27.103); and identified in *ZY*: no. 2627, as *Sonchus oleraceus* L. This plant was a regular seasoning in ancient Chinese cuisine, adding a pungent bitter taste to dishes. Han textual sources and the modern botanical identification are discussed in the transcription notes to the grave inventory document from Mawangdui tomb 1, which lists a beef stew and a dog stew flavored with *ku* (Hunan sheng bowuguan and Zhongguo kexueyuan kaogu yanjiusuo 1973, vol. 1: 133). *MWD*, vol. 4, "Transcription," n. 1, associates *ku* with *daku* 大苦, interpreted as a name for the fermented soybean condiment known as *shi* 豉. Ma Jixing gives three other possible identifications for *daku* (1992: 395, n. 3).

[4][1] *ji* 薺 is an unidentified herbal drug.

[5]The wound was probably caused by an arrow or weapon coated with aconite poison.

MSI.E.45 (C79)

Another. [?].

MSI.E.46 (C80)

Another. Moisten, spread salt on it, and have a cow lick it.

MSI.E.47 (C81)

Another. Seal it with *jili* (caltrop) and *baihao* (artemisia).

MSI.E.48 (CC82-83)

Another. Spit on it and spout: "Elder Brother and Father live on Tai Mountain. You dwell down in [1] Ravine.[1] [3] {2} [4] {1} Wind Bird [6] flee. Flee, and its beak[2] will bore your heart."[3]

MSI.E.49 (C84)

Another. "Father dwells in Shu. Mother is the Wind Bird who punishes.[4] Do not dare flee up or down. The Wind Bird bores your heart."[5]

---

[1]There is another occurrence of Tai Mountain 大山 (the Great Mountain) in *MSI*.E.229. In the latter recipe, the mountain is definitely the sacred peak of the east situated in present-day Shandong; perhaps this denotation applies to *MSI*.E.48 as well. Part of the incantation's efficacy derives from creating a magical space under the dominion of those who occupy the Great Mountain (hence the scorpion spirit blamed for the sting is at their mercy down below).

[2]彖 is used regularly in *MSI*.E to write *hui* 喙 (snout, beak) in the drug name *wuhui* 烏喙.

[3]*MWD*, vol. 4, "Transcription," n. 3, notes that *fengniao* 鳳鳥 (Wind Bird) is written in the text as a fusion graph 鳳 (the sign = indicates that 鳥 is to be repeated). The incantation in *MSI*.E.49 pairs the Wind Bird as Mother with a Father who dwells in Shu. Thus in both incantations it is the Wind Bird/Mother who eliminates the scorpion spirit with her lethal beak. Rather than understand the Wind Bird as the so-called Chinese phoenix, I suspect that it is the kite (*yuan* 鳶). A discussion of ritual banners used in funeral processions in *Liji*, 3.5a, mentions a banner with a "crying kite" emblem; the Zheng Xuan commentary explains the symbolism equating the crying of the kite with wind. A southern tradition of the kite as a wind spirit is indicated in the ca. tenth century *Qinjing*: "The Wind Bird is a kite. The people of Yue call it the Wind Elder. When it soars in flight there is a great wind in the heavens" (*Qinjing*, 11b). Known for its ability to drop from the sky like an arrow to attack its prey—and known as the Wind Elder among the people of Yue—the kite is a likely candidate for the Wind Bird in *MSI*.E.48-49. The extant rhyming words in the incantation are ***xun/*rjəm*** 尋 (flee) and ***xin/*sjəm*** 心 (heart).

[4]My guess is that Father controls the ground (specifying the southwestern region of Shu suggests a southern tradition of magic) and Mother/Wind Bird controls the air, making escape impossible for the scorpion spirit. Translating ***ru*** 蓐 as "punish" is based on reading the word as ***ru*** 辱, which in *SW*, 14B.30b is glossed as "humiliate." The *SW* etymologizes the word as signifying the execution of men who fail to observe the seasonal regulations for agricultural work. "The Wind Bird who punishes" undoubtedly reflects a popular religious belief similar to the belief in Rushou 蓐收, the bird-headed divinity of the east who punishes misdeeds (see Riegel 1989-90: 58).

[5]The rhyming words in the incantation are Shu/*Djuk 蜀 and ***ru/*njuk*** 蓐 (punish); and ***xun/*rjəm*** 尋 (flee) and ***xin/*sjəm*** 心 (heart).

MSI.E.50 (C85)

Leeches Bite a Person's Shin, Thigh, and Knee

When they appear in these places, combine glutinous panicled millet, soybeans, and glutinous spiked millet—three (substances). Cook them. Steam [4] ailment.

MSI.E.51 (C86)

Another. Mince *gui*[1] and spread (the *gui*) on it.

MSI.E.52 (C87)

Lizard[2]

Mince *lan* (eupatorium). Pour liquor over it. Drink the liquid and seal the wound with the dregs. Change it continually. {2} [?].

MSI.E.53 (C88)

Another. Press *ji* (thistle).[3] into the center of the crown of the head.

MSI.E.54 (C89)

Another. Rub it with a raw suckling pig snout.[4]

---

[1] *SW*, 13A.58b, glosses *gui* 蛫 as "crab." Song sources cited in *GM*, 45.17, identify *gui* as a poisonous crab with six legs.

[2] *MWD*, vol. 4, "Transcription," n. 1, identifies *yuan* 蚖 as the name of a poisonous snake. *Yuan* occurs as the name of a type of viper in *BL* (*GM*, 43.80), but this usage appears to be post-Han. Besides, the recipes to treat the ailment in *MSI*.E do not describe the kind of emergency treatment that would be expected if the ailment were the lethal bite of the viper. *SW*, 13A.43a, glosses *yuan* with *rongyuan* 蠑蚖 and *sheyi* 它醫. Both names are applied to various lizards. According to the fourth century *Gujinzhu*, 2.5b, *rongyuan* is the name for large lizards which can be as long as three *chi*; and the dark purplish black ones like to bite people. The Shuanggudui *Wanwu* also identifies *yuan* "lizard" as the name of an ailment (Fuyang Han jian zhenglizu 1988: 39).

[3] 葪 is an attested variant graph for *ji* 薊 (see *Shanhaijing*, 5.23a). *BL* lists a large and a small *ji* (*GM*, 15.34); the former identified as *Cirsium japonicum* DC (*ZY*: no. 0191), and the latter as *Cephalanoplos segetum* (Bge.) Kitam. (*ZY*: no. 0479). *MWD*, vol. 4, "Transcription," n. 1, reads the graph as *jie* 芥 (*Brassica juncea*; mustard), noting the use of mustard plasters as a counterirritant in medicine. The textual evidence is not convincing, and I do not accept the reading.

[4] *MWD*, vol. 4, "Transcription," reads 豙 as *yi* 藙, identified as a name for the herb *zhuyu* 茱萸. This reading is clearly justified in *MSI*.E.103 where 豙 occurs together with the drug name *zhuyu*. However, the weight of evidence in *MSI*.E.54 is far from convincing. Han ritual literature stating that a condiment of *yi* is eaten with the "three sacrificial animals" (cow, sheep, pig) is adduced in the "Transcription," n. 1, to explain the term "suckling pig *yi*." Ma Jixing offers a different argument—that *chan tun* 產豚 means "fresh and plump" (referring to the *zhuyu* fruit) not "raw suckling pig" (1992: 406, nn. 2-3). Despite additional circumstantial evidence concerning the later use of *zhuyu* as a drug, Ma's interpretation of *chan tun* remains unconvincing and I still question reading 豙 as *yi*. I provisionally adopt the argument in Qiu Xigui 1992: 531, and read the graph 豙 as *hui* 喙

MSI.E.55 (C90)

Another. Take one piece of *jin* and beat it into bits.[1] Seal it (with the medicine). Then incinerate deer horn and drink it with urine.

MSI.E.56 (C91)

Another. Blow: "Tsjar![2] Nien bites.[3] The killed man now cries out."[4] Repeat it again.

MSI.E.57 (CC92-93)

Another. Make gruel with blue choice millet grains.[5] Use fifteen parts water to one part grain to produce five *dou* of gruel.[6] Remove it, let the vapor steam away, and fill a new pottery water jar with it. Cover the mouth with three layers of cloth. Then seal it with mud

---

(snout) in *MSI*.E.54 (see *MSI*.E.48). Perhaps this treatment is similar to *MSI*.E.46, which treats a scorpion sting by having a cow lick it.

[1]"Beat into bits" translates *yang zhu* 陽筑. I am guessing that *yang* modifies *zhu* to indicate the manner in which the drug is beaten. Lacking an appropriate meaning for *yang* itself in this context, perhaps it can be read as *dang* 蕩 (broken apart, scattered). *KGS*, vol. 1: 178, n. 243, proposes this reading, but interprets *dang* to mean "clean" and translates *dang zhu* as "clean (the *jin*) and beat it." The identification of *jin* 堇 is uncertain. *MWD*, vol. 4, "Transcription," n. 1, equates it with *jincai* 堇菜. According to Miao Qiyu's commentary in *Qimin yaoshu* 28, 3.161, the plant denoted by this name is a viola, perhaps *Viola yedoensis* Makino or *V. verucunda* A. Gray. Several other possible identifications for *jin* are summarized in Ma Jixing 1992: 408, n. 1.

[2]*Jie/*tsjar* 嗟 is one of several incantatory utterances in the *MSI*.E incantations. In *MSI*.E.128, *yu/*gwjag* 吁 is the first word uttered in the incantation, followed by the name of an animal demon. The *locus classicus* for the compound utterance **gwjag *tsjar* is *Shijing*, Mao 11, 1C.7a; and Mao 25, 1E.8b. The themes of both poems concern auspicious animals—the *lin* 麟 in the former and the *zouyu* 騶虞 in the latter—and the utterances are followed immediately by the animal names. The purpose of the utterances is to conjure the animal spirits. In *MSI*.E these utterances are used in a specifically exorcistic manner to magically force the demon responsible for the ailment into submission.

[3]Although *nien* 年 is not attested as the name of a spirit in received literature, I suspect that in the incantations in *MSI*.E.56 and *MSI*.E.60 the lizard spirit blamed for the ailment is named Nien. The verb *he* 蓋 is used when a venomous bug or scaly creature delivers a bite or sting (*SW*, 13A.53b).

[4]I read *zi* 兹 in the text as *zi* 嗞 (cry out). The latter word is glossed in *SW*, 2A.25a, with *jie/*tsjar*. *Zi* is another word used in *MSI*.E to denote the action of calling upon spirits—I suspect in this case to call upon other spirits to aid the "killed man" (i.e. the wounded man). The rhyming words in the incantation are: *he/*hrjiag* 蓋 (bite) and *zi/*tsjəg* 嗞 (cry out). See Luo and Zhou 1958: 81, for evidence that these words rhymed in southern dialects in Han times.

[5]"Choice millet" translates *liang* 粱, which refers to the choicest grade of *su* 粟 (*ZY*: no. 4841, *Setaria italica* [L.] Beauv.; spiked millet). *BL* classifies the large seeds of *liang* according to color: white, yellow, and blue (i.e. a dark bluish-black hue; *GM*, 23.75).

[6]Ma Jixing interprets this to mean that one *dou* of millet is cooked in fifteen *dou* of water (1992: 410).

two *cun* thick. Bake until the mud is completely fired, and drink it. The wound desists.

*MS*I.E.58 (CC94-95)

Another. Boil two roosters that have been aged for three nights,[1] pouring three *dou* of water (into the kettle). Remove when done. Scoop out[2] the liquid and pour it over (the roosters) again. Set a [metal][3] [1] beneath a slotted steaming-pot[4] and cook the five grains.[5] Drop rabbit [1] flesh into the slotted steaming-pot.[6] Gradually pour the liquid on top, letting it collect in the bowl below. When done, drink the liquid.[7]

*MS*I.E.59 (C96)

Another. Spout and blow: "Hidden eater. Father's dwelling is at the north. Mother's dwelling is to the south. Together they gave

---

[1]*Su* 宿 means literally "pass the night." In *MS*IV.7 a drug is soaked in vinegar for "five nights (*su*)"; that is, for a five day period counted by nights. In *MS*I.E.58 I assume that the roosters are killed and then allowed to age for a three day period before cooking. A similar use of *su* occurs in *MS*III.54, which calls for "three-night-old rooster blood." Ma Jixing argues that *su* in *MS*I.E.58 refers to "years of age," and that the recipe calls for "three-year-old roosters (1992: 412, n. 2). But Ma does not provide sufficient evidence to support this interpretation of *su*.

[2]I read text *ji* 及 as *ji* 汲 (draw water, scoop).

[3]The graph in C94 is fragmentary and is transcribed as 食 in *MWD*, vol. 4, "Transcription." Qiu Xigui argues that the graph in the text looks like *jin* 金 (metal; 1992: 531). Comparing the fragmentary graph to other occurrences of 食 and 金 in *MS*I.E, I am inclined to agree with Qiu.

[4]At the end of the recipe the broth from the boiled roosters is poured into the steaming apparatus and drops into a bowl. I suspect that the graph missing in the preceding lacuna is *yu* 盂 (bowl). It appears that a metal bowl is set beneath the *yan* 甗 (slotted steaming-pot), which itself rests on top of the *fu* 釜 (kettle) holding the water for steaming. Sun Ji reviews the archaeological evidence for the steaming apparatus in Han times, which consisted of an upper pot with a slotted bottom that fit into the mouth of the kettle below (1991: 332).

[5]There are differing lists of which grains constitute the "five grains" in Han sources. The various identifications are discussed in Hayashi 1975: 10. Millet, barley, soybean, rice, and hemp could all be among the grains called for in *MS*I.E.58.

[6]I do not accept *MWD*, vol. 4, "Transcription," which reads *tuo* 陀 (drop) as *tuo* 他 (another). The graph in the lacuna is fragmentary. The "Transcription," n. 2, states that it might be *tou* 頭; and further speculates that *tutou* 兔頭 (rabbit head) might be the name of a kind of melon.

[7]The recipe involves rather complicated cookery to produce a rich broth. First the roosters are boiled; and when they are done, the broth is poured over them once again. Having placed a bowl beneath the slotted steaming-pot (perhaps attached to the bottom of the pot or resting on the kettle below), grain is cooked and "rabbit [1] flesh" is added to the cooked grain in the slotted steaming-pot. Finally, the rooster broth is poured over and the liquid collects in the bowl.

birth to three men who do not treat people virtuously. Desist. If you do not desist, *qing* (azurite) will be spread on it."[1]

*MS*I.E.60 (CC97-98)

Another. Put one cup of silted water into a large-bellied gourd.[2] Carry it in the left hand. Facing north, face towards the person and perform the Pace of Yu thrice.[3] Ask his name. Then say: "So-and-so was [1] by a certain Nien and now [1]."[4] Have (the person) drink one half cup and say: "Ailment [2] desist; slowly leave, slowly desist." Then cover the gourd flask and discard it.

*MS*I.E.61 (C99)

Another. Boil deer flesh or wild pig flesh. Eat it and drink the liquid. Superb.

*MS*I.E.62 (C100)

Another. Incinerate the skin of a *li* (raccoon-dog).[5] Smith the ash. Put it into liquor and drink. Large amounts are permitted and do not harm the person. Boil sheep flesh. Take the liquid and [1] it.

---

[1]*Qing* 青 refers primarily to azurite (*ZY*: no. 3062), but is applied to malachite and other copper ores. It is listed in *BC* (*GM*, 10.11). In addition to the natural ores, verdigris (*tongqing* 銅 青) was also used in medicine. *Qianjin yaofang*, 76.3a, provides a recipe for treating snake, reptile, and insect bites by simply spreading verdigris over the wound. In *MS*I.E.59 the incantation threatens the lizard spirit with the three rough men and in addition names the drug that will be applied to the wound to expel it. *Qing* itself was probably applied to the bite wound at the conclusion of the incantation. The incantations in *MS*I.E.233 and *MS*I.E.235 employ a similar strategy, concluding with the threat to apply feces to the skin to expel the spirit blamed for the ailment. The rhyming words in the incantation are: *shi/*djək* 食 (eater), *zai/*dzəg* 在 (is at), *zhi/*krjəg* 止 (is to), *de/*tək* 德 (virtuously), *yi/*rəg* 已 (desist), and *zhi/*tjəg* 之 (it).

[2]The *jili* 奚 蠡 (large-bellied gourd) is identified as a water vessel with a capacity of up to one *dou* in *Mozi* 52, 14.309. *Jili* is synonymous with *huli* 瓠 蠡 as a name for gourds used as containers. The gourd is either *hulu* 壺 盧 (*ZY*: no. 3683, *Lagenaria siceraria* [Molina] Standl. var. *depressa* Ser.) or *ku hulu* 苦 壺 盧 (*ZY*: no. 2653,*L. siceraria* [Molina] Standl. var. *gourda* Ser.). For another gourd container, see *MS*I.E.134.

[3]There are seven additional occurrences of the Pace of Yu 禹 步: *MS*I.E.67, 118, 120, 128, 225, 276, and *MS*III.83. See the discussion in the Prolegomena, Section Five, "Varieties of Magic."

[4]Based on the parallel with the incantation in *MS*I.E.56, the incantation might read: "So-and-so was [bitten] by a certain Nien and now [cries out]."

[5]I accept Schafer's judgment that *li* 貍 refers to the raccoon-dog (*Nyctereutes procyonoides*; 1987: 29). The Asian raccoon-dog is a small fox-like animal with dark fur by the eyes resembling raccoon markings (see Tate 1947: 162). In *Huainanzi*, 10.154, *li* is said to belong to the same category of animal as the fox (*hu* 狐), the two animals being easily mistaken for one another. *Li* is commonly identified as wild cat (*ZY*: no. 3904, *Felis bengalensis* Kerr).

MSI.E.63 (C101)

Take[1] mud from inside a well. Surround and seal the wound with it. It desists.

MSI.E.64 (C102)

Warts[2]

Take a worn-out cattail mat or the soft leaves of a cattail bedmat[3] and make them into a cord. Then light the tip and cauterize the tip of the wart with it. When it becomes hot, pluck off the wart and discard it.[4]

MSI.E.65 (C103)

Another. Have the person with warts clasp grain plants.[5] Have other people shout: "Why do you do this." Respond: "I am the wart." Set the grain plants down and leave without looking back.

MSI.E.66 (C104)

Another. On the last day of the month[6] go to an abandoned well that has water in it. Brush the warts twice seven times with a worn out broom and chant this incantation: "Today is the last day of the month. I brush the warts to the north."[7] Drop the broom into the well.

MSI.E.67

(CC105-107) Another. On the last day of the month at the end of the late afternoon,[8] take clods the size of a chicken egg—men seven and

---

[1]The usual "another" does not occur at the head of *MSI*.E.63.

[2]For the identification of *you* 疣 with warts, see Yu Yan 1972: 243.

[3]*Jie* 藉 (cattail bedmat) is synonymous with *jian* 薦, the doublefaced mat filled with straw used for sleeping. *SW*, 1B.14a, glosses *ruo* 蒻 as the soft young leaves of the cattail which are suitable for covering a bedmat. The ancient vocabulary for mats and relevant archaeological data are summarized in Hayashi 1976: 203–204.

[4]Judging from this description of how to perform cauterization and one other description in *MSI*.E.127, early cauterization treatment entailed touching the person's skin with a brand-like material: a burning cattail cord in *MSI*.E.64, and a kind of cigarette wrapped in *ai* (mugwort) leaves in *MSI*.E.127. Presumably the technique used was similar whenever cauterization is mentioned in the Mawangdui medical manuscripts. The mugwort cigarette in *MSI*.E.127 is not moxa, and its use should not be construed as moxibustion.

[5]*He* 禾 was a general term for grain plants in Han times. Perhaps it refers to spiked millet, as it did in Shang and Zhou times (see Hayashi 1975: 4).

[6]*Hui* 晦 denotes the day when the moon is darkest preceding the appearance of the new moon.

[7]The rhyming words in the incantation are: *hui/*hməg* 晦 (last day of month) and *bei/*pək* 北 (north).

[8]*Bu* 餔 refers the time of day when the sun is low on the western horizon and is used to designate a division of the day corresponding to 3:00–5:00 P.M. This is also the time of one

women twice seven. First set the clods[1] down behind the house, arranging them in a line from south to north. When dark, go to the place where the clods are. Perform the Pace of Yu thrice. Starting from the southern quarter, pick up a clod and say:[2] "Today is the last day of the month. I rub the warts to the north."[3] Rub the [1][4] once with the clod. After rubbing, set the clod back in its place and leave without looking back.

MSI.E.68 (C108)

Another. On the last day of the month, go behind the inner (chamber).[5] Say: "Today is the last day of the month. I rub the warts north of the inner (chamber)."[6] Rub the warts on the wall of the inner (chamber) twice seven times.

MSI.E.69 (CC109-110)

Another. On the first day of the month,[7] rub the warts twice seven times with *kui* (mallow) stalks. Say: "Today is the first day of the month. I rub the warts with a *kui* (mallow) halberd."[8] In addition, take *sha* root[9] or *jian* root[10] from the side of the road—twice seven in number—and toss them into a marsh or deep pool. If it is a "removal day," (wait until) after mid-month.[11]

---

of the standard meals. *Xiabu* 下餔 (end of the late afternoon) corresponds to a time around 5:00 P.M. (see Chen Mengjia 1965: 123).

[1] *MWD*, vol. 4, "Transcription," emends the text by adding *yi* 以 before the word for "clod." The meaning of the text is clear as written, and I do not accept the emendation.

[2] The phrase 塊言曰 is written twice in the text, an obvious scribal error.

[3] The rhyming words are the same as *MSI*.E.66.

[4] The lacuna is probably *you* 疣 (warts).

[5] I.e. the bedroom.

[6] The rhyming words are the same as *MSI*.E.66.

[7] *Shuo* 朔 denotes the day of the new moon.

[8] Presumably the mallow halberd represents the nature of the mallow stalks as an exorcistic weapon. The rhyming words in the incantation are *shuo/*sngrawk* 朔 (first day of month) and *ji/*kjiak* 戟 (halberd).

[9] *SW*, 6A.14a, describes *sha* 榝 as a plant that "resembles *zhuyu* (evodia) and comes from Huainan." Other sources simply identify *sha* as *zhuyu*. Ma Jixing discusses two additional identifications (1992: 423, n. 6).

[10] *MWD*, vol. 4, "Transcription," reads *jian* 前 as *jian* 葥. The latter graph is glossed with *wanghui* 王蔧 in *Erya*, 8.1b; and *wanghui* is an alternate name for *difu* 地膚, listed in *BC* (*GM*, 16.105) and identified as broomplant (*ZY*: no. 1635, *Kochia scoparia* [L.] Schrad.). The dried stalks of *difu* were commonly used to make brooms. Perhaps *jian* in *MSI*.E.69 refers to this plant.

[11] The reference to a "removal day" is to a hemerological system known as *jianchu* 建除 (establishment and removal). According to the description of the system in *Huainanzi*, 3.48, each of the twelve Branches of the sexagenary cycle is correlated with one of twelve

MSI.E.70 (C111)

Another. To treat warts by incantation, go to the north of the house on the last day of the month. Rub the warts—men seven times and women twice seven times. Say: "Today is the last day of the month. I rub the warts north of the house."[1] The warts desist within a month.

MSI.E.71 (CC112-13)

Seizure Sickness[2]

First have ready a white chicken and dog feces. When it occurs,[3] use a knife to cut open his head from the crown to the nape. Then moisten that with the dog feces and halve the chicken. [1] cover the place that was moistened with dog feces. Stop after three days. After stopping, cook the chicken that was used to cover and eat it. [1] desists.[4]

---

divinatory signs, among which *jian* "establishment" is the first in the sequence and *chu* "removal" the second. To give an example, the first lunar month is assigned the Branch *yin* 寅, making the Branch *yin* the sign of "establishment" and the following Branch *mao* 卯 the sign of "removal" during the course of the first month. If during the first month, a day which includes the Branch *mao* in its cyclical designation occurs, this day is a "removal" day and is unlucky. The earliest records of the *jianchu* system are in the Shuihudi and Fangmatan hemerological manuscripts. Kalinowski analyzes the Shuihudi evidence (1986: 198-99). In *MSI*.E.69 the restriction prohibits a person from performing the ritual and incantation on the first day of the month if that day happens to have a "removal" Branch in its cyclical designation for the month in question; as would be the case if the first day of the first month happened to be *guimao* 癸 卯. When this circumstance arises, the person must wait until after mid-month; i.e. after the fifteenth day which is the day of the full moon (*wang* 望).

[1]The rhyming words are the same as *MSI*.E.66.

[2]Yu Yan reviews references to *dian* 癲 in received literature, concluding that the ailment encompasses epileptic fits as well as fits of craziness (1972: 109-113). In *MSI*.E.71 the ailment name is written 顛, literally "crown of the head." There is evidently an etymological and etiological link between the ailment and the head, since the treatment described in the recipe involves making an incision from the crown to the nape of the afflicted person's head. *Dian* also means "fall over," which is often cited in explanations of the ailment in received literature and is the basis for Yu Yan's identification with epilepsy.

[3]I.e. when the seizure occurs.

[4]The graph in the lacuna is fragmentary. Ma Jixing writes *zhi* 致 without explanation (1992: 426). Having examined the manuscript, the fragments are not decipherable and I do not accept Ma's emendation.

*MS*I.E.72 (C114)

Another. For seizure sickness, take *quanwei*[1] and grain plants that are on the wall of the animal pen. Smith it, hammering. Drink with silted water.

*MS*I.E.73 (CC115-16)

Recipe for *Baichu*[2]

Take Guan *qing* (azurite), another name for which is Guan laminar[3]—using (an amount) like [2]; salt, one twentieth of a *dou*; and yellow earth from the stove,[4] one tenth of a *sheng*. Smith all and [2] {1} and drink it before eating. If it does not desist, repeat it again and [1] the Guan *qing* (azurite). Drink a second time and it desists. Excellent.

*MS*I.E.74 (CC117-29)

Another. [2] {1} [5] {3} [2]. To treat it, take one half *dou* of unbroken bird eggs,[5] [1] sweet salt [15] {1} [6] into it. The eggs come second. {1} [5]. Cover the water jar with four [layers] of cloth [16] three [6] {1}. After daubing (the medicine) on it, hang (the medicine) in the [place] for drying in the dark.[6] [20]. Cover the flesh

---

[1]*MWD*, vol. 4, "Transcription," n. 1, suggests that *quanwei* 犬尾 may be the same as *gouwei cao* 狗尾草 (*ZY*: no. 2959, *Setaria viridus* [L.] Beauv.) listed in later materia medica (*GM*, 16.120).

[2]The ailment name *baichu* 白處 is not attested in received literature. According to *MS*I.E.75, "whiteness and no webbed pattern (on the skin)" is a sign of the occurrence of the ailment. *Baichu* can be translated "white patches," and perhaps the ailment is vitiligo. However, the meaning of the ailment name is complicated by the fact that *MS*I.E.74-75 use three different graphs to represent the second word: 施, 瘧, and 虘. On the assumption that all four graphs are intended to represent the same word, I provisionally read them all as *chu*. The probability that *chu* itself denotes a specific ailment—and does not simply mean "patch"—is increased by the occurrence of the ailment name 疕 in *Wanwu*, where it is not preceded by *bai* "white" (Fuyang Han jian zhenglizu 1988: 37). 疕 and the variant graph 疟 occur in medieval rhyming dictionaries, but the meaning is uncertain (Morohashi 1957-60, vol. 7: no. 22101).

[3]It is likely that Guan 灌 is a toponym identifying the source of the mineral. The alternate name Guan *ceng* 曾 (laminar) indicates that the azurite to be used is a stratified variety.

[4]I.e. stove ash.

[5]Because the recipe below specifies the exact time in spring to gather the eggs, they may be the eggs of sparrows and other small wild birds, known generically as *que* 雀 (dickeybird). See *MS*III.16.

[6]The complete phrase *yinzao suo* 陰燥所 occurs below, so there is no difficulty filling the lacuna here with *suo* "place." The reference to a room for drying and storing drugs suggests that such rooms were to be found in elite households. Perhaps the *yinzao suo* in *MS*I.E.74 is related to the palace *pushi* 暴室 (drying chamber). The Yan Shigu commentary in *Hanshu*, 8.2a, derives the name from the activity of processing and dyeing silk, but his explanation has been discounted several times (cf. Goodrich 1966). The *pushi* was also

thickly, completely covering the areas with *chu* and no more. [5] {2} [4]. Stop when the heat is unbearable.[1] Having stopped, the *chu* [2]. Even though it responds,[2] do not remove the medicine. The medicine [2] {2} [1]. [2] {1} [1]. When roasting it, [1] eat very [3] {1}, and do not spread (the medicine) on it with the hands. Spread the medicine at dawn before eating. After spreading the medicine, drink good liquor, stopping when very sated. Then roast [1]. After roasting [1] it and rise. When you want to eat, eat. Goings and comings as well as drink and food are all as you wish. Apply the medicine at dawn. Beforehand, do not eat [1] for two to three days. While applying the medicine, do not eat fish. When the ailment desists, (you may do things) as before. While treating the ailment there are no temporal (restrictions).

Collect the bird eggs between the fifteenth and seventeenth of the second and third months. After [1], then use them. [2] bird. Even though the eggs have kernels[3] they are still usable. When this medicine is finished, even if it sits for over ten years up to [1] years, it continues to get better. [1] becomes dry and cannot be daubed on the body, take a small amount of the medicine—sufficient to daub on the *chu*—and [1] it in a shallow pottery bowl with fine gruel vinegar. Let it soak [1] and it can be blended, gradually returning to its regular (consistency). Boil gelatin.[4] Then set the bowl over a fire of grain chaff until the medicine is finished and remove it. After removing it [4] daubing, cover with cloth, use a shallow bowl as a

---

the infirmary and place of detention for the ladies of the palace, a use that would fit well with a place used primarily for processing drugs.

[1]Repetition of 而 止 in the text is an obvious scribal error. It becomes clear a little later in the recipe that the egg-base medicine is daubed on the skin with *chu*, which is then roasted over a fire. To help alleviate the pain of the roasting treatment the recipe tells the patient to first get drunk on good liquor.

[2]"Respond" translates *yu* 愈, which is one of two words used in *MSI*.E to indicate that the medicine or therapy has taken effect, and that the patient is moving toward full recovery. *MSI*.E.95 states that the ailment *yu* "responds" after one treatment, and that it is finally cured after three days of repeating the treatment once a day. In *MSI*.E.117 *zhi* 智 is the word used to mean that the ailment responds to the treatment.

[3]I.e. fertilized eggs. *Ren* 仁 (kernel) referring to the embryo in a fertilized egg also occurs in "Jie" in the first Shuihudi hemerological manuscript (*SHD*: 212; Harper 1990: 223).

[4]The gelatin must be added to the egg medicine after it boils. *BC* lists gelatin made from various animal hides (*GM*, 50.93) and gelatin made from deer horn (*GM*, 51.28). *MSI*.E.96 calls for adding gelatin in the form of sticks. The production of dried gelatin wafers is described in *Qimin yaoshu* 90, 9.550–52.

lid, and hang it in the place for drying in the dark. Medicine made ten years previous becomes dry.

MSI.E.75 (CC130-31)

Another. *Baichu*. When *baichu* occurs, there is whiteness and no webbed pattern. Take cinnabar granules and *zhanyu* (sturgeon) blood or chicken blood—either one is permissible. Leave a chicken to soak for two [2] it [1]. Scratch the *chu* with the claws until they redden, and [spread] (the medicine) on them.[1] Wash after two days and wipe thoroughly with new cloth. Spread (the medicine) again following this procedure, stopping after thirty days. Excellent.

MSI.E.76 (C132)

Dadai[2]

Incinerate *dang*.[3] Combine with old lard and spread (the medicine) on it.

MSI.E.77 (C133)

Another. Boil gelatin in clear (liquor).[4] Daub (the medicine) on it.

MSI.E.78 (CC134-36)

Recipe for *Ming* Ailment[5]

---

[1]It is not clear what is done with the chicken, unless it was soaked just to prepare the claws for scratching the affected skin.

[2]*Dadai* 大 帶 is not attested in received literature and we can only surmise that it refers to a skin ailment.

[3]𡍬 is unattested in received literature. *MWD*, vol. 4, "Transcription," n. 2, suggests that the right side may be a variant of *dang* 當, but 壋 is also unattested. The romanization *dang* is used for lack of another way to represent the unknown drug.

[4]*Qing* 清 refers to *qingjiu* 清 酒 (clear liquor), one of three grades of liquor listed in *Zhouli*, 5.6b. According to the Zheng Xuan commentary, clear liquor is brewed in winter and is ready to drink the next summer. The name also indicates that it is a filtered liquor (see Hayashi 1976: 74). *MWD*, vol. 4, "Transcription," n. 1, suggests an alternative interpretation that the recipe calls for boiling the liquor "until gelatinous" rather than boiling gelatin in liquor.

[5]*Ming* 螟 is one of two crop pests that are regularly paired in early literature, the second being *te* 螣. The modern identification of both insects is uncertain. Zhou Yao has proposed that *ming* may refer to *Diatraea shariinensis* or *D. venosata*, insects that infest millet and sorghum crops (1957: 43). *Te* has been identified with the locust, but this is clearly inapplicable to pre-Han and Han usage in which *te* is paired with *ming* (the locust constituted a category of pest unto itself). Neither *ming* nor *te* are attested as ailment names in received literature. Yet *MSI*.E.244 and *MSI*.E.248 treat damage caused by the *te* bug: the first for when the *te* chews at the mouth and nose, and the second for when it chews at the teeth. In addition, *Maishu*, "Ailment List," records the name *teshi* 螣 食 (chewing by *te*) for an ailment characterized by painful scabs on the nose (*MSSW*: 72). Identifying crop-destroying pests as the source of decay on the body is not merely figurative, but

Ming is a bug. The places where it chews holes [1]. It does not emerge at a regular spot. Sometimes it is located at the nose, sometimes at the side of the mouth, sometimes at the teeth and gums, sometimes at the hands and fingers [1]. It causes a person's nose to be gouged out and his fingers to break off. To treat it, take fresh raw fish [1] and blend a sufficient amount of salt with it. Spread (the medicine) where the bug has chewed [6] it, stopping when the ailment desists. Previously tested. There are no prohibitions. Excellent.

MSI.E.79 (C137)

[1] *Quan*[1]

[2] put one *quan* into an egg [4] it.

MSI.E.80 (CC138-39)[2]

Put in [?] rabbit skin [?].

MSI.E.81 (C140)

Another. Mince *lan* (eupatorium) [?].

MSI.E.82 (C141)

Another. Use pure liquor [?].

MSI.E.83 (C142)

Another. Pour hot water over [?].

MSI.E.84 (C143)

Yun[3]

---

reflects the belief that the very bugs that destroy crops also afflict the body. In applying the classical pairing of *ming* and *te* to ailments, it is evident in *MSI*.E that the *ming* ailment is the more major and life-threatening of the two. Based on the symptoms in *MSI*.E.78 it has been suggested that the ailment is leprosy, even though two names for an ailment that is definitely associated with leprosy are attested in Qin and Han texts: *li* 癘 (also a word for pestilence) and *eji* 惡疾 (foul sickness; also applied to disabling afflictions like blindness or deafness). I think the identification is plausible. For further analysis of the *ming*-bug ailment, see Harper 1990: 227-30.

[1] *MWD*, vol. 4, "Transcription," n. 2, notes that there is a break in the text following C137; it is not clear how many columns might be missing. *SW*, 13A.43b, glosses *quan* 蠸 as follows: "It is a bug. Another meaning is a major poisonous bite." *Erya*, 9.7a, glosses *quan* as *shougua* 守瓜 (melon guardian), a bug that infests melons. There are several possible ways to interpret the ailment name and the fragment of the one extant recipe. Assuming that the [1] *quan* ailment is similar to the *ming* ailment, it is another case of bug etiology. When the recipe calls for mixing a *quan* bug with egg, perhaps we have a case of homeopathic medicine in which the bug that caused the ailment is used to treat it. Alternatively, the ailment is some kind of poisonous bite that can be treated with its namesake, the *quan* bug.

[2] *MSI*.E.80-83 must belong to the unknown ailment category [1] *zhe* 者 listed in *MSI*.E.1.

Take *lan* (eupatorium) [?].

MSI.E.85 (C144)

Another. Roast *hua* (birch)[1] [?] *yun*.

MSI.E.86 (CC145-47)

To Make a Person Ailing from the Horse not Have Spasms[2]

[?]. Bathe the ailing person with it. If the ailing person is a woman [I], and if a man [?]. Then incinerate a woman's first (menstrual) cloth [?].

MSI.E.87 (CC148-49)[3]

[?] drink. Use cloth [?] in liquor and drink [?].

---

[3]疠 is not attested in received literature, and the reading *yun* is based on the phonetic 云. *MWD*, vol. 4, "Transcription," n. 1, offers two tentative identifications of the ailment name: perhaps it is equivalent to *yun* 殞, glossed in *SW*, 7B.27b, as "an ailment" and associated in later sources with dizzyness (Yu Yan 1972: 113); or it may be a scribal miswriting of *jie* 痎, identified in *SW*, 7B.31b, as a form of *nue* 瘧 (cold and hot syndrome; see *MSI*.B.1).

[1]*SW*, 6A.13b, glosses *hua* 槬 as follows: "A tree. The bark is used to wrap pine pitch." The Duan Yucai commentary adduces early sources to identify this name with *hua* 樺, the Chinese white birch (*ZY*: no. 3657, *Betula platyphylla* Suk.). *GM*, 35.58, includes references to the use of birch bark to make torches of the type described in *SW*. Ma Jixing offers a second identification as *shu* 樗 (1992: 441, n. 2); but the Duan Yucai commentary in *SW*, 6A.6b, indicates that the two graphs were confused for one another and that the identification is invalid.

[2]For *xian* 癇 (spasms) see *MSI*.E.26. According to *MSI*.E.1 there are four categories of *xian* ailments in this section of the text, all named after animals: horse, [I] (the name of the animal is not written in the text, a clear case of scribal error), sheep, and snake. *MSI*.E.86 is the only recipe that can be placed with certainty in the horse type of *xian*, and recipes for the latter three categories are no longer extant (unless the fragmentary phrases in *MSI*.E.87 represent recipes for a subsequent category). *Qianjin yaofang*, 10.15a, describes a classification of *xian* according to the six domestic animals: horse, cow, sheep, pig, dog, and chicken. The sounds emitted by the afflicted person and the contortions of his body during an attack of spasms are the basis for naming each type. The four categories of *xian* ailments in *MSI*.E seem to have a similar basis.

[3]*MWD*, vol. 4, "Transcription," n. 1, notes that there is a break in the text following C149; it is not clear how many columns might be missing. In addition to the three types of *xian*, two other ailment categories are lost: Various Eating Ailments and Various [I] Ailments.

MSI.E.88

(CC150-51)[1] [6] dried *cong* (onion) [?] salt the *duo* (navel)[2] and roast the buttocks.

MSI.E.89 (C152)

Another. Seal the *duo* (navel) and lesser abdomen with *chuohua*[3] [?].

MSI.E.90 (C153)

Another. Smith one third *sheng* of *ximing* (pennycress) and one [1] of old *kui* (mallow) seeds and [?].

MSI.E.91 (C154)

Another. Boil one bunch of *longxu* (bog rush) in three *dou* of silted water. [?].

MSI.E.92 (C155)

Another. Cauterize the middle toe of the left foot.[4]

---

[1]On the basis of *MSI*.E.1 and the fact that the recipes following *MSI*.E.88 open with the conventional "another," *MSI*.E.88 is the first extant recipe in the ailment category Urine Retention (*long* 癃). *Long* is identified as an ailment characterized by "prostration" in *SW*, 7B.34b, and this seems to be the meaning of *long* in *MSI*.E.120. *Suwen* 23, 7.8b, provides positive identification of *long* as retention of urine in the bladder. In *Maishu*, "Ailment List," inability to urinate is called *bi* 閉 (blockage; *MSSW*: 72). *Wanwu* records the name *long* along with the fact that it can be cured with *shiwei* (pyrrosia), the drug used to treat urine retention in *MSI*.E.109 (Fuyang Han jian zhenglizu 1988: 36). *Long* is also the name used in the Wuwei recipes, which record four types of urine retention also treated in *MSI*.E: bloody (*MSI*.E.108), stone (*MSI*.E.109), lardy (*MSI*.E.110), and rice slop (*MSI*.E.95 describes stones that come out "like rice slop" after treatment; *WWYJ*: 2a). The standard name for difficulty in urination in later medical literature is *lin* 淋 (Yu Yan 1972: 239).

[2]*Duo/*duarx* 隋 is not attested as an anatomical name in received literature. I accept Zhao Youchen's argument that it represents a word meaning "navel" (1981). *MWD*, vol. 4, "Transcription," reads it as a phonetic loan for *shui/*djəd* 脽 (buttock). Phonological evidence does not support the loan. Reviewing the related occurrences of *duo* in *MSI*.E.89, 97, 135, and 138, Zhao cites evidence from later medical literature to show that the navel is the logical referent of *duo* in these recipes. Additional support for Zhao's identification comes from *Maishu*, "Ailment List" (see the discussion of *cuo* in *MSI*.A.3). *Duo* has the meaning "oblong" (as in *MSI*.E.146), and this sense may account for its use as a name for the navel. Although unattested, the possibility of an anatomical application is suggested by the Zheng Xuan commentary in *Liji*, 16.13b, which glosses *dou* 竇 as a hole in the ground "with an oblong shape (*duo*)."

[3]*Chuohua* 追 華 is unknown. 追 is also unattested in received literature (the reading *chuo* assumes 𠂤 as phonetic).

[4]Performing cauterization on the middle toe of the left foot does not appear to be related to vessel theory.

MSI.E.93 (CC156-57)

Another. [Perform the Pace of Yu] thrice.[1] Take a cup of silted water. Spout and snort[2] three times. Say: "Above there is [10] spearhead. So-and-so [5] drink it and cover the cup.[3]

MSI.E.94 (CC158-60)

Another. Recipe for when [2] and dries up[4] so that it does not come out. Put pure liquor into a [1]. Boil gelatin, {1} [7] incinerate {1} [4] fire and quench in the liquor. When the bubbling stops, remove it. Have the ailing person drink the liquor. [8] drink it, until [3] and rise as you wish.[5] If it does not desist, repeat [it][6] again following this procedure. Excellent.

MSI.E.95 (CC161-65)

Another. Urine retention. There is pain in the bladder and the inside.[7] The pain is intense, and when urinating [1] the pain is even more intense. [4]. To treat it boil three *sheng* of black soybeans in three [1] of fine gruel vinegar. Cook rapidly. When it bubbles, stop the fire. When the bubbling subsides, cook again, stopping after it bubbles for the third time. Sieve to obtain the liquid. Use one portion of oysters and three of smithed *dujin*[8]—altogether two substances—[2]. Take one three-fingered pinch reaching to the

---

[1]The context clearly indicates that the two-graph lacuna is 禹步.

[2]"Snort" translates *gu* 鼓. *Gu* was used idiomatically to refer to blowing the nose in Han times, as attested in the *SW*, 2A.24a, gloss of *pen* 噴: "Another meaning is to blow (*gu*) the nose."

[3]The conclusion of the incantation is missing in the lacuna. It appears that the cup of silted water is used to magically remove the ailment (similar to the gourd of silted water in *MSI*.E.60).

[4]㿰 appears to be a variant graph for *bi* 㿰. *Bi* is listed in later dictionaries with a meaning of "withered" (Morohashi 1957-60, vol. 7: no. 22588). The word has been linked with *bi* 秕, which *SW*, 7A.49a, glosses as "unformed millet"; i.e. millet that shrivels on the stalk. I suspect that in *MSI*.E.94 *bi* refers to being unable to urinate because the urine "dries up" internally—perhaps forming the kind of bladder stones mentioned in *MSI*.E.95 and 109. *MWD*, vol. 4, "Transcription," n. 1, offers an alternative interpretation by simply reading the graph as a phonetic loan for *bi* 閉 (blocked).

[5]It appears that a solid object has been heated and plunged into the liquor to quench it. Then the person drinks the liquor.

[6]The graph in the lacuna ought to be 之.

[7]"Inside" probably refers to the lower abdominal region around the bladder.

[8]The herb *dujin* 毒 堇 does not appear in later materia medica. *MWD*, vol. 4, "Transcription," n. 4, suggests identifying it with *zijin* 紫 堇 (*ZY*: no. 4867, *Corydalis edulis* Maxim.; see *GM*, 26.84). The description of the herb at the end of *MSI*.E.95 supports rather than negates the identification, but it remains uncertain.

knuckles, put it into lukewarm gruel vinegar, [1] drink it. Drink before eating or after eating as you wish. After drinking it once the ailment responds. Drink it once a day. After three days the ailment desists and a stream of stones like rice slop[1] comes out of the front.[2] There are no prohibitions and no temporal (restrictions). Smith the oysters. Do not dry the *dujin* in the sun. On the day of the summer solstice go to [2] the *dujin*.[3] Dry it in the dark. Smith the leaves and fruits together and store in a leather pouch. When (you need to) use it, take it (from the pouch). Collect *dujin* again every year. *Dujin* [3] *jin* leaves are different and smaller.[4] The stalks are red and the leaves have vertical cords.[5] [1] leaves and fruit have a bitter taste. It forms fruit about six or seven days before the summer solstice. [4] by the side of a marsh. Excellent.

*MS*I.E.96 (C168)

Another. Boil one *dou* of *kui* (mallow) seeds in one *dou* of water. Sieve to obtain the liquid. Boil one and a half sticks of gelatin in the liquid to produce one third *dou* of liquid and [?].

*MS*I.E.97 (C169)

Another. Fill the *duo* (navel) with a small cup of Rong salt[6] or fine salt. In addition, daub it [1] the *duo* (navel) from the bottom reaching to the top,[7] and dry in the sun {1} [?].

---

[1] *Gan* 泔 (rice slop) is one of several words that refer to the liquid left over from cleaning grain to prepare it for cooking (see *SW*, 11A-2.33a).

[2] *Qian* 前 (front) refers to the genitals. See *MS*IV.3.

[3] *MS*I.E.95 provides the earliest testimony to the custom of gathering herbs on the day of the summer solstice, celebrated on the fifth day of the fifth month. In received literature the custom is first mentioned in the sixth century *Jing Chu suishi ji* (Moriya 1963: 353), although the gathering of artemisia to serve as a protective amulet on this day is attested earlier. The summer solstice is the day when the solar power culminates, and herbs gathered on this day swell with potency. Special notice is accorded to red colored plants. The red stalks of *dujin* mentioned below may account for the association with the solstice, although it is equally probable that the fruit is reddish.

[4] I suspect that *dujin* is being compared to another type of *jin* in this sentence; that is, the leaves of *dujin* are smaller than the leaves of the other unknown *jin*.

[5] *Xi* 繫 is literally the main-cord on a net (*SW*, 13A.25a). Here it refers to the distinctive veins on the leaves.

[6] Rong 戎 refers to the northwestern borderlands. This is the source of Rong salt, which is listed in *BC* (*GM*, 11.41).

[7] Because of the lacuna the grammar of the sentence and precise area to be coated with salt are uncertain, but it is somewhere in the vicinity of the *duo* (navel).

MSI.E.98 (C170)

Another. Boil *kui* (mallow) and drink the liquid. In the winter [2] the root. Pour [2].

MSI.E.99 (C171)

Another. Boil *kui* (mallow) and drink the liquid. Then [2] {1}, taking a large amount as the standard,[1] and [2] the buttocks.

MSI.E.100 (C172)

Another. Soak the neckband of an undershirt[2] and dandruff in one cup of liquor. Let it bubble and drink it.

MSI.E.101 (CC173-75)

Another. Urine retention. Recipe for when urination is difficult and the bladder is full. Take two *sheng* of coarsely flaked *zao* (jujube) seeds and one *sheng* of *kui* (mallow) seeds. Combine them, stirring. Divide into three portions. Boil one portion in one and a half *dou* of water. When done, remove the dregs and again boil one portion, proceeding like this until all three portions are used up. Sieve to obtain the liquid. Blend in honey until it is just sweet. When lukewarm [1] drink it. When the medicine is used up, make it again. Stop when the ailment desists. Excellent.

MSI.E.102 (CC176-77)

Another. Urine retention. Take one large bunch of one-*chi* long *jingtian* (stonecrop) and divide into three parts. Scald[3] it thrice in one half *dou* of pure liquor. When done, sieve to obtain the liquid, and drink it. If it does not desist, repeat it. After no more than the

---

[1]The same idiomatic phrase occurs in *MS*III.5, where *yan* 厭 (satiation) replaces *duo* 多 (large amount). The use of *gu* 故 to mean "standard" is attested in *Lüshi chunqiu*, 17.209.

[2]*Ru* 襦 is an undershirt that fits closely around the neck and goes down to the waist. For early text references and archaeological data, see Hayashi 1976: 9-10. *Jing* 頸 (neck) probably refers to the neckband of the undershirt. Another possibility is that *rujing* is a compound meaning "undershirt." *Fangyan*, 4.2b, gives *quling* 曲領 (neck wrapper) as a name for *ru* in the southwest region; and another synonym of *ru*, *yan* 褗, is glossed as *yanling* 褗領 (shirt that wraps around the neck) in *SW*, 8A.51b. However, one cup of liquor seems like too little liquid to soak the whole undershirt. *Hanshan* 汗衫 (sweatshirt) is listed in *GM*, 38.31.

[3]沕 is not attested in early literature, and it is difficult to determine a reading for it. Ma Jixing cites the graph in recent sources, but they are inapplicable to the occurrence of the graph in *MSI*.E (1992: 459, n. 4). *MWD*, vol. 4, "Transcription," n. 2, suggests that it be read as *zheng* 蒸 (steam), which is doubtful. The word appears to represent a method of boiling that contrasts with *fei* 沸 (bubble; i.e. a full bubbling boil) and *wen* 溫 (heat). Since *wen* probably refers to cooking a liquid until hot (see *MSI*.E.108-109), I suspect that 沕 represents a stage in between "heating" and "bubbling"; hence the provisional translation "scald."

third time of drinking, it desists. Do not eat the evening before. Drink the medicine at dawn. Excellent.

MSI.E.103
(CC178-79) Another. Urine retention. Make a square pit one and a half *chi* to a side and as deep as your elbow. Then burn old straw in it until the ash is not quite one half *chi* deep. Lightly sprinkle fine liquor on it. [1] one *zaojia* (honey locust), fourteen *zao* (jujubes), *yi* style *zhuyu* (evodia),[1] and *jiao* (zanthoxylum). Combine, deposit in one spot in the pit, and burn it. Drop the lower (body) into it. When it desists, rinse.

MSI.E.104 (C180)
Another. Urine retention. Incinerate old fodder or old kindling. Have the ailing person turn his back to the fire and roast it. Have two people rub his buttocks for him. The urine retention desists.

MSI.E.105 (C181)
Another. Boil one third *dou* of gelatin and one *sheng* of rice in one *dou* of water. When cooked, eat it. Do not eat at night.

MSI.E.106 (C182)
Another. Take snails, twice seven in number, and one small bunch[2] of *xie* (scallions). Boil them together in liquor and drink it.

MSI.E.107 (C183)
Another. At daybreak on a *jisi* day,[3] shout.[4] Face east and urinate. If it does not desist, repeat it.

---

[1]I follow *KGS*, vol. 1: 205, n. 399, in identifying *zhuyu* 茱萸 as Wu *zhuyu* 吳茱萸 (*ZY*: no. 2280, *Evodia rutaecarpa* [Juss.] Benth.), listed in *BC* (*GM*, 32.37). *Yi* 藙 in one usage refers to the *zhuyu* fruit, but most often is the name of a spicy condiment prepared from the fruit. In *MSI*.E.103 *yi* may refer to the condiment, but I suspect that it is part of the name of the herb itself. There is considerable confusion in materia medica between Wu *zhuyu* and *shi zhuyu* 食茱萸 (*ZY*: no. 3504, *Zanthoxylum ailanthoides* Sieb. et Zucc.), described in *GM*, 32.41. Ma Jixing argues for the latter identification in *MSI*.E.103 (1992: 461, n. 4).

[2]*SW*, 6B.9a, glosses *jian* 菅 as a "small bunch (*shu* 束)."

[3]*Jisi* 己巳 is the sixth cyclical designation in the sexagenary cycle of Stems and Branches. Two other cyclical days are indicated in *MSI*.E: *MSI*.E.124 specifies the day *xinsi* 辛巳 (eighteenth in the cycle) for an exorcistic cure; and *MSI*.E.126 specifies *xinmao* 辛卯 (twenty-eighth in the cycle). In all three cases I am unable to determine the precise symbolism of selecting these days. However, there must have been a reason for choosing them. The Shuihudi and Fangmatan hemerological manuscripts provide abundant data on calculations involving the sexagenary cycle (see *MSI*.E.69).

[4]I accept Qiu Xigui's argument that the graph transcribed as 屖 in *MWD*, vol. 4, "Transcription," should be 㞚, read as *ti* 嗁 (shout; 1992: 531).

MSI.E.108 (C184)

Another. Bloody urine retention. Boil *jing* (vitex). Heat it thrice, and drink it.

MSI.E.109 (C185)

Another. Stone urine retention. Boil *shiwei* (pyrrosia) and[1] liquor, heating it thrice, and drink it.

MSI.E.110 (C186)

Another. Lardy urine retention. Use *zaoshi* the size of a plum pit.[2] Drink it after eating.[3] If it does not desist, repeat it.

MSI.E.111 (C187)

Another. Female urine retention. Take three-year-old bean leaves.[4] Steam and obtain the liquid. [1] and drink it.

MSI.E.112 (C188)

Another. Female urine retention. Boil *yinfu mu*,[5] and drink it. Wait one day. Mince *yang* [1] and make it into a boiled-dish.[6]

MSI.E.113 (C189)

Another. Boil glutinous panicled millet and panicled millet in gruel vinegar and liquor, scalding thrice, and drink the liquid. All [2].

MSI.E.114 (C190)

Another. Use the hem-band from a robe[7] to bind the thumb of the left hand once. In three days [1].

---

[1] *Ruo* 若 functions as a conjunction in this sentence.

[2] The name *zaoshi* 澡石 does not occur in received literature. It might be an unattested name for *huashi* 滑石 (*ZY*: no. 5037, talc), which is listed in *BC* (*GM*, 9.77) and recommended for curing urine retention. Other identifications are proposed in Ma Jixing 1992: 466, n. 2; and in Wei and Hu, vol. 1: 92, n. 2. *KGS*, vol. 1: 207, n. 409, doubts that *zaoshi* is a drug name and translates the sentence literally: "Cleanse a stone the size of a plum pit."

[3] If *zaoshi* is a mineral drug, it is probably powdered first. If it is simply a "cleansed stone," perhaps it can be swallowed whole.

[4] *Huo* 藿 is a general term for the leaves of bean plants (see *Guangya*, 10A.42b). Perhaps soybean or adzuki bean are intended in *MSI*.E.111.

[5] The identity of *yinfu mu* 隱夫木 is not known. It appears to be a single drug, undoubtedly a tree. The compound *yinfu* occurs in *Hanshu*, 57A.34b, identified as two plant names in the Wang Xianqian commentary: *yin* 櫽 and *fu* 枎. Neither of these names can be identified with certainty; and the commentary may be incorrect in reading the graphs as two names rather than as a single compound name.

[6] *Yang* [1] 陽 occurs again in *MSI*.E.116 with the second graph still missing. Judging from the fact that it is made into a *geng* 羹 ("boiled-dish"), it may be a food plant.

[7] I interpret *renzi* 衽緇 as a compound meaning "the band that forms the hem of a robe." *Ren* refers to the band of cloth attached to the collar and front edge of a wrap-around robe (*SW*, 8A.51b). Archaeological evidence shows that the wrap-around robe had a long flap

MSI.E.115 (C191)

Recipe for When Urine Has [1] Sediment[1]

Take [6] {1} [4] {1} take *hao* from under a magpie dwelling.[2]

MSI.E.116 (C192)

Lard Urine[3]

This is called Internal Return.[4] Boil old *kui* (mallow) seeds in water and urine, and drink it. In addition, mince *yang* [1] and make it into a boiled-dish.

MSI.E.117 (CC193-94)

Swollen Scrotum[5]

When swollen scrotum occurs, the scrotum is black and distended, and it does not go away. To treat it, take three *dou* of coarse horse manure. Break it up thoroughly. Pour water over it, stopping when the water is clear. Sieve to remove the liquid. Pour in [1] *dou*

---

on the left that was wrapped across the right and around the back, which explains the association of *ren* with the fastening of the robe (Sun Ji 1991: 241). The identity of *zi* is problematic. *KGS*, vol. 1: 208, n. 418, reads *zi* in its original meaning "black"; and interprets the compound as "a band of black (material)." I suspect that *zi/*tsrjəg* is a phonetic loan for another word, most likely the word *zhi/*drjək* 幟 used in *Liji*, 29.6b, to denote the trim attached to ritual banners. This was evidently a rare usage because the Zheng Xuan commentary supplies a sound gloss and defines it as *yuan* 緣 (edge). *MWD*, vol. 4, "Transcription," n. 1, proposes a different solution to reading the compound *renzi* that I find unacceptable.

[1]This recipe and *MSI*.E.116 treat ailments where the discharge of urine is abnormal. One of the meanings of *lun* 淪 in *SW*, 11A-2.7a, is "sink." I follow *KGS*, vol. 1: 209, n. 420, in interpreting *lun* in *MSI*.E.115 as "sunken matter, sediment."

[2]The drug is unknown and the translation is conjectural. The main conjecture is reading *tang* 棠 (the name of a species of pear) as *tang* 堂 (dwelling), and guessing that this refers to the magpie nest. Perhaps the compound *quetang* 鵲堂 (magpie dwelling) is related to the magpie nest as a metaphor for the ideal conjugal dwelling, the *locus classicus* of which is *Shijing*, Mao 12, 1C.7b. *Hao* 蒿 might be artemisia in *MSI*.E.115, but perhaps it should be read as *gao* 稾 (straw)—and the drug is grassy material taken from the magpie nest. Other conjectures are possible.

[3]Whereas lardy urine in *MSI*.E.110 is a form of urine retention (perhaps the urine does not flow because it is congealed), lard urine suggests a thick, milky discharge. *Maishu*, "Ailment List," lists an ailment that may be related: "When the urine comes out and is white like hair-washing rinse—it is white conglomeration" (*MSSW*: 72).

[4]The meaning of the second name for the ailment is unclear. Perhaps *fu* 復 (return) represents *fu* 腹 (abdomen).

[5]橐 in *MWD*, vol. 4, "Transcription," should be transcribed as *nang* 囊 (the meaning "scrotum" is well attested for the latter). The same correction applies to the ailment name in *MSI*.E.1. Later medical literature usually includes this type of ailment under the category *tui* 穨 (inguinal swelling), which is the next ailment category beginning in *MSI*.E.118 (Yu Yan 1972: 225). A similar classification occurs in *Maishu*, "Ailment List": "When the scrotum has a swelling—it is blood inguinal swelling" (*MSSW*: 72).

of *suanjiang*.[1] Take *jie zhong jia*.[2] After using once, it responds. After using four or five times, the swelling goes away. There are no prohibitions and no temporal (restrictions). Excellent.

MSI.E.118
(CC195-97)

Inguinal Swelling[3]

Grasp a *bai* (arbor-vitae) pestle.[4] Perform the Pace of Yu thrice. Say: "Spouter expel the Hu once. Spouter expel the Hu twice. Spouter expel the Hu thrice.[5] The *bai* (arbor-vitae) pestle bores

---

[1]*Suanjiang* 酸漿 is a liquid added to the manure after the water is drained away. The compound might refer to a "vinegar beverage," similar to the *cujiang* 酢漿 (vinegar beverage) given in *SW*, 11A-2.34b, as a gloss for *jiang*; and related to the *suanjiang* listed among medicinal liquids in *GM*, 5.54. However, *suanjiang* is also the name of a herb identified as *Physalis alkekengi* L. var. *franchetii* (Mast.) Mak. (*ZY*: no. 5287), listed in *BC* (*GM*, 16.97). The liquid extracted from the plant is commonly used in medicine.

[2]The interpretation of *jie zhong jia* 芥衷莢 is problematic. *MWD*, vol. 4, "Transcription," n. 6, identifies *jie* as mustard (*ZY*: no. 2173, *Brassica juncea* [L.] Czern. et Coss.); and suggests that *jia* "pod" may refer to the fruit body, usually called *jiao* 角. To accept this interpretation one must assume that the recipe is incomplete, for there is no indication of how the newly introduced ingredient is used. *KGS*, vol. 1: 210, n. 431, reads *jie* in the sense of "refuse matter"—referring to the manure. For attestation of *jie* as "grassy matter, refuse," see *Zuozhuan*, Ai 1, 57.3b. In this interpretation, the recipe would have the person pick out the "pods" from the refuse/manure (either undigested pods that are still in the manure or pod-like pieces of the manure). The problem of whether the therapy is internal or external remains, since the recipe does not say.

[3]*Tui* 穨 means literally "drop down," and is attested first as a word for a fiery, descending wind in received literature (Harper 1990: 219). The Mawangdui and Zhangjiashan medical manuscripts provide the earliest attestation of *tui* as a name for various kinds of swellings in the inguinal region, including hernias. Several of the magical treatments in *MSI*.E provide evidence of a demonic etiology for *tui*. A naturalistic conception related to pathogenic vapor is also evident; e.g. in *MSI*.E.135, which recommends cauterizing the foot Great Yin and Great Yang vessels. For discussion of the ailment in Han and later received sources, see Yu Yan 1972: 225-29. The name of this ailment category as given in *MSI*.E.1 is *changtui* 腸穨 (intestine *tui*). Intestine *tui* is included in *Maishu*, "Ailment List": "When there is a screeching noise above and below the swelling—it is intestine *tui*" (*MSSW*: 72). *Yinshu* also describes an exercise routine to treat intestine *tui* and muscle *tui* (*YSSW*: 84). The description does not appear to match the illustration of the exercise to treat *tui* in *MSII*.C. Many of the recipes in *MSI*.E refer to the male genitals and possibly concern a scrotal hernia.

[4]The patient is beaten with the pestle at the end of the recipe. Arbor-vitae wood has associations with the east and solar potency that make it an appropriate material for an exorcistic instrument.

[5]The use of Hu 胡 in the incantation probably involves a pun. *KGS*, vol. 1: 211, n. 435, interprets the word literally as "cow dewlap"—the gloss in *SW*, 4B.31b. Hence the swellings to be exorcised are likened to the excrescent skin of the dewlap. At the same time, it appears that Hu designates a demon, and that the three Hu are the trio mentioned below ("there are only three"). Hu/*Gag was a generic term for northern barbarians, but I suspect that the pun involves the fox (*hu/*gwag* 狐). The earliest attestation of fox possession

through the mortar. There is one Mother and one [Father; Sons] there are only three.[1] Spouter, for these swellings[2] you use the *bai* (arbor-vitae) pestle seven times and let not a single one of so-and-so's inguinal swellings remain."[3] Members of the same clan must be made to carry [1] the person with inguinal swelling, set him down by an east-facing window looking out, and beat him with the exorcising rod.[4]

MSI.E.119 (C198)

Another. At the time of clear brightness[5] have someone whose foot has been cut off face east and stamp on the person twice-seven times with the amputee peg.[6]

---

in China is found in *MSI*.E.124 and 128, where a fox is named in the incantations as the cause of the inguinal swellings. Post-Han sources tell of were-foxes disguising their identity by adopting the surname Hu (see Groot 1892–1910, vol. 4: 195). Perhaps the Hu in *MSI*.E.118 represent fox demons.

[1]The two-graph lacuna is probably 父 子. The incantations in *MSI*.E.120 and 125 attribute inguinal swellings to the Sons born of a Mother and Father.

[2]潼 in *MWD*. vol. 4, "Transcription," should be written 穜, and read as *zhong* 腫 (swellings).

[3]The rhyming words in the incantation are: Hu/*Gag 胡 (all three occurrences) and *fu/*bjag* 父 (father); and *qi/*tshjit* 七 (seven) and *yi/*ʔjit* 一 (one).

[4]*Si chui* 敁 椎 (beat with an exorcising rod) refers in this case to beating the person with the pestle. *Si* occurs again as a verb in *MSI*.E.120, where the person is exorcistically beaten with an iron mallet; and in *MSI*.E.124, where a cloth is used. *Si* was already a rare word in Han times. The only attestation is the definition in *SW*, 3B.40a: "It is a *haisi* 毅 敁, which is a large *gangmao* 剛 卯 used to expel demonic apparitions." The definition indicates that *si* was only known as a member of the compound *haisi*, the name of an apotropaic amulet related to the *gangmao* amulet (for which see Bodde 1975: 304–306). The use of *si* in *MSI*.E to denote the action of exorcistic beating is an archaic usage that can be traced back to the Shang bone and shell inscriptions. Shirakawa demonstrates that *si* is to be identified with a Shang graph that depicts a hand holding a rod and beating a snake or bug-like creature (i.e. a demonic creature). In Shang inscriptions the word is used both as a verb and as a noun (meaning the rite of beating with an exorcising rod; 1974: 462–70). The word *chui/*tjəd* ("to hammer, mallet")—either as verb or noun—also has particular relevance to the treatment of the ailment *tui/*dəd*, since the two words are homophonous. The word magic involved in the pun on the name of the ailment and the instrument or method used to exorcise it may account for the prevalence of exorcistic beating to treat *tui* in *MSI*.E. The same kind of word magic figures in later magical treatments for inguinal swelling. *Qianjin yaofang*, 74.19b, includes recipes for treating inguinal swelling that make use of a treadle mill (*dui* 碓), another homophone of the name of the ailment.

[5]*Qingming* 清 明 (clear brightness) refers to dawn in this context. See the Kong Yingda commentary in *Shijing*, Mao 236, 16B.7a.

[6]*Tong* 筩 is glossed in *SW*, 5A.11b, as a tube of cut bamboo. In the context of *MSI*.E.119 it is clear that the graph is to be read as *yong* 踊 in the sense of the prosthetic device used by foot-amputees (foot amputation was one of the mutilation punishments). See *Zuozhuan*, Zhao 3, 42.6a.

MSI.E.120 (CC199-200)

Another. For prostration.[1] On the sixteenth day of the month when the moon first begins to deteriorate, perform the Pace of Yu thrice. Say: "Moon is matched against sun" and "Sun is matched against moon"—three times each. "Father is perverse, Mother is strong. Like other people they bore Sons, and only bore inguinal swelling bulges.[2] Perverseness desist. Grasp the hammering stone and strike your Mother."[3] Immediately, exorcistically beat and hammer the person twice seven times with an iron mallet. Do it at sunrise, and have the person with inguinal swelling face east.

MSI.E.121 (C201)

Another. Soak a woman's (menstrual) cloth. Boil meat in the liquid. Eat it, and drink the liquid.

MSI.E.122 (C202)

Another. Break an egg into a cup of gruel vinegar. Drink it.

MSI.E.123 (C203)

Another. Roast silkworm eggs until they sizzle and turn yellow.[4] Smith them. Put a three-fingered pinch reaching to the knuckles into one half cup of liquor. Drink it for three or four days.

MSI.E.124 (CC204-205)

Another. On a *xinsi* day utter this curse:[5] "The day is *xinsi*"—three times. Say: "Spirit of Heaven send down the sickness-

---

[1]In the context of the ailment *tui* it is probable that *long* 癃—which refers to urine retention above—should be understood in the sense glossed in *SW*, 7B.34b, "prostration ailment."

[2]尣 in *MWD*, vol. 4, "Transcription," should be transcribed as *gang* 亢. I understand the word in the sense of "high" (*Guangya*, 4B.7a), referring to the "bulges" of the ailment.

[3]I follow *KGS*, vol. 1: 213, n. 450, in interpreting *duanshi* 鍛石 as "a stone used for hammering." The rhyming words in the incantation are: *qiang/*gjang* 强 (strong) and *kang/*khang* 亢 (bulges); and *zi/*tsjəg* 子 (Sons), *yi/*rəg* 已 (desist), and *mu/*məg* 母 (Mother).

[4]Silkworm eggs (*luan* 卵) are silkworm larvae. In *MSI*.E.133 the recipe calls for "dark silkworm eggs (*zhong* 種)" and the measurement is stated in terms of the length of cloth on which silkworm larvae are cultivated. In later materia medica the measurement of silkworm larvae is by the sheets of paper containing the larvae (see *GM*, 39.78). I follow *MWD*, vol. 4, "Transcription," n. 1, in reading 簍 簍 as *shushu* 數 數, attested in *Zhuangzi* 1, 10, in the sense of "urgent, hasty." In *MSI*.E.123 it refers to the movement of the silkworm eggs as they roast.

[5]*Xinsi* 辛 巳 is the eighteenth cyclical designation in the sexagenary cycle (see *MSI*.E.107). The word *gu* 古 occurs again in *MSI*.E.178, and in both occurrences has the sense of "utter a curse." *MWD*, vol. 4, "Transcription", n. 1, identifies it with *gu* 辜, glossed in *SW*, 14B.22b, as *zui* 辠 (guilty of a crime). Duan Yucai traces the etymology of the word to

shield.[1] Spirit Maids according to sequence hear the spirit pronouncement.[2] A certain fox has seized a place where it does not belong.[3] Desist. If you do not desist, I hack you with an ax."[4] Immediately grasp a cloth and exorcistically beat the person twice seven times.

MSI.E.125
(CC206-207) Another. At sunrise have the person with inguinal swelling face east beneath the roof gutter.[5] Have another person grasp a rammer,[6]

---

execution by dismemberment, as attested in *Zhouli*, 36.8a; and the word is also associated with the exorcistic rite of dismembering an animal to neutralize demonic danger, as attested in *Zhouli*, 18.3b. The words of the incantations in *MSI*.E.124 and 178 are the verbal counterpart of exorcistic dismemberment. It is possible that the use of *gu* in *MSI*.E is related to a specifically southern tradition of exorcistic magic. According to *Hanshu*, 28A-1.30a, there were three cult sites established near Han-time Chang'an where Yue shamans performed their exorcisms, known as *gurang* 㐰 鄉. It has been argued that the graph 㐰 is an error for 𣧼, given as a variant orthography of 辜 in *SW*. However, the Yue shamans were renowned for their methods of incantation. I suspect that *gu* 㐰 refers to a type of malediction practiced by the Yue shamans and now attested in *MSI*.E. Another word for exorcistic malediction, *liu* 褶 (*SW*, 1A.12b), may be related to *gu* 㐰 (graphically if not phonologically).

[1]"Sickness-shield" translates *ganji* 干 疾. It is a verb-object compound functioning as a noun ("that which shields sickness"), similar to the well-known compound *bixie* 辟 邪 (that which wards off evil). Spirit of Heaven 天 神 is the same chief deity referred to as Yellow Spirit in *MSI*.E.178 and as Thearch of Heaven in *MSI*.E.233. On the relation between these names and the concept of a chief deity in Han popular religion, see Seidel 1987.

[2]The Spirit Maids (or perhaps Maid) appealed to in this incantation appear to be spirits associated with the cyclical designations; that is, the appeal is being addressed to the spirit(s) who presides over the *xinsi* day. The belief in spirits of the cyclical designations is attested in *Lunheng*, "Jieshu," 25.499 (Wang Chong makes disparaging remarks about the belief). Summoning Jade Maids of the cyclical designations for assistance is described in the *Baopuzi* and in many religious Daoist scriptures of the post-Han period (see Schipper 1965: 34-38).

[3]The incantations in *MSI*.E.124 and 128 are the earliest attestation of fox possession in China. The fox's demonic reputation is indicated in the gloss in *SW*, 10A.36a: "It is an ill-omened creature, one that demons ride." Malicious and cunning, the fox is frequently blamed for sickness and mental derangement in post-Han sources (see Groot 1892-1910, vol. 4: 188-96; and vol. 5: 576-600). I reject the argument in *MWD*, vol. 4, "Transcription," n. 2, that ***huzhao*** 狐 叉 should be read as ***hushan*** 狐 疝 (referring to a type of hernia). See *MSI*.B.8 for evidence that the ailment name ***hushan*** in the *Huangdi neijing* is a corruption of ***pianshan*** 偏 疝.

[4]The rhyming words in the incantation are: *yu/*ngjag* 語 (pronouncement), *suo/*skrjag* 所 (place), *yi/*rəg* 已 (desist; two occurrences), and *ruo/*njak* 若 (you). See *MSI*.E.56 for rhyming between **-əg* and **-ag*.

[5]"Roof gutter" translates *wuliu* 屋 霤. The compound must be the equivalent of *chengliu* 承 霤, which refers to rain gutters attached to the outer edge of the roof (see Hayashi 1976: 193, for discussion of *chengliu*). The symbolic significance of placing the person beneath the

face west, and chant this incantation: "Today [ ]. So-and-so's inguinal swelling bulges[1] today desist. So-and-so's inguinal swelling desist. [ ] your Father and Mother. Both are expired—*bai* (arbor-vitae) rammed them. Throwing down Father and hitting the Sons, how can there not be desistance."[2] Hit the inguinal swellings twice seven times with the rammer. After completion, immediately say: "So-and-so rise. Inguinal swelling desist."[3]

MSI.E.126 (C208)

Another. On a *xinmao* day,[4] stand at the foot of the hall facing east toward the sun. Have someone lift the person with inguinal swelling by both arms. Say: "Today is *xinmao*. His name is changed to Yu."[5]

MSI.E.127 (C209)

Another. Take *xi* (hemp) refuse[6] and wrap in *ai* (mugwort).[7] Use this to cauterize the center of the crown of the head of the person with inguinal swelling.[8] Let it blister and no more.

---

center of the house that constituted a central axis connecting the house to heaven and the spiritual realm.

[6]*Zhu* 築 (rammer) may refer to a pestle, or perhaps to the tool used in rammed earth construction.

[1]尢 in *MWD*, vol. 4, "Transcription," should be transcribed as *gang* 亢 (see *MSI*.E.120).

[2]I follow the punctuation of the incantation proposed by Qiu Xigui which is based on the sequence of rhyming words (1992: 532): *yi/*rəg* 已 (desist; two occurrences), *mu/*məg* 母 (Mother), *zhi/*tjəg* 之 (them), *zi/*tsjəg* 子 (Son), and *you/*gwjəg* 有 (there is).

[3]I place the words "inguinal swelling desist" within the incantation because of the continuation of the rhyming pattern: *qi/*khjəg* 起 (rise) and *yi/*rəg* 已 (desist). It is also possible that they belong outside the incantation as the conclusion to the recipe, indicating that the magical treatment will cure the ailment.

[4]*Xinmao* 辛 卯 is the twenty-eighth cyclical designation (see *MSI*.E.107).

[5]The incantation reveals yet another magical element in Yu's identity. The ritual of name changing, like the Pace of Yu, is an efficacious way to deal with demonic entities.

[6]*Xi* 枲 is a general name for hemp (see *SW*, 7B.1a, and Duan Yucai commentary). *Xi gou* 枲垢 must refer to the refuse produced when hemp is processed to obtain the fibers.

[7]*Ai* 艾 (mugwort) is associated with cauterization therapy in *Suwen* 14, 4.5b; and *Lingshu* 51, 8.6b. While the use of moxa (prepared *ai* leaves) which is burned on the skin is implied in *Lingshu* 51, there is no Han period description of moxa (Lu and Needham 1980: 175–76). The earliest description of a method of performing cauterization with *ai* is *MSI*.E.127, which describes not moxa but a kind of cigarette with hemp filling rolled in *ai* leaves. Yamada 1985a: 58–63, speculates that the use of *ai* in cauterization is related to its earlier use as an exorcistic fumigant (see *MSI*.E.155, which uses *ai* as a fumigant). Perhaps the use of *ai* leaves in *MSI*.E.127—in contrast to *MSI*.E.64 where warts are cauterized with a cattail cord—is related to the strong association between the ailment *tui* and demonic causation in *MSI*.E.

*MS*I.E.128 (C210)

Another. Have the person with inguinal swelling look north and lie down facing north in a hall with a four-slope roof.[1] Perform the Pace of Yu thrice. Shout: "Gwjag.[2] Fox *piao*"[3]—thrice. "You know so-and-so ails from fox [?].[4]

*MS*I.E.129 (C211)

Another. Inguinal swelling and goiter.[5] Steam the food sacrifice of a dead person and wrap it in new cloth.[6] Use a sack[7] [4] {2} [?].

*MS*I.E.130 (C212)

Another. Wrap hive-bee eggs[8] that have been dried in the dark in cloth [2].

---

[8]The center of the crown of the head is also used for a counter-irritant treatment in *MS*I.E.53. While this is the location of a well-known acupuncture point—the *baihui* 百會 (hundred convergence; see Lu and Needham 1980: 80-83)—there is no indication in *MS*I.E.127 that performing cauterization there is related to vessel theory, just as there is no evidence of vessel theory in *MS*I.E.53.

[1]For identification of *wu* 廡 as a building with a four-sloped roof, see Hayashi 1976: 190; and Sun Ji 1991: 164.

[2]See *MS*I.E.56 on the use of the utterance *yu/*gwjag* 吁.

[3]I assume that *hupiao* 狐 麃 (fox *piao*) is a compound name for a demonic animal (*piao* is attested as a variety of deer), but I have found no supporting references. It is also possible that *piao* should be read as another word that I am unable to identify.

[4]The fact that the rest of the incantation is missing makes it difficult to interpret the opening fragment. Other translations are possible.

[5]Early glosses consistently identify *ying* 瘿 as a growth by the throat, which Yu Yan shows refers to goiter (1972: 212). The identification is also confirmed by *Maishu*, "Ailment List": "When located beneath the chin—it is *ying*" (*MSSW*: 72). *MS*I.E.129 doubles as a treatment for goiter.

[6]*Zhui* 腏 is food prepared for a sacrificial offering (*SW*, 5B.15a, and Duan Yucai commentary). *MS*I.E.143 calls for millet food sacrifice as well as the head of a dead person. The earliest occurrences of *zhui* are in the Fangmatan resurrection account (the passage concerns the proper way to offer *zhui* to the dead in the graveyard; Li Xueqin 1990: 43; Harper 1994) and in the first Shuihudi hemerological manuscript (where setting out *zhui* forms part of a prayer ritual to the guardian deity of horses; *SHD*: 228). As distinct from the ritual feeding of ancestors in ancestor worship, *zhui* appears to have been part of the growing mortuary cult centered on the graveyard in the late Warring States period. This custom is reflected in *MS*I.E.129 when the recipe specifies the "food sacrifice of a dead person." *MS*I.E.143 identifies the source for *zhui* as the "offering niche by the entrance to the inner chamber," which might be a household offering site or a cult site (in the graveyard?).

[7]*Nang* 囊 (sack) might refer to the scrotum.

[8]I.e. the larvae.

MSI.E.131 (C213)

Another. When there are inguinal swellings as well as thigh abscesses and rat bellies,[1] [1][2] scratch twice seven times with the middle finger. It is invariably cured.

MSI.E.132 (C214)

Another. Use straw to make a bow, the cord handle from a slotted steaming-pot to make a bowstring,[3] *ge* (kudzu) to make arrows, and [feather them] with [1] feathers.[4] Shoot at dawn. At sunset [1] become small.

MSI.E.133 (CC215-16)

Another. Take a one-*chi* square (sheet) of dark silkworm eggs,[5] once seven clothes-eating *baiyu* (silverfish),[6] and twice seven *changzu* (spiders).[7] Scorch the silkworm eggs until they turn yellow and

---

[1]I follow *MWD*, vol. 4, "Transcription," in reading 復 as *fu* 腹 (belly). "Rat belly" describes the shape of a swelling, similar to the use of the term *yufu* 魚 腹 (fish belly) to refer to the calf (see *Suwen* 41, 11.8a). Ma Jixing reads the the graph as *fu* 伏 (crouch), citing *Suwen* 52, 14.3b, which uses the compound *shupu* 鼠 僕 (1992: 485, n. 2). The Wang Bing commentary explains the compound as "a swelling like the shape of a crouching (*fu*) rat." In *Suwen* 52 the "crouching rat" swelling is caused by improper acupuncture, whereas in *MSI*.E.131 the "rat belly" is a third type of swelling along with inguinal swelling and thigh abscess.

[2]The lacuna is probably 以.

[3]The compound *yanyi* 甗 衣—literally, "slotted steaming-pot garb"—must be equivalent to *zengdai* 甑 帶, the cord handle attached to the steaming-pot. *KGS*, vol. 1: 218, n. 481, argues that *yi*/*ʔjəd is a phonetic loan for *wa*/*ʔwjar 瓾. The latter word occurs in *Huainanzi*, 16.284, and is glossed in the Gao Yu commentary as *zengdai*. The argument is plausible. *Yanyi* occurs again in *MSV*.5. *Zengdai* is among the items listed in *Wanwu* (Fuyang Han jian zhenglizu 1988: 39). The item is also listed in later materia medica (*GM*, 38.50).

[4]The text is not clearly visible, but I suspect that there is a graph-repeat sign following *yu* 羽 (the first occurrence is the noun "feather" and the repeat is the verb "attach feathers"), and that the lacuna following 羽 is 之 "them." The kind of feather used is missing in the lacuna preceding *yu*. Exorcistic archery is also employed in *MSI*.E.137, which uses the peachwood bow attested in descriptions of formal exorcistic rituals in received literature (see Bodde 1975: 127, 134). See the Prolegomena, Section Five, "Varieties of Magic."

[5]The measurement "one-*chi* square" means that the silkworm larvae are measured by the length of the cloth on which the larvae are deposited (see *MSI*.E.123). The meaning of *ming* 冥 (dark) with reference to the silkworm larvae is uncertain. Ma Jixing proposes reading *ming* as *mu* 暮 (1992: 487, n. 1), but his argument is implausible.

[6]*BC* gives the names *yiyu* 衣 魚 (clothes fish) and *baiyu* 白 魚 (white fish; *GM*, 41.18). The "clothes-eating *baiyu*" in *MSI*.E.133 must represent a long form of the name for the silverfish.

[7]*Changzu* 長 足 must be equivalent to *changyi* 長 踦. The latter name occurs in *Erya*, 9.9a, and is glossed in the Guo Pu commentary as a kind of long-legged spider. For spiders in materia medica, see *GM*, 40.97.

grind. Smith the silkworm eggs. Also grind the *baiyu* (silverfish) and *changzu* (spiders). Measure the three proportionately and combine. Blend with two *sheng* of gruel vinegar. Drink it before eating. Infants use one *sheng*.

MSI.E.134 (CC217-20)

Another. Bore into a small gourd,[1] making the hole (large enough) to completely contain the testicles and penis[2] of the person with inguinal swelling. Then have the person with inguinal swelling cup[3] the gourd in his hands, face east, and kneel beneath an old eastern wall. Then insert his testicles and penis into the hole in the gourd. Make four-*cun* long pegs from *cai* (oak),[4] twice seven in number. Then chop at them with a *cai* (oak) mallet, once [2] and twice smoothing them.[5] After they are chopped, immediately poke the pegs (into the ground) beneath the wall, stopping when all twice seven pegs have been exhausted. Always do it when the moon is waning on the sixteenth day [2] exhausted.[6] Do it once a

---

[1]*Hu* 瓠 and *hu* 壺 are synonyms for a gourd used as a vessel (*SW*, 7B.5a, and Duan Yucai commentary). In *MSI*.E.134 they must represent a compound referring to a gourd similar to the one used in *MSI*.E.60.

[2]*Zui/*tsuad* ⿰月最 represents the same word as *zui/*tsuəd* 朘, which refers to the male genitals. Rhyming between words with final **-ad* and **-əd* in the *Huainanzi* corroborates the phonological identity in southern speech (Luo and Zhou 1958: 254). *SW*, 4B.40b, glosses *zui* as "the Yin (i.e. genitals) of the red infant." The *locus classicus* is *Laozi*, par. 55, as confirmed by the Mawangdui *Laozi* manuscripts (*MWD*, vol. 1: 105). The graph 最 is used in *MS*III.33; and the same graph is used in the medieval sex manual *Dongxuanzi* 洞 玄 子, cited in *Ishinpô*, 28.47b. *Zui* refers generally to the male genitals as well as more narrowly to the penis.

[3]I read text *fan* 煩 as *fan* ⿰⻊煩, which is given as a variant graph for *fan* 番 (animal paw) in *SW*, 2A.4a. The person is supposed to "cup" the large end of the gourd in his hands as a bear would hold something in its front paws.

[4]*Cai* 采 occurs in *Shiji*, 87.12b, and is glossed in the commentary as another name for *li* 櫟 (*ZY*: no. 5433, *Quercus acutissima* Carr.).

[5]"Chop at" translates *duo* 剟. The exact procedure described is unclear because of the lacuna, but the act of chopping at the pegs with a mallet of the same material must form part of the overall exorcistic ritual that culminates with the insertion of the pegs beneath the wall. *MWD*, vol. 4, "Transcription," n. 5, argues that *duo* means "knock, hit," even though this meaning is not attested for *duo*. I suspect that the instruction to "chop" with a mallet is intentional, and that it has magical significance. Perhaps the tips of the pegs are splintered with a chopping action and then the splintered wood is "smoothed."

[6]"Exhausted" may refer to the moon waning, meaning that the exorcistic treatment continues over the last half of the month.

day. [1] do it a second time.[1] Always do it when the stars come out. Wait for the inguinal swelling to desist and then stop.

MSI.E.135 (CC221-22)

Another. Inguinal swelling. First raise the testicles and pull down the skin. Pierce the side of the *duo* (navel) with a lancing-stone.[2] [2] liquid and lard [1] stir with pure [liquor].[3] In addition, cauterize the wound.[4] Do not allow the wind to reach it. For an easy cure,[5] cauterize the Great Yin and Great Yang [2].[6] Excellent.

MSI.E.136 (CC223-24)

Another. Recipe for treating inguinal swellings when they first erupt, and there is humping and cramping but they are not yet large.[7] Take one whole bug slough and [3] incinerate both.[8] [8] liq-

---

[1]I suspect that the lacuna is a negative indicating that the treatment is not to be performed twice in one day.

[2]*Bian* 砭 (lancing-stone) is discussed in *MSI*.C. The initial treatment in *MSI*.E.135 focuses on the *duo*. Although the treatment does not rely on vessel theory, Zhao Youchen (1981) cites later medical literature in which acupuncture points near the navel are used to treat *tui*—which at least lends credibility to identifying *duo* with the navel.

[3]From the context, the final lacuna must be 酒. The preceding lacunae make it impossible to follow the recipe at this point, other than to surmise that a salve is prepared and applied to the spot that was lanced.

[4]Presumably the spot that was lanced.

[5]The text writes 易瘳 ㄴ 而, placing the hook-sign after the phrase "easy to cure." In my reading, *er* 而 functions grammatically like *nai* 乃 (then; a common usage in early texts), and I understand the phrase "easy to cure" to be logically linked to what follows. Ma Jixing links "easy to cure" to what precedes in his translation and does not account for *er* (1992: 492). The hook-sign is used in the Mawangdui manuscripts mostly to break phrases where confusion might occur (e.g. in lists of drug names), not to mark the end of a sentence or logical unit. In the case at hand I suspect that the hook-sign marks "easy to cure" as a topic, followed by the statement concerning cauterizing the Great Yin and Great Yang vessels; that is, cauterizing the two vessels is represented as easier than the complicated procedure just described (Ma's interpretation is that the preceding treatment "makes the ailment easy to cure").

[6]Great Yin and Great Yang must refer to the foot Great Yin and Great Yang vessels. This is the only occurrence of vessel names in *MSI*.E, and the only clear instance of a treatment based on vessel theory. It is worth noting that *MSI*.A-B do not associate the foot Great Yin and Great Yang vessels with *tui* (nor is the association made in *Lingshu* 10). In *MSI*.B.8, *tui* is one of the ailments listed under the foot Ceasing Yin vessel. Perhaps *MSI*.E.135 reflects an earlier association between *tui* and these vessels that was already discarded in *MSI*.A-B; or perhaps it is simply a different medical tradition that found its way into *MSI*.E.

[7]I interpret "humping and cramping" as describing the condition of the swellings as they first erupt, before becoming large. Ma Jixing interprets "humping and cramping" as describing the body of the patient hunched over in pain; and "not yet large" as meaning that the ailment is "not yet severe" (1992: 493).

uor, drinking a sufficient amount to become intoxicated. Allowed for men and women. Excellent.

MSI.E.137

(CC225-26) Another. Inguinal swelling. Cover the testicles with a large-bellied gourd. Then take *tao* (peach) branches that face east and make a bow with them. Take [1] {1} [11] {1}. On the last day of the month shoot three arrows in one shot.[1] [2] drink the medicine. The medicine is called "yellow cow gall dried in the dark." When it has dried, gradually [9] drink it.[2]

MSI.E.138

(CC227-31) Another. Smith one *chi* of *jungui* (curled cinnamon)[3] and one *sheng* of *du* [1]. Smith them together and place inside a bamboo tube. Fill the bamboo tube [18]. Then cover with cloth. Spread it below the *duo* (navel) in two places. {3} [17] it. {6}. Wait for his body to become calm and stable. [18]. When inguinal swelling desists,[4] reverently perform the requital rite with a suckling pig.[5] If this

---

[8]The second ingredient is missing in the lacuna. Depending on the identification of 虫, the first drug is either the sloughed skin of a snake—the interpretation in *MWD*, vol. 4, "Transcription," n. 1, which reads the graph as *hui* "snake"—or the slough of an insect (reading the graph as *chong* "bug"); e.g. cicada slough (*chantuo* 蟬 蛻). Both are listed in materia medica: *GM*, 43.67 (snake slough), and *GM*, 41.10 (cicada slough). Fragment 1 of *MSI*.E (*MWD*, vol. 4: 76) records snake slough by the name *shetuo* 蛇 蛻 (it is uncertain in which ailment category the fragment belongs).

[1]See *MSI*.E.132 for exorcistic archery.

[2]The cow gall medicine is probably first mentioned in the long lacuna at the beginning of the recipe. Gall is listed along with other parts of the cow in *BC* (*GM*, 50.70). It is usually dried and then broken into pieces when used. The lacuna at the end of the recipe may describe how to process the gall.

[3]"Curled cinnamon" refers to the curled bark used as a drug.

[4]已 in *MWD*, vol. 4, "Transcription," should be transcribed as *yi* 已 (desist).

[5]The lengthy lacunae make it impossible to discern the treatment. The reference to the "requital rite" (*sai* 塞) indicates that at some point above there should be a "ritual requesting a favor from the spirits," called *dao* 禱. The purpose of the *sai* is to present spirits with the sacrificial offerings that were pledged to them when the person first requested a favor in the form of a *dao*. Thus the *dao* constitutes the promise of a bribe to the spirits, which must be paid when the spirits fulfill the requested favor. The use of *dao* and *sai* to deal with illness is documented in *Hanfeizi* 35, 14.253, where a cow is the promised offering. The earliest attestation of *sai* and *dao* in popular Warring States religion is in the fourth century B.C. divination records from Baoshan (Li Ling 1990: 84). The Shuihudi hemerological manuscripts include the text of a *dao* prayer to alleviate nightmares in which the spirit who controls nightmare demons is offered material goods as payment (Harper 1987a: 270).

is considered inhumane, use *bai* [19]. Hang the *mao* (woolly grass) in the place for the pig sacrifice[1] and requite the favor[2] {2} [?]

MSI.E.139 (CC232-34)

Another. [1]. Take a woman's menstrual cloth. Soak it, and roast[3] until it becomes warm [24] [vegetation] from the four up-turned slopes of the roof.[4] Incinerate *lianghuang*.[5] Smith five *cun* of *gui* (cinnamon). [?] {1} [?]

MSI.E.140 (C235)

Inguinal swelling [1].[6] Cauterize the left shin. [?]

MSI.E.141 (C236)

Another. Do not eat at night. At dawn take one bee egg. Soak it in one cup of fine gruel vinegar and give it to the person to drink.

MSI.E.142 (CC237-38)

Vessel Hemorrhoid[7]

---

[1]I follow *KGS*, vol. 1: 223, n. 515, in reading *bi* 比 as *bi* 祉, glossed in *SW*, 1A.9b, as "sacrificing a pig to the Director of the Life-mandate 司命." Other Han sources cited in the Duan Yucai commentary describe the cult of the Director of the Life-mandate in popular religion, including the pig sacrifice. Perhaps the *dao* prayer in *MSI*.E.138 is directed to him. *Mao* 茅 is *Imperata cylindrica* (L.) P. Beauv. var. *major* (Nees) C. E. Hubb. (*ZY*: no. 1435), listed in *BC* (*GM*, 13.64). The plant is commonly called *baimao* 白茅 (hence *bai* preceding the lacuna is undoubtedly followed by *mao*, naming the plant). For a study of the religious use of *mao* in the pre-Han period, see Mizukami 1977: 615-26. It was regarded as a receptacle for spirits, as evidenced in the *SW*, 14A.51b, definition of a roadway ritual known as *ba* 軷: "When a person is about to embark and engage in affairs on the roadway, he must first make a declaration to the spirit (of the roadway). The altar is placed at a crossroads. *Mao* is set up, thereby providing a prop for the spirit. This is *ba*." *MSI*.E.138 indicates that *mao* might be substituted for animal sacrifices in the event that the person is loath to kill an animal as an offering to the spirits.

[2]"Requite the favor" translates *saidao*.

[3]灸 in *MWD*, vol. 4, "Transcription," should be transcribed as *zhi* 炙 (roast).

[4]Qiu Xigui identifies the fragmentary graph following 四榮 (four up-turned slopes of the roof) as *cai* 蔡 (vegetation; 1992: 531). It appears to be the same material used in *MSI*.E.27.

[5]The drug *lianghuang* 量簧 is unknown.

[6]The customary "another" does not occur at the head of *MSI*.E.140.

[7]脈者 denotes the "vessel" type of hemorrhoid. The standard name for hemorrhoids is *zhi* 痔. Later medical literature recognizes five types: male hemorrhoid, female hemorrhoid, vessel hemorrhoid, intestine hemorrhoid, and bloody hemorrhoid (*Chaoshi zhubing yuanhoulun*, 34.14a). The name vessel hemorrhoid is probably derived from the appearance of the swollen vein of the hemorrhoid. Male hemorrhoid is the next ailment category in *MSI*.E; followed by female hemorrhoid, within which are recipes for bloody hemorrhoid as well as a condition called "nest" (i.e. anal fistula). *Maishu*, "Ailment List," also lists male and female hemorrhoids: "When it is located in the perineum and forms a swelling like a jujube—it is male hemorrhoid"; "When the swelling has holes that ooze liquid—it is female hemorrhoid" (*MSSW*: 72). Early etiological theories attribute the swollen veins of hemorrhoids to the chewing of bugs (Yu Yan 1972: 232). Worms are mentioned in the

Take equal amounts of the fur from five kinds of wild animals whose flesh is eaten. Incinerate and smith. Combine them, stirring [1]. Every dawn before eating take three large three-fingered pinches and blend in one cup of warm liquor. Drink it. At sunset drink it again before eating, following the previous procedure. Continue ingesting the medicine for twenty days. Even an old ailment invariably [1].[1] While ingesting the medicine it is prohibited to eat pork and fresh fish. Previously tested.

*MS*I.E.143 (CC239-40) Male Hemorrhoid

There is snail-like flesh protruding, sometimes like the shape of a rat teat.[2] The tip is large and the base small, and there is a hole in it. [1] it, heat it quickly using cauterization, grasp the small base, and twist until it breaks off. Take the millet food sacrifice from the offering niche by the entrance to the inner (chamber)[3] and incinerate the head of a dead person. Smith both, moisten with rancid lard, and put it into the hole.

*MS*I.E.144 (CC241-43) Another. For when there are many holes. Boil fatty black ewe[4] and use the liquid to soak three *dou* of fine glutinous panicled millet. Cook it, and moisten with (ewe liquid).[5] When done, divide into

---

description in *MS*I.E.149. The elaborate fumigation treatments described in several recipes in *MS*I.E are undoubtedly intended as vermifuges to kill the bugs.

[1]The lacuna must be one of the several words meaning "cured."

[2]The description is similar to that of male hemorrhoid in *Chaoshi zhubing yuanhoulun*, 34.14a: "On the side of the anus a rat teat appears and emerges outward."

[3]See *MS*I.E.129 on the food sacrifice. "Offering niche by the entrance to the inner chamber" translates 内户旁祠空中. *MWD*, vol. 4, "Transcription," n. 6, suggests that 空中 (niche) may be excrescent (perhaps a case of dittography since the two graphs conclude the recipe). But we are still left with an "offering (place) by the entrance to the inner chamber." If there were "offering places" near the bedroom in early China, this recipe is the first evidence of them. I suspect that there may be a technical denotation that is unknown to me. For example, *neihu* 内户 seems to mean "entrance to the inner chamber" (there are corroborative uses of *hu* in *MS*VII.A), but perhaps it is an unattested compound for a cult site. Because the recipe also calls for the head of a dead person, and *MS*I.E.129 calls for the food sacrifice of a dead person, the "entrance to the inner chamber" may refer to a structure located in the graveyard.

[4]"Black ewe" translates *yu* 羭, which is the gloss given in *SW*, 4A.34a.

[5]I read *xiu* 滫 as a verb meaning "moisten." According to *SW*, 11A-2.33a, *xiu* is the slop left over from cleaning grain to prepare it for cooking, specifically aged slop that has soured. The word is also used like *sou* 溲 to refer to moistening flour to make a paste; and is attested in the sense of moistening a dish with the addition of liquid (see the Duan Yucai commentary). *MWD*, vol. 4, "Transcription," n. 2, interprets *xiu* as a noun meaning

two portions. Use [3] {1} one portion. Then take copper bits[1] and the dregs of soybean sauce,[2] half and half. Pestle together. Spread (a layer) as thick as a *jiu* (leek) leaf on the holes. Then wrap with thick cloth. [2] warm it anew. In two days it desists.

MSI.E.145 (CC244-45)

Another. Recipe for male hemorrhoids lodged on the side of the anus—large ones like a *zao* (jujube) and small ones like a *zao* (jujube) pit. Use a small horn to perform horn treatment for the time it takes to cook two *dou* of rice and lift off the horn.[3] Bind it with a small cord and cut it open with a knife. Inside there is something like a *tu* fruit.[4] If hardened blood comes out like it is breaking open the tip (of the hemorrhoid), then it desists. Excellent.

"grain slop" and proposes that the sentence is missing a verb to indicate that the grain slop is added to the millet while it is cooking. Given the attested meaning of *xiu* as "moisten," the argument for the missing verb is weak.

[1]"Copper bits" translates *yumo* 鋊末. *Yu* is glossed as "copper flakes" in *SW*, 14A.7b; and the term refers specifically to the bits of copper scraped off coins. Copper flakes are listed in materia medica (*GM*, 8.9).

[2]The recipe specifies *shujiang* 菽醬, so it is clear that the main ingredient of the sauce is soybeans. Besides soybeans, fish and meat were also fermented to produce *jiang* in Han times; and it is possible that *jiang* was the name for a mixture combining these thick sauces with gruel vinegar (Hayashi 1975: 58–60).

[3]"Perform horn treatment" translates *jiao* 角. *Waitai biyaofang*, 13.9a, contains a description of cupping by Zhang Wenzhong 張文仲 (fl. 685) that uses *jiao* as the verb for cupping. The cups are short sections of bamboo that are boiled and then pressed on the skin. *MSI*.E.145 seems to concern the same general therapy, making it the oldest record of cupping in Chinese medical literature. The recipe indicates neither how to fashion the horn-cup nor how to apply it to the skin. Ma Jixing interprets the lack of details as a sign that cupping was already commonly practiced and did not require explanation (1992: 507). Given that *MSI*.E.145 provides the only evidence of cupping in early Chinese medicine, I am skeptical that it was a common therapy and am inclined to regard its use in *MSI*.E to treat a hemorrhoid as an exceptional case. There is no comparison between early Chinese medicine and Greco-Roman medicine, where the popularity of cupping is well documented from the fifth century B.C. Used most often in conjunction with blood-letting, the cups came to serve as symbols of the medical profession. In China, on the other hand, there is no evidence that cupping was integrated into medical theory and therapeutics. The most likely explanation of the cupping technique in *MSI*.E.145 that I have found is given by the first century A.D. Roman physician Celsus. Most Greek and Roman cups were bronze, but Celsus also describes a horn cup that is open at the large end with a small hole in the tip. The horn is placed on the skin, the air sucked out, and the small hole sealed with wax to make the cup adhere (Jackson 1988: 72–73).

[4]*MWD*, vol. 4, "Transcription," n. 3, reads [illegible] (unattested in received literature) as *shi* 實 (fruit), and compares the compound *tushi* 兔實 to *tuxi shi* 兔系實 in the Wuwei recipes (*WWYJ*: 2a). The latter drug can be equated with *tusi zi* 菟絲子, which refers to dodder seeds (*ZY*: no. 4125, *Cuscuta chinensis* Lam., *C. japonica* Choisy).

*MS*I.E.146
(CC246-47) Another. Recipe for male hemorrhoids the size of a *zao* (jujube) pit lodged on the edge of the anus which at times itch and at times are painful. First cut it off. If it cannot be cut off, [take][1] turtle brain and *didan chong* (oil beetles), half and half. Blend and spread on (the hemorrhoid). Burn small oblong stones. Quench them in gruel vinegar and use them to hot-press. If it does not desist, repeat it again following this procedure. Excellent.

*MS*I.E.147
(CC248-52) Female Hemorrhoid

Recipe for (female hemorrhoids) that are one *cun* inside the anus, are shaped like a cow louse, {1} [2] {1}, burst and ooze blood when defecating, and face upward when not defecating. Take five *dou* of urine. Use it to boil two large handfuls of *qinghao* (wormwood), seven *fuyu* (golden carp) the size of a hand, a six *cun* piece of smithed *gui* (cinnamon), and two nodules of dried *jiang* (ginger). Let it bubble ten times. Remove (the liquid) and put it in a water jar. Bury (the jar) under a sitting mat, make an opening in it, and fumigate the hemorrhoids. Stop when the medicine becomes cold. Fumigate thrice a day. When the throat becomes choked, drink medicinal beverage and do not drink anything else.

The recipe for making medicinal beverage. Take two *sheng* of the dried and smithed stalks of *qu*.[2] Soak it in two *dou* of *shuluo* (yam)[3] liquid to make a beverage. Drink it, stopping when the ailment desists. The Jing name for *qinghao* (wormwood) is *qiu*.[4] The Jing

---

[1]The lacuna must be 以 or 取.

[2]Identification of *qu* 蓲, which is not attested as a drug name in received literature, and its alternate name given below, *luru* 盧 茹, is problematic. *MS*I.E.253 uses the drug *quju* 屈居, which is glossed with *luru* in *Guangya*, 10A.24b. This drug is listed in materia medica. However, I doubt that *qu* in *MS*I.E.147 can be equated with *quju* in *MS*I.E.253; and given that *qu* is supposed to be the name with wider currency, I doubt that the Jing (i.e. Chu) name *luru* can be identified with the name attested in materia medica. *MWD*, vol. 4, "Transcription," n. 7, argues that *luru* is a scribal metathesis of *rulu* "madder" (*ZY*: no. 3276, *Rubia cordifolia* L.). *Rulu* occurs in *MS*I.E.252. Ma Jixing reviews other speculations regarding the alternate name and continues to regard *rulu* as the best (1992: 513, n. 23). I think it advisable to refrain from a positive identification.

[3]I accept the judgment of *MWD*, vol. 4, "Transcription," n. 5, that *shuluo* 署 蓏 is equivalent to *shuyu* 署 預 (*ZY*: no. 0319, *Dioscorea opposita* Thunb.). *Luo* refers to edible tubers (*SW*, 1B.3a, and Duan Yucai commentary), in this case the yams.

[4]Jing 荆 designates the region of Chu 楚. *SW*, 1B.28b, also glosses *qiu* 萩 as a variety of artemisia.

name for *qu* is *luru*. Its leaves can be boiled and are sour; its stalks have thorns. Excellent.

*MS*I.E.148 (C253)

Another. Recipe for female hemorrhoids that have holes, are curved, and ooze blood. Incinerate a woman's (menstrual) cloth. Set it in a vessel and fumigate the hemorrhoids with it, stopping after three days. Excellent.

*MS*I.E.149 (CC254-57)

Another. Recipe for female hemorrhoids that have numerous openings with *rao* (pinworms),[1] white and swarming, coming out. First introduce a slick *xia* (catalpa) rod[2] to let out the blood. Dig a hole in the ground one and a half *chi* deep, one *chi* long, and three *cun* across. Incinerate [1] charcoal in it. Dry[3] one third *dou* of *luoruan*[4] and distribute it on the charcoal. Cover the entire top with cloth and kneel to fumigate the anus. When the fumes are extinguished, take fatty [1] flesh and set it in the fire.[5] From time to time, (have the person) open the anus himself. [2] burn [1] {1} fire is extinguished [1] {1} [1]. Fumigate once a day. {1} [2] {1} [1] five to six days {1} [4]. Other names for *luoruan* are *baiku* and *kuqin*.

---

[1] *SW*, 13A.42b, glosses *rao* 蟯 as "a short worm inside the abdomen." The worm is the pinworm, *Enterobius vermicularis*. Several pinworm eggs were found in the lower intestinal tract of the corpse buried in Mawangdui tomb 1 (Hunan yixueyuan 1980: 202); and in *Shiji*, 105.18a, Chunyu Yi diagnoses an ailment he calls *raojia* 蟯瘕 (pinworm conglomeration). *MS*I.E.149 associates female hemorrhoids with the presence of the pinworms, reflecting the belief that chewing bugs cause hemorrhoids. *Chaoshi zhubing yuanhoulun*, 18.5a, explicitly names pinworms as the culprits: "Pinworms inhabit the colon. When numerous, they cause hemorrhoids."

[2] *Xia* 夏 should be read as *xia* 榎, a variant graph for *jia* 檟 (*SW*, 6A.8a, and Duan Yucai commentary). It refers to the catalpa (*ZY*: no. 4091, *Catalpa ovata* G. Don).

[3] "Dry" translates *xia* 煆, which is the gloss for *xia* in *Fangyan*, 7.5b (especially to dry something by heating it).

[4] *Luoruan* 駱阮 is not attested in received literature. Ma Jixing reviews arguments for identifying the plant based on the second of the two alternate names given below, *kuqin* 苦浸 (1992: 519, n. 12). Reading *qin/*tshjəm* as a phonetic loan for *shen/*tshəm* 參, the name is equivalent to *kushen* 苦參 (*ZY*: no. 2624, *Sophora flavescens* Ait.), listed in *BC* (*GM*, 13.54). The identification is plausible.

[5] Fat is added to generate more fumes.

*MS*I.E.150 (C258)

Another. For hemorrhoids. Pour sauce into a yellow hen until it dies on its own. Wrap it in *jian* (miscanthus),[1] daub mud on it,[2] and bake it.[3] When the mud has dried, eat the chicken. Use the feathers to fumigate the perineum.

*MS*I.E.151 (CC259-60)

Another. Smith *miwu* (lovage), *fangfeng* (saposhnikovia), *wuhui* (monkshood), and *gui* (cinnamon)—all in equal amounts. Soak in pure liquor and form them into balls the size of a black soybean. Then swallow them. At the beginning, eat one. If it does not respond, increase by one, with [1] as the upper limit. It may also be used[4] to master wounds.[5] Always eat them before eating.

*MS*I.E.152 (C261)

Another. For before there is a nest.[6] Boil one *dou* of *zao* (jujubes) and one *dou* of lard to produce four *dou* of liquid. Put it in a basin and squat in it. The worms come out.

*MS*I.E.153 (CC262-63)

Another. For when a nest obstructs the rectum. Kill a dog. Take its bladder and insert it through (the end of) a bamboo tube. Insert the tube into the rectum and blow on it. Draw it out and slowly cut off the nest with a knife. Smith *huangqin* (skullcap) and spread it on repeatedly. If the person's anus is prolapsed and cannot be put back inside, grease the part that is prolapsed with lard and suspend the person upside down. Throw cold water on his heart and abdomen and it will go back inside.

---

[1]Mizukami presents conclusive evidence that *jian* 菅 should be identified as *Miscanthus sinensis* (1977: 558-60). The grass is similar to *mao* "woolly grass," and the two are often confused.

[2]*MWD*, vol. 4, "Transcription," emends text *shang* 上 to *tu* 土, claiming scribal error. Since the meaning "to daub (something) with mud" is already implicit in the preceding word *tu* 涂, the emendation is unnecessary.

[3]"Bake" translates *bao* 炮, a popular Han method of baking whole animals wrapped in clay without removing the fur or feathers (*SW*, 10A.45a, and Duan Yucai commentary).

[4]以 in *MWD*, vol. 4, "Transcription," should be transcribed as *wei* 爲.

[5]The medicine in *MS*I.E.151 is similar to some of the medicines in the first ailment category, Various Wounds.

[6]I follow *MWD*, vol. 4, "Transcription," n. 1, in identifying *chao* 巢 (nest) as an anal fistula; and in associating the name with the presence of worms "nesting."

MSI.E.154 (C264)

Bloody hemorrhoid. Boil thoroughly one male rat in urine. Hot-press with the vapor.

MSI.E.155 (CC265-69)

Anus Itchiness[1]

For when hemorrhoids occur and small holes protrude like cones on the side of the rectum of the person with hemorrhoids. At times white worms emerge from the holes,[2] and the burning pain in the rectum is caustic. To treat it use one portion of *liuxun* (willow fungus)[3] and two of crumbled *ai* (mugwort),[4] altogether two substances. Dig a hole in the ground, making the width and depth the same size as a small saucer. Burn the earth inside the hole until it is dry, and put the *ai* (mugwort) in it. Put the *liuxun* (willow fungus) on top of the *ai* (mugwort) and burn the *ai* (mugwort) and fungus. Then take a small saucer. Bore a hole in the bottom one *cun* in diameter, and cover (the hole in the ground) with it. Mound up earth around the

---

[1] "Anus" translates 朐, for which *MWD*, vol. 4, "Transcription," n. 1, offers two possible readings. The first is based on the Mawangdui manuscript of the *Yijing* hexagrams. The text of the hexagram Jing 井 writes *gou/*kug* 句, whereas in the received *Yijing* the graph in the corresponding position is *lou/*lug* 漏. Since *lou* denotes anal fistula in medical usage (Yu Yan 1972: 120), perhaps the graph 朐 is a phonetic loan for *lou* and means "fistula." The argument is plausible, but flawed. In the Mawangdui *Yijing* text, *gou* is not a phonetic loan for *lou*, but is part of a phrase whose grammar and meaning differ from the received text. For the phrase 甕 敝 漏 ("the jar is worn out and leaks") in the received text, the Mawangdui text has 唯 敝 句. Han Zhongmin compares *bigou* 敝 句 to *bigou* 敝 笱 in the *Shijing*, in which case the phrase means, "it is a worn out fish-trap basket" (1992: 139). The second "Transcription" reading equates the graph 朐 with *gouzi* 鉤 子, a word meaning "anus" in Shaanxi dialect that is related to other similar vernacular terms for the buttocks and anus. I tentatively accept the second reading.

[2] The worms are undoubtedly the pinworms mentioned in *MS*I.E.149. The phrase 時 從 其 空 出 "at times emerge from the holes" is written twice in the text before and after 有 白 蟲 "there are white worms." The first occurrence is excrescent. I suspect that the scribe initially erred by not writing 有 白 蟲 before writing 時 從 其 空 出; and after correcting himself by writing the whole again, he then forgot to blot out the now excrescent phrase.

[3] *Xun* 蕈 is the fungus known as "wood ear" (*ZY*: no. 0701, *Auricularia auricula* [L. ex Hook.] Underw.). Wood ear is listed in *BC* (*GM*, 28.23). *Liu* 柳 (*ZY*: no. 3175, *Salix babylonica* L.) is one of five trees from which wood ears are harvested according to *GM*.

[4] "Crumbled" translates *nuo* 捼, glossed in *SW*, 12A.45a, as "break up by rubbing the hands together." Duan Yucai regards 捼 as a miswriting of 挼, but *MS*I.E.155 shows that first graph is also correct. *MWD*, vol. 4, "Transcription," n. 5, interprets *nuo* as a measure word for the amount of *liuxun* ("one *nuo* of *liuxun*"), in which case it does not modify *ai*. Ma Jixing proposes reading 捼 as *rui* 䅗, which is attested in medieval sources as a measure word meaning "four handfuls of grain" (1992: 529, n. 10). I am not convinced by either argument.

saucer, and seal it [so that][1] smoke cannot leak out. Then cover the saucer with a garment without covering the hole in the saucer. Then have the person with hemorrhoids squat on the saucer with his rectum directly over the hole in the saucer, and let the smoke fumigate the rectum. When fumigating the rectum, raise it when it gets hot and lower when it gets cold. Stop when exhausted.

*MS*I.E.156 (C270)

Another. Take stones the size of a fist, twice seven in number. Thoroughly burn them. Have two thirds *sheng* of well beaten rice[2] and eight times that amount of water, and put the stones into it.[3] [2] cooked, then drink it, and it desists.

*MS*I.E.157 (CC271-72) *Ju* Abscess Ailment[4]

Smith *bailian* (ampelopsis), *huangqi* (astragalus), *shaoyao* (peony), *gui* (cinnamon), *jiang* (ginger), *jiao* (zanthoxylum), and *zhuyu* (evodia)—altogether seven substances. For *ju* abscesses of the bone, double the *bailian* (ampelopsis). For *ju* abscesses of the flesh, double the *huangqi* (astragalus). For *ju* abscesses of the testicles, double the *shaoyao* (peony). Use one portion of each of the others. Combine, and put one large three-fingered pinch into a cup of liquor. Drink it five or six times a day. Wait for it to desist [?].

*MS*I.E.158 (C273)

Another. Boil *penglei* (raspberry),[5] scalding thrice. Use four *dou* of the liquid to wash the *ju* abscess.

---

[1]The lacuna is undoubtedly 令.

[2]*Fa* 伐 (beaten) is not attested as a term for grain preparation. It probably refers to polishing the rice.

[3]The hot stones cook the rice.

[4]According to *SW*, 7B.30a, *ju* 疽 refers to "an old *yong* 癰," *yong* being the more general term for an abscess. Duan Yucai interprets the gloss to mean that *ju* is an abscess that becomes *ju* 沮 (rotted, leaky). A separate ailment category for *yong* begins in *MS*I.E.225. The *SW* definition of *ju* as "an old *yong*" does not seem to apply in *MS*I.E because a number of recipes treat *ju* "when it first appears." The distinction between *yong* and *ju* in *Lingshu* 81, 12.10b, also cannot be applied to *MS*I.E. *MS*I.E.158 uses the compound *juyong*—meaning the "*ju* type of *yong*"—whereas *ju* is not mentioned in the section of recipes which treat *yong*. In light of this usage, and lacking better evidence, I adopt the expedient of translating *yong* as "abscess" and *ju* as "*ju* abscess."

[5]*Penglei* 蓬 虆 is listed in *BC* (*GM*, 18.6). There is much scholarly discussion over the question of whether the name refers to the vine and root or to the berries of the raspberry (*ZY*: no. 0964, *Rubus tephrodes* Hance). Tao Hongjing identifies it as the root.

MSI.E.159 (C274)

Another. When a *ju* abscess first occurs, soak *shanglao* (pokeweed)[1] in gruel vinegar, and hot-press the swollen spot with it.

MSI.E.160 (CC275-76)

Another. Take *bailian* (ampelopsis), *huangqi* (astragalus), *shaoyao* (peony), and *gancao* (licorice)—and boil the four substances. [1],[2] *jiang* (ginger), Shu *jiao* (Shu zanthoxylum), and *zhuyu* (evodia)—(use an amount of) the four substances equivalent to one of the (first four) substances. The first is bone [3] {1} [2] using one cup of liquor [4] muscle type, which glares and glitters. [2] {2} [5].[3] Drink four times a day. Once it is ready to burst, stop.

MSI.E.161 (CC277-79)

Another. Recipe for [25].[4] Use [2] *dou* [20] {1} wash the *ju* abscess [5] {2} [?].

MSI.E.162 (CC280-82)

Another. When a *ju* abscess has not yet [4] fourteen nodules of *wuhui* (monkshood). Use one half *sheng* of fine gruel vinegar [6] two thirds *dou* of grain-cleaning slop,[5] and put the medicine into it. [3] until it is like [5] roast[6] the hand {2} [3] spread [5] it. Seal with the remaining medicine and wrap [4] not be painful. When it desists[7] [2]. Excellent.

---

[1] *MWD*, vol. 4, "Transcription," n. 1, equates *shang lao/***lǝgw* 商牢 with *shang lu/***ljǝkw* 陸 (*ZY*: no. 4664, *Phytolacca acinosa* Roxb.; pokeweed), listed in *BC* (*GM*, 17.7).

[2] The lacuna must be the name of a drug because the recipe specifies that there are also four substances in the second list of drugs.

[3] The extensive lacunae prevent a clear understanding of the recipe. The latter part of the recipe appears to discuss two types of abscess—bone and muscle—and to give a description of the appearance of the muscle abscess. *Shu* 倏 (glare) is attested as an orthographic variant of 倏 (Morohashi 1957-60, vol. 1: no. 763). The reduplicated compound *shushu* is glossed in *Guangya*, 6A.8a, as "radiant." In *MSI*.E.160 and again in *MSI*.E.166, the compound describes the inflamed appearance of the abscess. The second compound, *didi* 翟翟 (glitter), represents a term for the glistening quality of light and is written with a number of related graphs: 曜曜, 耀耀, 燿燿, 濯濯. In *MSI*.E.160 *didi* refers to the shiny swollen surface of the abscess.

[4] The word "recipe" occurs near the bottom of C277, meaning that there must be an extended description of the kind of *ju* abscess being treated.

[5] *Shi* 釋 refers to the action of soaking and washing grain (*SW*, 7A.61a); and *gan* 泔 is the grain slop left over from the cleaning process (*SW*, 11A-2.33a).

[6] 灸 in *MWD*, vol. 4, "Transcription," should be transcribed as *zhi* 炙 (roast).

[7] 己 in *MWD*, vol. 4, "Transcription," should be transcribed as *yi* 已 (desist).

*MS*I.E.163 (C283)

Another. For a *ju* abscess of the throat. Smith together three portions of *bailian* (ampelopsis) and one portion of *bahe*.[1] [7] drink it.

*MS*I.E.164

(CC284-85) Another. Suppurating abscess. When a suppurating abscess [2] occurs and [8] and smith. Take pig lard that has not been rendered,[2] melt it by roasting,[3] and blend it with [1]. Spread (the medicine) on it. Spread the medicine once a day. Before spreading the medicine, wash with warm water. Apply the medicine for thirty days. [1] desists. Previously tested. Excellent.

*MS*I.E.165

(CC286-88) Another. When various *ju* abscesses first appear. Thoroughly scorch one *dou* of soybeans. Then quickly remove them and set in a slotted steaming-pot. [9] {2} [2]. Pour one *dou* of pure liquor over it. [2], then drink the entire amount of liquid. If after drinking once the ailment has not desisted, [11] drinking it is permitted.[4] After just several times of drinking (the medicine), the ailment desists. There are no prohibitions. Previously tested. Excellent.

*MS*I.E.166

(CC289-91) Another. When a blood *ju* abscess first appears, is glaringly[5] hot, and the pain is unrelenting. [6] *ju* abscess [12] *daishen* (astragalus),[6] *huangqin* (skullcap), and *bailian* (ampelopsis)—leaving them all for three days. [19] it, until sweat flows down to the feet. It desists.

*MS*I.E.167

(CC292-93) Another. When a vapor *ju* abscess first appears, forming a volatile callus[7] in the shape of a [1]. If rubbed [1] and [16], two nodules,

---

[1]*Bahe* 罷 合 is not attested in received materia medica. Ma Jixing equates *ba/*prəg* with *bai/*prak* 百—which is phonologically plausible (1992: 539, n. 2). *Baihe* 百 合 is listed in *BC* (*GM*, 27.121) and refers to *Lilium brownii* F.E. Brown var. *colchesteri* Wils., and other species (*ZY*: no. 1728).

[2]Evidently pig fat was usually rendered before being used in medicine.

[3]灸 in *MWD*, vol. 4., "Transcription," should be transcribed as *zhi* 炙 (roast).

[4]The lacuna probably details the increased dosages, including the maximum dosage permitted.

[5]倏 must be an orthographic variant of *shu* 倏 (see *MS*I.E.160).

[6]*Daishen* 戴 糁 is given as an alternate name for *huangqi* (astragalus) in *BC* (*GM*, 12A.85).

[7]I read the unattested graph 痹 as *pian* 胼. *Pian* occurs frequently in pre-Han and Han literature with the meaning "callus" (e.g. *Xunzi* 29, 29.348). While the graph in *MS*I.E.167 is not an attested variant for *pian*, the significs 疒 and 月 are often interchangeable (*you* "wart" is written 疣 and 肬). In *MS*I.E.167 *pian* refers to the layer of skin covering the abscess. "Volatile" translates *yun* 涓, attested in the sense of agitated, choppy water in Guo

until smashed;[1] soybeans, [1] scorched {1} [1]. Pour liquor over it, then sieve [16] comes out and stop.

*MS*I.E.168 (CC295-96)

Another. When a [1] *ju* abscess appears, protruding from the body like the [1] of a person who has died.[2] If someone jostles it, it is extremely [19] one half *dou*, and boil to produce three *sheng*.[3] Drink it. Dress warmly and lie down [?].

*MS*I.E.169 (C297)

Another. [10] {1} [?].[4]

*MS*I.E.170 (C298)

[?] although [?].

*MS*I.E.171 (CC299-300)

Another. [?] *ju* abscess. *Jiang* (ginger), *gui* (cinnamon), *jiao* (zanthoxylum), [1]—leaving them for four [?] one half *dou* of pure liquor. Boil until it produces three *sheng*.[5] [?].

*MS*I.E.172 (CC301-302)

Another. [?] three small bunches, and chop finely. One *dou* of pure liquor [?], then sieve and [drink] it.[6] Dress warmly [?].

*MS*I.E.173 (C303)

Another. [?] *gui* (cinnamon), *jiao* (zanthoxylum) [?].[7]

Pu's 郭璞 "Jiang fu" 江賦 (*Wenxuan*, 12.7b). *SW*, 6B.14a, glosses a related word, *yun* 䞫, as describing a chaotic, turbulent condition.

[1]I read the unattested graph ⿱⿰言勿手 as *hu* ⿰扌忽. The phonetic ⿰言勿 can be equated with *hu* 曶. The interchangeability of 曶 and 忽 as the phonetic in certain graphs is noted in the Duan Yucai commentary in *SW*, 5A.28b. Thus ⿱⿰言勿手 (the bottom represents hands) is probably a variant of ⿰扌忽. According to *Fangyan*, 10.9b, the latter word means "strike, beat" in southern Chu, which suggests that the use of ⿱⿰言勿手 in *MS*I.E.167 is an example of regional dialect.

[2]The abscess is being compared to some noticeable feature of a corpse.

[3]I.e. the liquid is reduced from one half *dou* (five *sheng*) to three *sheng*.

[4]*MWD*, vol. 4, "Transcription," n. 1, notes that there is a break in the text after C297; it is not clear how many columns might be missing.

[5]As in *MS*I.E.168 the liquid is reduced to three *sheng*.

[6]I suspect that the unattested graph ⿰氵㚇 is a scribal miswriting of *jun* 浚 (sieve); and that the lacuna is *yin* 飲 (drink). Ma Jixing reads the unattested graph as *zong* 㚇, with the meaning "gather" (1992: 546, n. 2). However, the context suggests that a liquid medicine is sieved and drunk (compare the fragmentary *MS*I.E.167, which mentions sieving; and several recipes in which the medicine for *ju* abscess is drunk).

[7]*MWD*, vol. 4, "Transcription," n. 1, notes that there is a break in the text after C303; it is not clear how many columns might be missing.

*MS*I.E.174 (C304)[1]

Another. Boil wheat.[2] When the wheat is cooked, wash it[3] with the liquid. [3] lard [?].

*MS*I.E.175 (C305)

Another. Roast[4] *zi* (catalpa) leaves, and warm it.[5]

*MS*I.E.176 (C306)

Recipe for [1] Burns[6]

Daub human sludge[7] on it, and seal with dog or sheep fur. If it does not desist, again use [?].

*MS*I.E.177 (C307)

Another. When a burn occurs, masticate malt, wring (in a cloth) to obtain the liquid,[8] and fry until it resembles gelatin. Then smith *houpu* (magnolia bark). Blend. Spread (the medicine on the burn).

*MS*I.E.178 (C308)

Another. When a burn occurs, utter this curse: "Sjit sjit, khwjət khwjət.[9] Come out from the stove and do not spread. The Yellow Spirit is about to speak with you."[10] Immediately spit on it thrice.

---

[1]According to *MS*I.E.1 there is one ailment category between *Ju* Abscesses and [1] Burns. The name is missing both in *MS*I.E.1 and in the body of the text. Since [1] Burns begins in *MS*I.E.176, and *MS*I.E.174-175 both open with the formula "another (recipe)," the latter two recipes must belong to the unknown ailment category.

[2]There is ambiguity as to whether *mai* 麥 refers to *damai* 大麥 (*ZY*: no. 0186, *Hordeum vulgare* L.; barley) or *xiaomai* 小麥 (*ZY*: no. 0474, *Triticum aestivum* L.; wheat). Based on archaeological evidence and received sources, Hayashi argues for barley (1975: 8). However, I am inclined to identify *mai* as wheat on the basis of a hemp sack labeled *mai* that was excavated from Mawangdui tomb 1 and that contained a quantity of *Triticum turgidum* L. mixed with which were a very few grains of *Hordeum vulgare* L. (Hunan nongxueyuan et al. 1978: 4-5). The occurrence of *mai* in recipes for liquors in *MS*III.10 and *MS*III.74 also suggests wheat. Wheat and barley are listed in materia medica (*GM*, 22.53, 58).

[3]I.e. wash the affected part of the body.

[4]灸 in *MWD*, vol. 4, "Transcription," should be transcribed as *zhi* 炙 (roast).

[5]I.e. use the roasted leaves to warm the affected part of the body.

[6]*MWD*, vol. 4, "Transcription," n. 1, states that judging from the remaining fragment of the graph in the lacuna it might be *huo* 火 (fire). In any case, *lan* 爛 is attested meaning a skin burn in *Zuozhuan*, Ding 3, 54.5a.

[7]*Renni* 人泥 (human sludge) is not attested in materia medica. *MS*I.E.198 calls for "sludge (*ni*) from old urine," which can be equated with a urine product in received materia medica. *MWD*, vol. 4, "Transcription," n. 2, suggests that "human sludge" might refer to body sweat and grime. Dandruff occurs elsewhere in *MS*I.E, but other waxy, grimy matter that collects on the body might all come under the heading "human sludge." Compare *GM*, 52.86 (ear dirt, dirt from the kneecap); and 52.102 (dental detritus, body sweat). *KGS*, vol. 1: 245, n. 660, suggests feces as one referent for "sludge," but given other words for feces in *MS*I.E I doubt the identification.

[8]On wringing a medicine through a cloth, see *MS*I.E.13.

MSI.E.179 (C309)

Another. Boil a sufficient amount of glutinous spiked millet. When just cooked, sieve, and scorch it until it becomes ash. Spread (the ash) on it for several days. If (the ash) becomes dry, beat liquid into it.

MSI.E.180 (C310)

Another. Beat a chicken egg into rabbit fur, and spread (the medicine) on it.

---

[9]The utterance *xi xi, qu qu* 肸 肸 詘 詘 (represented in reconstructed form in the translation) must be related to the utterance *xi xi, chu chu* 譆 譆 出 出 recorded in *Zuozhuan*, Xiang 30, 40.3b. The utterance is shouted anonymously in the Great Temple of the state of Song. According to the commentary, *xi* signifies a fire omen and *chu* is monitory ("get out"); and in the *Zuozhuan* narrative the utterance anticipates a conflagration in Song. In *MSI*.E.178 the phrase is written using the repeat-graph sign, mistranscribed in *MWD*, vol. 4, "Transcription," as 肸 詘 肸 詘. Qiu Xigui notes the *Zuozhuan* parallel and corrects the "Transcription" (1992: 532). In *MSI*.E.178 *xi* 肸 refers literally to a swarm of bugs rising like a cloud (*SW*, 3A.6a, and Duan Yucai commentary), an image that might also suggest fire. *Qu* probably has the sense of "submit." In context, the utterance seems to express the idea that "the burn submit"; which is then explicitly stated in the following line of the incantation: "Come out from the stove and do not spread." The connection between the use of the utterance to treat a skin burn in *MSI*.E.178 and its premonitory use in the *Zuozhuan* is obvious. Together with a similar four syllable utterance in *MSI*.E.265 (in an incantation that also names the Yellow Spirit) we have evidence of multi-syllabic utterances that belonged to a common stock of incantatory speech.

[10]The rhyming words in the incantation are: *yan/*ran* 延 (spread) and *yan/*ngjan* 言 (speak). The incantation in *MSI*.E.265 also invokes the Yellow Spirit 黄 神. The Yellow Spirit is the same deity as the Yellow Thearch 黄 帝 (see *Huainanzi*, 6.96), whose identity in received literature as a mythical culture hero and patron of esoteric arts is being expanded through archaeological evidence that reveals him as a supreme deity in popular religion. Seidel discusses the nature of the Yellow Spirit as a supreme deity as it is currently known from Han archaeological evidence, which is mostly related to mortuary customs (1987: 28-34). The invocations in *MSI*.E.178 and 265 clearly relate to the religious aspects of the Yellow Spirit identified by Seidel. Another reference to the Yellow Spirit in *MSVII*.B.1 in a dialogue concerning sexual hygiene serves to indicate that the images of supreme deity and patron of esoteric arts are not independent traditions, and that they can probably be traced to a common magico-religious source. It is also noteworthy that the Yellow Thearch as culture hero has the name Yellow Progenitor 黄 宗 in the cosmo-political writings that precede the second Mawangdui edition of *Laozi*, where the Yellow Thearch's emergence in the world is described as an act of cosmic self-creation (*MWD*, vol. 1: 61). While a complete understanding of the multifaceted Yellow Thearch in pre-Han and Han belief still eludes us, the archaeological and manuscript evidence regarding his role in religion sheds new light on the subject.

*MS*I.E.181 (C311)

Another. Smith malt, blend breast milk[1] into it, and spread (the medicine) on it. It is not painful and does not scar.

*MS*I.E.182 (C312)

Another. Incinerate *yuyi* (algae),[2] and spread the ash on it.

*MS*I.E.183 (C313)

Another. Incinerate worn out plaited hemp[3] and smith. Spread (the ash) on it with a cloth.

*MS*I.E.184 (C314)

Another. Soak a menstrual cloth, and spread the liquid on it.

*MS*I.E.185 (C315)

Another. Steam alkaline soil[4] and wrap. Hot-press it with (the wrapped soil).

*MS*I.E.186 (C316)

Another. When a burn from scalding bath water occurs, scorch pig feces, soak in gruel vinegar, and seal it (with the medicine).

*MS*I.E.187 (C317)

Another. When a serious burn from scalding water occurs, scorch pig feces, moisten with liquor, and seal it (with the medicine).

*MS*I.E.188 (CC318-19)

Another. For scars. Use two portions of mercury, four portions of a man's muck,[5] and one portion of cinnabar. Blend together, and set

---

[1]*Ruzhi* 乳汁 (breast milk) is a general term for milk, as attested in *SW*, 11A-2.40a, which glosses *dong* 湩 with *ruzhi*. It is probable that *ruzhi* in *MS*I.E.181 refers specifically to milk from a woman's breast.

[2]The Zheng Sinong commentary in *Zhouli*, 6.1b, identifies *tai* 箈 as "*yuyi* 魚衣 (fish garment) which is in the water." *SW*, 1B.32b, glosses *tai* similarly as "*qingyi* 青衣 (green garment) in the water." *Tai* also refers to moss and lichens, but it is evident that in Han times algae was the primary referent; and that *yuyi* was one of several names comparing the algae to a garment. The algae called *zhili* 陟釐 in *BL* (*GM*, 21.17) appears to represent the type denoted by such names. It is described as a hair-like algae usually found growing on submerged rocks. Although the name *zhili* is also applied to some seaweeds, it is unlikely that *yuyi* in *MS*I.E.182 is a seaweed.

[3]*He* 褐 is glossed in *SW*, 8A.65a, both as plaited hemp footwear and as a coarse garment. Hayashi identifies the hemp footwear mentioned in *SW* as a shoe sole, and shows that the hemp garment was also made of plaited material rather than woven fabric (1976: 43-44, 141).

[4]圂 is a variant of *lu* 鹵. Wei and Hu cite Li Xueqin, who states that the identification is confirmed by occurrences of the graph in Zhangjiashan manuscripts and pottery inscriptions (1992, vol. 1: 124, n. 1). The name *lutu* 鹵土 suggests that the substance is raw alkaline soil and not the salt purified from it. *Lutu* is also listed in *Wanwu*, where it is recommended for treating drowsiness (Fuyang Han jian zhenglizu 1988: 38).

on the stove flue for two or three days.[1] When it is finished, then [3] sack, and spread (the medicine) on it. (During the time the medicine) is being spread, remain indoors. Block the windows, bar the entry, and do not go out. Perform private functions in the inner (chamber),[2] and do not look at the stars and moon for one month.[3] In a hundred days, it desists.[4]

*MS*I.E.189 (CC320-21)

Another. To remove old scars, carefully split open a large melon and (?) the seeds.[5] Cut the melon, and use the [1] the size of two fingers to rub the scar until [2] it. Use [2] to spread on it. When dry, spread again. After the third time it desists. One must carefully observe ritual abstinence and restrictions[6] without [1] and it desists.

*MS*I.E.190 (C322)

Another. For [2]. {1} [2] {1} [1]. Spread the liquid on it, and skin grows.

*MS*I.E.191 (C323)

Another. For a scar [12]. Incinerate it until ashed. Use it to [2] like the old skin.

*MS*I.E.192 (C324)

Another. [?].

---

[5]*E* 惡 is used in *Wu Yue chunqiu*, 7.6a, to denote human feces (the passage concerns diagnosis by tasting feces). Perhaps "a man's muck" in *MS*I.E.188 refers to feces. *MWD*, vol. 4, "Transcription," n. 1, argues that the name denotes semen; and that it is related to the name "a man's slime" in *MS*I.E.11. The basis for the identification is the use of semen to treat scars in later medical literature, which is not incontrovertible proof of the meaning of *e* in *MS*I.E.188. The early textual evidence favors feces, but I would not rule out semen as a possible identification. *SW*, 13B.25b, glosses *e* 堊 as "white daub" (the white plaster applied to walls); perhaps semen is the corresponding male substance.

[1]月 in *MWD*, vol. 4, "Transcription," should be transcribed as *ri* 日 (day).

[2]*Si* 私 (perform private functions) is glossed as "urinate" in the commentary in *Zuozhuan*, Xiang 15, 32.13b.

[3]The prohibition on looking at the night sky might be related to a belief that scar tissue, like the growths in *MS*I.E.34, is affected by the essence from the stars and moon.

[4]己 in *MWD*, vol. 4, "Transcription," should be transcribed as *yi* 已 (desist).

[5]I am unable to offer a grammatical analysis of the sentence as written, and I suspect that the scribe omitted the verb from the phrase 而 其 瓣 (attempting to link the phrase as written with the sentence that follows also results in syntactic difficulty). The missing verb must indicate that the seeds are to be removed.

[6]*Zhaijie* 齋 戒 is the standard term for ritual purification preceding sacrifices to the spirits.

*MS*I.E.193 (C325)

Another. Boil autumn bamboo,[1] and fumigate the wound with the vapor. It desists.

*MS*I.E.194 (C326)

Shin Burns

To treat shin burns, smith old glutinous panicled millet and soybeans. Blend with dog bile, and spread it (on the burn).

*MS*I.E.195 (C327)

Another. Smith the pits inside *wuyi* (stinking elm fruits). Heat the firm[2] lard of a castrated pig and pour it into the smithed (pits). Blend, and spread it (on the burn).

*MS*I.E.196 (C328)

Another. Thoroughly boil two pheasants at a very fast boil. When the bird quill feathers loosen on their own and drop from the tail [5]. Incinerate both and smith. Blend the ash with pig lard, and spread.

*MS*I.E.197 (C329)

Another. On summer days use *jin* leaves, and on winter days use the root. Chew either one in the mouth and seal it. When it dries, immediately seal on top of that. This is all already proven.[3]

*MS*I.E.198 (CC330-31)

Shin Wounds

Carefully pick out the grass and grit from old urine sludge.[4] Put the sludge in a vessel. At dawn, use bitter liquor [2].[5] Spread the sludge on the wound. Spread [2] it, and the wound desists. Already used.[6]

---

[1] Autumn must refer to the season in which the bamboo is gathered.

[2] "Firm" translates *man* 糒, which is attested in medieval rhyme dictionaries with the meaning "congealed gruel" (see Morohashi 1957-60, vol. 8: no. 27099). *Man* occurs again in *MS*I.E.218, where it also refers to the firmness of castrated pig lard.

[3] *Yiyan* 已驗 (already proven) is one of the terms for tauting recipes mentioned in *Lunheng* (see *MS*I.E.15).

[4] *Niaozhong ni* 溺中泥 (urine sludge) can be equated with *niao baiyin* 溺白沍 (white sediment in urine) in materia medica (*GM*, 52.93). It is the sediment that precipitates out of human urine (*ZY*: no. 0056).

[5] *Kujiu* 苦酒 (bitter liquor) refers to vinegar—because vinegar has a bitter taste according to Tao Hongjing (*GM*, 25.23).

[6] I.e. the recipe has been used previously with good results.

MSI.E.199 (CC332-36)

Another. Old shin wound.[1] When an old shin wound becomes abscessed, the abscess bursts, and the liquid is like gruel. To treat it, boil two *dou* of water. Have one third *dou* of *yu* (tumeric), one third *dou* of *zhu* (atractylodes), and one third *dou* of [1]—altogether three substances—and smith both the *yu* (tumeric) and the *zhu* (atractylodes). [Put][2] them into the hot water and heat. When the water cools sufficiently to permit putting the foot into it, set a small piece of wood in the water. Then [2] {1} [2]. Put the foot into the water, step on the piece of wood, and slide [1].[3] When the water gets cold, heat it; and when it is hot, stop the fire and wait for the temperature to adjust itself. Put (the foot) into the water in the morning after eating, and remove it in the late afternoon.[4] The ailment will then be cured. If the ailment is not [severe],[5] it is cured after putting it into the water once. If severe, it is cured after putting it into the water five or six times. When it is cured, [1] abscess. [1] abscess and new flesh grows. When new flesh grows, stop putting (the foot) into the water. Then it will close itself and be cured. When applying the medicine there are no prohibitions, and in treating the ailment there are no temporal (restrictions). Excellent.

MSI.E.200 (C337)

Scabies[6]

---

[1] *Jiu* 久 occurs in several other recipes to indicate ailments that persist for a long time. Ma Jixing favors reading the graph as *jiu* 灸 (cauterize), and understands the ailment as "cauterization wounds on the shin" (i.e. eschars that do not heal following cauterization; 1992: 567, n. 1). Eschar scars are mentioned in a description of a corpse in the Shuihudi *Fengzhen shi*: "On his belly were old scars from cauterization in two places" (*SHD*: 157).

[2] Judging from the context, the lacuna should be *ru* 入.

[3] It appears that the person slides the piece of wood with his foot in order to move the shin around in the water while it soaks.

[4] "Late afternoon" translates *bushi* 餔 時, which corresponds to 3:00–5:00 P.M. (see *MSI*.E.67).

[5] Judging from the context, the lacuna should be *shen* 甚.

[6] By translating *jia* 痂 as "scabies," I understand scabies in the older sense of a scabby itch, not as the parasitic skin disease caused by the itch mite *Sarcoptes scabiei*. *MSI*.E.208 does refer to expelling bugs from the scabies, and many of the treatments in *MSI*.E are clearly vermifugal. But associating the ailment with bugs does not necessarily indicate early Chinese knowledge of the itch mite. *MSI*.E evidences a similar association between hemorrhoids and bugs, including vermifugal treatments and observation of pinworms (see *MSI*.E.149). *Chaoshi zhubing yuanhoulun*, 50.9a, provides more definite evidence of the observation of the itch mite when discussing *jie* 疥 (the standard name for the ailment in later medical literature): "The *Discourse on the Nine Bugs* states that pinworms undergo

Soak the feces of a black ram in the urine of an infant. Leave for one whole day.[1] Spread (the medicine) on it.

*MS*I.E.201 (C338)

Another. Smith realgar. Moisten with pig lard, and blend in a little gruel vinegar. Let (the medicine) [cool] to lukewarm,[2] and spread it on it. When (the medicine) is spread, do not clean it off. First wash the scabies thoroughly with hot water, and then spread (the medicine).

*MS*I.E.202 (C339)

Another. Smith *pulei*.[3] Work hub grease into it,[4] and spread (the medicine on the scabies). Spread and then roast it, spreading for three or four times.[5]

*MS*I.E.203 (C340)

Another. Slit the throat of a red lizard,[6] and daub the blood on it.

---

manifold transformations, and that they also transform to become *jie*. There are tiny bugs in the sores that are extremely hard to see." While *jie* and *jia* were synonymous in Han times (*SW*, 7B.30b), *jie* replaced *jia* as the name for the ailment in the post-Han period; and *jia* came to refer only to a scab that forms on a wound (Yu Yan 1972: 128, 235). *Jia* is the name for scabies recorded in *Maishu*, "Ailment List": "When it is located on the body, the scabs spread in channels, and it itches—it is *jia*" (*MSSW*: 72). *MS*I.E includes a separate category for other types of itch beginning in *MS*I.E.249.

[1] *Zu qi shi* 卒其時 is equivalent to *zu shi* 晬時, which is defined by Tao Hongjing as "the period of time from dawn today until dawn tomorrow" (*GM*, 1.40).

[2] Judging from the context, the lacuna must be *han* 寒. The literal meaning of the whole phrase is "let it be balanced between cold and warm."

[3] It is not certain whether *pulei* 僕鼺 is an herbal or animal drug. *MWD*, vol. 4, "Transcription," n. 1, identifies it as one of the alternate names of *mai mendong* 麥門冬 (*ZY*: no. 2082, *Ophiopogon japonicus* Ker-Gawl.), listed in *BC* (*GM*, 16.84). However, *pulei* is also attested in *Shanhaijing*, 5.6b, and *Guanzi* 58, 19.314 (written 僕累), as the name of a kind of snail.

[4] Hayashi shows that *gang* 釭 refers to an iron ring placed inside the hub to reduce friction between the axle and the hub (1976: 300). *MS*I.E.253 calls for "old grease from a carriage." Carriage grease (*chezhi* 車脂) is listed in materia medica (*GM*, 38.48). *Shan* 饍, which I have translated as "work in," is attested as a variant of *shan* 膳 (Morohashi 1957-60, vol. 12: no. 44390); but the word is not attested in an appropriate meaning in received literature. The translation is based on my conjecture that *shan* refers to mixing a liquid or soft substance into a medicine to make it malleable, the sense which it appears to have in *MS*I.E.202 and other occurrences in *MS*I.E.204, 207, 208, 211.

[5] As in the treatment in *MS*I.E.74, a medicine is first applied and then that part of the body is roasted.

[6] I have not found specific reference to a red lizard in received literature, nor does materia medica mention lizard blood as a drug.

MSI.E.204 (C341)

Another. Smith *tingli*[1] and *wuyi*.[2] Scorch soybeans [2]. Using equal amounts of all, work in male [pig][3] lard and *zhan* (sturgeon) blood. First wash (the scabies) with liquor. Burn bark[4] to roast it, and then spread (the medicine).

MSI.E.205 (CC342-43)

Another. Smith *niuxi* (achyranthes) and the ash of incinerated loose hair[5] in equal amounts, and combine [2]. Thoroughly wash the scabies and spread (the medicine) on it. Roast beef, and daub the old suet on top of (the medicine). Even when it desists, spread (the medicine) again without stopping.

MSI.E.206 (C344)

Another. Use [1] suet or leopard lard. [1][6] and roast it. [3] and is not painful. Repeat it over and over again. First drink fine liquor until the body becomes warm, then [?].

MSI.E.207 (C345)

Another. Carefully wash, and rub to make it bleed. Spread mercury on it. Also take equal amounts of smithed bronze and copper bits,[7] work in pig lard, and spread (the medicine) on it.

MSI.E.208 (C346)

Another. Pound *qianglang* (dung beetles), and work in gruel vinegar. Seal (the scabies with the medicine) and roast it. The bugs come out from all sides.[8]

---

[1] *Tingli* 葶 藶 is listed in *BC* (*GM*, 16.111). The seeds are the drug. *ZY*: no. 4818, lists several plants in the genus *Lepidium* as well as several other genera. *KGS*, vol. 1: 256, n. 715, names *Draba nemorosa* and various species of the genus *Brassica*. It is not clear which plants were the source of *tingli* in early medicine.

[2] The identity of the drug *wuyi* 莁 荑 is not known. In materia medica it has been treated as an alternate name for *wuyi* 蕪 荑 (stinking elm fruit; see *MSI*.E.195). However, the two names are glossed separately in *Erya*, 8.4a and 9.3a. Evidently the names originally referred to two different plants and were conflated in later materia medica.

[3] Judging from the context, the lacuna should be *zhi* 彘.

[4] "Bark" is the gloss for *pu* 朴 in *SW*, 6A.22b. *MWD*, vol. 4, "Transcription," n. 2, plausibly equates the word with *pumu* 朴 木, the magnolia from which the drug *houpu* 厚 樸 is obtained (see *MSI*.E.177).

[5] *SW*, 9A.26a, glosses *rong* 髶 as "disheveled hair" (*luanfa* 亂 髮). In materia medica, *luanfa* is the loose hair that drops from the head and collects in brushes and combs (see *MSI*.E.5).

[6] Based on other recipes for scabies, the lacuna might be *fu* 傅 (spread).

[7] Since the recipe specifies equal amounts of two substances, *jin* 金 must refer to a second source of metal in addition to *yu* 鋊 (copper bits; see *MSI*.E.144). The translation "bronze" reflects my speculation that the metal bits are obtained from bronzeware.

*MS*I.E.209 (C347)

Another. Remove the carapace and feet from one *dou* of *qianglang* (dung beetles), and combine with five nodules of *wuhui* (monkshood) and a piece of *yu* (arsenopyrite) the size of a plum. Boil in [1] *dou* of vinegar until the liquid evaporates.[1] Spread (the medicine) on it.

*MS*I.E.210 (C348)

Another. Cover with large-bark *tong* (paulownia)[2] and bind. Superb.

*MS*I.E.211 (C349)

Another. Incinerate the feces of a male rat and smith. Work in good vinegar, and seal it.

*MS*I.E.212 (C350)

Another. Incinerate *yu* (arsenopyrite). Smith one *ge* each of *wuhui* (monkshood), *lilu* (black veratrum), Shu *shu*,[3] *zhe*,[4] Shu *jiao* (Shu zanthoxylum), and *gui* (cinnamon). Blend them together. Take dandruff [3] cloth. Roast, and hot-press with it.[5] Stop when exhausted.

---

[8]Perhaps the conclusion to *MS*I.E.208 indicates that the itch mite was already observed in early Chinese medicine, but I remain skeptical. Several other recipes conclude with similar statements that following the treatment, "the bugs come out" (of a wound in *MS*I.E.15, and of hemorrhoids in *MS*I.E.152). Like hemorrhoids, the etiology of *jia* is grounded in early Chinese ideas about bugs and disease that do not correspond to modern parasitology. Without additional evidence it is difficult to determine what bugs are seen coming out in *MS*I.E.208.

[1]*Dai* 截 as a Han word for vinegar is discussed in *MS*I.E.9.

[2]I agree with *MWD*, vol. 4, "Transcription," n. 1, that *dapi tong* 大皮桐 may refer to a kind of *tong* (paulownia), but the name "large-bark paulownia" is not attested in received literature.

[3]Identification of Shu *shu* 蜀叔 is problematic. Presumably *shu* is to be read as *shu* 菽, referring to some kind of bean. Ma Jixing reviews several proposed identifications, concluding that the name refers to a bean from the region of Shu and that its identity is not known (1992: 581, n. 4). I tend to agree with Ma in rejecting the proposed equation between Shu *shu* and Ba *dou* 巴豆 (*ZY*: no. 1028, seed of *Croton tiglium* L.), listed in *BC* (*GM*, 35.63). The geographic proximity of Shu and Ba is insufficient evidence to justify equating the two different drug names.

[4]*MWD*, vol. 4, "Transcription," n. 1, proposes reading *zhe* 庶 as *zhe* 蔗 (*ZY*: no. 1190, *Saccharum sinensis* Roxb.; sugar cane; *GM*, 33.58). However, Liu Junzheng (1989) proposes reading it as *zhe* 䗪 (*ZY*: no. 5633, *Eupolyphaga sinensis* Walker; cockroach), listed in *BC* (*GM*, 41.21). Liu cites several occurrences of *zhe* "cockroach" in the Wuwei recipes to support his identification.

[5]It appears that the medicine is wrapped in cloth, roasted until hot, and then used to hot-press the scabies.

MSI.E.213 (C351)

Another. Soak *lingji* (water chestnuts) in the urine of a young boy. Put it in a pottery vessel, cover with cloth, and place it on the stove flue for five or six days. [1] spread (the medicine) on it.

MSI.E.214 (C352)

Another. Smith *wuyi* and *kuhu* (bitter gourd) seeds. Combine, and beat in pig lard. Spread (the medicine) on it. Wrap with cloth and bind.

MSI.E.215 (C353)

Another. Smith four nodules of *wuhui* (monkshood) and one and a half *sheng* of *lingji* (water chestnuts). Combine with one and a half *dou* of the urine of a male youth and [1]. Boil until done. Put in one *sheng* of [1] grain, and stir. Spread (the medicine) on it.

MSI.E.216 (C354)

Another. Smith *wuhui* (monkshood). Roast black ram suet and beat (it in). Spread (the medicine) on it while hot.

MSI.E.217 (C355)

Another. Incinerate old *kui* (mallow) stalks and smith. Blend rancid pig lard into it, beating. Spread (the medicine) on the wound.

MSI.E.218 (CC356-57)

Another. Moist scabies. Smith one sixth *dou* of *wuyi*. Take castrated pig lard that is fatty, firm, and glistening [1] {1} [7]. Wash the scabies well with water. When dry, spread (the medicine) on it and bind with cloth. [2] the shinbone of a dead person. Incinerate and smith it. Using rancid lard [?].

MSI.E.219 (C358)

Another. Fresh scabies.[1] First wash well with water; and roast snake lard until it melts, and spread. Spread thrice [?].

MSI.E.220 (C359)

Another. Recipe for scabies. Spread three-year-old rancid pig lard on it. Incinerate a rotted *jing* (vitex) winnowing basket. Take the ash [2] {1} [2] desists. Excellent.

MSI.E.221 (C360)

Another. Dry scabies. Smith *shechuang* (cnidium) fruits, and work in male pig lard. First scrape the scabies. When it bursts, then spread (the medicine) and [2] {2} [1] {1} [?].

---

[1]I am uncertain of the sense of *chan* 産, which means "live, grow, raw, fresh." Perhaps it refers to a fresh outbreak of scabies.

*MS*I.E.222 (C361)

Another. Blend mercury with *gu* (paper mulberry) liquid,[1] and spread (the medicine) on it. First use vinegar to cleanse[2] [3] spread.

*MS*I.E.223 (C362)

Another. Recipe for scabies. Smith a sufficient amount of *lilu* (black veratrum). Blend it with bee larvae,[3] beating. Then thoroughly [4] scabies [1] and it desists. Previously tested. There are no prohibitions.

*MS*I.E.224 (C363)

Snake Bite

Daub *sang* (mulberry) liquid on it.[4]

*MS*I.E.225 (C364)

Abscess[5]

Take [2] feather [1] {1} [1] {1}. Perform the Pace of Yu thrice. [2] one cup [?].[6]

*MS*I.E.226 (C365)

Another. When an abscess appears on its own, take about one joint of *tong* (paulownia) root. Boil in grain-cleaning slop [?].

---

[1]I follow Ma Jixing (1992: 589, n. 2) in reading *gu* 縠 as *gu* 榖, paper mulberry (*ZY*: no. 4754, *Broussonetia papyrifera* [L.] Vent.), which is listed in *BC* (*GM*, 36.78). *MWD*, vol. 4, "Transcription," n. 1, plausibly interprets *guzhi* 縠 汁 as referring to "grain" cooking liquid; but occurrences of the term in *MS*III.38 and *MS*IV.5-6 suggest that the substance is a liquid prepared from the tree not from cooked grain. Whether the liquid is sap or a decoction is not certain.

[2]脩 in *MWD*, vol. 4, "Transcription," should be transcribed as *xiu* 滫. Qiu Xigui notes that this is the only instance in *MS*I.E where the signific for water is written with three short bars rather than with the older seal-script style water signific (氵; 1992: 532). Qiu speculates that the scribe initially wrote the graph without the water signific, and when he corrected the graph there was only room to write the abbreviated three bar form. For attestation of *xiu* in the sense of "cleanse," see *SW*, 3B.9b, where *zhi* [鬲+攴] is glossed as "the vessel for cleaning (*xiu*) grain."

[3]I read 駘 as *tai* 胎, literally "embryo." I accept the suggestion in *MWD*, vol. 4, "Transcription," n. 1, that the word refers to the same substance as the "bee eggs" already used in *MS*I.E.130 and 141. Twenty wasp *tai* are used in *MS*III.12. It has been argued that the graph should be read as *yi* 飴 (malt sugar), and that the substance is bee sugar (i.e. honey). I agree with Ma Jixing that wasps do not produce honey, therefore the word cannot be *yi* (1992: 590, n. 4).

[4]The liquid is probably mulberry sap, but it could also be a decocted liquid.

[5]For identification of *yong* 癰 with abscess, see Yu Yan 1972: 238. Etymologically the word connotes a "walled-up" place where pus collects.

[6]The "feather" might be related to exorcistic archery preceding the Pace of Yu.

MSI.E.227 (CC366-67)

Another. When abscess swellings occur, smith *wuhui* (monkshood) and *lilu* (black veratrum). [10] it. Use it to hot-press the places with swellings.[1] {2} [2] {1}, making the abscess swellings all desist.

MSI.E.228 (C368)

Another. Head abscess. Chop finely one half *dou* of *zi*,[2] and using six *dou* of good vinegar [6] {2} [2] {5} [?].

MSI.E.229 (CC369-71)

Another. When there is an abscess on the body, say: "Kəgw. I dare to [declare] to the Tai Mountain Barrow.[3] So-and-so [un]fortunately[4] ails from an abscess. I direct the [1] of the hundred illnesses. With the bright moon I irradiate you;[5] with the cold [4]

---

[1]潼 in *MWD*, vol. 4, "Transcription," should be transcribed as 穜, and read as *zhong* 腫 (swellings).

[2]*Zi* 茈 is glossed as *zicao* 茈 艸 in *SW*, 1B.19b, which is listed in *BC* (*GM*, 12B.26; *ZY*: no. 4863, *Lithospermum erythrorhizon* Sieb. et Zucc. and several other plants). *MWD*, vol. 4, "Transcription," n. 1, reads *zi* as referring to *chaihu* 柴 胡 (also written 茈 胡). *Chaihu* (*ZY*: no. 3763, *Bupleurum chinense* DC. and other spp.) is listed in *BC* (*GM*, 13.43). Either identification is plausible.

[3]自 in *MWD*, vol. 4, "Transcription," should be transcribed as *yue* 曰 (say); and 取 should be transcribed as *gan* 敢 (dare). Qiu Xigui (1992: 532-33) compares the opening formula of the incantation to an incantation recorded in the Shuihudi hemerological manuscripts (translated and studied in Harper 1987a: 270-71; the same formula occurs in other incantations). I agree with Qiu's speculation that in *MSI*.E.229, the scribe omitted the word *gao* 告 (declare), which invariably follows *gan* "dare" in the formula (in incantations as well as in the speech of government officials addressing superiors). The scribe left out another word in the following sentence. The scribe also omitted a word from the incantation in *MSI*.E.233, but there he corrected the omission. The utterance at the beginning of the incantation, *gao/*kəgw* 皋 (also written 睾), is attested both in Han ritual literature and in the Shuihudi hemerological manuscripts. Zheng Xuan glosses **kəgw* as "an extended cry" in the commentary in *Yili*, 35.2b, where the utterance forms part of the ritual of summoning back the soul of a person recently deceased. In *MSI*.E.229 the "extended cry" is directed toward Tai Mountain Barrow 大 山 陵, the sacred peak of the east located in present-day Shandong. For the role of the spirit of Tai Mountain in Han popular religion, see Seidel 1987: 30; and Ngo 1976: 111. Tai Mountain was regarded as the abode of the dead, and the presiding deity was one of the arbiters of human fate who could be entreated to intervene in matters concerning illness and death. The appeal to Tai Mountain in *MSI*.E.229 is similar to the one made to the Spirit of Heaven in *MSI*.E.124; and in both cases the request for help is followed by cursing the demonic agent responsible for the ailment.

[4]The scribe omitted 不 in the text.

[5]炻 is not attested in received literature, and the translation "irradiate" is based on my judgment that the word probably has the sense of attacking the demon with moonrays. The phonetic indicates a pronunciation *shi/*djiak*. *KGS*, vol. 1: 264, n. 771, suggests

with a *zuo* (oak) rod I stab you;[1] with tiger claws I gouge and grab you;[2] with a knife I butcher you; with *wei* (reeds) I sever you.[3] [Today] [1].[4] If you do not depart, it will be bitter." Spit. [5] at dawn before [eating], face [east] and spit on it.[5]

*MS*I.E.230
(CC372-75) Another. *Baizhi* (angelica), *baiheng*,[6] *jungui* (curled cinnamon), dried *jiang* (ginger), and *xinzhi* (magnolia bud)[7]—altogether five substances in equal amounts. After smithing the five substances [3]. Take beef suet [3] fine cloth. Combine and bake in a metal chafing

---

reading the graph as *yi/*dag* 燡 (shine), which is phonologically plausible but unlikely because the word is attested just once in Han literature. Ma Jixing argues that the graph is a scribal miswriting of *zhao* 炤 (i.e. 照; 1992: 595, n. 5), but I think *KGS* must be basically correct in proposing a phonological solution to the identity of the graph.

[1]棯 is not attested in received literature. I propose the pronunciation *shi/*djək*, perhaps a phonetic loan for *zhi/**tjək 樴 (pole, rod). 柱 in *MWD*, vol. 4, "Transcription," should be transcribed as *zhu* 柱. *Zhu* is commonly used for *zhu* 拄 in Han literature (see *SW*, 6A.31b, and Duan Yucai commentary); and the latter word is attested in the sense of "strike, stab" in *Hanshu*, 67.5b.

[2]Tiger claws symbolize the punishment inflicted on demons by the tiger (*hu* 虎), the demon-queller par excellence in early China (Bodde 1975: 129). In analyzing *wei* 畏 (fearsome), *SW*, 9A.43a, identifies the top as the head of a demon and the bottom as an abbreviation of 虎. The significance of its composition is explained as follows: "To have a demon head and tiger *claws* is to be something that can be feared."

[3]The common reed, *wei* 葦 (*ZY*: no. 2191, *Phragmites communis* Trin.), played a significant role in Han exorcistic practices, including the New Year's customs of presenting reed halberds at the Great Exorcism and hanging reed cords over doorways (Bodde 1975: 82, 128-30). The Shuihudi "Jie" states that a spirit who harasses a woman can be expelled by striking it with reeds, followed by bathing in feces (*SHD*: 215). The punctuation of this part of the incantation in *MWD*, vol. 4, "Transcription," is incorrect. Each phrase should end with the word *ruo* 若 (you).

[4]肉 in *MWD*, vol. 4, "Transcription," should be transcribed as *jin* 今 (today). The bottom part of the graph is missing, but enough remains to compare with other occurrences of the two graphs in *MS*I.E and to confirm the correct identity. The lacuna below might be *qu* 去 (depart), making the incantation read: "Today depart. If you do not depart, it will be bitter." Compare the formula using "today" in *MS*I.E.125. Li Xueqin (private communication) suggests that perhaps the silk fragment should be moved up slightly, leaving no lacuna between 今 and 若 (in which case the incantation would read, "Today if you do not depart it will be bitter").

[5]Based on remaining fragments of the first graph and on the context, Qiu Xigui fills the two-graph lacuna with *shi* 食 (eat) and *dong* 東 (east; 1992: 533).

[6]*Baiheng* 白 衡 is not attested in materia medica. *MWD*, vol. 4, "Transcription," n. 1, suggests identifying the name with *duheng* 杜 衡 (*ZY*: no. 2094, *Asarum forbesii* Maxim.; *GM*, 13.70).

[7]*Xinzhi* 薪 雉 is attested for *xinyi* 辛 夷 in *Wenxuan*, 7.3a (*zhi/*drjid* and *yi/*rəd* are homophones).

dish over *sang* (mulberry) charcoal.[1] When it barely bubbles, uncover and let the vapor escape. Once again bake and allow to bubble like this [3] cloth to remove and obtain the liquid.[2] Then crumble mercury in the palms and blend it into the medicine. Spread. At dawn use {3} [3] {1} [5]. While spreading the medicine do not eat [1] pork and fish, and do not (have intercourse) with women. When it desists, the face resembles that of [2].[3]

*MS*I.E.231 (CC376-77)

Another. Recipe for when there are abscess swellings on the body. Take one male [1] and gut it.[4] {1} [8]. Cook it. Watch for when the broth is reduced to just under one *dou*. Remove and store it. Use a small amount to daub on the places on the body where there are swellings, and roast it. [6] the abscess swellings entirely depart, and it desists. Previously tested. Excellent.

*MS*I.E.232 (CC378-79)

Another. When a chin abscess occurs, combine in a caldron one portion of smithed *banxia* (pinellia), two of rendered beef suet, and six of gruel vinegar. [3] {1} [1] {1}. Spread (the medicine). Do not spread it all over, but rather make a ring that extends for one *cun*. When dry, spread (the medicine) on it again, and wash off the medicine with hot water. It will desist.

*MS*I.E.233 (C380)

Lacquer[5]

Spit and say: "Pən, Lacquer"—thrice. Then say: "The Thearch of Heaven sent you down to lacquer bows and arrows.[6] Now you

---

[1]Archaeological evidence indicates that the *diao* 銚 was a shallow, flat-bottomed bowl that could be placed directly on the fire to warm food and drink (Hayashi 1976: 230-31).

[2]The cloth is probably used to strain the cooked medicine as in *MS*I.E.13.

[3]Evidently the recipe concerns an abscess on the face.

[4]I read 夸 as *ku* 刳. For examples of *ku* in the sense of cutting out the inside of something, see *SW*, 4B.45a, and Duan Yucai commentary.

[5]*SW*, 6B.8a, glosses *xiu* 髹 with *qi* 桼 (*ZY*: no. 0131, *Rhus verniciflua* Stokes), the tree that produces the sap for lacquer. Duan Yucai cites evidence that *xiu* refers to applying lacquer to objects. Thus the ailment category in *MS*I.E probably refers to the rash caused by working with lacquer, a reflection of the lacquer industry in the region of Changsha.

[6]The incantation portrays a pantheon in which the Thearch of Heaven 天帝 presides over lesser nature spirits like the lacquer spirit. On the Thearch of Heaven in Han popular religion, see Seidel 1987: 28.

cause scabby sores[1] for the people down below.[2] I daub you with pig feces."[3] Rub and slap[4] it with the sole of a shoe.[5]

*MS*I.E.234 (C381)

Another. Chant this incantation: "The Thearch possesses the five weapons.[6] You, begone. If you do not go, I will spew knives to coat you."[7] Then spit on it, men seven times and women twice seven.

*MS*I.E.235 (C382)

Another. "Pən, Lacquer King. You are incapable of lacquering armor and weapons, and have caused so-and-so to be wounded. Chicken feces and rat detritus are daubed on the Lacquer King."[8]

*MS*I.E.236 (C383)

Another. [3] rat [1] {1}. Drink the [1], one cup. It will make a person not have lacquer (rash) for his whole life.

*MS*I.E.237 (C384)

Another. [12]. Spread (the medicine) on it.

---

[1] *Bi* 疕 refers to thin scabs that spread across the skin (Yu Yan 1972: 117). *Bi* occurs as a separate ailment category beginning in *MS*I.E.257.

[2] *Min* 民 (people) was initially omitted by the scribe, who then corrected the error by writing the graph in tiny script on the left beside the graphs between which it should be inserted.

[3] The rhyming words in the incantation are: *shi/*hrjəd* 矢 (arrow), *bi/*pjiəd* 疕 (scabby sore), and *shi/*hrjəd* 矢 (feces).

[4] The text writes *di* 抵, but apparently means *zhi* 抵, glossed in *SW*, 12A.51a, as "strike with a sideways blow." Duan Yucai notes that the use of 抵 to write *zhi* is a common error in received editions of Han texts; *MS*I.E.233 suggests that the error may have already been a scribal convention in Han times.

[5] It is likely that the incanted threat to daub feces on the lacquer spirit was fulfilled by actually slapping feces on the lacquer rash after the incantation. On the exorcistic nature of feces in early magico-religious belief, see Harper 1985: 495.

[6] There are several different lists of the five weapons. One legend has it that weapons were invented by the war-like Chiyou 蚩尤, who was defeated by the Yellow Thearch. The pairing of the two figures and the role of Chiyou as a demon-queller are examined in Bodde 1975: 120-27; and Lewis 1990: 185-95. Seidel 1987: 34-39, examines the parallel relationship between the Thearch of Heaven and his weapon-bearing envoy in popular Han religion.

[7] The incantation likens the exorcistic saliva to knives. The rhyming words in the incantation are: *bing/*pjiang* 兵 (weapon), *wang/*mjang* 亡 (begone), and *zhuang/*tsrjang* 裝 (coat).

[8] As in *MS*I.E.233, chicken feces and rat detritus are probably daubed on the lacquer rash following the incantation. *Rang* 壤 (detritus) refers to the soil from a rat burrow. The rhyming words in the incantation are: *wang/*gwjang* 王 (king; two occurrences), *bing/*pjiang* 兵 (weapon), *shang/*hrjang* 傷 (wound), and *rang/*njang* (detritus).

MSI.E.238
(CC385-87)

Another [31]. Spread at dawn before eating. [21]. The ailment desists and (the body) is as it was before. When treating the ailment there are no temporal (restrictions). When treating the ailment it is prohibited to [?].

MSI.E.239
(CC388-89)

Another. [2]. Cook five *dou* of rice using wood kindling. When done, [1] it. Then [17] {1}, use *langya* root.[1]

MSI.E.240
(CC390-97)

Chewing by Bugs[2]

[2] located on the throat or located at another place. The place where the ailment is located is called [9] {4} [2] {1} [2]. Wash it with [1] until irritated,[3] then spread (the medicine). When spreading [9] hot water, and rub with a feather [5]. Then spread the medicine. When spreading the medicine, let it just fill the holes and no more. [9]. The next day wash again with hot water and spread the medicine as before. Wash once a day, and spread the medicine once a day. In three [9] {1} flesh grows {1} [2] flesh and stop. Then wash off the medicine. After washing off the medicine, use pig [11] the scabs are cured and stop. [2] three days and flesh grows. In about eight or nine days, the wound is level. When the wound is level [7]. In somewhat more than ten days it is cured and (the body) is as it was before. The wound [2]. If one wants to wrap it, then wrap it. If one [1] want [1], do not [9].[4] When spreading the medicine, first at dawn before spreading [2] spread the medicine. If one wants to eat, eat. While the medicine is being applied [9].

---

[1]*Langya* 狼牙 is listed in *BC* (*GM*, 17.11). Its botanical identification is uncertain. Ma Jixing offers two possibilities: *Potentilla cryptotaenia* Maxim.; and *Agrimonia pilosa* Ledeb (1992: 605, n. 2).

[2]*MSI*.E.244 and *MSI*.E.248 specifically mention *te* 蟘 as the bug that damages the mouth, nose, and teeth with its chewing. It appears that this chewing is of the same nature as, but less serious than, the chewing by the *ming* bug in *MSI*.E.78. Other recipes are less specific, but clearly reflect the belief that bugs chew holes into the surface of the body. Treatment in *MSI*.E.240 consists of filling the chew-holes with medicine and getting new flesh to grow. As noted in *MWD*, vol. 4, "Transcription," n. 1, later medical literature deals with a similarly broad range of body decay ailments under the category *ni* 匿(hidden bugs).

[3]*Pupu* 僕僕 is used in *Mengzi* 5B, 10.423, to refer to feverish activity. In *MSI*.E.240, the term must refer to scrubbing until the skin is irritated.

[4]While it is difficult to guess the exact words of the phrase preceding the nine-graph lacuna, it must state that not wrapping the wound is also all right.

*MS*I.E.241 (C398)

Another. Incinerate *loulu*,[1] and smith it. Use male pig lard [?].

*MS*I.E.242 (CC399-400) Another. Incinerate rooster feces, and fumigate the wound with it. [10] rat until it dies on its own. Boil in water. [1] cloth in the liquid and spread (the liquid) on it. Do not rub the wound with the hands.[2]

*MS*I.E.243 (C401)

Another. When there is chewing by bugs, take Yu stove [2][3] to fill the wound. [8]. Excellent.

*MS*I.E.244 (C402)

Another. When the *te* eats the mouth and nose, smith *jinkui*[4] [3] incinerate using *sang* (mulberry) kindling. [2] {1} [2] until the liquid comes out. Use a feather to take [?].

*MS*I.E.245 (C403)

Another. Quickly split a carriage's lacquered *guo* [?].[5]

*MS*I.E.246 (CC404-405) Another. [1] eating. Use fatty pork [?] {1} [?].

*MS*I.E.247 (C406)

Another. Smith old *kui* (mallow). Use [?].

*MS*I.E.248 (C407)

Another. When the *te* eats the teeth, take *yu* (elm) bark, *bai* [1], and fine *gui* (cinnamon), and combine [4]. Spread (the medicine) on the holes [?].

*MS*I.E.249 (CC408-409) Recipe For Dry Itch[6]

---

[1]*Loulu* 漏蘆 is listed in *BC* (*GM*, 15.38). *ZY*: no. 5397, gives two principal identifications, *Rhaponticum uniflorum* (L.) DC.; and *Echinops latifolius* Tausch. *BL* (*GM*, 15.39) identifies *loulu* as an alternate name for *feilian* 飛廉 (*ZY*: no. 0567, *Carduus crispus* L.), also listed in *BC*.

[2]I.e. the medicine must be applied with the cloth just mentioned (the lacuna preceding "cloth" should be a verb meaning to dip the cloth into the liquid).

[3]I suspect that the first graph in the lacuna belongs to the name of the preceding substance; and that the substance may be another form of stove ash. *MS*IV.7-8 record the name Yu *xun* 禹熏, which may be stove soot.

[4]Ma Jixing discusses several possible identifications for *jinkui* 堇葵 (1992: 611, n. 4). None permit certain identification of the drug in *MS*I.E.244.

[5]*KGS*, vol. 1: 273, n. 827, suggests reading *guo* 桲 as *kuo* 鞹; and conjectures that the next missing graph might be *hong* 鞃. *Kuohong* is the name for a horizontal leather piece that is attached to the front of the carriage chassis.

Use two *liang* of realgar, one third *liang* of mercury, and one *sheng* of dandruff. [1] the realgar, and crumble the mercury [in][1] the hands [6] the realgar and stir it thoroughly. First thoroughly wash the itch with hot water so that the washed places burst. Wipe with a cloth until [2] and spread (the medicine) on it. For one night and one [?].

*MS*I.E.250 (C410)

Another. Scorch one third *dou* of *lingji* (water chestnuts) until they yellow. Boil in one half *dou* of pure liquor. Let it bubble thrice and stop. Clarify[2] the liquid. In the evening do not eat, and drink (the liquid).

*MS*I.E.251 (C411)

Another. Use *fuling* (pine truffle). Select one that is large and pound it. Pound in a mortar, beat in suet, and form into large balls. Rub (the itch with the balls).

*MS*I.E.252 (C412)

Another. Mince *rulu* (madder) root, and soak in liquor. After[3] a day and a night, daub (the medicine) on it. It desists.

*MS*I.E.253 (CC413-14)

Another. Take two measures of *lilu* (black veratrum), one measure of *wuhui* (monkshood), one measure of *yu* (arsenopyrite), [1] measure of *quju*,[4] and one measure of *yuanhua* (daphne). Blend them together using old carriage grease. {1} [3] wrap.[5] Carefully wash and dry. Then roast the wrapped medicine and rub the itch with it. [1] rub suet [2] suet. The itch then desists.

---

[6] *Sao* 瘙 means literally "scratch" (*SW*, 12A.36a), and by extension refers broadly to skin itch (Yu Yan 1972: 128). *Sao* is included in *Maishu*, "Ailment List": "When the body ails from itch and pus oozes—it is *sao*" (*MSSW*: 72).

[1] Judging from the context and from the parallel in *MS*I.E.230, the lacuna should be 中.

[2] The reading for 蛪 is problematic. Based on *SW*, 13A.53a, and Duan Yucai commentary, I propose the pronunciation *che/*thrjat*. I suspect that the graph is a phonetic loan for *shui/*sthjuad* 涗, which refers to a filtration process using ash that is mentioned in Han ritual literature (*SW*, 11A-2.31a, and Duan Yucai commentary; and Hayashi 1975: 77). Ma Jixing proposes a phonetic loan for *che/*thrjat* 澈 (clear), understanding the word to mean "clarify" in *MS*I.E.250 (1992: 615, n. 3). I am skeptical of Ma's reading because the word is rare and is not attested in Han sources, whereas *shui* is well attested in the sense of "clarify."

[3] 後 in *MWD*, vol. 4, "Transcription," should be transcribed as 后.

[4] *Quju* 屈 居 is identified as *luru* 盧 茹 in *Guangya*, 10A.24b. *Luru* can be identified with *lüru* 藘 茹, which is listed in *BC* (*GM*, 17.12). *ZY* does not give a botanical identification.

[5] The itch is rubbed with the roasted, wrapped medicine below. The lacuna probably describes wrapping the medicine to prepare it for use in hot-pressing.

MSI.E.254

(CC415-16) Another. Take one *sheng* of *lan* (eupatorium) root and of *baifu*[1] chopped into small pieces. Pound, and pour vinegar and grain rinse[2]—half and half—into it until just [2]. Set in a warm place for three days, and put one *ge* of pig lard that is [2] into it. Then cook, letting it bubble thrice. Spread (the medicine) on the rash and roast it. When dry, spread again [1]. Leave for two days, then bathe. The rash desists. Excellent.

MSI.E.255 (C417)

Another. Boil *tao* (peach) leaves, scalding thrice, to make hot bath water. Go to a warm inner (chamber), drink hot liquor, and afterward get into the hot bath water. Drink hot liquor again in the bath. Even old itch desists.

MSI.E.256 (C418)

Another. Dry itch. Boil two *dou* of urine until it reduces to two *sheng*. Combine with one *sheng* of pig lard and two *sheng* of *lilu* (black veratrum), and spread (the medicine) on it.

MSI.E.257 (C419)

Body Scabbing[3]

When there is no name for the scabbing but it itches, scorch and smith *lingji* (water chestnuts). Blend with dog bile, and spread (the medicine) on it. When spreading (the medicine) for a long time, always stop for three days.[4] After the third time, the scabbing desists. Previously tested. Excellent.

---

[1]The identification of *baifu* 白付 is problematic. *MWD*, vol. 4, "Transcription," n. 1, offers two suggestions. First, it may be *bai fuzi* 白附子, which is listed in *BL* (*GM*, 17.50). Tao Hongjing already does not know what the drug is. In later materia medica it is sometimes identified as a variety of *fuzi* (g. *Aconitum*), but Li Shizhen pointedly notes that it is not an aconite. Alternatively, the drug in *MSI*.E.254 may be *baifu* 白符, which belongs to the so-called *wuse fu* 五色符. The name is associated with the *wuse shizhi* 五色石脂, five kinds of clay classified by color that are listed in *BC* (*GM*, 9.80). The red and white varieties of *fu* occur in *MSIII*.62.

[2]*Mu* 沐 is the verb for washing the hair, but also denotes the grain-cleaning liquid used for hair-washing (see *Shiji*, 49.6a).

[3]In received literature *bi* 疕 refers broadly to any rash that forms scabs. Yu Yan associates the word with conditions like eczema (1972: 117). *MSI*.E.266-270 concern chilblain, which is not classified under *bi* in received medical literature.

[4]I.e. spread the medicine, stop for three days, and spread again.

MSI.E.258 (C420)

Another. Scabbing. Mince *kui* (mallow), and soak in water. During summer days do not soak. Spread (the medicine) on it. The hundred types of scabbing all desist.

MSI.E.259 (C421)

Another. Blend two portions of *lilu* (black veratrum) with one portion of *yu* (arsenopyrite), and *suo*.[1] Hot-press the scabbing with it.

MSI.E.260 (C422)

Another. When old scabbing does not desist, soak the dry matter scraped from the stove.[2] Spread (the medicine) on it. It desists.

MSI.E.261 (C423)

Another. When scabbing like cow eyes appears on the body while traveling in the mountains, this is called "day [?].

MSI.E.262 (C424)

Another. Exposed scabbing.[3] Incinerate the charred crust of cooked rice.[4] Smith, blend with old lard, and spread.

MSI.E.263 (C425)

Another. [?].

MSI.E.264 (C426)

Another. Use the east-facing root, branches, and leaves of *huai* (pagoda tree). Boil, scalding thrice. Use the liquid [?].

MSI.E.265 (C427)

Another. The incantation is: "Tsjəm tsjəm, hjəkw hjəkw bugs.[5] The Yellow Spirit is in the stove. [2] {1}. Yellow Spirit arise. [?].[6]

---

[1]膝, which I pronounce *suo*, is not attested in received literature. It must be a verb describing what is done with the medicine. *MWD*, vol. 4, "Transcription," n. 1, simply reads the graph as *suo* 索 in the sense of "gather up"; and interprets the line to mean that the medicine is gathered in something so that it can be used for hot-pressing.

[2]This appears to be another form of stove ash.

[3]"Exposed" translates *lou* 露. I am uncertain of the meaning of "exposed scabbing." Perhaps *lou* refers to a kind of open sore; perhaps it has the sense of "protruding," describing a pattern of raised bumps with scabs.

[4]Ma Jixing associates the name *fanjiao* 飯焦 with *guojiao* 鍋焦 in later medical literature, which refers to the charred crust of rice that sticks to the cookpot (1992: 626, n. 1).

[5]熇 is not attested in received literature. It may be related to *chu*/**hjəkw* 滀, which is the basis for the pronunciation. The utterance *qin qin, chu chu* 浸浸熇熇 is similar but not identical to the utterance in *MSI*.E.178 (the repetition of syllables in *MWD*, vol. 4, "Transcription," should be corrected as in *MSI*.E.178). I am not able to identify the symbolic significance of the choice of words for the utterance. 虫 is read *chong* "bug" here, as confirmed by the rhyming words.

MSI.E.266

(CC428-30) Another. Chilblain.[1] First wash the chilblain thoroughly with glutinous panicled millet slop. Then incinerate straw that is several years old. [Take][2] the ash and smith. [3] spread on the chilblain. After spreading the ash, soak the ash entirely [3] and wipe to scrape it away.[3] After scraping, immediately spread ash again and scrape as before. When the liquid is used up, then even old chilblain will be cured. When spreading the medicine it is prohibited [4].[4] Previously tested. Excellent.

MSI.E.267 (C431)

Another. Steam frozen earth, and use (the earth) to hot-press it.

MSI.E.268 (C432)

Another. Daub fresh rabbit brain on it.

MSI.E.269 (C433)

Another. Chew *xie* (scallions), and seal it.

MSI.E.270 (C434)

Another. When being barefoot results in chilblain, burn the inside of a pit in the ground and put the foot into it for the time it takes to eat and no more. Then [1] *cong* (onions) and seal it, or hot-press it with steamed *cong* (onions).

MSI.E.271 (C435)

[1] *Gu*[5]

---

[6]The extant rhyming words in the incantation are: *chong/*drhəngw* 虫 (bug), *zhong/*trkəngw* 中 (in), and *xing/*hjəng* 興 (arise). On the Yellow Spirit, see *MSI*.E.178.

[1]*SW*, 7B.32a, glosses *zhu* 瘃 as "swollen lumps due to being struck by coldness." For identification with chilblain, see Yu Yan 1972: 67, 136.

[2]The lacuna should be 取 or 以.

[3]I read *li* 捚 as *li* 梩 (also pronounced *si*), given as a variant graph for *si* 梠 in *SW*, 6A.42a. It is the name of kind of spade (see Sun Ji 1991: 2, for archaeological artifacts). In *MSI*.E.266, the word is used verbally to denote the action of "scraping away" the layer of ash.

[4]I suspect that the "liquid" and the "medicine" refer to the same thing. The two three-graph lacunae earlier in the recipe must identify the medicine, which is applied simultaneously with the ash.

[5]The Shang bone and shell inscriptions provide the first attestation of *gu* 蠱, pictographically a representation of bugs in a vessel. If later explanations of *gu* are applicable to Shang usage, the etymology of the word goes back to a demonic potion prepared from bugs that the manufacturer uses to sicken chosen victims. See, for example, *Chaoshi zhubing yuanhoulun*, 25.1a: "They mostly use kinds of bugs and serpents, and keep them in a vessel until they eat one another. There is just one creature remaining, which is then called the *gu*." By extension, *gu* refers to demonic evil and to black magic in general. Shirakawa 1976, vol. 1: 250-51, discusses Shang and later evidence. *Zuozhuan*, Zhao 1, 41.13b, records the

Incinerate a bat using *jing* (vitex) kindling, then feed it to the accursed person.

MSI.E.272 (C436)

Another. Incinerate a woman's (menstrual) cloth, and have (the person) drink it.

MSI.E.273 (C437)

When someone ails from [1] *gu*, incinerate a north-facing paired talisman.[1] Then steam sheep buttock, drop (the buttock) into hot bath water, and toss in the talisman ash.[2] Then [2] the ailing person, and wash the hair and body to treat the *gu*.[3]

MSI.E.274 (CC438-40)

Another. When ailing from *gu*, combine one black rooster and one snake in a red pottery kettle. Then cover, and use [2] to cook it on an east-facing stove until the rooster and snake are completely charred. Then remove and smith.[4] Have the ailing person put three three-fingered pinches of the medicine into one cup of liquor or gruel every morning at dawn, and drink it. Drink once a day. When the medicine is used up, it desists.

---

diagnosis of the ruler of Jin 晉 by Physician He 醫和, who declares that the ruler has an ailment caused by sexual excess that is "like *gu*." The passage includes Physician He's etymology of *gu* ("bugs inside a vessel") and two denotations: the bugs that are generated from grain, and delusions arising from female seduction. The idea of internal bugs is the basis for the *SW*, 13B.5b, gloss: "*Gu* is when the abdomen is attacked by bugs." Lu and Needham suggest schistosomiasis as one identification for *gu* (1967: 225), but associating the ailment with a modern parasitic disease is highly questionable given early Chinese notions about bugs and illness. The aspect of female seduction in *gu* etiology is very much alive in Han accounts that associate *gu* with female witchcraft and with the use of voodoo-like objects to harm victims (see Loewe 1974: 81-90). The recipes in *MSI*.E do not describe *gu*, but demonic bugs or female witchcraft are likely factors in the identity of the ailment.

[1]"Paired talisman" translates *bingfu* 并符. It seems likely that talismans of wood, bamboo, or fabric inscribed with magical images and script are involved, similar to talismans of later times. The earliest archaeological specimens of talismanic writing occur on burial writs dating to the Later Han period (Sun Ji 1991: 404-407; and Wang Yucheng 1991).

[2]"Toss" translates *dui* 敦, which is attested in this sense in *Huainanzi*, 15.266, in the phrase 敦六博 "toss (the die to play) *liubo*."

[3]It is possible that the lacuna has the patient first drink the water, followed by bathing with it. Water containing talisman ash anticipates the *fushui* 符水 (talisman water) used to cure ailments in the second century A.D. politico-religious movement headed by Zhang Jue 張角 (see *Hou Hanshu*, 71.la); and widely used in later religious Daoism.

[4]The medicine seems to be an antidote whose production imitates the production of the *gu* potion.

*MS*I.E.275 (C441)

Another. *Gu*. Soak the menstrual cloth of a woman who has never had a husband [2] cup. Smith *gui* (cinnamon), put it in until the odor is gone, and give the [1] to the person to drink.

*MS*I.E.276 (C442)

Child Sprite[1]

Perform the Pace of Yu thrice. Take a branch from the east side of a *tao* (peach). In the middle separately fashion [3] figurines, and fasten them above the doorway, one on each side.[2]

*MS*I.E.277 (CC443-45)

Another. Chant this incantation: "Spouter. Child Sprite Father. Child Sprite Mother. Do not hide [3] north. [1] Shamanka Mistress searches for you and certainly catches you. She [1] your four limbs, plaits your ten fingers, and casts you [1] water. Being human, being human—you join demons."[3] Each time travel [1] with large-bellied gourds[4] for axles and a worn out winnowing basket for the chassis. Harness it to the person's black pig and travel through the person's home. [9] {1} [2] {2} child sprite [1] child sprite [4] place.[5]

---

[1] *SW*, 9A.41b, glosses *qi* 鬾 as "child demon." A number of Han sources identify the child demon as the third of Zhuan Xu's 顓 頊 three children who died after birth and became disease demons. Whereas the first two demons inhabit rivers, the child demon occupies the home and likes to frighten people, especially children (see the Duan Yucai commentary in *SW*; and *Lunheng*, "Dinggui," 22.450). Both of the recipes in *MS*I.E involve exorcistic magic performed in the home, confirming the received account of the child demon.

[2] 俏 in *MWD*, vol. 4, "Transcription," should be transcribed as *kuai* 儈. *Kuai* is not attested in the sense of "figurine," but it must represent a word similar to *geng* 梗, which is attested in pre-Han and Han sources as the term for a figurine of wood or clay. Perhaps the figurines in *MS*I.E.276 are like the apotropaic peachwood figurines placed in the coffin in Mawangdui tomb 1, which are made from short pieces of peach branch cut in half lengthwise. The upper end of each piece is carved into a triangular shape, and painted with a nose and two eyes (Hunan sheng bowuguan and Zhongguo kexueyuan kaogu yanjiusuo 1973, vol. 1: 100). *MS*I.E.276 is the earliest account of hanging peachwood figurines over the doorway (see Bodde 1975: 127-38, for further discussion of the custom).

[3] The Shamanka Mistress is invoked to apprehend the child sprite, perhaps with assistance from the "parents." Disposing of demons in water is a common device. I cannot claim to have understood the conclusion of the incantation. The rhyming words are: *mu/*məg* 母 (Mother), *bei/*pək* 北 (north), *de/*tək* 得 (catch); and *ti/*hliəd* 體 (limb), *zhi/*krjid* 指 (finger), *shui/*hwrjid* 水 (water), *gui/*kwjəd* 鬼 (demon).

[4] *MWD*, vol. 4, "Transcription," n. 2, argues that *cai* 采 is a scribal error for *ji* 奚. I accept the emendation. For *jili* 奚 蠡 (large-bellied gourd) see *MS*I.E.60.

[5] I suspect that a second incantation is lost in the lacunae in the latter part of the recipe.

MSI.E.278 (CC446-48)

Recipe for Removing a Person's Horse Warts[1]

Take iron forging ash,[2] three [20]. Boil in a wide-mouthed kettle. Cook gently, without letting it bubble rapidly. When about one *sheng* of the [1] remains, [3] {2} [10] and remove it. Spread it over and over again on this spot, and it desists. Previously tested. There are no prohibitions. Excellent.

MSI.E.279 (CC449-50)

Another. Removing a person's horse warts. The tip of the wart is large and the base is small. [2], take *jia* [1] and *baifu*[3] [1]. Tie with a cord, binding it firmly. [2] {2} [3] warts will go away. There are no prohibitions. Previously tested. Excellent.

MSI.E.280 (CC451-53)

Treating Facial Pustules[4]

When facial pustules occur the abscess is painful and bursts. If the pustule is situated on the right, [use] the right cheekbone of a horse; if situated on the left, [use] the left cheekbone.[5] Incinerate and smith. Boil soybeans, and wash the [1] with the liquid.[6] Anoint it with already rendered pig lard, and take the smithed horse cheekbone [3] spread on a cloth [1] lard [3] and wrap again.[7] Again anoint (with lard), spread (the medicine), and wash with the soybean liquid. In twenty days the facial pustules desist. Previously tested. Excellent.

---

[1]*Mayou* 馬疣 (horse wart) probably refers to some kind of tumor or polyp. *MWD*, vol. 4, "Transcription," n. 1, cites a passage from the *Huangdi hama jing* 黃帝蝦蟆經 that mentions the ailment name alongside abscess and fistula, but *mayou* is otherwise unattested in received medical literature.

[2]Ma Jixing (1992: 639, n. 3) equates this substance with *tieluo* 鐵落 (*ZY*: no. 3812, oxidized iron produced during forging), listed in *BC* (*GM*, 8.29).

[3]*Baifu* 白柎 may represent the same substance as *baifu* 白付 in *MSI*.E.254 (identity uncertain).

[4]*SW*, 7B.28b, lists three denotations for *ma* 瘍: an eye ailment, noxious vapor adhering to the body, and a festering wound. Because of the use of horse cheekbone as a drug in *MSI*.E.280 as well as the reference to facial *pao* 皰 in *MSI*.E.281 (*pao* is well attested for acne-like pustules), *ma* evidently denotes facial pustules in *MSI*.E.

[5]The two lacunae should be either 以 or 取. The use of horse (*ma* 馬) cheekbone to treat the *ma* ailment exemplifies the same homeopathic principle as *MSI*.E.79 where the *quan* insect is used to treat the *quan* ailment. Using the cheekbone also suggests that the ailment is located on the patient's face.

[6]The lacuna must contain a reference to the pustules.

[7]Perhaps the horse cheekbone medicine is applied with a cloth.

*MS*I.E.281
(CC454-55) Another. Facial pustules. There are female and male types of facial pustules. In the male type the skin swells. The female type has a hole. Treat it with cinnabar [10] {2}. Combine, stirring, and blend in rancid pig lard. Spread (the medicine) on it. If some comes off, immediately reapply it. Do not wash [10]. The redness of the facial pimples desists.[1]

*MS*I.E.282
(CC456-57) Another. Facial pustules. When facial pustules occur there is an abscess that bursts. Use good soybeans and *leishi* (bamboo truffle), each [10] and pound them. Spread it in the hole of the abscess. When spreading the medicine, (the abscess) must first be washed. Wash and spread the medicine once a day. After spreading the medicine for sixty days, the facial pustules [?].

*MS*I.E.283
(CC458-62) [1] Bite[2]

[1] take *mei* (berry) vine.[3] Dry it in the sun [?]. Do not [2]. After drinking this he should go to sleep. When he awakens, he should again [6] {3} [9] dried *mei* (berry) {2} [2] root. Dry it. Peel to obtain the skin. [2] {2} [?] ten *dou*. Use fine [?].

---

[1] *Pao* 靤 (pimple) is attested as an orthographic variant of *pao* 皰, which is glossed in *SW*, 3B.31a, as "an outbreak of vapor on the face" (see Yu Yan 1972: 72-73, for identification with acne).

[2] *MWD*, vol. 4, "Transcription," n. 1, notes that the graph in the lacuna may be *she* 它 (snake). CC458-62, as well as fragments 7-19 (*MWD*, vol. 4: 79-81), are in the hand of a different scribe and were evidently added at the end of the silk sheet subsequent to the original redaction of the text. The ailment names are also not recorded in *MS*I.E.1.

[3] *Mei* 莓 is glossed as *mamei* 馬 莓 in *SW*, 1B.10a, but this name is not found in later sources and its identity is unknown. *Mei* 莓 is a general term for berry vines, and perhaps the reference to *mei* in *MS*I.E.283 is also nonspecific.

*MS*II.A

QUEGU SHIQI

却穀食氣

ELIMINATING GRAIN AND EATING VAPOR

*MS*II.A (CC1-9)

Those who eliminate grain eat *shiwei* (pyrrosia).[1] On the first day of the month eat the base. Daily add one joint, stopping on the fifteenth day.[2] On the sixteenth day begin to decrease. Daily [1] one

[1]"Eliminate grain" translates *quegu* 却穀. The term refers to a dietetic regimen that shuns ordinary foodstuffs, which are replaced by drugs and by breath cultivation. Comparable terms in received literature of the Han period are *bigu* 辟穀 (avoid grain) and *juegu* 絶穀 (abstain from grain). The former is attested in *Shiji*, 55.12a-b, in the account of Zhang Liang 張良 d. 187 B.C.), who is said to have practiced "avoidance of grain," "guiding and pulling" (*daoyin* 道引), and "lightening of the body" (*qingshen* 輕身). The latter is attested in Lu Jia's 陸賈 (fl. 200-180 B.C.) *Xinyu*, 1.11a, which criticizes the man who, hoping to achieve *shenxian* 神仙 (divine transcendence), "abstains from the five grains" and "strains his body and exhausts his physique" while abandoning parents and family. I regard *MS*II.A and the other Mawangdui medical texts that treat of macrobiotic hygiene to be representative of a medical tradition of macrobiotic hygiene which was related to, but not identical with, Daoist ideas and *xian*-cult hygiene in the third and second centuries B.C. These matters are discussed in the Prolegomena, Section Four, "Intellectual Background" and "Body and Spirit."

Shiwei (pyrrosia) is used in *MS*I.E.109 to treat urine retention; eating the drug in *MS*II.A is surely intended to ameliorate some of the physical effects of not eating regular foodstuffs, which include abnormal urination. Descriptions of initial symptoms experienced by the adept who eliminates grain while ingesting vapor in later religious Daoist literature are relevant to *MS*II.A. Here, for example, is the description of the first two decades of a hundred day regimen from *Yunji qiqian*, 57.10b: "During the first decade essence and vapor are weak and slight; facial coloration is wan and yellow. During the second decade movements are lurching, the limbs and joints ache, defecation is difficult, and urine is red-yellow. At times there is dysentary that at first is firm and then turns to muck."

[2]The precise denotation of *zhi* 質 (base) and *jie* 節 (joint) in relation to the herb *shiwei* (pyrrosia) is uncertain. *MS*I.E.226 uses *jie* as a measure for the root of a herb, and *jie* is sometimes used as a measure for sections of the stalk. *Shiwei* (pyrrosia) grows mainly in rocky places, spreading by means of a rhizome that sends out single leaves at intervals. I suspect that *zhi* refers to the end of the rhizome—the "base"—as the primary unit of the herb, and that the *jie* are the sections between leaves. Perhaps a whole herb was measured out in this fashion at the time of use, but it seems likely that there was an established equivalence between this form of measurement and a volumetric measurement.

joint,[1] returning to the base on the last day of the month. Advance and retreat together with the moon. If the head becomes heavy, the feet become light, and the body has itchy swellings,[2] practice *xu* exhalation and *chui* exhalation—stopping when the benefit is realized.[3] Those who eat grain eat the base and [1]; those who eat vapor practice *xu* exhalation and *chui* exhalation when they first go to bed and first arise.[4] Whenever doing *xu* exhalation, in mid-breath change to *chui* exhalation. A twenty year old does it twenty times at dawn, twenty times at dusk, and two hundred times every second

---

[1]The lacuna is a word meaning to decrease the amount of the drug.

[2]"Itchy swellings" translates *zhen* 軫. *Zhen* is attested for *chen* 疹 in *Suwen* 64, 18.7a. For discussion of early glosses of the ailment name, see Yu Yan 1972: 196 (Yu gives hives as one identification).

[3]*Xu* 呴, *chui* 吹, and *hu* 呼 are the three methods of exhaling vapor in early breath cultivation. The manner of executing them is not described in the Mawangdui and Zhangjiashan medical manuscripts, but passages in the *Yinshu* indicate certain characteristics of each. When the body is affected by heat, it is vented by *xu* exhalation; when affected by dampness, by *chui* exhalation; and when affected by dryness, by *hu* exhalation. When a person is joyful, Yang vapor is abundant; and the somatic disharmony is corrected by venting the excess Yang vapor using *xu* exhalation. Anger represents an excess of Yin vapor; and *chui* exhalation restores balance. As part of a daily regimen of breathing, a person should adhere to the following seasonal schedule: in spring, *xu* twice, and *hu* and *chui* once each; in summer, *hu* twice, and *xu* and *chui* once each; in winter, *chui* twice, and *xu* and *hu* once each (autumn is not mentioned in the text; *YSSW*: 86). Summing up the data, *xu* is associated with heat, Yang, and spring; *chui* with dampness, Yin, and winter; *hu* with dryness and summer. Ma Jixing discusses several later explanations of *xu* and *chui* in connection with breath cultivation (1992: 825, n. 17). Ma notes that *xu* is performed with a round open mouth while *chui* is performed with lips spread flat. I suspect that *hu* exhalation is with the mouth in a regular breathing position. The illustrations of exercises in *MS*II.C depict many mouth positions from wide open to closed, which undoubtedly represent *xu*, *chui*, and *hu* exhalation (precise identification is, however, not possible). In *MS*II.A, heavy head, light feet, and itchy body are to be treated with *xu* or *chui* (the text below describes a combination beginning with *xu* exhalation and changing midway to *chui*).

[4]The "base" must refer to *shiwei* (pyrrosia). The outcome of eating the herb for "those who eat grain" (*shigu zhe* 食穀者) is lost in the lacuna. The sentence probably underscores the difference between the ordinary use of the herb and its use as part of a program of breath cultivation cum grain-elimination diet. The contrast between grain-eaters and "those who eat vapor" (*shiqi zhe* 食氣者) is made again below, where it is stated in cosmological terms: eating grain is linked to the symbolism of square and earth; eating vapor to round and heaven. The contrast parallels the "Heshang gong" 河上公 commentary to *Laozi*, par. 6, which identifies heaven with the nose and earth with the mouth. Thus, according to the commentary, "heaven feeds man with the five vapors which enter through the nose and are deposited in the heart," while "earth feeds man with the five tastes which enter through the mouth and are deposited in the stomach" (*Daode zhenjing zhu*, 1.5a). *Shiqi* "eating vapor" is the usual term for breath cultivation in *MS*VI.A, and does not assume simultaneous grain-elimination dietetics (see Prolegomena, Section Four, "Techniques").

day at dusk. A thirty year old does it thirty times at dawn, thirty times at dusk, and three hundred times every third day at dusk. Use this calculation to extrapolate.

For spring eating, eliminate entirely Turbid Yang; blend with Waning Light and Dawn Aurora.[1] Dusk and dawn are allowed. For

---

[1]The remainder of *MS*II.A concerns a tradition of breath cultivation for which parallels exist in Han received literature. This first paragraph specifies five vapors in the external atmosphere to be avoided and six to be ingested during each season. The next two paragraphs describe first the five harmful vapors (four of the five also occur in *MS*VI.A.4), and next the six vapors to be ingested. The five harmful vapors are not attested in received literature, but the other set of six can be associated with the *liuqi* 六氣 (six vapors) in Han sources. *Chuci*, "Yuan you" 遠遊, 5.4a, incorporates them into the narrative of the poem: "I will follow Wang Qiao to find pleasurable entertainment. Consume the six vapors and drink Drifting Flow (*hangxie* 沆瀣), ah! Rinse the mouth with True Yang (*zheng* Yang 正陽) and swallow Dawn Aurora (*chaoxia* 朝霞)." The Wang Yi commentary identifies the six vapors by quoting the lost *Lingyang Ziming jing* 陵陽子明經 (Lingyang Ziming is a personage associated with the Han *xian* cult; see Kaltenmark 1953: 183). According to the *Lingyang Ziming jing*: "In spring eat Dawn Aurora; Dawn Aurora is the red-yellow vapor when the sun is just about to rise. In autumn eat Sunken Yin (*lun* Yin 淪陰); Sunken Yin is the red-yellow vapor after the sun has set. In winter eat Drifting Flow; Drifting Flow is the midnight vapor of the northern quarter. In summer eat True Yang; True Yang is the midday vapor of the southern quarter. Together with Heaven's and Earth's Dark and Yellow vapors, these are the six vapors." In the *Lingyang Ziming jing* each of the vapors corresponds precisely to one of the four seasons, heaven, and earth—the final two vapors being Heaven Dark (*tianxuan* 天玄) and Earth Yellow (*dihuang* 地黄).

The parallel with *MS*II.A is obvious, but the correspondence is not complete. Both texts share the names Dawn Aurora, Drifting Flow (*hanggai* 行暨 in *MS*II.A, which is equivalent to *hanggai* 沆漑 in *Hanshu*, 57A.21b), and True Yang (*duan* Yang 端陽 in *MS*II.A). They are the vapors of dawn, midnight, and midday respectively. That leaves three names in *MS*II.A without direct counterparts in the *Lingyang Ziming jing*: Resurgent Yin (*shu* Yin 輸陰), Resurgent Yang (*shu* Yang 輸陽), and Waning Light (*kuangguang* 銧光). I agree with Ma Jixing (1992: 833, n. 5) that 銧 should be read as *kuang* 匡 in the sense of "wane, decrease." Waning Light is probably a vapor produced as the sun declines in the sky. In translating *shu* as "resurgent" I rely on the interpretation in Ma Jixing 1992: 838, n. 13. *Shu* connotes renewal, and Ma suggests that Resurgent Yin is the vapor produced as day shifts to night and Yin is ascendant; in contrast, Resurgent Yang is the vapor produced as night turns to day. I further agree with Ma (1992: 839, n. 17) that Resurgent Yin is probably equivalent to Sunken Yin in the *Lingyang Ziming jing*; and that it is probably the vapor produced after sunset.

While it is reasonable to associate the four vapors Dawn Aurora, True Yang, Resurgent Yin, and Drifting Flow with seasons and times of day, their use does not match with the *Lingyang Ziming jing*. For example, Drifting Flow is not consumed in winter, but in summer; and True Yang is consumed in winter rather than in summer. The differences are greater than simple seasonal switches, for in *MS*II.A at least two vapors are consumed in each season, and as many as four in winter. In short, *MS*II.A does not exhibit the kind of formal cosmo-seasonal correspondence that is laid out in the *Lingyang Ziming jing*. The understanding of the vapors and their cultivation in *MS*II.A may predate the categorical correspondences of the *Lingyang Ziming jing*. Moreover, the *Lingyang Ziming jing* was most summer eating, eliminate entirely Scalding Wind; blend with Dawn Aurora and Drifting Flow. Dusk and dawn are allowed. For autumn eating, eliminate entirely [Cool Wind] and Frost Mist;[1] blend with Resurgent Yang and Waning [Light].[2] Dusk and dawn are allowed. For winter eating, eliminate entirely Frozen Yin; blend with True Yang, Waning Light, Resurgent Yang, and Resurgent Yin. Dusk and dawn are allowed.

[3] As for [Cool Wind],[3] [1] permeates the four directions.[4] Cool Wind (is a vapor) that snaps the head. Frost Mist [7]. As for Turbid Yang, black permeates the four directions. It is heaven's chaotic vapor, and becomes mist when the sun rises. Scalding Wind is [1] wind. It is (a vapor) that is hot and strikes people. {1} [1]. Frozen Yin enters the bones [2]. These five cannot be eaten.

Dawn Aurora [13]. As for [Resurgent Yang],[5] when the sun ascends the height of two poles[6] it becomes turbid [5][7] clouds are like

---

likely associated with *xian*-cult hygiene. Explaining unclear parts of the admittedly fragmentary text of *MS*II.A by making its contents conform to the *Lingyang Ziming jing* is, in my judgment, unwise. I am skeptical of the equation that Ma makes between Resurgent Yang in *MS*II.A and Earth Yellow, as well as between Waning Light and Heaven Dark (1992: 840). Until more manuscripts are discovered that might shed additional light on the subject of early breath cultivation, the most that I would conclude is that *MS*II.A lists the names of six vapors to be ingested in different combinations in each season, that three of the names correspond to names in the lost *Lingyang Ziming jing*, and that a fourth can be correlated as well.

[1]I follow Ma Jixing (1992: 837, n. 11) in filling the lacuna with Cool Wind (*qingfeng* 清風). The emendation is tentative, but justifiable. Cool Wind is the first vapor named in the paragraph below. Unless the first of the five harmful vapors is not mentioned in this paragraph (which is unlikely) it can only occur here.

[2]I emend the text by adding *guang* 光 (light), which was clearly omitted by the scribe.

[3]I follow Ma Jixing (1992: 842, n. 2) in filling the final two graphs of the five-graph lacuna in *MWD*, vol. 4, "Transcription," with 清 風. The other four harmful vapors are all listed below. The formulaic language used to introduce the other vapor names corroborates the emendation.

[4]Comparison with the description of Turbid Yang indicates that the lacuna is a color word. *Sisai* 四 塞 (permeates the four directions) is attested in connection with the reporting of portentous mists in the *Hanshu*. See, for example, *Hanshu*, 27C-1.6a: "On the night of *xinchou* (of the fourth month, in the year corresponding to 32 B.C.) there was something like fire light in the northwest. At dawn on *renyin*, a great wind arose from the northwest. The cloud vapor was red-yellow and *permeated* under-heaven *in the four directions*. After a whole day and night, what dropped to the ground was yellow dust." The precise knowledge of atmospherics necessary for the practice of breath cultivation no doubt paralleled the expertise of the portent interpreters.

[5]I follow Ma Jixing (1992: 845, n. 2) in filling the final two graphs of the fifteen-graph lacuna in *MWD*, vol. 4, "Transcription," with 輸 陽. The name of a third vapor between Dawn Aurora and Resurgent Yang is lost in the lacuna. The emendation is tentative, but I

a cover that veils [4] {2} [2] {2} [6][1] is the cool wind of summer dusk.

Whenever eating [19]. Those who eat grain eat what is square; those who eat vapor eat what is round. Round is heaven; square is earth. [3] {1} face north [8] eat a large amount.[2] [21] then blend with True Yang. {3} [13] is mostly Yin. Day and night are divided [31] [is][3] the blue adjunct. The blue adjunct is mostly Dawn Aurora. The dispersed vapor of dawn is the white adjunct. The white adjunct is mostly Waning Light. The dispersed vapor of dusk is the black adjunct. The black adjunct is mostly Resurgent [10] {2} [?].[4]

---

agree with Ma that the reference below to a time when the sun has risen above the horizon can only match Resurgent Yang.

[6]I follow Ma Jixing (1992: 845, n. 3) in reading *gan* 干 as *gan* 竿 (pole). Ma adduces several medieval sources in which the height of the ascending the sun is measured in "poles." *MS*II.A indicates that this form of measurement was already in use by the second century B.C.

[7]The name of the fourth vapor is lost in the lacuna. Ma Jixing conjectures that it is Waning Light (1992: 845, n. 5), but I am skeptical of the identification.

[1]The names of the fifth and sixth vapors are lost in the lacunae. Ma Jixing conjectures that the sixth vapor is Drifting Flow (1992: 846, n. 9). As with the fourth vapor, I remain skeptical.

[2]There is a large dot in the text at this point, indicating a change of topic. It appears that discussion of the manner of eating vapor is lost in the lacunae.

[3]I fill the last graph of the thirty-two graph lacuna in *MWD*, vol. 4, "Transcription," with 爲, which is clearly indicated by the grammatical parallels below.

[4]Color-coded "adjuncts" (*fu* 附) that designate the "dispersed vapor" (*yiqi* 佚氣) of different times of the day are clearly related to the six vapors, since the composition of each adjunct is "mostly" one of the six vapors. And there is probably a "yellow adjunct" and a "red adjunct" in addition to the blue, white, and black adjuncts. However, the idea of "dispersed vapor" and "adjuncts" has no counterpart in received literature, and the text of *MS*II.A is too fragmentary to interpret. Wei and Hu offer a tentative interpretation based on cosmo-seasonal correspondences in *Huainanzi* (1992, vol. 2: 9), but I am skeptical of their reasoning.

*MS*II.C

DAOYIN TU

導引圖

DRAWINGS OF GUIDING AND PULLING

*MS*II.C.1[1]

(The caption is missing. The figure is in profile and is bent at the waist, performing a toe-touch.)

*MS*II.C.2

(The caption is fragmentary. Little of the drawing remains.)

*MS*II.C.3

(The caption is fragmentary. The figure is in profile and is standing upright, arms pressed against the sides.)

*MS*II.C.4

(The caption is missing. The figure is in half profile and is standing upright with the right arm bent back level with the shoulders. The left arm is missing.)

*MS*II.C.5

(The caption is missing. The figure is standing upright, forearms bent up in front of the chest.)

*MS*II.C.6

Snapping Yin (The figure is in half profile. The head and arms are missing; the left foot appears to be behind and raised.)[2]

*MS*II.C.7

(The caption is missing. Little of the drawing remains.)

---

[1]The forty-four human figures are arranged in four registers, eleven figures in each register. For each drawing I translate the caption, if extant, and provide a brief parenthetical description of the figure. *MS*II.C.1-11 are drawn in the first register of the manuscript.

[2]*Zhe* 折 means "snap" or "bend sharply." *Yinshu* includes a "snapping Yin" exercise, but it is performed by bending down with hands clasped (*YSSW*: 82). *MS*II.C.6 is a different exercise.

*MS*II.C.8

[1] *lang* (The figure is standing with arms raised above the head, the upper body twisting backward, and the face looking down at an oval object behind, perhaps a lacquer dish.)[1]

*MS*II.C.9

(The caption is missing. The figure is standing, but most of the drawing is missing.)

*MS*II.C.10

(The caption is fragmentary. The figure is in profile and is standing upright with the left arm hanging down by the side and the right arm raised straight up.)[2]

*MS*II.C.11

(The caption is missing. The figure is standing with the left arm curved down and away from the body. The right arm is missing, but evidently curves up.)

*MS*II.C.12[3]

(The caption is missing. The figure is in profile and the arms are raised straight overhead. The left leg is missing except for the tip of the foot, but evidently it is striding forward or kicking.)

*MS*II.C.13

Pain [1] (The figure is in half profile and is stepping forward with arms extended straight in front. The mouth is open wide.)[4]

---

[1]Fragments of the first graph remain. *MWD*, vol. 4, "Transcription," writes *tang* 螳, giving the caption *tanglang* 螳 狼. Ma Jixing reads the caption as homophonous 螳 螂 (praying mantis), and argues that the exercise *dulang* 度 狼 in the *Yinshu* represents the same name (1992: 850). Tang Lan suspects that the first graph is *hu* 虖; the exercise name would then be "shouting wolf" (1979: 7). Given the high degree of uncertainty about the graph, I treat it as illegible and mark a lacuna. The *Yinshu* exercise *dulang* is performed by placing the hands in the armpits (*YSSW*: 83). *MS*II.C.8 is a different exercise. The oval object appears to belong to *MS*II.C.8 rather than to *MS*II.C.19 beneath it. Assuming it is a lacquer dish, there may be a connection with the Han style of dance performed with dishes placed on the ground (for archaeological evidence, see Hayashi 1976: 395).

[2]Li Xueqin thinks the exercise depicted might be the exercise named *zhiluo* 支 落 (meaning uncertain, perhaps "limbs dropping") in the *Yinshu*; and Li suspects that the fragmentary caption might be *zhiluo* (1991: 9). The *Yinshu* text is fragmentary, but does refer to placing one hand at the waist and raising the other arm (*YSSW*: 82).

[3] *MS*II.C.12-22 are drawn in the second register of the manuscript.

[4]The second graph is written *ming* 明 in *MWD*, vol. 4, "Transcription," giving the name *tongming* 痛 明 (meaning uncertain). Tang Lan writes *le* 肋 for the second graph, glossed in *SW*, 4B.23b, as "bones of the sides" (i.e. the ribs); the exercise name would then be "pain in the ribs" (1979: 8). Examining the fragments of the graph in question, Tang Lan's transcription appears to be the more plausible one; but the graph is best treated as illegible.

*MS*II.C.14

(The caption is missing. The figure is in profile and is bending forward from the shoulders with arms hanging down in front.)

*MS*II.C.15

Pulling Inguinal Swelling (The figure is standing with legs spread and knees slightly bent. The arms are hanging away from the body.)[1]

*MS*II.C.16

(The caption is missing. The figure is standing, but most of the drawing is missing.)

*MS*II.C.17

(The caption is missing. The figure is in profile and is standing with hands in front of the chest holding a pole vertically.)

*MS*II.C.18

Inside the Abdomen (The figure is standing. The arms are missing, but evidently they are stretched out on either side.)[2]

*MS*II.C.19

(The caption is missing. The figure is in profile and is standing with arms pressed against the sides.)

*MS*II.C.20

Pulling Deafness (The figure is standing with legs apart. The arms are missing except for a small fragment of the right arm, but evidently they are stretched out on either side.)[3]

*MS*II.C.21

(The caption is missing. The figure is in half profile and is bending over at the waist with the left arm reaching straight up and the right arm reaching straight down. A round object, perhaps a ball, is beneath the figure.)[4]

---

[1]See *MS*I.E.118 for the ailment. The *Yinshu* includes an exercise with the same name, but the description does not relate to the drawing in *MS*II.C.15 (*YSSW*: 84).

[2]The *Yinshu* includes exercises for both abdomen pain and bloated abdomen, but neither is related to the drawing (*YSSW*: 84).

[3]An exercise of the same name is included in the *Yinshu*, but it is not related to the drawing (*YSSW*: 85).

[4]The position of the arms does not seem to represent a throwing motion. It is not clear how the round object—if it is indeed a ball—is used.

*MS*II.C.22

Feverishness (The figure is evidently standing, but little of the drawing remains.)[1]

*MS*II.C.23[2]

Pulling Knee Pain (The figure is in profile. Only the front part remains, minus the legs and arms. The figure might be kneeling.)[3]

*MS*II.C.24

Pulling Upper Side Accumulation (The figure is in profile and is standing with the left foot placed behind, hands holding an object by the waist, and head looking down.)[4]

*MS*II.C.25

Crane [1] (The figure is in half profile and is standing with the left foot placed slightly behind, arms stretched horizontally to the front and rear, and head looking up.)[5]

*MS*II.C.26

(The caption is fragmentary. The figure is in half profile and is standing with the right arm reaching up at an angle and the left arm exactly opposite stretching back.)

*MS*II.C.27

Dragon Ascending (The figure is standing with arms raised at an angle on either side.)[6]

*MS*II.C.28

Bending Down for Reversal (The figure is in profile and is bending over from the waist with the back rigid and the arms touching the ground in front.)[7]

---

[1] *Fan* 煩 (feverishness) may be related to "feverishness of the heart" (see *MS*I.A.4).

[2] *MS*II.C.23-33 are drawn in the third register of the manuscript.

[3] An exercise of the same name is included in the *Yinshu*, but it does not seem to be related to the drawing (*YSSW*: 83).

[4] *Ji* 積 (accumulation) probably refers to a blockage, perhaps of vapor.

[5] The second graph is fragmentary. The left side is 言. Tang Lan suspects that the graph is *ting* 聽 (listen; 1979: 9); i.e. that the right side is 悳, which is unlikely. Shen Shou thinks the graph is *tan* 譚, meaning the sound of the crane as represented by the onomatopoetic word *li* 唳 in the *Lunheng* and later sources (1980: 72). Ma Jixing accepts the transcription *ting*, and also argues that it should be read as *li* (1992: 855, n. 1). The graph probably represents a word for the call of the crane, rather than the crane "listening," but the transcription of the graph itself remains uncertain.

[6] The *Yinshu* includes an exercise with a similar name, but it is not related to the drawing (*YSSW*: 82).

[7] 備 is not attested in received literature. I tentatively accept *MWD*, vol. 4, "Transcription," which identifies the graph with *mian* 俛. The latter graph is given as an

*MS*II.C.29

Pulling the Nape (The figure is in half profile. The right arm is extended downward in front; the left arm is missing as are the lower legs, which may be bent.)[1]

*MS*II.C.30

Penetrating Yin and Yang with a Pole (The figure is in half profile and is bending over at the waist with the hands gripping a pole at either end. The left arm is missing, but it is surely reaching straight up and the right arm straight down.)[2]

*MS*II.C.31

Swinging the Upper Arms (The figure is standing with the arms stretched out at shoulder level on either side.)[3]

*MS*II.C.32

Stretch (The figure is in profile and is bending over from the waist with the back rigid and parallel to the ground, and the arms hanging down in front.)[4]

*MS*II.C.33

(The caption is missing. The middle section of the figure is missing, including the arms, but it is evident that figure is standing in half profile and that the arms are in front.)

---

orthographic variant of *mian* 頫 in *SW*, 9A.10a, glossed as "lower the head." *Jue* 欮 (reversal) is an ailment caused by vapor moving contrary to the proper direction of flow (see *MS*I.B.1). The exercise for treating the reversal ailment (written 瘚) in the *Yinshu* is not related to the drawing (*YSSW*: 84).

[1]The exercise for treating nape pain in the *Yinshu* is not related to the drawing (*YSSW*: 83).

[2]The exercise position is similar to *MS*II.C.21, with the addition of the pole.

[3]The first graph in the caption is *yao* 䍃. The second graph is fragmentary; and is written *bei* 北 in *MWD*, vol. 4, "Transcription," read as *bei* 背 (back). Li Xueqin (1991: 9) compares *MS*II.C.31 to the *Yinshu* exercise written *yaohong* 榣 弘, read as *yaohong* 搖 肱 (swinging the upper arms; *YSSW*: 83). It is probable that the fragmentary second graph in the caption should be written 弘, as in the *Yinshu*. The *Yinshu* exercise may be related to the drawing: "Swing both upper arms in front, like the hitting position."

[4]The caption is the single word *shen* 信 (stretch). Ma Jixing suspects that the scribe omitted *niao* 鳥 above *shen* (1992: 859, n. 1). While I would not emend the caption, the exercise is probably related to the *niaoshen* 鳥 伸 (bird stretch) mentioned in *Zhuangzi* 15, 237; and *Huainanzi*, 7.105. The Cheng Xuanying commentary in *Zhuangzi* explains *niaoshen* as an imitation of a bird in flight with feet extended. The *Yinshu* includes an exercise named *jishen* 鷄 信 (chicken stretch), which it says "benefits the shoulder and ham" (*YSSW*: 86). Although the text does not describe how to execute the exercise, the therapeutic indications seem relevant to the figure in *MS*II.C.32.

*MS*II.C.34[1]

Looking Up and Shouting (The figure is in profile and is standing with both arms flung straight back over the head. The face is looking straight ahead with mouth open.)

*MS*II.C.35

Monkey Bawling to Pull Internal Hotness (The figure is in half profile and is standing with fisted hands held near the belly. The mouth is open wide.)[2]

*MS*II.C.36

Pulling the Warm Ailment (The figure is standing with arms crossed above the head.)[3]

*MS*II.C.37

Sitting and Pulling the Eight Radial-cords (The figure is in half profile and is kneeling in a sitting position with both arms held away from the body.)[4]

*MS*II.C.38

(The caption is missing. The lower body is missing except for the feet. The figure is in profile and is standing with the arms extended down in front away from the body.)

*MS*II.C.39

Pulling Ham Pain (The figure is in profile and is sitting with knees tucked up against the chest and arms wrapped around the knees.)[5]

---

[1] *MS*II.C.34-44 are drawn in the fourth register of the manuscript.

[2] 熱 in *MWD*, vol. 4, "Transcription," should be transcribed as 炅, which is scribal error for *jiong* 炅 (hotness; see Tang Lan 1979: 10). *Jiong* is often used synonymously with *re* 熱 in the sense of hot. *Jiongzhong* 炅 中 (internal hotness) in *MS*II.C.35 is equivalent to *rezhong* 熱 中, which occurs as an ailment name in *MS*I.B.8 (see also the occurrence of *jiongzhong* for *rezhong* in *Suwen* 62, 17.4a).

[3] *Wenbing* 溫 病 (warm ailment) occurs as a generic term for ailments that arise due to unseasonal warmth in *Suwen* 71, 21.3b. The ailment in *MS*II.C.36 may be related to *wen* as described in *Maishu*, "Ailment List": "When the head and body are painful and sweat dries up before coming out—it is *wen*" (*MSSW*: 72).

[4] "Radial-cord" translates *wei* 維. The eight radial-cords denote the eight compass directions in terms of the analogy between net-cords radiating from a center and the axial structure of the cosmos. The cosmological exercise in *MS*II.C.37 must be related to the exercise named *bajing zhi yin* 八 經 之 引 (pulling the eight warps-strings) in the *Yinshu* (the manner of performing the exercise is not described; *YSSW*: 86). The exercise also forms part of an allusion to macrobiotic hygiene in the poem "Zibei" 自 悲 in the poem cycle "Qijian" 七 諫 in *Chuci*, 13.15a: "I pull the eight radial-cords to guide myself, ah! I swallow Drifting Flow to prolong life."

[5] I read 髀 as *bi* 髀 (ham); the same usage is attested in *MS*I.B.2.

*MS*II.C.40

Gibbon Shouting (Little of the drawing remains except for a fragment of the left side of the face and of the right hand, which is reaching at an angle above the head.)[1]

*MS*II.C.41

Bear Ramble (The figure is standing with arms at the sides away from the body and bent at the elbows.)[2]

*MS*II.C.42

[1] *hen*[3] (The figure is in half profile and is standing with arms extended straight in front at shoulder level.)

*MS*II.C.43

(The caption is missing. The hands and trunk of the figure are extant; the head, arms, and most of the lower body are missing. The figure appears to be bending at the waist and shoulders, with the arms hanging in front.)

*MS*II.C.44

Merlin (Much of the drawing is missing. The figure is in profile and appears to be springing forward with the left leg extended in front and bent at the knee, and the right arm curving back above the head.)[4]

---

[1] I read [illegible] as *hu* 謼 (shout). *Huainanzi*, 7.105, includes an exercise named *yuanjue* 蝯躩 (gibbon jumping). Perhaps the graph in *MS*II.C.40 should be read as a word meaning to jump, but I do not know what the word might be and the drawing is too fragmentary to help in determining the nature of the exercise.

[2] The *xiongjing* 熊經 (bear ramble) is mentioned in *Zhuangzi* 15, 237; and in *Huainanzi*, 7.105. Commentators have identified the exercise as imitating a bear climbing a tree (Cheng Xuanying in *Zhuangzi*) or as bear-like movement (Gao Yu in *Huainanzi*). Judging from the figure in *MS*II.C.41, the exercise imitates a bear's gait.

[3] The transcription of the first graph in the caption is uncertain. Tang Lan surmises that the first graph is the name of an animal (1979: 10). Ma Jixing identifies the graph as a variant of *gui* 龜 (turtle), but gives no philological demonstration of the identification (1992: 865, n. 1). The second graph is *hen* 恨, meaning uncertain.

[4] "Merlin" translates *zhan* 鸇, glossed in *SW*, 4A.52a, as *chenfeng* 鷐風, literally "bird of the morning wind." The rapid flight of the *chenfeng* is the opening image in *Shijing*, Mao 132, 6D.4b. Commentaries all identify *zhan/chenfeng* as a type of hawk that preys on pigeons and other small birds, undoubtedly a merlin. The exercise in *MS*II.C.44 evidently imitates a merlin in flight.

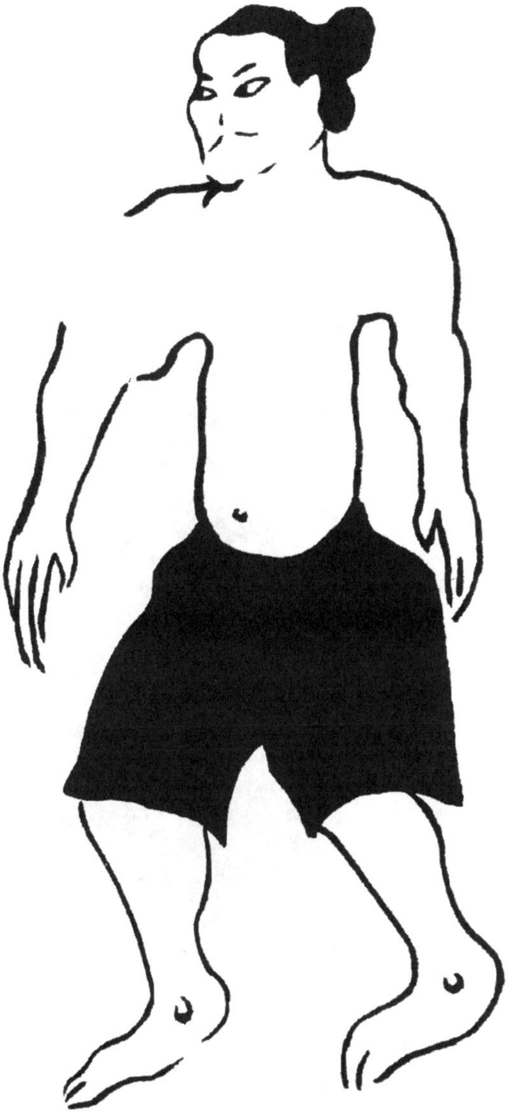

Fig.2 Facsimile of *MS*II.C.15

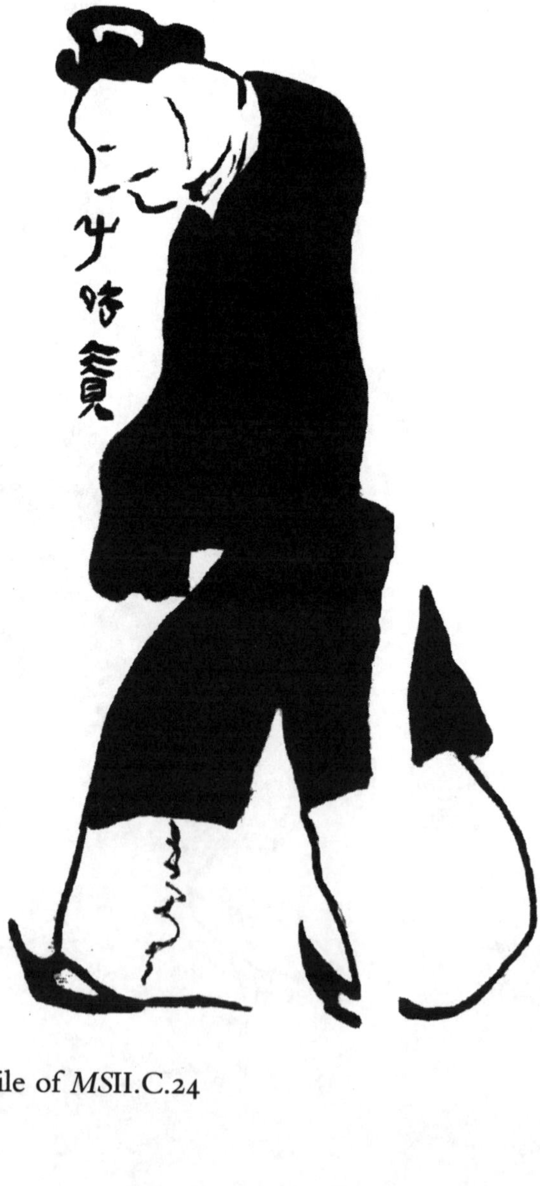

Fig. 3 Facsimile of *MS*II.C.24

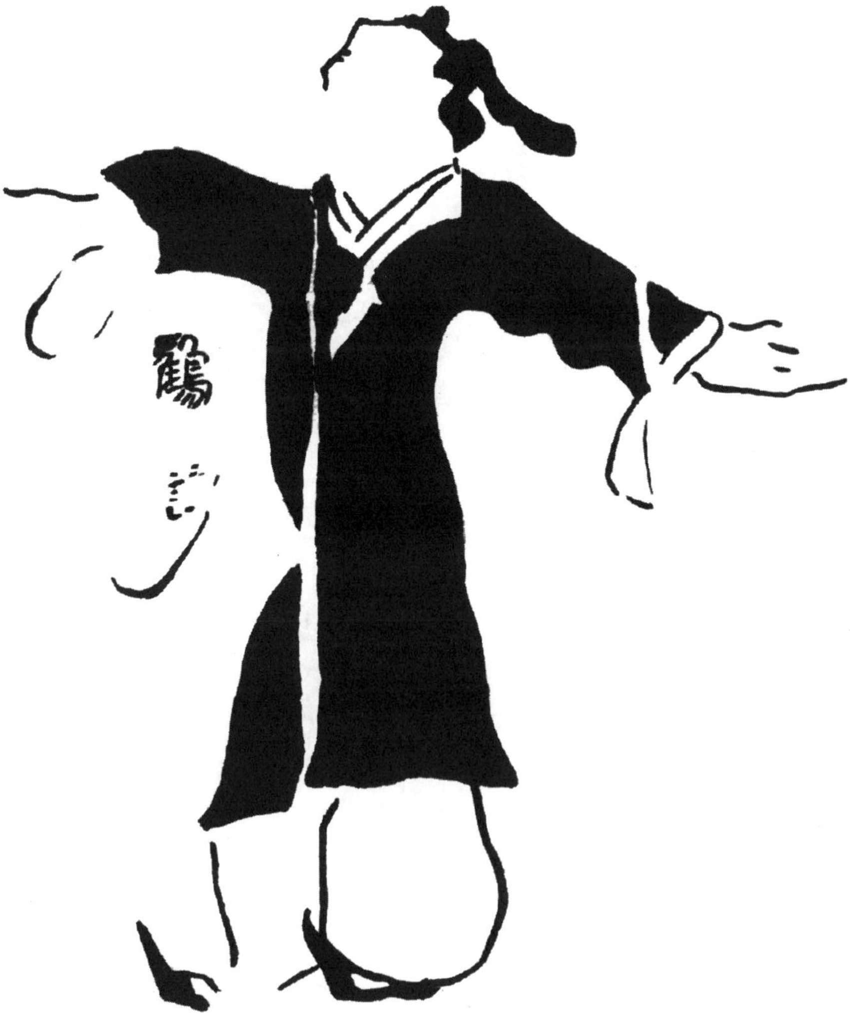

Fig.4 Facsimile of *MS*II.C.25

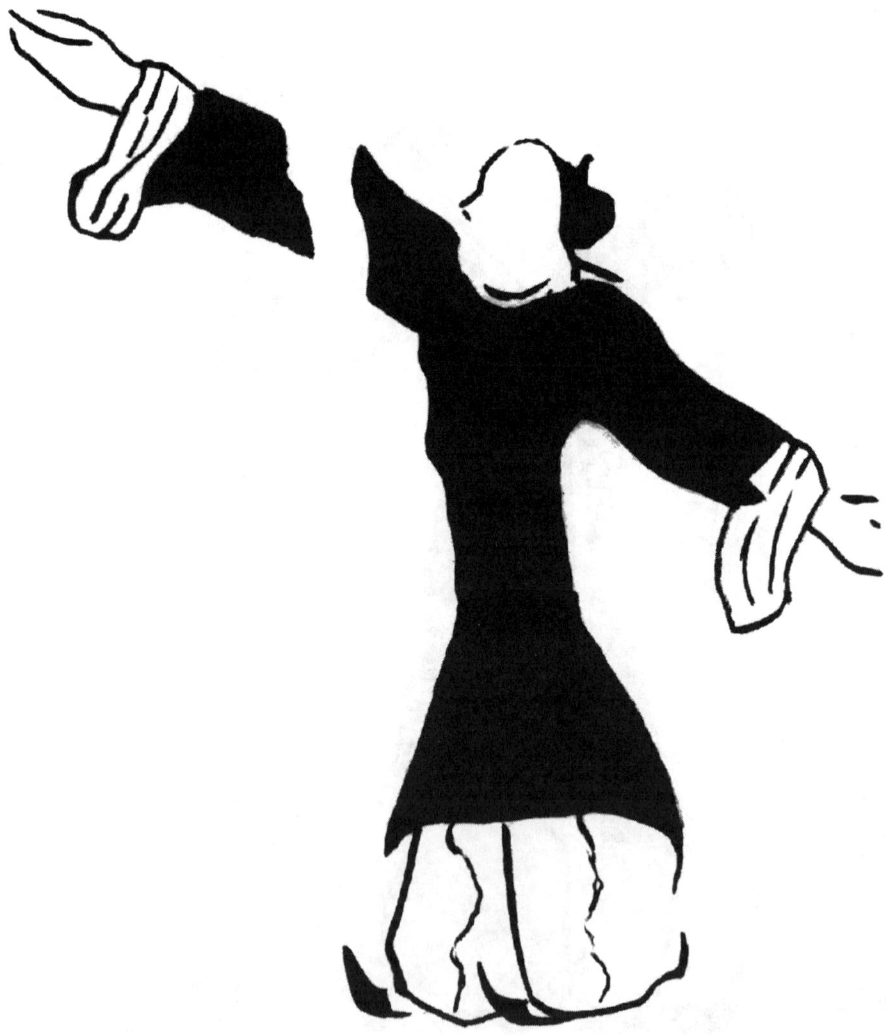

Fig. 5 Facsimile of *MS*II.C.26

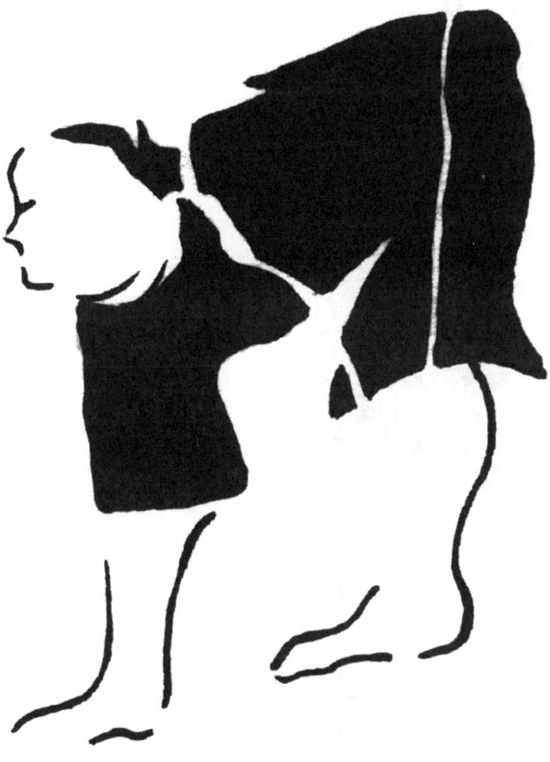

Fig.6 Facsimile of *MS*II.C.28

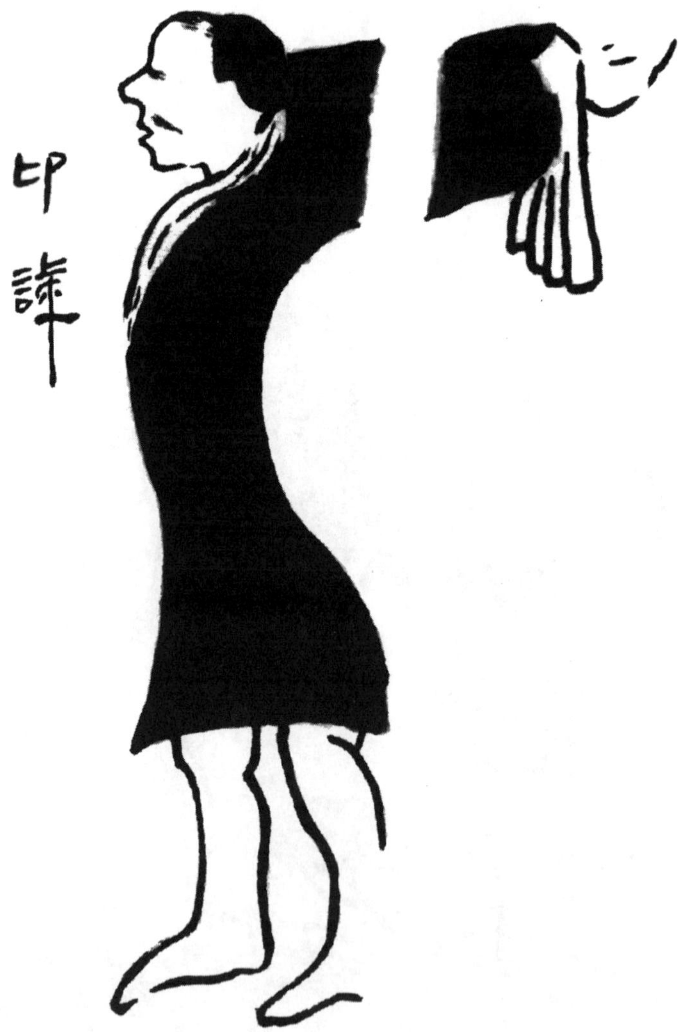

Fig.7 Facsimile of *MS*II.C.34

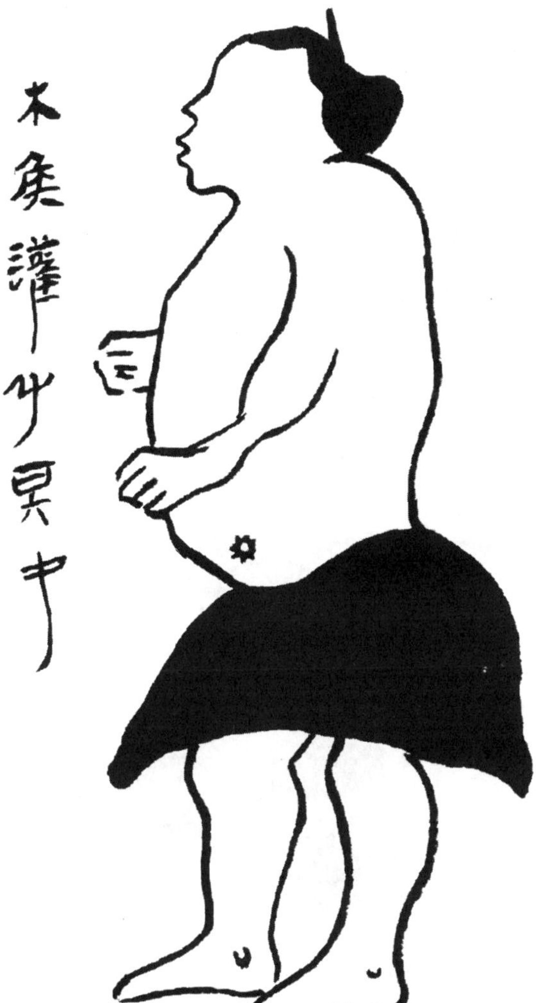

Fig.8 Facsimile of *MS*II.C.35

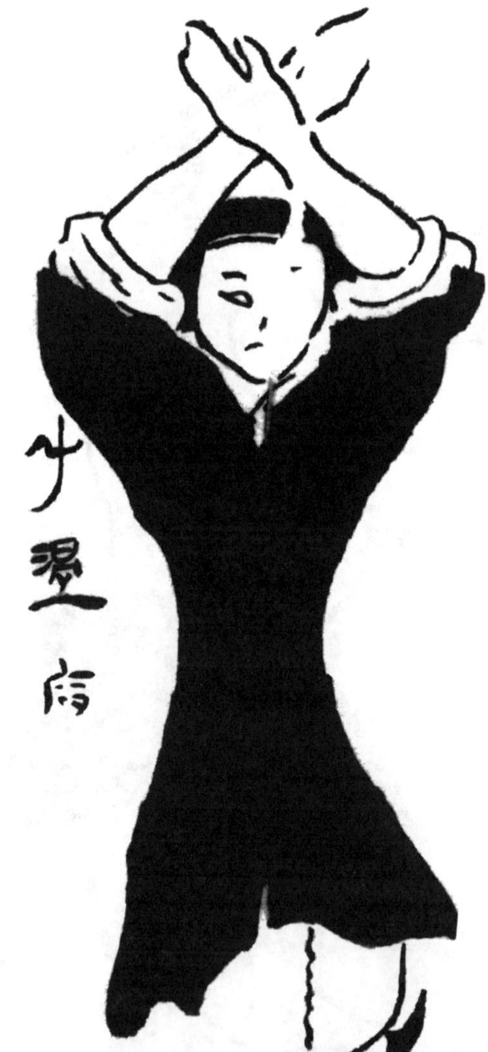

Fig.9 Facsimile of *MS*II.C.36

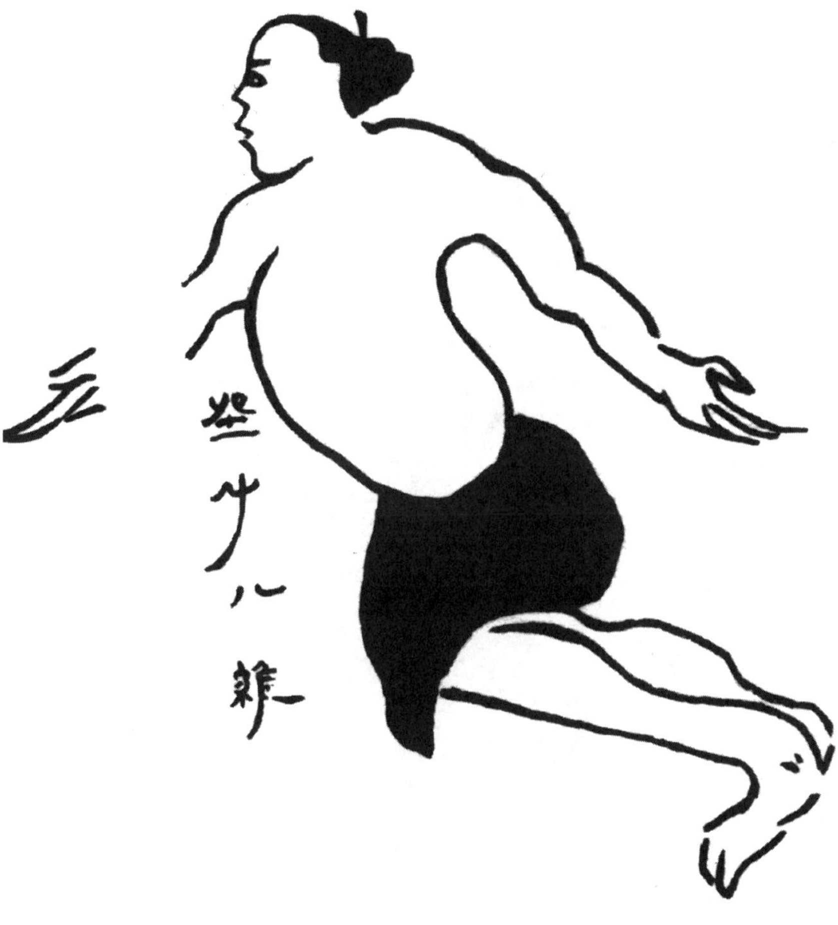

Fig. 10 Facsimile of *MS*II.C.37

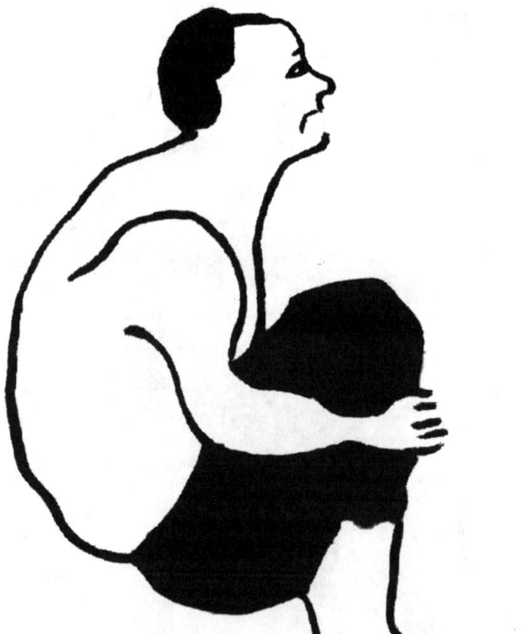

Fig. 11 Facsimile of *MS*II.C.39

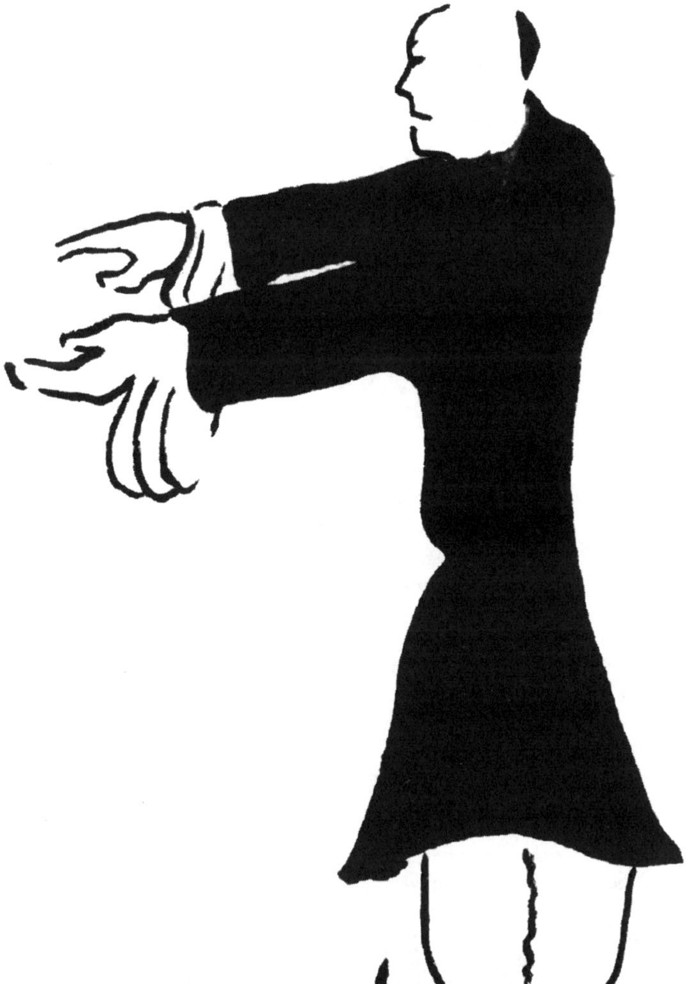

Fig. 12 Facsimile of *MS*II.C.42

*MS*III

YANGSHENG FANG

養生方

RECIPES FOR NURTURING LIFE

*MS*III.1 (CC1-2)

Non-erection Due to Agedness[1]

[9] aroma[2] {1} [29] blended, then [1] then [6] {1} [?].

*MS*III.2 (CC3-8)

Another. [2], recipe for making fermented beverage[3] with *dianji* (asparagus).[4] Cut up three *dou* of *dianji* (asparagus) into one-*cun* long [1] segments [8] it. Cook using firm reeds with close-set joints (as fuel).[5] When it comes to a full boil, stop the fire. When the boil subsides, cook again. If you do not wish to do it like this, two and a

---

[1]*MWD*, vol. 4, "Transcription," n. 2, notes that the right end of the silk sheet is damaged. It is not certain if *MS*III.1 is the first recipe; and the numbering of columns begins with the first extant fragments of text. The "Transcription" adds the heading for the first recipe category at the beginning of C1 based on the list in *MS*III.92. The headings are written above the first column of text of the first recipe in a given category. "Non-erection" translates *buqi* 不起. *Buqi* is a standard term for impotence in later medical literature. For example, a recipe for pills to bolster the vapor of the kidneys in *Qianjin yaofang*, 60.22b, includes "when the Yin (i.e. penis) shrivels and does not become erect (*buqi*)" among the many conditions treated by the pills.

[2]The reference to "aroma" suggests that the recipe concerns a fermented beverage as in *MS*III.2.

[3] 醬 in *MWD*, vol. 4, "Transcription," should be transcribed as *jiang* 漿. *Jiang* (fermented beverage) is named as one of the "four beverages" in *Zhouli*, 5.7a. According to the Zheng Xuan commentary, "*jiang* is the vinegar beverage (*daijiang* 截漿) of today (second century A.D.)."

[4]Tao Hongjing identifies *dianji* 顛棘 as an alternate name for *tian mendong* 天虋冬, which is listed in *BC* (*GM*, 18.37). *Dianji* is evidently synonymous with *dianle* 顛勒, which is given as an alternate name in *BC*. *Tian mendong* is asparagus (*ZY*: no. 0645, *Asparagus cochinchinensis* [Lour.] Merr. and other spp.). The use of *tian mendong* in Han *xian*-cult dietetics is attested in the *Liexian zhuan* (Kaltenmark 1953: 136).

[5]*Huan* 雚 is a reed (genus *Phragmites*) that is smaller than *wei* 葦 (*GM*, 15.59, and Li Shizhen commentary).

half *dou* [6].[1] Put into an old pottery vessel. [1] prepare two *dou* of glutinous spiked millet, cooking vigorously, and wring it.[2] When the vapor is spent, [1] ten days [1] cold [1], then dry [5] and pour over it. Let it sit for two days and [1] fermented beverage, and then it is finished.[3] Drink one *sheng* of this fermented beverage when approaching the inner (chamber).[4] The fermented beverage [13]. Store the liquid. {2} [2] and pour over it, until the sourness and sweetness [2] and drink it. Even [20]. It makes a man immediately have an erection. {2} [?].

*MS*III.3 (CC9-10)

Another. [5] {2} [?] {2} [?].[5]

*MS*III.4 (CC11-12)

To Make Sweet-liquor[6]

To make sweet-liquor take glutinous panicled millet and rice [24] rice. When the sweet-liquor is done, then every morning drink your fill. [6] {1} [?].

*MS*III.5 (CC13-17)

Non-erection

To treat non-erection, at dawn prepare gruel made with excellent water and [2]. Take satiation as the standard.[7] [15], and [1] take it out. Twice like this, and it will become erect. Do not [2] {6} [2] {1} [1] water [1] it. [6] handful, use [2]. After that, drink one (dose) a second time. And after that [1] a third time, not exceeding three drinks. After it becomes a jade rod,[8] engage in intercourse[9] [2].

---

[1]Presumably the recipe gives an alternative method for preparing the *dianji*, and two and a half *dou* refers to the amount of the drug.

[2]I read 足 as *zhuo* 捉 (wring). A cloth is used to separate the liquid from the millet by wringing (see *MS*I.E.13).

[3]Presumably the millet and boiled *dianji* are combined and left to ferment for two days.

[4]I.e. before sexual intercourse (see *MS*III.34).

[5]*MWD*, vol. 4, "Transcription," n. 1, notes that there is a break in the text between C9 and C10; it is not clear how many columns might be missing.

[6]"Sweet-liquor" translates *li* 醴. *SW*, 14B.34b, describes *li* as a liquor that is ready to drink after fermenting overnight. *Zhouli*, 5.6a, includes *li* as one of five liquors known as *ji* 齊 (a reference to the "proportionate measuring" of the grain and other ingredients); and the Zheng Xuan commentary describes *li* as a sweet, unfiltered liquor.

[7]I.e. drink until sated. For the idiomatic use of *gu* 故 meaning "standard," see *MS*I.E.99.

[8]*Ting* 珵 is attested as an orthographic variant of *ting* 珽. See *SW*, 1A.25a, and Duan Yucai commentary. The *SW* glosses *ting* as follows: "It is a large scepter (*gui* 圭), three *chi* long and tapered on the upper part, with a hammer-shaped head." The ritual "jade rod" with its hammer-shaped head denotes the erect penis in *MS*III.5.

[9]I suspect that *yong* 用 has the sense of engaging in intercourse here (see *MS*III.23).

When drinking it, do not follow with [8] drink. If (the semen) is already spent, splash with cold water,[1] without [2] you must drink again. Drink and food [3]. After eliminating water,[2] you must use [5] the vapor, make the mouth round[3] and raise it, {1} [1]. Gradually exhale the vapor through the nose. [2] {2} [1] {2} [?].

*MS*III.6 (CC18-20)

Augmentation[4]

Collect *lai* (chenopodium) and *xian* (eupatorium)[5] in the fifth month on the full-moon day.[6] Dry them in the dark and smith. Also smith *bai songzhi* (white pine rosin)[7] that is [14], using half of each. Wrap well in leather. Drink it once a day. Each time you drink, put a three-fingered pinch into liquor. [13] strength and excel in traveling. Drunk either at dawn or at dusk, (both) are permissible.

*MS*III.7 (CC21-23)

Pliancy[8]

---

[1]"Spend" translates *shi* 施, denoting ejaculation. The sexual denotation of *shi* is common in later sexual literature; see, for example, the passage concerning the number of ejaculations permitted depending on the man's age and physical condition in *Ishinpô*, 28.23b. *MS*IV.3 describes washing the penis to cause detumescence after having used an aphrodisiac to make it erect, which probably explains the use of cold water in *MS*III.5.

[2]*Qishui* 棄 水 (eliminate water) is an idiom for urination attested in the *Yinshu* (*YSSW*: 82).

[3]I read *gou* 鉤 as synonymous with *gui* 規 (compass, round). The usage is attested in *Hanshu*, 87A.4a. *MWD*, vol. 4, "Transcription," n. 3, suggests reading the graph as *xu* 呴. While the end of *MS*III.5 is concerned with some kind of breathing exercise, *xu* does not make sense grammatically here.

[4]I agree with Li and McMahon that *jia* 加 (augmentation) refers to increasing the size of the erect penis (1992: 151), rather than to increasing vitality with tonics as suggested in *MWD*, vol. 4, "Transcription," n. 1. This denotation is unmistakable in the recipes for *neijia* 内 加 (inside augmentation) in *MS*IV.3-7. The references to "strength" and "traveling" at the end of *MS*III.6 suggest that what is good for the male organ is also good for male vitality in general.

[5] 蕳 in *MWD*, vol. 4, "Transcription," should be transcribed as *xian* 閒. I nevertheless agree that the graph is to be read as *xian* 蕑, another name for *lan* 蘭 (eupatorium).

[6]I.e. the fifteenth day of the lunar month. The fifth month is the time of the summer solstice when Yang potency peaks, making it an optimal time to collect drugs possessing Yang properties (see *MS*I.E.95).

[7]For the use of pine rosin in Han *xian*-cult dietetics, see Kaltenmark 1953: 54, n. 2.

[8]The recipe category is entitled *suan/*suan* 筭. I suspect that the graph is to be read as a phonetic loan for *sun/*sjuan* 巽, in the sense of "pliant." Confirmation of this loan usage occurs in the Mawangdui manuscript of the *Yijing* hexagrams, which writes *suan* 筭 for the name of the hexagram written *sun* 巽 in the received *Yijing* (Han Zhongmin 1992: 175). References to a position "beneath the bed" in the hexagram text hint at a possible sexual

Collect swarming beetle larvae[1] in the fifth month on the full-moon day. Put them in a bamboo tube[2] [1] full. The length of the bamboo tube should be five [15] it. Set it in a slotted steaming pot, laid on [1],[3] and cook. When moisture rises [2] and take it out. Once again [16]. If it does not take effect, then take some medicine the size of a grain of glutinous panicled millet from inside the bamboo tube [?].[4]

*MS*III.8 (CC24-25)

Another. In the fifth month [1] *fuling* (pine truffle) that is just yellowed. Then [22] {4} [?].

*MS*III.9 (CC26-27)

Another. To cultivate the inside, pound *wu* [27] {2} [?].[5]

---

connotation for *suan/sun*. And a textual variant in the Mawangdui manuscript makes a sexual interpretation entirely plausible. The explanation of the bottom line of the hexagram in the received *Yijing* is, "In advancing and retreating (*jintui* 進 退) it is beneficial to have the rectitude of the military man." The corresponding text in the Mawangdui manuscript is, "In advancing inside (*jinnei* 進 内) it is beneficial to have the rectitude of the military man." The words "advance inside" suggest sexual intercourse; and in this context perhaps *zhen* 貞 should be rendered "erection" rather than "rectitude." Coming after Augmentation, which concerns increasing the size of the penis, the category Pliancy is concerned with impotence. Significantly, *suan* occurs in *MS*I.E, fragment 7 (*MWD*, vol. 4: 79), in a recipe to treat *wei* 痿 (impotence). The recipe is one of several added to the end of *MS*I.E after the original redaction. The meaning of *suan* is not clear in the fragment, but I would guess that it is related to *suan* in *MS*III.7.

[1]I read *xiang* 鄉 as *xiang* 蠁; and *rong/*njung* 軵 as a phonetic loan for *yong/*rung* 蛹. The compound *xiangyong* is not attested in received literature, but I suspect that it refers to the larva of an insect, probably the scarab beetle. *Guangya*, 10B.11a, glosses *tuyong* 土 蛹 (earth *yong*) with *xiangchong* 蠁 蟲 (*xiang* bug). *GM*, 41.3, associates these names with a type of grub that is cultivated by digging a pit and filling it with grain and manure; the larva produced is comparable to *qicao* 蠐 螬, the larva of the scarab beetle (*ZY*: no. 4934, *Holotrichia diomphalia* Bates). The method is first described in *Huainan wanbishu*, 1.11a: "In autumn and winter put mixed glutinous millet in a ditch and *qicao* are produced." The adjective *cheng* 蝱 (swarming) constitutes additional confirmation that *xiangyong* in *MS*III.7 is an insect drug; *SW*, 13A.53a, glosses *cheng* as "bugs swarming."

[2]*MWD*, vol. 4, "Transcription," erroneously transcribes 籥 入 籥. The first *yao* 籥 is not written in the text and should be excised from the transcription.

[3]*MWD*, vol. 4, "Transcription," writes 笩 for the fragmentary graph in the lacuna, which it reads as *ce* 策 (bamboo strip). Both the transcription and reading are doubtful. Qiu Xigui suggests that the graph in question might be *ji* 箕 (winnowing basket; 1992: 534). I treat the graph as illegible and mark a lacuna.

[4]Presumably it may be necessary to use the medicine more than once before the desired effect (an erect penis) is achieved.

[5]*MWD*, vol. 4, "Transcription," n. 1, notes a break in the text between C27 and C28; it is not clear how many columns might be missing.

*MS*III.10 (CC28-29)

To Make Mash-liquor[1]

Use three *dou* of fine liquor to soak wheat [16] it becomes mash-liquor, and drink it. A man [3] boil *xie* (scallions) in formula sweet-liquor[2] [?].

*MS*III.11 (CC30-31)

Cultivation[3]

Take[4] one rooster, pluck it alive, and [1] wash it. [9]. Dry in the dark and smith, using the same amount as the chicken.[5] [1], making them the size of [9][6] medicine. [1] the liquid to soak dried-meat slices for three days. Eat four *cun* of the dried-meat slices. Sixty-five.[7]

---

1 "Mash-liquor" translates *laozhuo* 醪酌. *Zhuo* is a verb meaning "pour liquor," but here it is a generic term for liquor. *SW*, 14B.35a, describes *lao* as a liquor in which the liquid and dregs are combined. Judging from the recipes for making *bailao* 白醪 in *Qimin yaoshu*, 7.394, the liquor is filtered after an initial period of fermentation, then a mash of freshly cooked grain is added. The liquor is ready to drink when the mash floats to the surface of the fermentation jar. According to one recipe, the liquor is "sweet like milk." *MS*III.74 provides a recipe for *lao* that is a potent herbal cordial unlike the *Qimin yaoshu* recipes.

2 "Formula sweet-liquor" translates *chengli* 稱醴. I suspect that *cheng* refers to the fact that the ingredients of the liquor are balanced according to a formula; and that *chengli* is synonymous with *liji* 醴齊, the name for *li* as one of the five *ji* (liquors made with "balanced proportions") in *Zhouli*, 5.6a (see *MS*III.4).

3 *MWD*, vol. 4, "Transcription" restores the recipe heading *zhi* 治 to the text based on the list in *MS*III.92. In *MS*III.92, the scribe evidently forgot once again to record this recipe category, since the graph is written in smaller script above the first register between the names of the sixth and eighth categories. Besides *MS*III.11-14, *MS*III.75 also belongs to the category Cultivation. The recipes concern increasing Yang vitality—as indicated by the use of substances like roosters and wasps—but it is not entirely clear whether the intended result is related to physical strength or to sexual prowess. I suspect that the two are not distinguished.

4 以 in *MWD*, vol. 4, "Transcription," should be transcribed as *qu* 取.

5 The drug or drugs used in the recipe are lost in the lacuna.

6 The medicine is probably formed into balls of a certain size.

7 Despite the lacunae, it is evident that dried meat is soaked in a medicinal liquid and eaten. The number sixty-five probably refers to people. *MWD*, vol. 4, "Transcription," n. 4, speculates that the number is related to sexual prowess and refers specifically to multiple female partners, citing a recipe in *Ishinpô*, 28.40b, entitled, "recipe for cultivating the man with the goal of vigorously engaging in bedroom activity so that in one night he (has intercourse) over ten times without stopping." The conclusion to the recipe states that, "Sire Cao consumed this and in one night passed through seventy women" (cf. Wile 1992: 101). The speculation is plausible. Similar use of numbers occurs in *MS*III.12, 14, and 75. The wording in *MS*III.75 suggests that physical strength to overpower opponents is the objective, which indicates to me that the category Cultivation concerns both physical strength and sexual prowess.

*MS*III.12 (C32)

Another. Take twenty wasp larvae[1] and place them in one cup of sweet-liquor. [2] and drink it at midday. Ten.[2]

Yi[3]

*MS*III.13 (C33)

Another. Soak one hundred wasps in one cup of fine sauce. Remove them after one day and one night. Use the liquid to soak two-ninths *sheng* of thick roasted-grain meal.[4] Each time you eat (the medicine), drink a three-fingered pinch in liquor.

*MS*III.14 (C34)

Another. Pingling Lü's way of pleasure.[5] Dry in the dark snails (removed) from the shell and smith. If you want twenty, use seven pinches; if you want ten, use three pinches—and one cup of liquor.[6]

*MS*III.15 (CC35-36

Wheat-and-egg[7]

At dawn regularly break a chicken egg and put it in liquor. Drink before (the meal). The next day, drink two (eggs), and the next drink three. Then begin anew drinking one (egg), the next day two, and the next three. In this fashion use up forty-two eggs. It makes a man strong and increases the beauty of his complexion.[8]

---

[1]I read 駘 as *tai* 胎 (embryo, larva; see *MS*I.E.223).

[2]I.e. the tonic is good for entertaining ten partners, for sex or physical combat.

[3]*Yi* 易 is written in large script below the recipe. The graph occurs again at the bottom of C44 in *MS*III.21. A second large-script graph, which is unidentified, is written at the bottom of C115 in *MS*III.55. I do not know why the graphs are written on the manuscript in the way that they are, nor do I know what *yi* means—other than to guess at a meaning like "easy."

[4]According to *SW*, 7A.62b, *qiu* 糗 is a food made by first roasting and then grinding various grains. *Shiming*, 4.129, describes *qiu* as grain that is cooked, dried, and ground, which is probably another Han-time method for preparing *qiu*. This type of converted grain provision played an increasingly important role in the Han diet (Ying-shih Yu 1977: 76-77). Former Han measuring spoons of a type that could have been used to measure two-ninths *sheng* have been recovered archaeologically (Qiu et al. 1984: 78).

[5]Pingling 平陵 must refer to the Dong Pingling 東平陵 recorded in *Hanshu*, 28A-2.72b; and situated east of present-day Jinan, Shandong. I interpret Pingling Lü 吕 as the moniker of a Mr. Lü from Pingling; and *ledao* 樂道 as his "way of (sexual) pleasure." *MWD*, vol. 4, "Transcription," n. 1, interprets Lü Le as the man's name, and understands *dao* as "say, state"; giving the translation, "Lü Le of Pingling states."

[6]A three-fingered pinch must be understood. The dosage is determined by the anticipated number of sexual partners.

[7]The recipe category concerns vitalizing tonics based on eggs and several other ingredients.

[8]The raw egg immersed in liquor and swallowed whole has a place in many cuisines. In North America it is the "prairie oyster," especially recommended for hangover. In

*MS*III.16 (CC37-38)

Another. In the eighth month collect *tulu* (dodder) fruit. Dry in the dark. When dry, split and remove the grains. Smith and wrap in leather. When spring arrives, beat in virile-bird egg liquid.[1] Make balls the size of rat feces and dry in the dark. [1] put eight balls into soybean sauce and eat.

*MS*III.17 (C39)

Another. [1] one spring-bird egg.[2] Break, and toss it into roasted-grain meal made from malt. Make it into balls the size of a large cow-louse. Eating many is good.

*MS*III.18 (CC40-41)

Another. [?].[3] {1} [1] {1} [1] {1} [?].

*MS*III.19 (C42)

Another. To cultivate Yin, use sauce to soak [18] in it.

*MS*III.20 (C43)

Washing the Male Organ[4]

[16] three *dou*, and soak one *dou* of *zi* (catalpa) fruit for five days. Wash the male organ with it, and the male organ becomes strong.

*MS*III.21 (C44)

To Cause Burning[5]

---

*MS*IV.23 the eggs are drunk in an ascending and descending progression (1:2:3:2:1), and are stirred.

[1]*MWD*, vol. 4, "Transcription," n. 2, surmises that *muniao* 牡鳥 (virile-bird) refers to *que* 雀 (dickeybird). The identification is plausible. *MS*III.17 and *MS*IV.4 call for "spring-bird eggs"; and *MS*VI.A.2 for "spring dickeybird eggs." *Que* flesh and eggs are associated with male potency in later materia medica (*GM*, 48.97-98), which perhaps accounts for the name "virile-bird" in *MS*III.16.

[2]I.e. a dickeybird egg.

[3]*MWD*, vol. 4, "Transcription," n. 1, notes a break in the text between C40 and C41; it is not clear how many columns might be missing.

[4]*Nan* 男 denotes the male genitals. The usage occurs again in *MS*III.41-42.

[5]I follow the interpretation in *MWD*, vol. 4, "Transcription," n. 1, that 勺 be read as *zhuo* 灼 with the sense of a "burning" sensation. The reading depends largely on the context of *MS*III.21-23, all of which describe medicines that stimulate sexual excitement by causing an itchy, burning sensation. Li and McMahon argue for reading the graph as *yue* 約 with the sense of "contract" (1992: 152). The latter interpretation is supported by *MS*IV.8-12 in which *yue* refers to contracting the vagina (the counterpart to *MS*IV.3-7 which deal with penile erection). However, in addition to the contextual evidence for associating *MS*III.21-23 with "burning," *MS*III.23 describes inserting the medicine in a nostril, which has little connection with tightening the vagina and could be applied to the man as well as the woman.

Collect snails[1] in the fifth month on the full-moon day. Soak [5] cloth [1] {1}. Dry in the dark. Use [2] becomes hot.

Yi[2]

MSIII.22 (CC45-46)

Another. Take dried *jiang* (ginger), *gui* (cinnamon), *yaotiao*,[3] *shechuang* (cnidium), and [2]. Smith all of them. (Taking) equal amounts of each, blend with honey or *zao* (jujube) fat[4] and make balls the size of a fingertip. Wrap in loose-weave cloth and insert into the inside.[5] The hotness is subtle.

MSIII.23 (CC47-50)

Another. In the fifth month collect three *dou* of snails and two *dou* of *tao* (peach) fruits. Stir together and put into a crock. Pour in three *dou* of fine vinegar. Cover and seal with mud. Bury inside the stove, making it [2] three *cun*. Fill in the top until level with the ground.[6] Cook over it during the day; the fire [1] be extinguished.[7] Remove after four days. Filter[8] and discard the dregs. Use the liquid to dye a three *chi* piece of cloth. Dry in the dark, then immediately dye again. When the liquid is used up, wrap the cloth well—do not

---

[1]The name *boluo* 勃蠃 is equivalent to *fuluo* 蚹蠃 in *Erya*, 9.12a, identified in the Guo Pu commentary as "snail." Two variations on the name are used in *MS*III: 蛂蠃 (*MS*III.23) and 弗選 (*MS*III.42).

[2]See *MS*III.12.

[3]*MWD*, vol. 4, "Transcription," n. 1, reads *yao* 要 as *piao* 蔈, and cites *Erya*, 8.9b: "*Tiao* 苕 is *lingtiao* 陵苕. With yellow flowers it is called *piao*; with white flowers it is called *ba* 茇." *Piao* is glossed in *SW*, 1B.34a, as "*tiao* with yellow flowers," but Duan Yucai suspects textual corruption and argues that the original gloss read "a plant with yellow flowers." In either case, if one accepts the "Transcription" reading *piao*, *piaotiao* in *MS*III.22 could be interpreted as a compound for a variety of *tiao* with yellow flowers. The botanical identity of *tiao* is based on *BC*, which gives *lingtiao* as an alternate name for *ciwei* 紫葳 (*GM*, 18.23; *ZY*: no. 3947, *Campsis grandiflora* [Thunb.] Loisel.). The "Transcription" identification is plausible, but uncertain. *Ciwei* occurs in *MS*III.73, which suggests that *yao/piaotiao* is not the same plant. While I am inclined to agree that the two graphs are a compound drug name, *yao* 葽 and *tiao* are each glossed as plant names in *SW*, 1B.31a, and 1B.51b, respectively.

[4]I.e. a paste prepared from jujube fruits.

[5]*Zhong* 中 (inside) refers to the vagina. The usage occurs again in *MS*III.24.

[6]The pot is buried so that the top is three *cun* lower than the ground, and the space is then filled with soil.

[7]The lacuna must be an injunctive negative: "do not" let the fire be extinguished.

[8]*MWD*, vol. 4, "Transcription," reads *lü* 閭 as *lü* 濾 (strain, filter), which would be plausible were it not for the fact that the latter word is not attested before the Tang period. I read *lü*/**gljag* 閭 as a phonetic loan for *shi*/**srjag* 釃, glossed in *SW*, 14B.34b, as "send down (i.e. filter) liquor." *Shi* occurs in *MS*III.74, and 麗 in *MS*III.37 should probably be read as *shi* as well.

let it be loosely [1]. When engaging in intercourse,[1] take a piece the size of the palm and insert it in a nostril. It itches slightly and is hot. If pressed on the arm, the arm itches greatly and is fiercely hot. Do not let it touch the face. If it touches the face, the itching is unbearable.[2] Whatever amount of cloth you make, use this to determine the proportions.

*MS*III.24 (CC51-52)

Increasing Craving[3]

[1] *fuling* (pine truffle) and discard the dregs.[4] Use the liquid to fatten a suckling pig. Feed it to the woman.[5] It makes her increase in sweetness and makes her inside[6] become fine. Incinerate and smith the inner part of cow horn. [1] dried *jiang* (ginger) and *jungui* (curled cinnamon). Combine them [3] put in a sack. Soak it in gruel vinegar and insert into the inside.

*MS*III.25 (C53)

Another. Blend [1] liquid with choice beef or venison.[7] Have the woman insert it herself deep inside her prohibited part.[8] [?].

---

[1]"Engage in intercourse" translates *yong* 用, which is used idiomatically to refer to having sexual intercourse in several recipes in *MS*III, as well as in *MS*IV, *MS*VI.A, and *MS*VII.B. The usage is attested in *Suwen* 5, 2.7a, where the Wang Bing commentary explains *yong* as having a sexual meaning. In *MS*III.35, 38, and 43 the expression 用之 occurs, which seems to have a double sense of "using" the prepared sexual excitant to "engage in intercourse." *Yong* occurs in the text with its usual meaning as well, and it is sometimes difficult to be certain when the idiomatic usage applies.

[2]"Itch" translates *yang* 癢, referring to the itching associated with sexual excitation.

[3]The recipe category concerns increasing the woman's sexual desire. *Gan* 甘 in the sense of "crave" is common in early literature; e.g., in *Huainanzi*, 6.97, where those who eat human flesh, pickle the human liver, and drink human blood are said to "crave it more than grass and grain fed animals." At the same time, *gan* "sweet" connotes succulence; and the recipes are probably intended to stimulate the woman to produce an abundant flow of sexual fluids during intercourse.

[4]The drug must be boiled.

[5]I agree with Ma Jixing that the phrase 以汁肥豯 means that liquid is fed to the pig, which is then cooked and fed to the woman (1992: 681). *MWD*, vol. 4, "Transcription," n. 2, interprets the phrase as an elliptical way of saying that the suckling pig is cooked in the liquid.

[6]I.e. vagina.

[7]For the translation of *niu* 朋 as "choice," see *MS*I.E.35.

[8]"Prohibited part" translates *jie* 戒, referring to the vagina. The usage is also attested in *Maishu*, "Ailment List," where it denotes either the male or female genitals: "When it is located in the prohibited part and the person cannot urinate—it is blockage" (*MSSW*: 72).

*MS*III.26 (CC54-56)

Another. Pare *xu* (oak) wood, removing the bark and bad spots, and hurriedly chop it. Boil in water [2] vapor [12] and becomes clear. Take the liquid and discard the sediment. Once again boil the clear liquid until it is evaporated.[1] When dry, [16] {1}, for the time it takes to eat, and wash with water. It keeps for seven or eight [3].[2] Previously [?].[3]

*MS*III.27 (CC57-58)

Another. Take a stillborn chick.[4] {5} [24] moisten, and dry in the dark. When dry [?].[5]

*MS*III.28 (CC59-60)

Play[6]

[2], take a gecko [1] {1} [3] deep.[7] When finished, bury it beneath the mouth of the stove, in depth [5] water, and dye it in the

---

[1]Other drugs are probably lost in the lacuna above. A purified medicine is produced by continuous boiling and clarifying until the liquid has boiled away.

[2]Judging from other contexts, the period of time the medicine keeps is probably measured in years.

[3]試 is probably the first graph in the lacuna. *Changshi* 嘗試 occurs several times in *MS*I.E to praise the effectiveness of a recipe.

[4]I interpet the phrase 烏產不㲉 to mean a chick that was born but did not live to be nurtured by its mother, understanding *kou* 㲉 as glossed in *SW*, 4A.56a, "a chick whose food is chewed and fed to it." *MWD*, vol. 4, "Transcription," n. 1, interprets *kou* in the sense of a chick about to hatch from the egg, citing the term *kouyin* 㲉音 in *Zhuangzi* 2, 30. Despite the commentary that defines the term as "the sound of a chick emerging from the egg," it is better understood as the sound of chicks chirping for their food. Thus I am not convinced by the "Transcription" argument that the phrase in *MS*III.27 refers to an unhatched egg.

[5]*MWD*, vol. 4, "Transcription," n. 3, notes a break in the text between C58 and C59; it is not clear how many columns might be missing.

[6]The two recipes in this category corroborate the recipes for a gecko and cinnabar compound used to detect illicit sexual activity in *Huainan wanbishu*, 1.4b. While we cannot know how often and in what circumstances the compound was actually used, the recipes suggest that marking a woman's skin with the compound was an ordinary feature of private life. The recipes should also dispel the skepticism of many later Chinese scholars concerning the veracity of received accounts of the practice.

[7]The name used for the gecko is *shougong* 守宮 (guard of the palace), referring both to the gecko's habit of climbing walls and to its application in preventing the occurrence of illicit sexual activity in the sleeping quarters. Because of the lacunae it is not clear whether cinnabar is also added in this recipe (some of the *Huainan wanbishu* passages only use gecko to produce the potion).

liquid. Dye the woman's arm with it.[1] If the woman plays with a man, the [1] then cracks and breaks. If [1] sleeps, then it vanishes.[2]

*MS*III.29[3]

Take a gecko, place it in a new jar, and place cinnabar in the jar. Have the gecko eat it. Wait for it to die, then smith. [1] to paint the woman's arm or body. If she plays with a man, it instantly loses its brightness. [?]

*MS*III.30 (C61)

To Remove Hair[4]

If you want to remove hair—when (a woman) who has newly given birth shaves[5] for the first time, if she first shaves the lower (body) and then shaves her hole, the hair will be removed.[6]

*MS*III.31 (C62)

Another. Fry white-necked earthworms.[7] Blend in spider webs and *kuhu* (bitter gourd), and quench iron (in the liquid).[8] Then spread the liquid on it.

---

[1]The lacuna makes the meaning unclear, but I suspect that a cloth is dipped in a liquid preparation of gecko and then the dyed cloth is applied to the woman's arm.

[2]The recipe distinguishes between sexual play and actual intercourse; in the former case the compound on the arm has cracks, and in the latter it disappears entirely.

[3]The recipe is written in the space beneath the main text in CC60-63, and is blocked off from the main text by a horizontal line. It was evidently added after the original redaction of the text.

[4]The recipe category concerns the removal of body hair, especially pubic hair. *Ishinpô*, 28.34b, testifies to the disapproval of body hair with the statement that a man should not have intercourse with a woman who "has hair on her thighs and lower legs"; and also warns of the harm a man suffers if he has intercourse with a woman whose pubic hair is "both coarse and stiff, and mostly grows in the opposing direction." Ideally, according to *Ishinpô*, 28.33b, the woman's "genitals and underarms should not have hair; and if there is hair, it must be made to be fine and smooth."

[5]"Shave" translates *mu* 沐. From a literal meaning of "cleanse the hair (on the head)," *mu* has the extended meaning of clearing away plants or debris (*SW*, 11A-2.36b, and Duan Yucai commentary). Since the goal in *MS*III.30 is hair-removal—and given the reference to "plucking" the hair in *MS*III.32—*mu* is best interpreted in its extended meaning.

[6]"Hole" translates *xu* 洫, here referring to the female genitals. *Xu* is glossed in *SW*, 11A-2.17b, as a ditch with specified dimensions; my translation is based on *Guangya*, 9B.14b, which groups *xu* together with words all meaning "hole in the ground." My understanding of the recipe is that removing the hair from her lower body and genitals after childbirth is supposed to keep the woman free of this unwanted hair.

[7]According to Tao Hongjing, old earthworms have white necks (*GM*, 42.40).

[8]Water must be added to the earthworms, spider webs, and bitter gourd at some point before the iron is quenched in the medicine.

*MS*III.32 (C63)

Another. Pluck out (the hair) in the fifth month, and spread formula sweet-liquor on it.[1]

*MS*III.33 (C64)

Ailing from Genital Swelling[2]

Beat *liufu* (willow catkins).[3] Combine with rancid lard and knead until blended. Spread it on the swellings. When finished, wrap with cloth.

*MS*III.34 (CC65-69)

To Facilitate Approaching the Inner (Chamber)[4]

Recipe to facilitate approaching the inner (chamber). Cut up two thirds *dou* of *dianji* (asparagus) root into pieces one *cun* long, and wash well. Also take a whole black rooster, closing the wings to make [3] the heart, brain, and breast of three chickens. Pour two *sheng* of water into an old iron kettle, and boil them together. Cook using firm reeds with close-set joints (as fuel). Let it come to a full boil once, then [3] and discard the dregs.[5] Use the clear liquid to boil the heart, lung, liver, and [1] of a black male dog that is one whole year old or older. Use firm reeds with close-set joints [8] *jue*[6] [4] five substances [2] {1} [6]. Eat it at the late afternoon meal,[7] in whatever amount you wish. [?].

*MS*III.35 (CC70-73)

Another. To approach the inner (chamber) [29] *wuhui* (monkshood)[8] that are large, four [19]. Take two large handfulls of

---

[1]See *MS*III.10 for formula sweet-liquor.

[2]For *zui* 最 (also written 朘) as a term for the male genitals, see *MS*I.E.134. Li and McMahon express the opinion that in *MS*III.33 *zui* denotes the female genitals (1992: 152), but do not offer a supporting argument. Occurrences of *zui* in received literature and in *MS*I.E.134 all indicate that the referent is the male genitals.

[3]I follow Ma Jixing (1992: 688, n. 2) in reading *fu* 付 as *fu* 柎; and identifying it as a term for a catkin. The identification is based on *Shanhaijing*, 2.12b, and Guo Pu commentary.

[4]*Jinnei* 近 内 (approach the inner chamber) as a euphemism for sexual intercourse also occurs in *MS*I.E.18, where intercourse is one of the prohibited activities during treatment for an ailment. It is likely that *nei* has a double reference that includes the female genitals.

[5]I.e. the decocted medicine is strained.

[6]Ma Jixing identifies *jue* 芵 as part of the drug name *beijue/xie* 萆 薢 (1992: 691, n. 17; see *MS*III.50).

[7]*Bu* 餔 refers to a time in the late afternoon between 3:00-5:00 P.M. (see *MS*I.E.67).

[8]In the text there is a twenty-eight graph lacuna in C70 and a one graph lacuna at the top of C71. *MWD*, vol. 4, "Transcription," n. 1, notes that there may be a break in the text between C70 and C71.

fresh steamed *chejian* (plantain).[1] The vapor [12] *chejian* (plantain) [3]. Put it in a cloth sack or (?).[2] When you want to engage in intercourse, then eat [1] it.

*MS*III.36 (CC74-76)

Another. To cultivate the inside.[3] Collect bulging fungi[4] that have just started to bulge forth, and dry them in the dark [without][5] letting them see the daylight. Wait until they are dry. [1] take five *bai* [1],[6] two *mendong*,[7] and one *fuling* (pine truffle). Then pestle them together. Soak in water, using just enough to cover. [1] and press[8] to obtain the liquid. Use it to soak the bulging fungi, again using just enough to cover. Then remove and dry them. Let them become completely dry, then smith. Drink a three-fingered pinch in one half cup of [1].

*MS*III.37 (CC77-80)

[?] Napkin[9]

---

[1]*MWD*, vol. 4, "Transcription," n. 2, equates the drug name *chejian* 車踐 with *cheqian* 車前.

[2]The grammar of the sentence, in which *ruo* 若 means "or," indicates that words naming the alternative to the cloth sack were omitted from the text by the scribe.

[3]*Zhong* 中 (inside) occurs in *MS*III.46, 71, and *MS*IV.23 referring to the inside of the body as a region to be cultivated, not necessarily for the purpose of sexual intercourse.

[4]I follow *MWD*, vol. 4, "Transcription," in reading 囷 as *jun* 菌; and identifying *fenjun* 汾菌 as the name of a type of mushroom (*fen* is well attested in the sense of something that swells and bulges).

[5]Judging from the context the lacuna should be an injunctive negative.

[6]*Bai* 稗 is glossed in *SW*, 7A.44a, as "grain of a different sort" (i.e. a grain-like plant; see Duan Yucai commentary). *Bai* is listed in materia medica (*GM*, 23.80; *ZY*: no. 5199, *Echinochloa crusgalli* [L.] Beauv.). Ma Jixing reads *bai* as *bei* 萆; and identifies *bei* [1] as the drug name *beixie* (1992: 692, n. 5; see *MS*III.50).

[7]*Mendong* 門冬 is the same drug name written *mandong* 滿冬 in *MS*III.52 and *mendong* 虋冬 in *MS*III.70. *Mendong* is the gloss given for *qiangmi* 蘠蘼 in *Erya*, 8.7a; and in *SW*, 1B.29a. According to the Duan Yucai commentary it is not certain whether the gloss refers to *tian mendong* 天虋冬 (i.e. the same drug already identified with the name *dianji*; see *MS*III.2) or to *mai mendong* 麥虋冬. *Mai mendong* is listed in *BC* (*GM*, 16.84; *ZY*: no. 2082, *Ophiopogon japonicus* Ker-Gawl., and plants in the genus *Liriope*). Primarily because of the occurrence of *dianji* in *MS*III, I suspect that *mendong* refers to *mai mendong*.

[8]I read *bi*/**pjiəd* 泌 as a phonetic loan for *bi*/**bljət* 滭, glossed in *Guangya*, 2B.12b, as a synonym for "strain." The Wang Niansun commentary supplies additional glosses indicating that *bi* refers to "pressing" the liquid out of something.

[9]"Napkin" translates *jin* 巾, which according to *SW*, 7B.44b, is a napkin worn at the waist. The Duan Yucai commentary outlines the use of the *jin* to wipe things (its use as a head covering is later). The recipe category concerns cloth saturated with medicine and used to rub the body—in particular the genitals—as a sexual stimulant.

Take a chicken that is just able to produce eggs.[1] Pluck it alive, completely removing the feathers except at the tip of both wings. Tie it so it hangs from a pole, [4] the chicken rub against a large bee hive, and let the bees sting it. When (the bees) are spent, shift the chicken again until it is stung to death.[2] When it dies, remove and discard its [4] its flesh, and smith well. Sift through cloth.[3] When finished, mix it with *yi zao* (jujube) fat,[4] and daub it on a cloth napkin. Then rub the feet with the napkin [3] four or five and then repeat. Stop after using two napkins. [1] the feet have little vapor, this makes a person have an abundance of vapor.[5]

*MS*III.38 (CC81-84)

Another. To prepare napkins. Take one *sheng* of *yangsi*,[6] one *sheng* of red ants, and twenty *banmao* (blister beetles). Soak them together in one half *dou* of fine [1], covering [4] the liquid. Soak one *chi* of finely woven cloth in it. After it has soaked, dry over heat. When dry, soak again. When the liquid is gone, take *gu* (paper mulberry) and *yitong* (paulownia) liquid [5], and daub it on the cloth that was soaked. Dry it, then store well. When engaging in inter-

---

[1]"Produce eggs" represents my interpretation of *juan* 卷. The phonetic *juan* 𢍏 is glossed in *SW*, 3A.37a, as "rolling cooked grain into a ball (*zhuanfan* 摶飯)." The practice of serving oneself by taking a handful of cooked grain from the pot and rolling it into a ball is attested in *Liji*, 2.12a, where it is prohibited. I suspect that in *MS*III.37 the sense of *juan* is extended to a bird laying eggs. It is equally likely that *juan/*kwjian* is a phonetic loan for *wan/*gwan* 丸 (ball), which is attested in the sense of "egg" in *Lüshi chunqiu*, 14.141. The speculation in *MWD*, vol. 4, "Transcription," n. 1, that *juan/*kwjian* is a phonetic loan for *huan/*gwan* 讙 (shout, cry) is phonologically possible, but in my judgment is the less likely alternative.

[2]I.e. set the chicken against another bee hive.

[3]I read 麗 as *shi* 釃, the word for filtering a liquid in *MS*III.74. In *MS*III.37, it is likely that the chicken flesh has been dried or incinerated before being smithed; and then it is sifted through a cloth before being mixed with jujube fat. This is the only reference to sifting a drug powder in the Mawangdui medical manuscripts. *MWD*, vol. 4, "Transcription," n. 2, reads the graph as *shai* 曬 (dry in the sun), which is possible but unlikely in my judgment.

[4]I am uncertain of the meaning of *yi* 邑. The same graph modifies bird eggs in *MS*III.41. *MWD*, vol. 4, "Transcription," n. 3, suggests that *yi/*ʔjəp* may be a phonetic loan for *za/*dzəp* 雜 (mixed, assorted); *ji/*dzjəp* 集 (collected, gathered) is another possibility.

[5]Increasing the vapor in the feet may be related to the idea expressed in *MS*I.C that vapor should flow towards the feet and that the feet should be warm.

[6]From the description at the end of the recipe *yangsi* 楊思 refers to a bug, but the name is not attested in received literature and its identity is not known.

course, rub the jade whip with it, and the horse will then be startled.[1] *Yangsi* [5]. Its shape is like a small [2] and bites[2] people.

*MS*III.39 (CC85-87)

Another. [2] *shechuang* (cnidium), two ninths *dou*; *lin* root,[3] two and a half *dou*; *fanshi*,[4] one three-fingered pinch; one-*chi* long *gui* (cinnamon), five sticks; [5] {3} [2], one small bunch. Use grass-filtered vinegar produced in the third month[5] to [1], and boil until done. Let it come to the boil, and steep[6] the cloth napkin in the [3] liquid. When having intercourse[7] [12] it. It makes the skin taut and not sag. Moreover, it makes the man {1} [?].

*MS*III.40 (C88)

Another. Take two *zaojia* (honey locust fruits).[8] Smith, and pour one third *dou* of water onto it. Stir well, then soak a napkin in it. Leave for one whole day and take it out. [3] dry, immediately soak it again.

---

[1] "Jade whip" translates *yuce* 玉 策, denoting the penis. The tèrm, which is not attested in received literature, occurs four more times in the Mawangdui medical manuscripts: *MS*III.43, *MS*VI.A.2, *MS*VI.A.10, and *MS*VI.B.6. The female counterpart to the jade whip in *MS*III.38 and 43 is *ma* 馬 (horse), denoting the female genitals (the term also occurs in *MS*III.44 where it is paired with *pin* 牝, which denotes the female genitals as well). *Ma* is attested for female genitals in Yuan to Ming drama and fiction; see, for example, the Ming collection *Gujin xiaoshuo*, 3.7b, where sexual intercourse is referred to as *ruma* 入 馬 (entering the horse). The analogy between horseriding and intercourse evident in *MS*III.38 and 43 also occurs, but the word for the whip/penis is *bian* 鞭. The Yuan drama *Shanshenmiao Pei Du huan dai*, 46a, plays on the image of the male horserider holding a silk whip, who after dismounting is promptly seduced—at which point the whip image shifts to the penis: "When (the women) got a glimpse of the First Candidate's whip those in the front of the hall were delighted." Given the horseriding analogy in *MS*III.38 and 43, the Han term *yunü* 御 女 clearly refers to the man "riding the woman/horse" (see *MS*VI.B.1).

[2] *MWD*, vol. 4, "Transcription," transcribes 䖒, read as *he* 齕 (bite, chew). Qiu Xigui suggests the transcription 赦, read as *shi* 螫 (bite, sting; 1992: 534).

[3] Identification of *lin* 藺 is uncertain. *MWD*, vol. 4, "Transcription," n. 1, suggests equating it with *lin* 菻, glossed as a plant related to artemisia in *SW*, 1B.28a.

[4] Identification of *fanshi* 潘 石 is uncertain. The same mineral name is written *fanshi* 蕃 石 in *MS*IV.8, 9, 11, and 12. *MWD*, vol. 4, "Transcription," n. 1, reads *fan* as *fan* 礬, identifying the mineral as alunite (*ZY*: no. 1383; *GM*, 11.68). However, *BL* gives *fanshi* 番 石 as an alternate name for *huashi* 滑 石 (*GM*, 9.77), which is talc (*ZY*: no. 5037).

[5] "Grass-filtered" translates *you* 莤, glossed in *SW*, 14B.40b, as a ritual of preparing liquor for sacrifices by filtering it through *mao* 茅 (woolly grass). *MS*III.39 testifies to the use of this filtering process outside of religion.

[6] I read 曼 as *man* 漫, glossed in *Fangyan*, 13.4a, as "soak until decomposed."

[7] 爲 之 is another expression meaning to have intercourse, similar to 用 之.

[8] *MWD*, vol. 4, "Transcription," n. 1, identifies 萩 莢 as equivalent to *zaojia* 皂 莢 (*qiu*/*tshjəgw* 萩 is a phonetic loan for *zao*/*dzəgw* 皂). The name occurs written 蕉 莢 in *MS*IV.5.

*MS*III.41 (C89)

Another. Dry rat testes in the dark, and smith. Crack open *yi* bird eggs,[1] combine (with the smithed testes), and daub it on a new cloth napkin. When going to bed,[2] wipe the male organ and the female organ with it.[3]

*MS*III.42 (CC90-91)

Another. Take one *dou* of snails and divide into two portions. Soak one portion in vinegar and dry in the sun. During the winter set it on the stove until it bubbles very rapidly, then remove the snails. [4] the remainder as before. Then soak a napkin in it until the liquid is gone. When finished, use a soaked napkin when going to bed to wipe the male organ. It also makes the female organ [?].[4]

*MS*III.43 (CC92-95)

Another. Four *dou* of snails; four *dou* of fine fermented milk; one fourth *sheng* of *tianmu*;[5] *taoke* (peach fuzz)[6] the size of a *zao* (jujube); twice seven *mulou* heads;[7] [9], one half *sheng*. Soak together in the fermented milk. When finished, take the liquid and use it to [3] cloth [2] soak, stopping when the liquid is gone. [1] engaging in intercourse, dampen [2] and rub the jade whip, and the horse will then become unrestrained. The substance called *tianmu* is [3] and eats *tao* (peach) and *li* (plum) flowers. *Taoke* is the fuzz from peach fruits when they are small. As for *mulou*, *jiequan* [12] {2} [2] is the shape of the skin of a *gan* (Job's tears fruit).[8]

---

[1]See *MS*III.37 for a possible interpretation of *yi*.

[2]I.e. having sexual intercourse.

[3]The genitals are referred to as *nan* 男 and *nü* 女 respectively.

[4]The genitals are referred to as *nan* 男 and *pin* 牝 respectively.

[5]Identification of *tianmu* 天牡 is uncertain. *MWD*, vol. 4, "Transcription," n. 2, proposes reading *mu* 牡 as a scribal error for *she* 社 and identifying the drug as the insect *tianshe chong* 天社蟲, listed in *GM*, 41.14 (a kind of beetle).

[6]Identification of *taoke* 桃可 is based on the description at the end of the recipe. *Taomao* 桃毛 is the name for peach fuzz in *GM*, 29.48, and is the name used in *MS*IV.3.

[7]Identification of *mulou* 牡螻 is uncertain. *MWD*, vol. 4, "Transcription," n. 4, associates the name with *bai mugou* 白牡狗 in *MS*V.6; and cites *Fangyan*, 11.2a, where *dugou* 杜狗 is given as a Southern Chu name for *lougu* 螻蛄. *Lougu* is the molecricket (*ZY*: no. 5477, *Gryllotalpa africana* Pal. de Beauvois; *GM*, 41.15). The identification is plausible, but at the end of the recipe the unidentified bug name *jiequan* 頡蠸 occurs in a context where it might form part of a definition of *mulou*, which in turn casts doubt on the identification with *lougu*.

[8]I follow *MWD*, vol. 4, "Transcription," n. 5, in reading 贛 as *gan* 藾, an alternate name for *yiyi* 薏苡 (*ZY*: no. 5548, *Coix lachryma-jobi* L.; *GM*, 23.83). The reference to the

*MS*III.44 (CC96-97)

Another. Incinerate [1] *fu*. Spread out a napkin in the [11] {1} [5]. Rub[1] the female organ with the napkin, and the horse just then [?].[2]

*MS*III.45 (CC98-101)

[To Lighten the Body and Increase Strength][3]

Another. If you wish to lighten the body, take {2} [24] {1} [1]. Use after the meal. In spring and autumn [29] them, four *dou* each, {1} [3] {1} [?].

*MS*III.46 (C102)

To Purge the Inside and Increase Vapor[4]

[2] *zi* meat[5] that is fat [3] lard. Dry them all in the dark and smith. Use one three-fingered pinch [?].

*MS*III.47 (CC103-104) Another. [1] {2}. The medicine uses bird [3], *zixie* (water plantain), *sui*,[6] *suanzao* (sour jujube), [12] in equal amounts, and smith. Then blend with *songzhi* (pine rosin) and make balls. Use after the meal, the amount as you [?].

"skin" must be to the outer covering of the fruit; thus it is the fruit that is denoted by *gan* in *MS*III.43.

[1] 玩 in *MWD*, vol. 4, "Transcription," should be transcribed as *wan* 抏. The graph is attested in the meaning "rub" in *Shiji*, 105.3b (the graph is erroneously written 抗 in the *Shiji* edition cited).

[2] *MWD*, vol. 4, "Transcription," n. 1, notes that there is a break in the text between C97 and C98; it is not clear how many columns might be missing.

[3] All other recipes in this cateogry are lost in the preceding break in the text. I add the category name from the list in *MS*III.92 for reference purposes only.

[4] *MWD*, vol. 4, "Transcription," provisionally adds the name of this recipe category from the list in *MS*III.92 to the beginning of *MS*III.46. The recipes seem to be primarily concerned with tonics for bolstering physical vitality, but several are sexual (*MS*III.51, 58).

[5] *MWD*, vol. 4, "Transcription," n. 2, suggests reading *zi* 兹 as *zi* 牸, listed in *Guangya*, 10B.37b, as one of the words for the female of animals. The "Transcription" note argues that the word denotes a female cow in *MS*III.46, but both the reading of the graph in the text and the interpretation are uncertain.

[6] *MWD*, vol. 4, "Transcription," n. 1, argues that *sui/*sdjəd* 蓫 represents the same plant name as *shu/*djət* 述 in *MS*III.52; and that both should be understood as *zhu/*djət* 术 (atractylodes). The argument is plausible but uncertain.

*MS*III.48 (CC105-106)

Another. In spring and fall collect *yuan*.[1] Dry it in the dark and smith. Take winter *kui* (mallow) seeds and smith. Combine them. Use a three-fingered pinch [12] increases the inside.

*MS*III.49 (C107)

Another. [2], *fangfeng* (saposhnikovia), and [1]—all three in equal amounts. Use *jie*[2] in an amount that matches the three substances. Smith. Use a three-fingered pinch after the meal [?].

*MS*III.50 (CC108-109)

Another. Slice beef thinly. Then take a one *cun* piece of *beixie* (yam)[3] and set [2] in the beef. Cook until it bubbles, stop, cook again until it bubbles, and stop again. After the third time remove the meat and eat it. Store the liquid and *beixie* (yam) to reuse for boiling meat, discarding them after the third use. [2] the person's ring becomes increasingly strong[4] and it does not harm a person. You may eat whatever amount of meat you wish.

*MS*III.51 (C110)

Another. Take *baiyuan* (daphne) root. Dry in the dark and smith. Blend with horse sauce. [1] balls, the size of a finger-tip. [6] hole. It swells and becomes large.[5]

*MS*III.52 (C111)

Another. *Mandong*,[6] *shu*,[7] and *fangfeng* (saposhnikovia): smith separately in equal amounts. Combine them [?].

---

[1]*MWD*, vol. 4, "Transcription," n. 1, reads *yuan* 宛 as *wan* 菀 and identifies the plant as *ziwan* 紫菀 (*ZY*: no. 4866, *Aster tataricus* L. f.; *GM*, 16.82). However, *SW*, 1B.19b, glosses *yuan* 蒬 as *jiyuan* 棘蒬, which is equivalent to *jiwan* 棘菀 (*ZY*: no. 2087, *Polygala tenuifolia* Willd.; *GM*, 12B.15). Materia medica assigns tonic properties to both drugs; which one is the referent of *yuan* in *MS*III.48 is uncertain.

[2]*MWD*, vol. 4, "Transcription," n. 1, suggests reading *jie* 界 as *jie* 芥 (*ZY*:no. 2173, *Brassica juncea* [L.] Czern. et Coss.; *GM*, 26.62). The identification is plausible.

[3]I follow *MWD*, vol. 4, "Transcription," n. 1, in reading 萆芙 as equivalent to *beixie* 萆薢 in *MS*III.70. The drug is listed in *GM*, 18.44 (*ZY*: no. 4120, *Dioscorea hypoglauca* Palib., and other spp.). The name is written 萆薁 in *MS*III.60.

[4]"Ring" translates *huan* 環, which I believe is an idiomatic term for the waist region in the Mawangdui medical manuscripts (see *MS*I.C). It is also possible that in *MS*III.50 *huan* means "all around" (i.e. the whole body).

[5]The end of the recipe suggests that the medicine is used to stimulate the penis. Perhaps the hole is the navel (see *MS*IV.5).

[6]See *MS*III.36.

[7]See *MS*III.47.

*MS*III.53 (C112)

Another. Take two portions of *jungui* (curled cinnamon), four of *xixin* (asarum), one of *qiu* (wormwood),[1] one of oyster, and two of Qin *jiao* (Qin zanthoxylum). Use a three-fingered pinch after the meal. It makes a person strong.[2]

*MS*III.54 (CC113-14)

Another. Grind *ru*[3] while wet and put it in a container. Eat and drink liquor until full, [2], and sniff it. [2]; smith well, separately, and combine both. Three-night-old rooster blood [6].[4] Pack it in silk. {3} [1] {2} [1] {1} [1] {1} [3] {1}. One section of bamboo with widely spaced joints and a diameter of three *cun* [?].

*MS*III.55 (C115)

Another. In autumn collect [*ban*]*mao* (blister beetle)[5] [2] head [5] three [3] it. You become strong.

[1][6]

*MS*III.56 (C116)

Another. Take [16] strong.

*MS*III.57 (C117)

Another. [2] liquid and set it in a bamboo tube. Virile-bird [9][7] put it in water, and drink it.

*MS*III.58 (CC118-19)

Another. Use pig lard the size of a hand. Have bees [17] four *dou* of pure liquor lees. Smith well [1]. When you do not want it, wash it off.[8]

---

[1]See *MS*I.E.147.

[2]Being strong might refer to penile erection in addition to physical strength (see *MS*III.20).

[3]*MWD*, vol. 4, "Transcription," reads *ru* 如 as *ru* 茹, which n. 1 identifies as *rucao* 茹草 (*GM*, 13.43; *ZY*: no. 3763, *Bupleurum chinense* DC. and other spp.). However, *ru* occurs in other plant names; e.g. *rugen* 茹根, which is the name for the root of *baimao* 白茅 (*GM*, 13.64; *ZY*: no. 1435, *Imperata cylindrica* [L.] P. Beauv. var. *major* [Nees] C.E. Hubb.).

[4]The two-graph lacuna must name two drugs, which are mixed with rooster blood. It is not clear how this preparation relates to the *ru* above or to the end of the recipe.

[5]I fill the lacuna with *ban* 盤 based on the context (see *MS*III.38).

[6] 盾 is written in large script beneath the text in C115 (compare *MS*III.12 and 21). Perhaps the graph is a variant of *dun* 盾, but this seems unlikely.

[7] *MS*III.16 calls for "virile-bird egg liquid," possibly dickeybird eggs.

[8]The instruction to wash the medicine off suggests that the recipe concerns stimulation of the penis (see *MS*IV.3).

*MS*III.59 (C120)

Another. [5] in equal amounts. Also take [2], and use after the meal.

*MS*III.60 (CC121-23)

Another. [3] large male rabbit. Skin and remove the intestines. Take four-*cun* long *beixie* (yam), one handful; *zhu* (atractylodes), one handful; and *wuhui* (monkshood), ten [3] pare the skin and chop finely. Add the large male rabbit meat to the medicine, mix completely, and dry without letting it see the sun. After one hundred days wrap in [1]. Use one three-fingered pinch after the meal for one hundred days. It keeps for six or seven years. [1] eating it is allowed. Use as you wish.

*MS*III.61 (CC124-25)

Another. Take *xixin* (asarum); dried *jiang* (ginger); *jungui* (curled cinnamon); and *wuhui* (monkshood)—altogether four substances. Smith separately. Take four parts of *xixin* (asarum) to two each of dried *jiang* (ginger), *jungui* (curled cinnamon), and *wuhui* (monkshood). Combine them. Use a three-fingered pinch after the meal. It increases the vapor, and also makes a person's face lustrous.

*MS*III.62 (CC126-30)

Another. Take two *liang* each of *baifu*, *hongfu*,[1] and *fuling* (pine truffle); ten nodules of *jiang* (ginger); and three *chi* of *gui* (cinnamon). Smith each separately. Blend them with two *dou* of fine gruel vinegar. Then take butchered horse loin, ten [1]. Prepare fine dried-meat slices with it, making them the thickness of three fingers. Then soak in gruel vinegar, stirring over and over again. Then drain. After draining, dry in the dark over heat. [4] bubble. Once again soak and dry over heat as before, stopping[2] when the liquid is gone. Dry over heat [1] jerky.[3] Then pound with a mallet until thin

[1]*Baifu* 白符 and *hongfu* 紅符 represent the white and red varieties of the *wuse fu* 五色符 (*fu* of the five colors). Wu Pu 吳普 (d. 250 A.D.) equates *wuse fu* with *wuse shizhi* 五色石脂, which is a name for five varieties of clay classified by color (*GM*, 9.80). However, Tao Hongjing lists *wuse fu* in a separate entry under mineral drugs, noting that the substance was no longer used and that no one in his time had knowledge of it (see *Bencaojing jizhu*, 2.33). Since *MS*IV.2 calls for [1] *shizhi* ([1] clay), it is possible that *fu* in *MS*III.62 represents a different, unidentified mineral.

[2]止 in *MWD*, vol. 4, "Transcription," should be transcribed as *yi* 已.

[3]"Jerky" translates *xiu* 脩, glossed in *SW*, 4B.33a with *fu* 脯 (dried-meat slice). According to the Duan Yucai commentary, *fu* is the basic term for a slice of dried meat while *xiu* refers to meat strips that are beaten and coated with ginger and cinnamon.

and lustrous, and again dry over heat [3] them, until [1] lustrous. [13] lacquer it with *qi* (lacquer). When dry, then store them well. Eat three *cun* at each of the dawn, daytime [1], and evening meals, always before the meal [15] smith separately in equal amounts. Use after the meal.[1]

*MS*III.63 (CC131-32)

Scantness When Engaging in Intercourse[2]

If a man experiences scantness when engaging in intercourse and (semen) is clear, [16] male bird. Blend with the blood of the two to make balls the size of a *suanzao* (sour jujube).[3] Use after the meal. {2}, then [?].

*MS*III.64 (CC133-34)

[7] *dou* [15]. Use [1] *hua*, one half *dou*, *mula* [9] *sheng* [?].[4]

*MS*III.65 (CC135-36)

To Cultivate Strength[5]

[30] the body seems to itch but does not itch,[6] {1} [?].

*MS*III.66 (CC137-40)

To blacken the hair and increase the vapor, take [25] {7} [23] {1}, without letting the fire go out. Thirty [2] smith. Use [2] to wrap. [18]. Prepare the medicine in the eighth month.

---

[1]The lacuna evidently contains a second medicine that is eaten after the meal (the dried meat is eaten before the meal).

[2]The heading *yongshao* 用少 is elliptical. *MWD*, vol. 4, "Transcription," n. 1, explains the sense by comparison with a passage in *Qianjin yaofang*, 60.18b, listing the "seven injuries" associated with intercourse, among which the second is "essence/semen (*jing* 精) is clear" (see the first line of the recipe below) and the third is "essence/semen is scant." The list of the seven injuries in a parallel account in *Waitai biyaofang*, 17.3a, is different, but still gives "essence/semen is clear" and "essence/semen is scant" as the third and fourth injuries.

[3]The drugs used to make the medicine are lost in the lacuna. The reference to *xiong* 雄 (male bird) and to blending the drugs with the "blood of the two" suggests that the blood of two birds is used.

[4]The occurrence of the volumetric measure *sheng* as the final extant graph in *MS*III.64 suggests that the listing of drugs and amounts continues at least to this point. *MWD*, vol. 4, "Transcription," n. 1, notes that there is a break in the text between C134 and C135; it is not clear how many columns might be missing.

[5]*MWD*, vol. 4, "Transcription," provisionally adds the heading for this recipe category from the list in *MS*III.92. The next few category names are missing both in the main body of the text and in *MS*III.92, until *MS*III.72 which can be restored based on *MS*III.92. The "Transcription" provisionally marks lacunae for the missing headings, which I omit.

[6]I.e. there should be a stimulating sensation of itching. The same phrase occurs again in *MS*III.68.

*MS*III.67 (CC141-43)

To prepare sweet-liquor.[1] Use one and a third *jin* of *shigao* (gypsum); *gaoben* (lovage), *niuxi* (achyranthes), [21] two *dou*. {1} [1] the liquid. {1} [?].

*MS*III.68 (CC144-45)

To increase strength and thoroughly purge foul vapor from the [1], heart, and chest. Take the fruits inside *huai* (pagoda tree) pods. Set on the stove [13] five fruits. The itching is intense. [1] it and there is no itching, increase it until the body seems to itch but does not itch. [13].

*MS*III.69 (CC146-47)[2]

[1] valley, are the places named Great Chamber and Lesser Chamber.[3] There are stones there named *pianshi*.[4] Take small ones [13] illness and increases longevity.

*MS*III.70 (CC148-51)

Take a butchered horse, dress it, and prepare dried-meat slices. Pound one *sheng* of *wuhui* (monkshood)[5] and soak it in pure liquor. [1] discard the dregs.[6] [10] *yu*, *mendong*,[7] each [2]; *beixie* (yam) and *niuxi* (achyranthes), five small bunches of each; [1] *jia*, *jiegeng* (balloon flower), and *hou* [1], two *chi*; and *wuhui* (monkshood), ten nodules. Combine and smith. Soak in four *dou* of pure liquor. Do not discard the dregs. Use [2] {2}. [3] wrap in a leather sack. Eat a three-fingered pinch after the meal. Ingesting it makes the six extremities[8] strong and increases longevity.

---

[1]See *MS*III.4.

[2]*MWD*, vol. 4, "Transcription," treats CC144-47 as one entry. I follow Ma Jixing in making CC146-47 a separate recipe (1992: 721).

[3]Great Chamber 泰室 and Lesser Chamber 少室 designate the site of Song Mountain 嵩山 in present-day Henan, which is the central peak in the system of the five sacred peaks. See *Huainanzi*, 4.64.

[4]The term *pianshi* 駢石 is attested in *Guanzi* 58, 19.312, where it refers to stones that are joined to form a solid layer. Perhaps in *MS*III.69 *pianshi* refers to some kind of conglomerate, or perhaps it is a technical term whose meaning is unknown. In any case, the recipe calls for stones that come from Song Mountain.

[5]"Pound" translates *tuan* 段. Ma Jixing argues that *duan* could also be read as *duan* 煅, and understood as a heating process used to cook the monkshood (1992: 722, n. 2). The argument for cooked monkshood is more plausible in *MS*III.72, where the word is *xun* 熏.

[6]The recipe probably states that the dregs should not be discarded.

[7]See *MS*III.36.

[8]*Simo* 四末 (four extremities) is a standard term for the arms and legs; *liumo* 六末 is not attested in received literature. *MWD*, vol. 4, "Transcription," n. 3, identifies the additional two extremities as the genital and anal regions.

*MS*III.71 (CC152-53)

Smith *yunmu* (mica)[1] and melt *songzhi* (pine rosin) in equal amounts. Combine with whole-wheat flakes[2] to make balls, without [1] the hands, making them the size of a *suanzao* (sour jujube). [1] it. Swallow[3] one ball. Daily increase by one ball until the tenth day. The day after, daily eliminate one ball until the tenth day. The day [6] increase and decrease [5]. It makes a person longlived and not become aged.

*MS*III.72 (CC154-58)

Mash-liquor to Benefit the Inside[4]

Take *qi* and [1] stalks[5] in equal amounts and [13] four and a half *dou* of the clear liquid [3] {5} [17] and ferment it. Take blackened *wuhui* (monkshood), eight nodules;[6] [1] take *qi* and *jie*[7] [16] beneath the fermented (grain).[8] Seal the mouth of the jar well, so that [25] it is done {3} [26].

*MS*III.73 (CC159-61)

Another. [1], nine *dou*. First [26], two *sheng*, in it for ten days. Smith [10] remove from the vessel [9] {1}. When ingested for one hundred days, it makes the intestines be without ailments.

---

[1] *MS*III.71 provides the earliest documentation of mica ingestion in Chinese macrobiotic dietetics. See Kaltenmark 1953: 59, for mica in *xian*-cult dietetics; and Schafer 1955: 282, for discussion of the earliest references in the received literature.

[2] "Whole-wheat flakes" translates *maizhi* 麥 麱. *Zhi* refers to coarsely milled whole grains of wheat, including the bran (*SW*, 5B.34a, and Duan Yucai commentary).

[3] 各 in *MWD*, vol. 4, "Transcription," should be transcribed as *tun* 吞.

[4] See *MS*III.10 for an earlier recipe for *lao* 醪. Of the three recipes in this category, only *MS*III.74 is well enough preserved to provide a fair description of the method of production.

[5] Based on *MS*III.74, the lacuna might be *jie* 節. See below for the possible identity of *qi* 漆 and *jie*.

[6] "Blackened" translates *xun* 熏. *Xun* usually means "fumigate," but is attested in the sense of "sear, roast" (*Shijing*, Mao 258, 18B.11a, and Mao commentary). In *MS*III.72 *xun* refers to preparatory cooking of the monkshood.

[7] In *MS*III.74, *MWD*, vol. 4, "Transcription," n. 1, suggests identifying *qi* 漆 as *zeqi* 澤 漆; and *jie* 節 as *dijie* 地 節. For *zeqi*, see *GM*, 17.15 (*ZY*: no. 3047, *Euphorbia helioscopia* L.). *Dijie* is probably the plant listed in *GM*, 12.105 (*ZY*: no. 1156, *Polygonatum odoratum* [Mill.] Druce var. *pluriflorum* [Miq.] Ohwi.). However, it may also refer to the plant listed in *GM*, 36.107 (*ZY*: no. 1640, *Lycium chinense* Mill.).

[8] In *MS*III.74 the herbal ingredients are set in the fermentation jar first and the fermented grain is placed on top. *MS*III.72 probably describes a similar procedure.

*MS*III.74 (CC162-68)

Another. To prepare mash-liquor. Finely chop *qi* and *jie*, one *dou* of each. Use water, five [4] sieve. Use the liquid to boil *ziwei* (trumpet-flower) [8] sieve again. Yeast and wheat yeast, one *dou* of each, [3]. Leave for one whole day, then sieve.[1] [4] glutinous panicled millet, rice [3], one *dou* of each. Combine [1], and rinse it with the yeast liquid, like the usual method for cooking grain.[2] Take *wuhui* (monkshood), three nodules; dried *jiang* (ginger), five; and *jiao* [2]—altogether three substances. Chew[3] [2] and toss them in. First put the [1] in the jar, and then the fermented glutinous millet on top of that. [1] liquid and pour over it evenly; then pour ten *dou* of fine liquor over it. Do not stir, [3] daub it with mud.[4] In eleven [1] it will be done. Then open and do not filter. Gradually [2] the clear liquid is gone. Once again use [2] liquor to pour over it. Do it like this thrice, and [2].[5] Drink one cup at the late afternoon meal. After drinking, rub any places on the body that itch. When ingested for one hundred days, it makes the eyes bright and ears perceptive; the extremities all become strong; and [2] ailments and withering on one side.[6]

*MS*III.75 (CC169-70)

Cultivation

Soak four *dou* of snails in vinegar for two days. Remove the snails and use the liquid to soak [1] meat that has been pounded.[7] [1] dog dried-meat slices [2], and soak again in the liquid [2]. Eat one *cun* of

---

[1]This appears to represent the first stage of production. A decoction of *qi* and *jie* is used to cook trumpet-flower, and two kinds of yeast are left to ferment in the second decoction for twenty-four hours.

[2]In the second stage millet and rice are prepared using the fermented yeast brew. Combining cooked grain with a partially fermented brew is characteristic of mash-liquor (see *MS*III.10).

[3]I follow Ma Jixing in reading 甫 as *fu* 哎 (1992: 729, n. 13). The compound *fuju* 哎 咀 (chew) occurs in *MS*IV.3.

[4]In the third stage a layer of chewed herbs is placed in the fermenting jar first, followed by the grain and the liquid in which it was fermenting, and finally by a quantity of liquor. At this point the fermentation jar is sealed.

[5]Evidently the fermentation jar is opened and the liquid allowed to drain naturally without filtration. Then more liquor is poured into the jar and the process of sealing and fermenting is repeated a second time. After the third time the mash-liquor is ready to drink.

[6]For *pianku* 偏 枯 (withering on one side), see *MS*I.B.8.

[7]The meat is probably dog meat, which is then used to prepare the dried-meat slices mentioned below.

the dried-meat slices to overcome one person, and ten *cun* to overcome ten people.[1]

*MS*III.76 (C171)

To Snap Horns[2]

Incinerate *chou*[3] and smith. Wrap the ash to [1] a bull, and it can snort [flagons][4] and snap horns. Increases strength.

*MS*III.77 (CC172-74)

Striding[5]

Feilian,[6] *fangkui*,[7] *shiwei* (pyrrosia), *jiegeng* (balloon flower), and *ziwei* (trumpet-flower), one small bunch each; *wuhui* (monkshood), three nodules; [9] large [3] bamboo skin, five *cun*; *bai tengshe* or *zang gengshe* that is three to four *cun* long,[8] or [8]. Smith separately, and combine with [1] or *zao* (jujube) fat to make balls the size of sheep

---

[1]See *MS*III.11 on the connection between dosage and the number of people whom the user can successfully encounter.

[2]Evidently a reference to fighting bulls, since the recipe indicates that the medicine is used on a bull. For animal combat and man-animal combat in early China, see Hayashi 1976: 411-12; and Lewis 1990: 157-60. The end of the recipe indicates that the medicine can also be used by humans.

[3]The insect *chou* 蝪 is unknown.

[4]Qiu Xigui suggests that the fragmentary graph marked as a lacuna in *MWD*, vol. 4, "Transcription," may be *hu* 壺 (flagon; 1992: 534). My translation is based on the guess that a raging bull "snorting flagons" is intended to suggest its brute energy.

[5]The recipe category is principally concerned with speeding travel by foot. *MS*III.77-80 all include monkshood in the medicine, which is the drug mentioned in *Wanwu*: "Ingested for one hundred days *wuhui* improves a person's ability to run" (Fuyang Han jian zhenglizu 1988: 38). According to *Huainan wanbishu*, 1.7b, one ball of medicine containing monkshood and crane embryo enables a person to travel one thousand *li* in one day. *MS*III.83-84 concern magic to secure a campsite at night.

[6]*MWD*, vol. 4, "Transcription," n. 2, reads *feilian* 非廉 as *feilian* 蜚蠊 (*GM*, 41.22; *ZY*: no. 5625, *Blatta orientalis* L.; flying cockroach). It is equally likely that the name refers to *feilian* 飛廉 (*GM*, 15.39; *ZY*: no. 0567, *Carduus crispus* L.; thistle).

[7]*Fangkui* 防葵 is listed in *GM*, 17.10 (not identified in *ZY*).

[8]*Bai tengshe* 白縢蛇 is unknown, but may be a southern dialect name. Most early glosses of *tengshe* identify it as a fantastic, flying dragon-like serpent. However, the Guo Pu commentary in *Erya*, 9.13a, seems to indicate that in Huainan dialect *tengshe* referred to *mangshe* 莽蛇 (python; my uncertainty is due to the possibility that *mang* is a textual error for *ben* 奔). *Huainan wanbishu*, 1.7b, lends support to the identification by recommending that *tengshe* bile be added to the monkshood and crane medicine for rapid travel (python bile is highly tauted in materia medica; *GM*, 43.68). *Zang gengshe* 蒼梗蛇 is unknown. Perhaps both names refer to snakes, although the short length (three to four *cun*) suggests something besides a snake.

feces. Eat once every fifty *li*. Dark fungus comes from Luo [8].[1] Seven hundred.[2]

*MS*III.78 (CC175-77)

Another. *Wuhui* (monkshood), five parts; *longkai*,[3] three parts; *shiwei* (pyrrosia), *fangfeng* (saposhnikovia), and *futu*,[4] each [1]. Dry in the dark [8] remove the {1} [2] smith the five substances. Put into liquor for one day and one night. Sieve and discard the dregs. Use the liquid to soak saturated cooked-grain for the time it takes to eat.[5] [2] dry. When dry, once again [2] dry. When the liquid is used up, it is finished.

*MS*III.79 (CC178-81)

Another. *Wuhui* (monkshood), two parts; north-south facing Yang [1] *gu*, one part. Smith. Combine and wrap in three layers of finely-woven new white cloth. Horse lard [4] {1} fat chicken [4]. Then boil roof-tile lichen[6] that is the length of the middle finger. Put [4] liquid. Remove the lichen and put it in a sack. [4] days discard and bury [2] dregs. When traveling, soak it, scoop[7] one cup of east-flowing water, put [14] {3} [3] see the sun, drink it.[8]

*MS*III.80 (CC182-84)

Another. [2] dog {2} [?] *wuhui* (monkshood), one half. Smith them. [?] {1} [?].

---

[1]The fungus must have been mentioned in one of the lacunae above. Luo 雒 probably refers to the region of the Luo River 洛水 in present-day Henan.

[2]Presumably the number of *li* that the medicine balls enable a person to travel in one day.

[3]The identity of *longkai* 龍慨 is uncertain. *MWD*, vol. 4, "Transcription," n. 1, suggests equating the name with *longkui* 龍葵 (*GM*, 16.95; *ZY*: no. 1286, *Solanum nigrum* L.). But the name is not attested in materia medica before the Tang.

[4]*Futu* 伏兔 is probably another name for *fuling* 茯苓 (pine truffle) as indicated in *GM*, 37.2. However, *futu* is also an alternate name for *feilian* (thistle; see *MS*III.77).

[5]"Saturated cooked-grain" translates *xiufan* 餷飯. The compound is written 脩飯 in *SW*, 5B.6b, where it occurs as the gloss for *fen* 饙. *Fen* is a thick porridge made by saturating cooked-grain with additional liquid. In *MS*III.78 the grain is saturated with the medicinal liquid, allowed to dry, and then saturated again until there is no more liquid.

[6]I follow *MWD*, vol. 4, "Transcription," n. 1, in reading *chi/*khrjəg* 茝 as a phonetic loan for *tai/*hrəg* 苔. *Tai* is a general term for various mosses and lichens, and several algae (*GM*, 21.17; roof-tile lichen is described in *GM*, 21.21).

[7]揃 is not attested in received literature; the graph is used to write *jian* 菅 (small bunch) in *MS*III.39. The translation "scoop" is a guess based on the idea of using the hand to gather a bunch of something, or in this case to scoop water.

[8]Perhaps the medicine is drunk at sunrise before setting off on the day's journey.

*MS*III.81 (CC185-86)

Another. For striding, take a woman's [28][1] {1} one *dou*. Take [?].

*MS*III.82 (CC187-88)

Another. [2] {1} [20]. Soak it during the night and dry it during the day. Having used up [3] travel one hundred *li*.

*MS*III.83 (CC189-90)

Another. When traveling and stopping overnight, call out to yourself: "The Yang side of Tai Mountain. Heaven [5] first [1]. Walls and ramparts that are not intact, [seal] with the metal bar."[2] Then perform the Pace of Yu thrice and say: "With a stick of fresh *jing* (vitex) two *cun* long I draw a circle around the inside."[3]

*MS*III.84 (C191)

Face east and shout: "I dare to declare to the East Lord and Bright Star.[4] The person who [1] comes and dares to reach the encircled place, and who beds down on those broken tiles—who is he?" Then return inside the circle.

---

[1]The missing drug at the beginning of the lacuna is probably a menstrual cloth.

[2]A similar incantation is recorded in *Baopuzi*, 17.89, where it also forms part of a magical ritual to secure a campsite for the night: "The Yin side of Heng Mountain. The Yang side of Tai Mountain. Let robbers and plunderers not arise. Let tigers and wolves not move. Walls and ramparts that are not intact, seal with the metal bar." The incantation in *MS*III.83 is clearly the antecedent to the *Baopuzi* incantation; and the latter incantation can be used to fill the final lacuna with *bi* 閉 (seal). For Tai Mountain, see *MS*I.E.229. The rhyming words in the incantation are: *wan/*gwan* 完 (intact) and *guan/*kwran* 關 (bar).

[3]The person states aloud that he is creating a magic circle as he draws the circle on the ground. In the *Baopuzi* the person draws a square on the ground with a knife, and after the incantation is finished the knife is laid on the square at the astrological position of the White Tiger 白虎.

[4]East Lord 東君 is a solar deity in the seventh of the "Jiuge" 九歌 in *Chuci*, 2.16a. However, I suspect that East Lord and Bright Star 東君明星 is a name for Taiyi 太一, who is called the Shining One of the East and Grand Monad 東皇太一 in the first of the "Jiu ge" in *Chuci*, 2.2a. In heaven, Taiyi is a polar star whose nature is revealed astrologically in the movement of the Big Dipper. Recent archaeological evidence indicates the existence of a Taiyi cult in the Chu region in the third to second centuries B.C., most strikingly the Mawangdui painting of Taiyi flanked by the Rain Master 雨師 and the Thunder Sire 雷公 (Li Ling 1991; the best photographic reproduction of the painting is Fu and Chen 1992: 35). Inscriptions on the Mawangdui painting are related to military astrology, which represents a significant aspect of the Taiyi cult. Among powerful spirits to whom a person might announce the securing of a campsite, Taiyi would be a logical choice.

*MS*III.85 (CC192–93)

Another. If while striding you are in a hurry and wish to stay ahead, take the cloth of a woman who has never been with a man.[1] Tie with hemp and keep it by your breast. When you see a whirling wind, throw (the cloth) at it. When the wind stops, [2] and attach it to your waist.

*MS*III.86 (C194)

To Travel Quickly[2]

Take the hemp thill-rope from an ox-cart and attach it to your waist. If you wish to hurry, bind it once around.[3]

*MS*III.87 (CC195–96)

Another. If while traveling you wish to have your feet not hurt, face south, perform the Pace of Yu thrice, and say: "Whatever the water, no disaster; whatever the way, no withering. Give[4] me [2]." When finished, take chimney soot [5] and insert it inside the shoe.

*MS*III.88 (CC197–204)[5]

[4] Under-heaven [10] {1}. Possessing vapor you live; lacking[6] vapor you die. This [6]. When it is angered yet not large, skin has not arrived;[7] when large yet not firm, muscle has not arrived; when firm yet not hot, vapor has not arrived. If you engage in intercourse when skin has not arrived, it droops. If you engage in intercourse when muscle has not arrived, it retreats. If you engage in intercourse when vapor has not arrived, it collapses. Therefore, the sage must [2] it.

Tang journeyed to the Blue-gem Terrace.[8] Chen [2] at the South Palace,[9] and (Tang) asked: "When man and woman achieve unison

---

[1] I.e. the menstrual cloth of a virgin.

[2] *Wanwu* uses the same term when it states that using spiders enables a person to "travel quickly" (*jixing* 疾行; Fuyang Han jian zhenglizu 1988: 37).

[3] I.e. tie a loop of rope all the way around the waist.

[4] *Xi* 氣 means "give provisions"; the graph was subsequently used to write *qi* "vapor" (*SW*, 7A.63b, and Duan Yucai commentary).

[5] *MS*III.88 represents the third from last category in the *MS*III.92 list. The entry is a pastiche of information on sexual cultivation. In every instance there is a fuller account in *MS*VI.B or *MS*VII.B.

[6] 無 in *MWD*, vol. 4, "Transcription," should be transcribed as 无.

[7] The "it" with which the remainder of the paragraph is concerned is the penis. The closest parallel to this passage on the arousal of the penis is *MS*VII.B.2; there is a partial parallel in *MS*VII.B.18.

[8] *Yao* 搖 (move) should definitely be read as *yao* 瑤 (blue-gem) in *MS*VI.A.4. However, the original graph may be intended in *MS*III.88, giving the translation Moving Terrace. The

and are a matched pair, how can it be accomplished without injuring the body?"[1] (Chen) replied: "What assists life is eating; what diminishes life is lust. Therefore, the sage must have a model.[2] The first is 'river deer [butting]';[3] the second is 'gibbon grabbing': the third is 'cicada clinging'; the fourth is 'toad'; the fifth is 'fish gobbling'; the sixth is '[dragonfly].' The first is 'cloud stone';[4] the second is 'dry gourd';[5] the third is 'glistening plug';[6] the fourth is 'crouching [1]';[7] the fifth is '[2].' The first is 'go up';[8] the second is 'go down'; the third is 'go to the left'; the fourth is 'go to the right'; the fifth is 'enter deeply'; the sixth is 'enter shallowly'; the seventh is

---

name occurs as Blue-gem Terrace in *Huainanzi*, 8.118, explained in the Gao You commentary as a structure decorated with blue-gem. It is one of several royal structures associated in received literature with the legendary degenerate rulers Jie 桀 of the Xia and Zhou 紂 of the Shang (rather than with Tang 湯, the Shang founder). The Gao You commentary additionally gives *yao* 搖 (move) as a textual variant of *yao* 瑤 (blue-gem), along with the alternative explanation of the structure as a marvel of mechanical engineering. Similarly, the chamber mentioned in *MS*III.89 occurs in received literature in forms that mean either a chamber of precious stone or a revolving chamber. Whether constructed of precious materials or engineered to move in harmony with the cosmos, these structures symbolized the ideal site for a ruler—conceptually identical to the Bright Hall 明堂 (Rickett 1985: 149). While received literature treats the Blue-gem Terrace as an example of royal excess, *MS*III.88 presents it as the natural site for a ruler.

[9]Chen 陳 is probably the surname of a master of sexual cultivation. In the exchange that follows I assume that Tang seeks instruction from Chen, which is the rhetorical pattern of the dialogues in *MS*VI.A.

[1]I.e. how can intercourse fulfill the goal of macrobiotic cultivation?

[2]There is a parallel to these lines in *MS*VII.B.8, which is a fuller statement of the need for a program of sexual cultivation.

[3]This begins a list of six names of sexual positions. Two lacunae have been filled on the basis of the parallel in *MS*VI.B.3 (a list similar to *MS*VI.B.3 also occurs in *MS*VII.B.10).

[4]This begins a list of five names for parts of the female genitals. There is a labeled drawing of the female genitals in *MS*III.91 in which seven names are extant; and a list of twelve names in *MS*VII.B.19. None of the names in *MS*III.88 have exact counterparts in *MS*III.91 or *MS*VII.B.19; and the connection between the names in *MS*III.88 and in later sexual literature is extremely uncertain. Reading *yun* 云 in the sense of "cloud" is merely a guess. The name *yunshi* 云石 may be related to *zaoshi* 磲石 in *MS*VII.B.19.

[5]I read 拈 as *ku* 枯, again merely a guess. The name *jianhu* 澗瓠 occurs in *MS*VII.B.19 and may be related.

[6]"Glistening plug" is a literal rendering of *zhuogua* 濯昏.

[7]The first graph is *fu* 伏; the name may be related to *fu* [1] 付 in *MS*III.91.

[8]This begins a list of seven ways for the man to move his penis inside the vagina. Parallels occur in *MS*VI.B.4 and *MS*VII.B.12. "Rabbit bolting" appears to be out of place in *MS*III.88, since it is given as the name of a sexual position in *MS*VI.B.3 and *MS*VII.B.10.

'rabbit bolting.' The first is 'blowing'; the second is 'biting.'[1] The first is '[2]'; the second is 'shaking.'[2] The first is 'secure the taste';[3] the second is 'bring vapor'; the third is 'exercise the fruit';[4] the fourth is 'attend to the joints.' "[5]

*MS*III.89 (CC205–217)

[1] Discourse[6]

[1] {1} the auspicious day[7] of the third month at [1]. Yu then [2] and entered the Circular-jade Chamber.[8] His shape was transformed and his complexion was extremely virile and beautiful, like someone in the vigor of manhood. The flock of beauties[9] beheld him [16] {3} [1] {4} [1] {10} [21]. My whiskers and eyebrows had already changed, blood and vapor was not sufficient, and I felt no pleasure.[10] [25] {5} [1] {1} [29] at dusk awoke. South Beauty [4]

---

[1]These refer to the woman's state of arousal as exhibited by signs coming from the mouth. "Blowing" and "biting" are given along with three other signs in *MS*VI.B.6, *MS*VII.B.15, and *MS*VII.B.20.

[2]"Shaking" is one of eight ways the woman moves her body during intercourse as described in *MS*VI.B.5 and *MS*VII.B.16.

[3]The final list of four has a parallel in *MS*VII.B.11 which names ten aspects of intercourse that the man must master. *MS*VII.B.11 places "bring vapor" first and "secure the taste" second.

[4]"Exercise the fruit" is fourth in *MS*VII.B.11.

[5]*Shijie* 侍 節 (attend to the joints) corresponds to *zhijie* 治 節 (control the joints) in *MS*VII.B.11.

[6]Despite the extensive lacunae, the general format of *MS*III.89 is discernible. Yu 禹, who has regained the vigor of youth, engages in a discussion of sexual cultivation with the females at his court. The passage is notable for presenting women in the role of the experts who instruct their lord. While this is a standard form for later sexual cultivation literature, it occurs nowhere else in the Mawangdui medical manuscripts.

[7]The *jiri* 吉 日 can refer to any auspicious day chosen in accordance with hemerological principles, but it also denotes the first day of the month (*Zhouli*, 12.5a).

[8]*Xuanfang* 璇 房 is equivalent to *xuanshi* 琁 室 in *Huainanzi*, 8.118; like the Blue-gem Terrace it exemplifies the architectural excesses of Jie and Zhou in received literature. I follow *MWD*, vol. 4, "Transcription," which reads the original 璇 as 琁, but 旋 is also possible. Both readings are indicated in the Gao You commentary in *Huainanzi*, which identifies the chamber either as decorated with a jade-like stone called *xuan* or as built to revolve (*xuan* 旋; see *MS*III.88).

[9]I follow *MWD*, vol. 4, "Transcription," n. 2, in reading *he/*gar* 河 as a phonetic loan for *e/*ngar* 娥. The compound *jing'e* 娙 娥 is glossed in *SW*, 12B.11b, as a term for a beautiful woman; and the same compound occurs written 娙 何 in *Shiji*, 49.13a, where it refers to one of the grades of consorts at the court of Thearch Wu (r. 141–87 B.C.).

[10]Yu is evidently describing a time when old age descended on him, before his rejuvenation.

{3} [31] not able to desist. West Beauty [12] {2} [16][1] severe ailment and [1] and did not desist. I feared suffering excess and not awakening. Young Beauty [1] {3} [15] {1} [1] {8}. Young Beauty came forward and replied: "The woman's [pleasure][2] is [13] suffer illness in youth. If you advance violently and withdraw violently, the good vapor is not maintained."[3] Yu said: "Well spoken, indeed![4] [16]. I wish to conjoin vapor so that man and woman propagate.[5] How is it to be accomplished?" Young Beauty said: "The way of conjoining vapor must always [11][6] {2} [1] {1}, vapor is not [1] clogged." Yu said: "Well spoken, indeed! Now my blood and vapor collect outside [11][7] said: "Why does Milord not make a boiled-dish of *mao* (woolly grass) and *ai* (mugwort), take the broth {7} [15] {7}. Ascend on the left and descend on the right; and do not reach completion violently."[8]

---

[1]It is probable that South Beauty and West Beauty both speak to Yu, their words lost in the lacunae.

[2]I follow Qiu Xigui in filling the lacuna with *le* 樂 based on the fragments of the graph (1992: 534).

[3]I.e. aggressive behavior by the man during intercourse nullifies the possible benefits of sexual cultivation.

[4]也 in *MWD*, vol. 4, "Transcription," should be transcribed as *hu* 虖.

[5]"Conjoin vapor" translates *heqi* 合 氣, which is attested in *Lunheng*, "Wushi," 3.68, in two senses: the union of the vapor of heaven and earth (which by coincidence engendered humankind); and the union of the vapor of man and wife (which by coincidence engenders offspring). As evidenced by *MS*III.89, *heqi* was one of several standard terms for sexual intercourse in the third to second centuries B.C. *Guanzi* 39, 14.236, also speaks of "essence and vapor conjoining" 精 氣 合 when intercourse between a man and a woman leads to the conception of a child. *Heqi* acquired special meaning in later religious Daoism, where it was the name of a group sexual rite practiced by Daoists as early as the Later Han (Rao Zongyi 1991: 142; Maspero 1981: 533-41; Schipper 1969: 27-31; and Kalinowski 1985: 781-85).

[6]The lacuna extends to the bottom of C215. After C215 *MWD*, vol. 4, "Transcription," erroneously omits an entire column of text. My transcription of the missing column (C215a) is based on Qiu Xigui (1992: 534-35): 必 至 [1] 思 氣 不 [1] 鬱 禹 曰 善 戋 言 虖 今 我 血 氣 外 揖 [11].

[7]The lacuna extends to the bottom of C215a. Since the lacuna begins at the same point on the manuscript as the eleven-graph lacuna in C215, I estimate the same number of missing graphs in C215a. It is evident that Yu has finished speaking and that one of the females now begins to speak.

[8]The final sentence refers to procedures for sexual intercourse. I do not know the significance of ascending on the left and descending on the right.

*MS*III.90 (CC218-19)

Eating and Pulling[1]

To assist in increasing vapor, when eating and drinking always shift the Yin and move it. When in bed once again pull it.[2] Thus it is said: "Give it drink [2]; and also instruct and counsel it."[3] Pull on the right and bend the left foot.[4]

*MS*III.91[5]

(Right side, inside the drawing)
red bead[6]
[1] strings[7]

---

[1] *MS*III.90 joins diet with exercise (*yin* 引) in cultivating the Yin element of the body. The genitals are a prime but not the sole referent of Yin in the passage.

[2] Compare *MS*VI.A.6, which describes the cultivation of "penile vapor" through diet and exercise. *MS*VI.A.8 mentions a morning exercise called "pulling Yin" (*yin* Yin 引 陰) which serves to "refine the muscles." It seems to refer to an exercise rather than to sexual activity; that is, Yin does not simply denote the genitals. Cultivating the Yin element of the body is the object of two techniques for "pulling Yin" described in the *Yinshu*, one a simple toe-touch and the other a procedure involving anal constriction (see the Prolegomena, Section Four, "Techniques," for details).

[3] In the parallel in *MS*VI.A.5 the "it" in the quotation is indisputably the penis.

[4] The sentence seems to be a fragment from a description of an exercise (for cultivating Yin?).

[5] Following C219 a heavy vertical line separates the main text from the list of recipe categories in *MS*III.92. The line ends about eight centimeters above the bottom of the silk sheet; a full-face drawing of the female genitals with names identifying the parts occupies the space directly beneath it (C218 contains a short column of text in order to make room for the right side of the diagram; see Fig. 13). Only one name is partially extant inside the drawing on the left side of the diagram. On the right side there is evidence of seven names: two inside the drawing; and five outside the drawing, one now completely illegible. Because of the parallel in *MS*VII.B.19 which lists twelve names, *MWD*, vol. 4, "Transcription," n. 1, suggests that the diagram in *MS*III.91 might originally have included twelve names as well. Li and McMahon argue that the diagram originally contained nine names (1992: 164); but this is based on the symbolic significance of the number nine in connection with vaginal penetration in later sexual literature that I doubt is applicable to *MS*III.91. Li and McMahon provide a table comparing names for parts of the female genitals in *MS*III.91 and *MS*VII.B.19 with later sexual literature. Ma Jixing also provides a table of all of the names that occur in the manuscripts and in received sexual literature; and speculates on possible identifications of the manuscript names (1992: 1063-65).

[6] *Chizhu* 赤 珠. "Red bead" is written at the top beside two dots drawn on either side of what must represent the labia major. I assume that the dots represent the two corpora cavernosa of the clitoris. Li and McMahon also identify *chizhu* as the clitoris (1992: 164). The name occurs in later sexual literature.

[7] [1]*xian* 弦. The name is written beneath "red bead." There is no counterpart in *MS*VII.B.19, but based on the occurrence of *qinxian* 琴 弦 (zither strings) in later sexual literature the lacuna is probably *qin*. Li and McMahon identify "zither strings" as the labia minor (1992: 164); Wile concurs (1992: 236, n. 73).

(Left side, inside the drawing)
attached [1][1]
(right side, outside the drawing)
hairpin light[2]
[1] rat[3]
[2][4]
wheat teeth
grain fruit[5]

*MS*III.92[6]

Non-erection Due to Agedness (*MS*III.1-3)
To Make Sweet-liquor (*MS*III.4)
Non-erection (*MS*III.5)
Augmentation (*MS*III.6)
Pliancy (*MS*III.7-9)
To Make[7] Mash-liquor (*MS*III.10)

---

[1]*Fu*[1] 付. Li and McMahon identify this as a name for the labia major (1992: 164). The identification is plausible.

[2]The names outside the drawing represent points inside the vagina. In later sexual literature such names identify successively deeper points and serve as landmarks for the depth of penile penetration (see the table in Li and McMahon 1992: 164). I translate the names in a sequence from upper right to lower left, beginning with *jiguang* 笄光 (hairpin light) and concluding with *gushi* 穀實 (grain fruit), written two columns to the left near the base of the drawing. *Jiguang* is the first of the twelve names in *MS*VII.B.19, but is not attested in later sexual literature. In later sexual literature *maichi* 麥齒 (wheat teeth) is the first interior point after passing the labia minor, and *gushi* is deeper than *maichi* (see Wile 1992: 255, n. 42; and Li and McMahon 1992: 164). If one assumes that *MS*III.91 follows a sequence from shallow to deep and that this sequence corresponds to later sexual literature, the names in *MS*III.91 ought to be listed beginning with *maichi* on the left and concluding with *jiguang*. That would make *jiguang* the deepest point in the vagina. The list in *MS*VII.B.19 does not help resolve the matter, since the names there do not follow any particular sequence. I leave the question of the location of *jiguang* inside the vagina and the sequence of the names written outside the drawing in *MS*III.91 unresolved. It occurs to me that the names may not be written in a strict shallow to deep or deep to shallow sequence.

[3][1]*shu* 鼠. The name is written in a column to the left of *jiguang*. The compound *shufu* 鼠婦 (rat wife) in *MS*VII.B.19 may be related to "[1] rat." Several names with "rat" as the second word of the compound occur in later sexual literature. The lacuna in *MS*III.91 may be *chou* 臭 (odorous) or *yu* 俞. *Choushu* is identified in later sexual literature as the next point deeper than *gushi*; *yushu* is a point between *maichi* and *gushi*.

[4]The two graphs written beneath [1]*shu* are illegible.

[5]*Maichi* 麥齒 (wheat teeth) and *gushi* 穀實 (grain fruit) are written in a column to the left of [1]*shu*. Both names occur in *MS*VII.B.19 and in later sexual literature. For discussion of the meaning of "wheat teeth" (which refers to irregular teeth, and by extension to a similar-appearing part of the vagina) see Wile 1992: 243, n. 129.

[6]The recipe categories of *MS*III are listed in four registers.

Cultivation (*MS*III.11-14)
Wheat-and-egg (*MS*III.15-19)
Washing the Male Organ (*MS*III.20)
To Cause Burning (*MS*III.21-23)
Increasing Craving (*MS*III.24-27)
Play (*MS*III.28-29)
To Remove Hair (*MS*III.30-32)
Ailing from Genital Swelling (*MS*III.33)
To Facilitate Approaching the Inner (Chamber) (*MS*III.34-36)
[?] Napkin (*MS*III.37-44)
To Lighten the Body and Increase Strength (*MS*III.45)
To Purge the Inside and Increase Vapor (*MS*III.46-62)
Scantness (*MS*III.63-64)
To Cultivate Strength (*MS*III.65)
[?]
[?]
[?]
[?]
Mash-liquor to Benefit the Inside (*MS*III.72-74)
Cultivation (*MS*III.75)
To Snap Horns (*MS*III.76)
Striding (*MS*III.77-85)
To Travel Quickly (*MS*III.86-87)
[?] (*MS*III.88)
[1] Discourse (*MS*III.89)
Eating and Pulling (*MS*III.90)

[7]I follow Ma Jixing (1992: 654, n. 3) in reading *sui/*stjəd* 虽 as a phonetic loan for *wei/*rəd* 惟; and understanding it as synonymous with *wei* 爲 (make) in the heading as written in *MS*III.10.

Fig. 13 Facsimile of *MS*III.89 (partial) - 92

*MS*IV

ZALIAO FANG

雜療方

RECIPES FOR VARIOUS CURES

*MS*IV.1 (CC1-2)

[18] bird egg [1] {1} [19] {2}.[1]

*MS*IV.2 (C3)

[2] increase vapor. Take *bai songzhi* (white pine rosin), *duyu*,[2] and [1] *shizhi* (clay)[3] in equal amounts. Smith and mix together. Then put a large three-fingered pinch [?].

*MS*IV.3 (CC4-7)

Inside augmentation and contraction.[4] Take two *dou* of *konglei*,[5] chew, and pound. [2] {2} or soak it in two *dou* of fine gruel-vinegar. [4] and remove the palms. Put two *sheng* of *tao* (peach) fuzz into [1] and stir [1]. Soak two *chi* of excellent cloth in the [1]. Dry in the dark. [7] cloth. When engaging in intercourse rub the mid-body and the front with the cloth.[6] When (the penis)

---

[1]*MWD*, vol. 4, "Transcription," n. 1, notes that the right end of the silk sheet is damaged. The numbering of columns begins with the first extant fragments of text.

[2]Ma Jixing (1992: 750, n. 3) argues that *duyu/*ngwjag* 杜虞 is *duruo/*njak* 杜若 (listed in *GM*, 14.23, botanical identity uncertain). The argument is phonologically plausible.

[3]*Wuse shizhi* 五色石脂 is listed in *GM*, 9.80, and refers to five types of clay classified by the five colors blue, yellow, black, white, and red. The lacuna must be the word for the color of the clay.

[4]I.e. recipes for increasing the size of the erect penis (augmentation) and reducing the size of the vaginal opening (contraction; see *MS*III.6, 21). *MS*IV.3-7 concern the penis and *MS*IV.8-12 the vagina.

[5]*Konglei* 空壘 is unknown.

[6]I interpret the term *zhongshen* 中身 (mid-body) to refer to the region between the waist and the navel; and *qian* 前 (front) to refer to the genitals, in this case the male genitals. *Zhongshen* is attested in *Zhanguoce*, 25.1a, in a passage that compares the strategic position of Liang 梁 to the body of a snake: "Using the example of a snake, strike the tail and the head comes to the rescue; strike the head and the tail comes to the rescue; strike the mid-body (*zhongshen*) and the head and tail both come to the rescue. At present the King of Liang is the mid-body of Under-heaven." The ancient division of the body into head, foot, and waist is indicated in the *SW*, 3A.39b, gloss of *yao* 要 (waist) as *shenzhong* 身中

rises, remove it. If you wish to stop it, wash with glutinous panicled millet slop or flowing water.[1]

*MS*IV.4 (C8)

Inside augmentation. Put spring-bird eggs between *sang* (mulberry) branches and steam them. [1] in glutinous panicled millet and eat. Consume one egg; do not eat more. If you eat more [?].

*MS*IV.5 (CC9-10)

Inside augmentation. Take *gui* (cinnamon), *jiang* (ginger), *jiao* (zanthoxylum), and *zaojia* (honey locust)[2] in equal amounts. Smith all of them, and mix together. Make balls using *gu* (paper mulberry) liquid, and roll them with *yu* (elm) [1] the size of [3]. Store in a bamboo tube and do not let them lose their moisture. Then put them into the mid-body hole.[3] When (the penis) rises, remove.

*MS*IV.6 (C11)

Inside augmentation. Soak two *chi* of excellent white cloth in one *dou* of *gu* (paper mulberry) liquid. [2] steam until the liquid is gone. Store well until ready to engage in intercourse. Moisten[4] the mid-body with the cloth. When (the penis) rises, remove.

*MS*IV.7 (CC12-15)

Inside augmentation. Put a dog liver in a bee hive and let the bees [1] sting it on all sides, running through over ten hives.[5] Smith

---

(middle of the body). *MS*IV.5 refers specifically to the *zhongshen kong* 中身空 (mid-body hole), which is the navel. I do not accept the argument in Li and McMahon (1992: 161) that *zhongshen* denotes the "shaft of the penis"; and *zhongshen kong* the "urinary opening" (the passage cited from *Ishinpô*, 28.12a, to support the latter identification does not contain the term *zhongshen kong*; the *Sunzi* passage adduced for *zhongshen* parallels the *Zhanguoce* passage quoted above, and the denotation "penis" is implausible). *Zunsheng bajian*, 860 (高子論房中藥物之害), lists four aphrodisiac drugs that are put in the navel and two that are applied to the waist. Thus there is no need for concern that the waist and navel are improbable locations for the application of aphrodisiacs in the Chinese tradition. Since *MS*IV.3 is concerned with penile erection, *qian* is best understood as male genitals; *qian* refers to the vagina in *MS*IV.8-11 and *MS*IV.17.

[1] *Ishinpô*, 28.40b, also recommends washing the penis with water if an aphrodisiac-induced erection does not stop. Napkins impregnated with aphrodisiac drugs and applied to both male and female genitals are described in *MS*III.38-39 and *MS*III.41-44.

[2] I follow *MWD*, vol. 4, "Transcription," in reading *jiao/*tsjagw* 焦 as a phonetic loan for *zao/*tsəgw* 皂.

[3] I.e. the navel.

[4] "Moisten" translates *wen* 搵, glossed in *SW*, 12A.53b, as "immerse." Perhaps the cloth remains moist with the aphrodisiac like the wadding in *MS*IV.7. Alternatively, the word may simply mean "rub" (attested in Song and later sources).

[5] Compare *MS*III.37.

one *sheng* of *linggao* (spurge). Soak in one *sheng* of fine gruel-vinegar for five nights, and remove the *linggao* (spurge). Then take one large three-fingered pinch each of Yu soot[1] and [2]. Combine with the liver in gruel-vinegar. Then [5] good wadding [6] the gruel-vinegar is gone.[2] Store well in a bamboo tube and do not let it lose its moisture. When engaging in intercourse, wrap the mid-body with it. When (the penis) rises, remove.

*MS*IV.8 (CC16-17)

Contraction. Take *fanshi*,[3] *zaojia* (honey locust), and Yu soot—the three substances in equal amounts. [3] one substance. Smith all of them, and mix together. When having intercourse, prepare a small sack. Insert it into the front[4] for the time it takes to eat, and remove.

*MS*IV.9 (CC18-19)

Contraction. Take one part each of *gui* (cinnamon) and dried *jiang* (ginger); two parts of *fanshi*; and three parts of *zaojia* (honey locust). Smith all of them and mix. Wrap in plain silk, making it the size of a finger. Insert into the front. When it takes effect, take it out.

*MS*IV.10 (CC20-21)

Contraction. Take three parts of Ba *shu* (croton);[5] two parts of *shechuang* (cnidium); one part each of *gui* (cinnamon) and *jiang* (ginger); and four parts of *zaojia* (honey locust). Smith all of them and mix together. Blend with honey or *zao* (jujube) fat. Make balls the size of a *gan* (Job's tears fruit) to insert into the front. When having intercourse, put them in a small sack and stuff into the front. When it takes effect, take it out.

*MS*IV.11 (CC22-23)

Contraction. Take two parts each of incinerated dog bone and *fanshi*; one part each of *gui* (cinnamon) and *jiang* (ginger); and three parts of *zaojia* (honey locust). Smith all of them and mix together. Use *zao* (jujube) fat [3] the front. When it takes effect, take it out.

---

[1]Yu *xun* 禹熏 may be the same substance as Yu *zao* [1] 禹竈 in *MS*I.E.243, probably stove soot.

[2]The wadding is soaked in the aphrodisiac until the liquid is completely absorbed.

[3]The mineral denoted by *fanshi* 蕃石 is uncertain (see *MS*III.39).

[4]I.e. the vagina.

[5]Ba *shu* 巴菽 is synonymous with Ba *dou* 巴豆.

*MS*IV.12 (CC24-25)

Contraction. Take one part each of *fanshi* and *tao* (peach) fuzz; and two parts of Ba *shu* (croton). Smith all three substances and mix. Blend with *zao* (jujube) fat. Make balls the size of a *gan* (Job's tears) fruit. Insert [4] for the time it takes to cook a meal.[1] Then [8] in the recess.[2]

*MS*IV.13 (CC26-27)

[1] excitation.[3] Sheep head [9].[4] Dry in the sun until solidified. Blend with honey, making them the size of [5] fingertip [?].

*MS*IV.14 (C28)

[14] {1}. The woman feels pleasure and desires it.

*MS*IV.15 (C29)

[?].[5]

*MS*IV.16 (C30)

[?] it.

*MS*IV.17 (CC31-32)

[?] all in equal amounts. Mix together. Yin [?] pinch. Insert into the front. The woman feels intense pleasure and desires it.

*MS*IV.18 (CC33-34)

[?] half. Smith all of them and mix together, making them the size of [1]. Put into good gruel [?].

*MS*IV.19 (C35)

[?] fine gruel-vinegar [1] and eat. {2} [4] do not eat more than thrice [?].

*MS*IV.20 (C36)

[?] three *cun*. Incinerate and smith. [4], for the time it takes [to eat].[6] [?].[7]

---

[1]I assume that 熟食 refers to cooking food, undoubtedly grain. Alternatively, 熟食頃 refers to an "extension" 熟 of the "time it takes to eat" 食頃.

[2]"Recess" translates *bi* 庳, glossed in *SW*, 9B.16b, as "house with a sunken area in the center." In *MS*IV.12 it is evidently another name for the vagina.

[3]I follow Ma Jixing in reading 痒 as *yang* 癢, referring to the excitation associated with sexual arousal (1992: 761, n. 1).

[4]Sympathetic magic based on punning between *yang* 癢 (itching) and *yang* 羊 (sheep) is probably the reason for using sheep head in the aphrodisiac.

[5]*MWD*, vol. 4, "Transcription," n. 1, notes that there is a break in the text between C29 and C30; it is not clear how many columns might be missing.

[6]Judging from the context the lacuna must be *shi* 食.

[7]*MWD*, vol. 4, "Transcription," n. 1, notes that there is a break in the text between C36 and C37; it is not clear how many columns might be missing.

*MS*IV.21 (CC37-39)

[4] {2} [24]. When finished, take the [1] {1} [9] three days [14]. If {5}, a small three-fingered pinch is also all right. Already tested.[1]

*MS*IV.22 (C40)

The method of the afterbirth-burial chart for entombment according to Yu.[2] When burying the afterbirth, avoid the location of the Small Period and the Great Period. According to the month of birth, look for the number that is highest to bury the afterbirth [1].[3]

*MS*IV.23 (CC41-42)

After having given birth, thoroughly wash the afterbirth with clear flowing water and well water. Wipe thoroughly until there is

---

[1]*Yishi* 已 試 is the same kind of term as *changshi* 嘗 試 (previously tested; see *MS*I.E.15).

[2]"Afterbirth" translates *bao* 胞, strictly speaking the placenta (see *SW*, 9A.38b; *bao* 包 is the original graph for the womb). *MS*IV.22-23 concern proper burial of the afterbirth, which is essential to the well-being of the newborn infant. *MS*V.2 is a drawing of the chart referred to in *MS*IV.22, identified there as "Entombment according to Yu, with south orientation" (南 方 禹 臧). Yu is also the recipient of the teaching on gestation in *MS*V.3. Yu's association with childbirth continued into the medieval period as reflected in a quotation from the pre-Tang *Chanjing* 産 經 (Childbirth canon) in *Ishinpô*, 23.19a: "In the past when Yu was at Thunder Marsh there was a woman who approached him sorrowfully wailing. Yu asked the reason and she replied, 'Your maid has given birth to numerous children who all died young. Not one is alive, and that is why I am sorrowfully wailing.' Yu taught her this method, and her children were all long-lived. None were lost young." The method subsequently described is similar to *MS*IV.22 and *MS*V.4-7. In all, quotations from the *Chanjing* on afterbirth burial occupy *Ishinpô*, 23.18b-23a.

[3]Small Period (*xiaoshi* 小 時) and Great Period (*dashi* 大 時) refer to calendro-astrological calculations based on the rotation of the Big Dipper and the Jupiter cycle respectively. The compass points on earth that correspond to the positions of the two astrological bodies for each month are unlucky. The chart in *MS*V.2 consists of twelve small squares arranged around the perimeter of a large square. Each small square represents one of the twelve months and is marked with twelve compass points. Two of the points are labeled *si* 死 (death), representing the positions of Small Period and Great Period for the month in question, and ascending numbers are written by the other points. As explained in *MS*IV.22, the afterbirth should be buried in the direction indicated by the point with the highest number; it should never be buried in the direction indicated by a point labeled "death" (see *MS*V.2 for further explanation of the calendro-astrological symbolism and use of the chart). A similar method was still in use in medieval times, as indicated in *Ishinpô*, 23.22b: "Whenever you wish to bury the afterbirth you should first examine the chart of the twelve months. The location with the highest number means (the infant) will be long-lived. The location with the lowest number means (the infant) will not be long-lived. If a place with the highest number is simultaneously occupied by an ill-omened spirit, you must avoid it. If you choose the location with the next highest number that will also be lucky."

no liquid. Put it in an old pottery slotted steaming-pot[1] that is free of grime. Cover very tightly with a pottery bowl so that bugs cannot enter. Bury it in unspoiled ground in a Yang position at a place where the sun shines long. This ensures that the infant has excellent heart-knowledge,[2] a good complexion, and few ailments.

*MS*IV.24 (CC43-47)

To increase the inside and benefit the interior. Warm one half cup of pure liquor without letting it get hot. Break a chicken egg and pour the liquid into the liquor. Stir, and drink it. Always drink it at dawn before eating. When you begin to drink, drink one egg; the next day drink two eggs; and the day after drink three eggs. On the day after that again drink two eggs, and the next day drink one egg. Always decrease after reaching three eggs; and after decreasing to one egg, again increase.[3]

Always begin ingesting (the eggs) on the first day of the eighth and second months. Drink [5]. Ingesting in these two seasons[4] makes a person's face not become wizened;[5] the mouth and lips are not dry; and it benefits the interior and increases the inside.

Always ingest [?].

*MS*IV.25 (CC48-53)

[3] tonic sweet-liquor.[6] Take {1} [69] {1} the amount [2] *sheng* and boil [2] {1} [1] above it. [11] to make five *sheng*. Combine the five substances with *bi* [1] root, set in a slotted steaming-pot, and collect the liquid in the small cup below.[7] [11] the taste is completely extracted and stop.[8] Then boil the liquid. When it bubbles once, the sweet-liquor is finished. Then drink it gradually, until [1]

---

[1]It is curious that the slotted steaming-pot (*yan* 甗) is specified, since the afterbirth is supposed to be tightly sealed inside. I suspect that the kettle (*fu* 釜) that sits beneath the slotted steaming-pot is the intended vessel (see *MS*I.E.58).

[2]I.e. a bright mind.

[3]Compare *MS*III.15.

[4]I.e. autumn and spring.

[5]"Wizened" translates *jiao* 焦, attested in *Suwen* 1, 1.3b, as the dark, wrinkled appearance of the face that comes with age.

[6]A recipe for *li* 醴 (see *MS*III.4).

[7]I read 贛 as *gan* 匴 (small cup), as in *MS*I.E.97. I am guessing that the solid ingredients from the preceding decoction are put into the slotted steaming-pot and the liquid allowed to drain into a cup placed below. *MWD*, vol. 4, "Transcription," n. 2, reads the graph as *gan* 韝, glossed in *SW*, 14B.36a, as liquor with a potent taste; giving the translation, "collect the potent-tasting liquid below."

[8]Perhaps liquor is poured over the ingredients in the steaming-pot to extract their essence.

body [8] the inside, and at the same time the interior has an abundance of essence-fluid.[1] {2} [?].

*MS*IV.26 (CC54-55)[2]

[?] {1} [?] {2} [1] {1} [?].

*MS*IV.27 (CC56-57)

[?] {1} [?]

*MS*IV.28 (CC58-60)

[2] arrive at a place where the *yu*[3] [9] name is *nüluo*.[4] {1} [9] {3} [12]. Yi makes you not[5] [8] {1} makes the *yu* not shoot.

*MS*IV.29 (C61)

To make the *yu* not shoot. When you arrive at water, throw a handful of grain at it.[6]

---

[1]"Essence-fluid" translates *jingzhi* 精汁, which refers to vital juices generated inside the body as the result of drinking the liquor.

[2]*MWD*, vol. 4, "Transcription," n. 1, notes that there is a break in the text between C53 and C54, and again between C55 and C56; it is not clear how many columns might be missing on either side of CC54-55. The "Transcription" does not note another aspect of the silk sheet, which is that after C53 there are about six blank ruled columns before the break. Moreover, the calligraphy beginning in CC54-55 is different. The blank columns and change of calligraphy indicate that *MS*IV.26-42 were added to the silk sheet by another scribe after *MS*IV.1-25.

[3]*Yu* 蜮 is the name of a deadly water creature that was an ever-present hazard for inhabitants of Chu and Yue. *SW*, 13A.58b, glosses *yu* with one of its several names, *duanhu* 短狐 (short fox); describes it as "resembling a turtle with three legs"; and notes that it "shoots vapor to injure people." Early *yu* lore is summarized in Eberhard 1968: 193-95. It was believed to have a mouth in the form of a bow, from which it shot vapor "arrows" at its victims. And shooting someone's reflection in the water was sufficient to mortally wound the person standing on the bank. The notion of the *yu* as an evil omen is first indicated in *Zuozhuan*, Zhuang 18, 9.8a. In the first century B.C. Liu Xiang expressed the opinion that the *yu* was locally generated from chaotic vapor in Southern Yue, and that it was a manifestation of the excessive sexuality of the women of Yue (*Hanshu*, 27C-1.13b). There is little solid information regarding its biological identity. *SW* gives 蟈 as an orthographic variant of *yu*. The same graph was understood as a name for the toad, but that does not mean that the *yu* was considered to be a toad (see the Duan Yucai commentary). In medieval times—when the southern *yu* was still feared—many regarded it as a kind of water insect (Schafer 1967: 111). The recipes in *MS*IV.28-35 focus on preventing the *yu* from shooting, no doubt because its wound is believed to be mortal and prophylaxis is the best remedy.

[4]*Nüluo* 女羅 is the name of a parasitic plant, probably tree moss (*GM*, 37.12). Its use in *MS*IV.28 is not clear.

[5]Yi 羿 refers to the master archer who appears in a number of early legends associated with exorcistic themes. His image in myth is reviewed in Eberhard 1968: 80-87. The direct form of address "you" indicates that these words belong to an incantation.

[6]The purpose of throwing grain is probably twofold: to appease the *yu* with an offering, and to break the smooth surface of the water so that the *yu* cannot shoot at the person's reflection.

*MS*IV.30 (C62)

Another. Every morning chew two or three nodules of *suan* (garlic),[1] and ingest them.

*MS*IV.31 (C63)

Another. Every morning chew three *lan* (eupatorium) fruits, and chew *lingji* (water chestnut).

*MS*IV.32 (C64)

Another. Wear a silkworm cocoon or a silk-trimmed garment.

*MS*IV.33 (C65)

Another. Dress in a red coarse-silk garment and a black alum-dyed garment.[2] Trim the collarband and sleeves with horsehair,[3] or use [1] and [1] to fill in the underarms.

*MS*IV.34 (C66)

Another. Trim the collarband and sleeves of the garment with wild[4] pig bristles. It makes the *yu* and venomous snakes not dare to shoot.

*MS*IV.35 (CC67-70)

If by misfortune you are shot by the *yu*, venomous snakes, and bees, chant an incantation and spit at it thrice. Name the creature that did the shooting with its name, saying: "So-and-so. You five brothers, so-and-so knows all your names.[5] You who dwell in the water are the fish-*qi*. You who dwell on the land are the bug-*qi*.[6]

---

[1]I read 蒜 as *suan* 蒜. For the use of 林 as a signific element in place of 艹 in Warring States script, see He Linyi 1989: 207 (the example given is 荤 to write *xun* 葷). I do not accept the reading *nai* 柰 (crab apple) in *MWD*, vol. 4, "Transcription," n. 1. Also, *suan* refers to the native Chinese garlic, *Allium scorodoprasum* L. (*ZY*: no. 0478), not to *A. sativum* L., the garlic with multiple-clove heads that was introduced from the West.

[2]This prophylactic attire must be related to the black upper garment and red lower garment worn by the chief exorcist in the Great Exorcism (*Hou Hanshu*, "Zhi" 志, 5.10a; cf. Bodde 1975: 81). Similar black and red attire is used to clothe the body of the deceased in *Yili*, 40.6b. According to the Zheng Xuan commentary the colors symbolize heaven and earth.

[3]*Lai* 㾢 is glossed in *SW*, 2A.11a, as bristly hair used to pad clothing. The horsehair is probably stuffed inside the collarband and sleeves.

[4]"Wild" translates 田 暘 (I read *chang* 暘 as *chang* 場 in the sense of "unarable land"; see *SW*, 13B.39a, and Duan Yucai commentary).

[5]The first "so-and-so" represents the name of the creature, the second the name of the person.

[6]*Qi* 蚑 is given as an alternate name for *zhi* 蛭 (leech) in *BL*; and Tao Hongjing notes that there are many varieties of *qi* both in the water and out (*GM*, 40.104). Perhaps the unattested graph 鮁 in *MS*IV.35 (which I render as "fish-*qi*") signifies the leech; and 蚑 "bug-*qi*" signifies another blood-sucking creature on land.

Those lodged in trees are the bee and *ransi* (catepillar).[1] The one who flew to Jing-in-the-South is the *yu*. You advance[2] [1] not [1]. You instruct the clan grandsons. So-and-so is a murderer. If you do not cause so-and-so's ailment to desist, once again [14].[3]

*MS*IV.36 (C71)

[19] root, one third *dou* and add it. Sieve thoroughly, and drink.[4]

*MS*IV.37 (CC72-73)

[?] dry. When dry, smith [?].

*MS*IV.38 (CC74-75)

Another. Take [11] fish. Do not eat that evening, and eat it at dawn.[5] Take satiation as the standard. Do not drink the liquid.

*MS*IV.39 (C76)

Another. Butcher a *bie* (soft-shelled turtle), and drink the blood. Steam the flesh and eat it.

*MS*IV.40 (C77)

Another. Soak yellow earth from the stove in gruel-vinegar. Steam, and hot-press the spot with it.

*MS*IV.41 (C78)

Another. Pound *lan* (eupatorium) leaves while fresh. Steam, and hot-press it.

*MS*IV.42 (C79)

Another. Steam earthworm excrement, and hot-press the spot with it.

---

[1]Tao Hongjing states that the hair on the *ransi* 蛅蟖 stings (*GM*, 39.77).

[2]I translate *jin* 晉 as glossed in *SW*, 7A.4b, "advance." *MWD*, vol. 4, "Transcription," n. 5, argues that *jin/*tsjin* is a phonetic loan for *jian/*tsjan* 箭 (arrow). The loan usage is phonologically plausible, but the following lacunae make it impossible to determine whether the meaning "arrow" is justified by the context.

[3]The first "so-and-so" is the creature, the second the person. *Qianjin yifang*, 30.357, records a similar incantation that first identifies the stinging creatures by their location and then concludes: "You five brothers, I know you all. Collect your five poisons, let no one transmit them. If you do not collect the poison, (I) destroy your clan." Several incantations in *MS*I.E also liken the agents blamed for the ailment to a family (for example, *MS*I.E.120).

[4]*MWD*, vol. 4, "Transcription," n. 1, notes that there is a break in the text between C71 and C72; it is not clear how many columns might be missing. It is also no longer clear what the recipes in *MS*IV.36-42 are intended to treat.

[5]I understand this to mean that the person should not eat a meal the night before taking the medicine; and that he should eat the medicine the next morning at dawn.

MSV

TAICHAN SHU

胎産書

BOOK OF THE GENERATION OF THE FETUS

MSV.1 (upper half, right side)

Explanation

The two human figures are placed sideways on the manuscript; each one stands with legs spread and arms raised (Fig. 14). Despite the poor preservation of the drawing, the extant Branch signs can be seen to be written on top of the head, by the sides of the head, by the shoulders, on the hands, by the underarms, beneath the feet, and in the crotch. Comparing *MSV*.1 with the drawing in the first Shuihudi hemerological manuscript (*SHD*: 206), the arrangement of Branch signs on the top figure matches the Shuihudi figure representing spring and summer; the bottom figure matches the Shuihudi figure representing fall and winter. The child's fortune is determined by consulting the figure for the appropriate season and locating the Branch sign in the cyclical designation of the date of birth on it. According to the explanatory text in the Shuihudi manuscript, if the Branch sign is atop the head the child will be extremely wealthy; by the neck (the Branch signs written by the sides of the head in *MSV*.1), noble; in the crotch, wealthy; by the underarms, the child will be loved; at the hands, he will be a thief; beneath the feet, ignoble; and on the "outside" (*wai* 外; the Branch signs written above the arms on the Shuihudi figures and by the shoulders on the *MSV*.1 figures), he will be a vagabond. Thus, a child born on a *mao* 卯 day in summer will be wealthy (*mao* is atop the head of the top figure); a child born on a *mao* day in winter will be a vagabond (*mao* is by the right shoulder of the bottom figure).

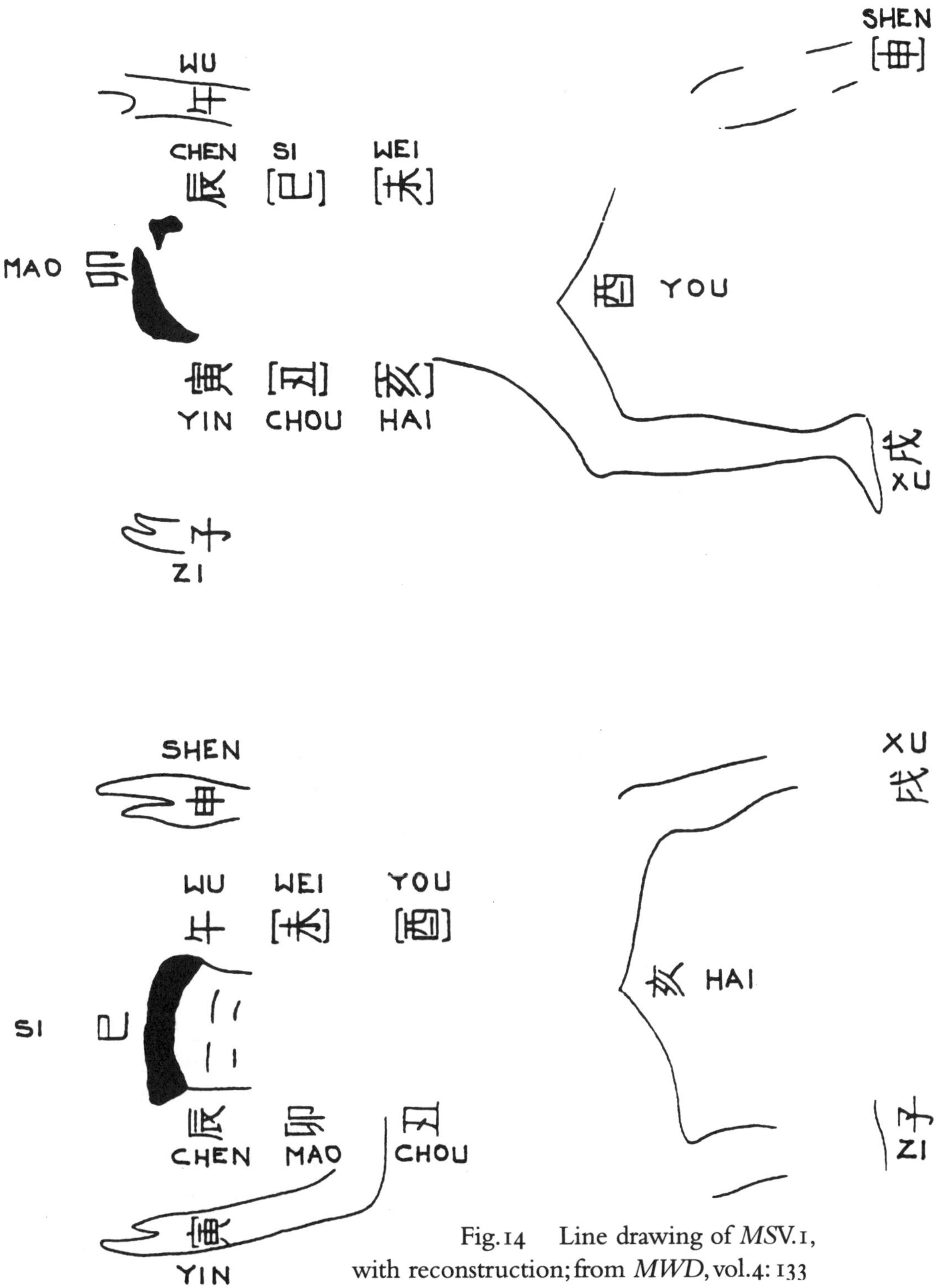

Fig. 14 Line drawing of *MSV*. I, with reconstruction; from *MWD*, vol. 4: 133

*MS*V.2
(upper half, left side)

Explanation

The name of the chart is written in the center: "Entombment according to Yu, with south orientation" 南方禹臧 (Figs. 15-16). Its use in the method for burying the afterbirth is explained in *MS*IV.22. Looking at the chart, each square representing a month is marked with twelve points corresponding to the twelve Branch signs and compass directions (south is at the top): *zi* 子 (N), *chou* 丑 (N-NE), *yin* 寅 (E-NE), *mao* 卯 (E), *chen* 辰 (E-SE), *si* 巳 (S-SE), *wu* 午 (S), *wei* 未 (S-SW), *shen* 申 (W-SW), *you* 酉 (W), *xu* 戌 (W-NW), *hai* 亥 (N-NW). According to *MS*IV.22 the directions corresponding to Small Period (*xiaoshi* 小時) and Great Period (*dashi* 大時) must be avoided when burying the afterbirth. These points are labeled *si* 死 (death) on the chart. As explained in *Huainanzi*, 3.42, Small Period corresponds to the handle of the Big Dipper, which shifts clockwise one position per month beginning at *yin* (E-NE) in the first month. The points marked "death" on the chart corresponding to the positions of Small Period are: first month, E-NE; second month, E; third month, E-SE; fourth month, S-SE; fifth month, S; sixth month, S-SW; seventh month, W-SW; eighth month, W; ninth month, W-NW; tenth month, N-NW; eleventh month, N; twelfth month, N-NE. Having established the positions of Small Period on the chart, the positions of Great Period are: first month, E; second month, S; third month, W; fourth month, N; fifth month, E; sixth month, S; seventh month, W; eighth month, N; ninth month, E; tenth month, S; eleventh month, W; twelfth month, N. The *Huainanzi* passage just cited identifies Great Period as another name for one of the cycles associated with *taisui* 太歲 (Grand Year). In calendro-astrological calculations Grand Year represents a planet that moves clockwise in opposition to counter-clockwise rotating *suixing* 歲星 (Year Star; i.e. Jupiter). However, the Great Period cycle described in *Huainanzi* moves counter-clockwise, beginning from *mao* (E) in the second month and shifting to the successive cardinal compass points in subsequent months (N in the third month, W in the fourth month, etc.). Later sources show that the *Huainanzi* text is corrupt and that the cycle should begin at *mao* (E) in the first month rather than in the second month, in agreement with the chart in *MSV*.2 (Zhang Peiyu 1989: 137–38). But the later sources still indicate a counter-clockwise direction for the Great Period cycle, rather than the clockwise direction in the chart. The Great Period cycle indicated in *MSV*.2 does, however, correspond to the cycle of *sui* (Jupiter) described in the first Shuihudi hemerological manuscript (*SHD*: 190).

I know of no other examples of the numbering system used on the chart. The lowest number is 20, and the numbers increase clockwise by tens until interrupted by a "death" point, after which the numbering begins again with 20. There are three exceptions to this pattern. In the second month the number 40 appears at S-SW, followed by 30, 40, and 50 on the west side of the square (the numbers are missing in *MSV*.2, but can be restored based on the sequence 60, 70, 80 on the north side of the square). This is clearly scribal error, writing 卌 (40) instead of 廿 (20). In the ninth month, the number 30 appears at E-SE instead of 20 following the position of Great Period at E, and the numbering continues 40, 50, 60 on the south side of the square. Similarly, in the first month 20 appears at E-SE, followed by 40, 50, 60 on the south side. According to the regular progression, 110 is the highest number that can be reached in the chart, but the first month records a 120 at N-NE. There must be a reason for skipping from 20 to 40 in the first month in order to reach a high number of 120; and the ninth month sequence beginning with 30 at E-SE is probably also intentional, not scribal error. Besides choosing the highest number to determine the burial site for the afterbirth, I do not know what other significance the numbers may have. I doubt that they represent a prediction of the lifespan of the child as suggested in Ma Jixing 1992: 820. The appropriate burial sites by month are: first month, 120 (N-NE); second month, 90 (E-NE); third month, 70 (E); fourth month, 70 ((N-NW); fifth month, 90 (E-NE); sixth month, 110 (S-SE); seventh month, 110 (S-SW); eighth month, 90 (W-SW); ninth month, 80 (W); tenth month, 70 (S-SE); eleventh month, 90 (W-SW); twelfth month, 110 (N-NW).

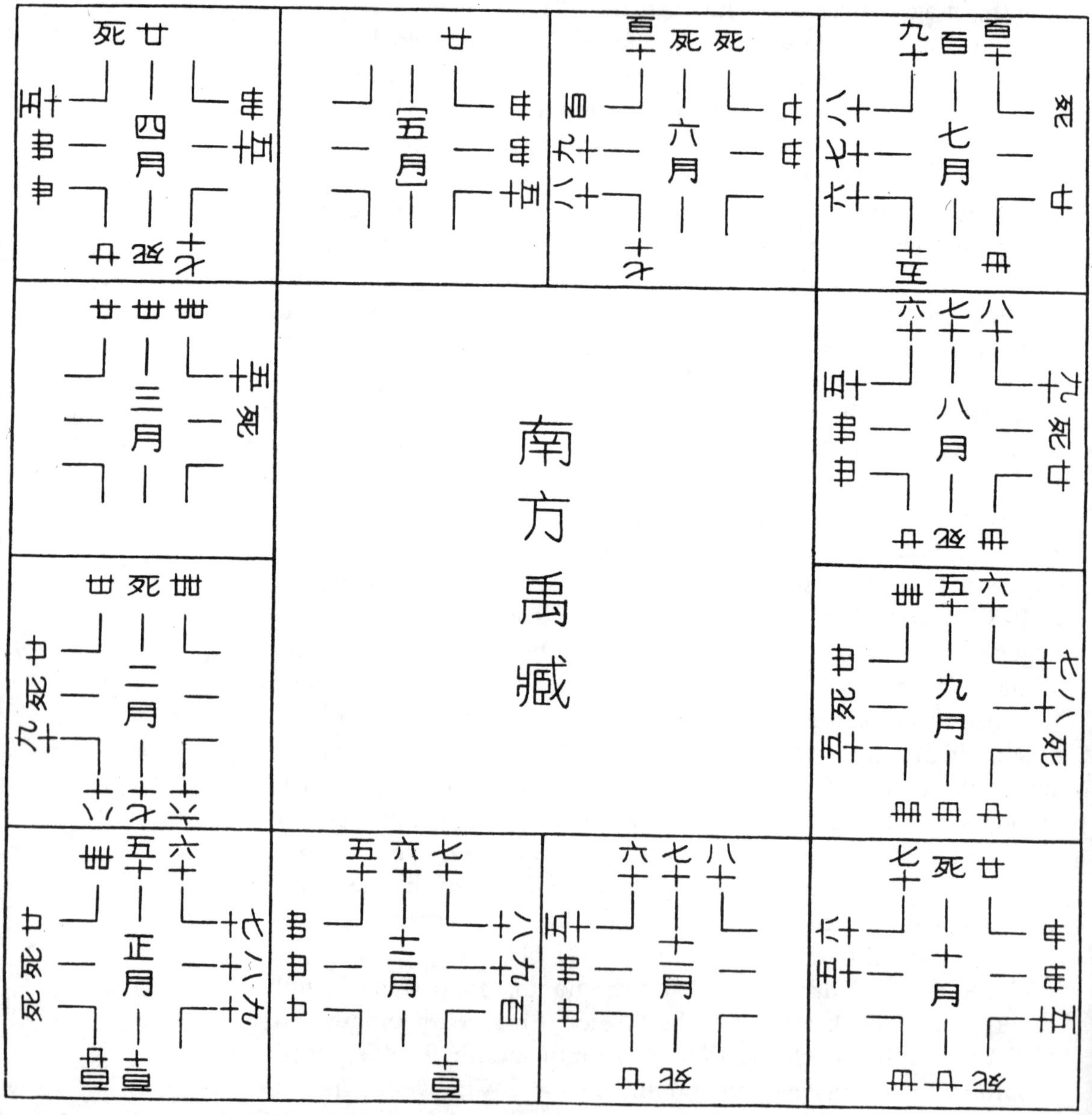

Fig. 15 Line drawing of *MSV*.2, from *MWD*, vol. 4: 134

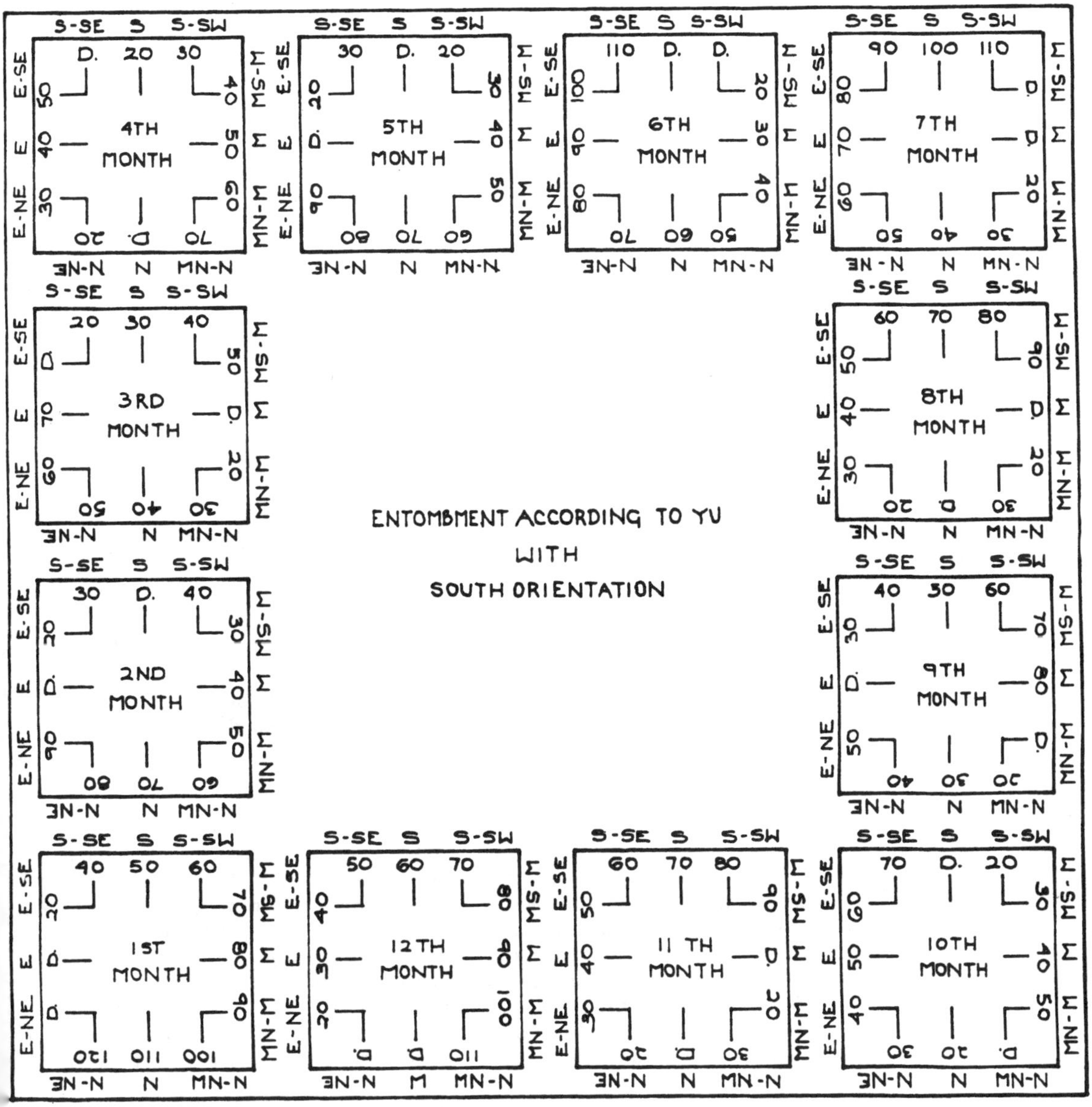

Fig. 16 Line drawing of *MSV*.2, with reconstruction and compass points

MSV.3
(lower half, CC1-13)

Yu asked Youth Multiplier:[1] "I wish to propagate people and engender children. How is it that this occurs?"

Youth Multiplier replied: "After menstruation[2] is finished and the fluid [1],[3] have intercourse with her over the next three days and there will be a child. If on the first day, it is a boy; if on the second day, a girl.[4] Thus when human beings are engendered, having entered into obscure darkness and exited from obscure darkness, they first become humans.[5] In the first month it is called 'flowing into the form.'[6] Food and drink must be the finest; the sour boiled dish must be thoroughly cooked. Do not eat acrid or rank foods. This is called 'initial fixture.' In the second month it first becomes lard.[7] Do not eat acrid or stinking foods. The dwelling place must be still. For

---

[1]A literal translation of the name You Pin 幼 頻, which suggests someone who produces a continuous line of offspring. I assume that Youth Multiplier is a male expert on childbirth. *MWD*, vol. 4, "Transcription," emends lacunae in *MSV*.3 based on the *Chaoshi zhubing yuanhoulun* and *Qianjin yaofang* parallels (printed in *MWD*, vol. 4: 140-41).

[2]"Menstruation" translates *yueshuo* 月 朔, which is related to the term *shuoshi* 朔 事 used for menstruation in the Shuihudi *Fengzhen shi* (*SHD*: 162). *Yueshi* 月 事 (menstrual activity) is the term used in *Shiji*, 105.18a. The use of *shuo* in the Mawangdui and Shuihudi manuscripts specifically correlates menstruation with the spring tide that accompanies the new moon.

[3]The fluid must be the menstrual blood, which no longer flows.

[4]There is probably a symbolic connection between odd numbers which are Yang and a male birth; and between Yin, even numbers and a female birth. *Waitai biyaofang*, 33.3b-4a, states that insemination on the first, third, and fifth days after menstruation produces a boy; insemination on the second, fourth, and sixth days produces a girl.

[5]"Obscure darkness" translates *mingming* 冥 冥. *Mingming* forms part of an epithet for *dao* 道—Way as the source of all phenomena—in *Shiji*, 130.6a. A writing entitled "Daofa" 道 法 (Model of Way) preceding the second Mawangdui *Laozi* edition also uses the compound: "The empty and formless its central seam is obscurely dark (*mingming*); it is the place from which the myriad creatures come into being" (*MWD*, vol. 1: 43). Perhaps "entering and exiting obscure darkness" alludes to the action of the penis in the vagina. In any case, conception is likened to the emergence of living things from the empty place that is Way.

[6]The "it" is the newly conceived entity inside the womb. *Liuxing* 留 刑 occurs written 流 形 in *Guanzi* 39, 14.236, where it introduces the passage on gestation: "The essence and vapor of man and woman conjoin and water flows into the form (*liuxing*)." The term likens the creation of the embryo to the flowing of fluid into a mold where it acquires its distinctive shape.

[7]I.e. the embryo is a soft mass like lard (*gao* 膏). Lard is the term for the first month of gestation in *Huainanzi*, 7.99.

a boy there must be no exertion, lest the hundred joints all ail.[1] This is called 'first deposition.'[2] In the third month it first becomes suet, and has the appearance of a gourd. During this time it does not yet have a fixed configuration, and if exposed to things it transforms. For this reason lords, sires, and great men must not employ dwarves. Do not observe monkeys. Do not eat *cong* (onion) and *jiang* (ginger); and do not eat a rabbit boiled dish.[3] [1] you wish to give birth to a boy, set out bow and arrow, [1] male pheasant, mount a male horse, and observe the male tiger. If you wish to give birth to a girl, wear hairpins and earrings at the waist, and wear a pearl belt.[4] This is called 'inner imaging to complete the child.'[5] In the fourth month Water is bestowed on it, and blood first forms.[6] The ap-

---

[1]Presumably the pregnant woman already has an idea about the gender of the child to be born, and must take care not to exert herself if she is expecting a boy.

[2]I.e. a matrix now exists for the growth of the fetus.

[33]As explained in *Bowuzhi*, 2.1b, the prohibition of rabbit and ginger during the malleable third month is to prevent harelip and hand deformities: "A pregnant woman can neither eat rabbit nor look at a rabbit, for it causes the infant to have a split lip; moreover, she cannot eat fresh ginger, which causes the infant to have many fingers."

[4]I follow *MWD*, vol. 4, "Transcription," in reading *shen* 呻 as *shen* 紳, glossed in *SW*, 13A.20b, as "large belt." *SW*, 1A.34b, glosses *zhu* 珠 as "Yin essence inside the oyster," making pearls an ideal material for inducing the development of a female in the fetus. It is possible that *shen/*stjin* 呻 is a phonetic loan for *tun* 吞 (swallow; the graph is also pronounced like its phonetic *tian/*thin* 天). This usage occurs in *MSV*.9; and is also attested in *MWD*, vol. 3: 68. However, all of the other items used to induce male or female gender affect the fetus from the outside; none are ingested by the pregnant woman. Thus it is more likely that she wears the pearls rather than swallowing them. The parallels in the later descriptions of gestation use the verb *long* 弄 (fiddle with).

[5]The impressionability of the fetus during the third month is also evident in *MSV*.9 10, which specify that medicines to guarantee the birth of a boy should be taken no later than the third month of pregnancy.

[6]From the fourth to eighth months the fetus receives the Five Agents, each of which is responsible for a physiological constituent: Water produces blood; Fire produces vapor; Metal produces muscle; Wood produces bone; Earth produces skin. Underscoring the elemental nature of the Agents, a sixth material Stone follows Earth in the ninth month to produce hair. The enumeration of the Five Agents in *MSV*.3 follows the order of the "conquest sequence" given in Han sources, which usually begin with Wood: Wood conquers Earth; Earth conquers Water; Water conquers Fire; Fire conquers Metal; Metal conquers Wood (Kalinowski 1991: 247). The first Shuihudi hemerological manuscript lists the "conquest sequence" in the order: Metal conquers Wood; Fire conquers Metal; Water conquers Fire; Earth conquers Water; Wood conquers Earth (*SHD*: 223). It is interesting that *MSV*.3 applies the "conquest sequence" to the formulation of a cosmo-physiological model of creation (the "generation sequence" of Wood, Fire, Earth, Metal, Water was known in the third century B.C.). There is a definite logic to the correlations between Agents and constituents. Water producing blood and Fire producing vapor situates the Yin Yang duality of blood and vapor at the beginning of the process. The reasons for associat-

propriate foods are rice, wheat, *shanyu* (mud eel) [2], which clarify the blood and brighten the eyes. In the fifth month Fire is bestowed on it, and vapor first forms. Rise late and [1] wash the hair. Wear a thick layer of clothing and remain inside the house. At dawn inhale heaven's rays and avoid harm from the cold. The appropriate foods are [rice] and wheat;[1] the appropriate boiled dishes are beef and mutton, mixed with *zhuyu* (evodia); and do not eat [1], thereby nurturing the vapor. In the sixth month Metal is bestowed on it, and muscle first forms. Exercise [3]; [go out] to wander [in the countryside; frequently][2] observe running dogs and horses. You must eat [2] without [3]. This is called 'changing the skin's webbed pattern and [1] muscle.' [4]. In the seventh month Wood is bestowed on it, and [bone] first forms.[3] Occupy heated places, and do not become [immobilized].[4] [12]. [With drink and food][5] avoid (things that have a) cooling effect. [9] and fine teeth. In the eighth

---

ing Metal with muscle, Wood with bone, and Earth with skin can also be deduced without stretching the imagination. By implication, the correlations described for the fetus ought to apply to human physiology. However, such correlations are not mentioned in the Mawangdui medical manuscripts; and there are few counterparts to *MSV*.3 in extant writings related to physiology. Later received literature on physiology also correlates the constituents differently; for example, Fire is correlated with muscle, Metal with bone, and Wood with hair and skin (Kalinowski 1991: 222). In the *Huangdi neijing*, constitutents like muscle and bone are subsumed under the larger category of the vessels and the internal organs; and the primary correlates of the Five Agents are the Five Depots (liver, heart, lung, kidney, spleen; these correlations are also not in evidence in the Mawangdui medical manuscripts). Antecedents to the *Huangdi neijing* emphasis on internal organs occur in *Guanzi* 39, 14.236, which describes gestation as a process in which the Five Tastes produce the Five Depots, which in turn produce constituents like bone and flesh (the Five Agents are not mentioned); and in third century B.C. calendars that include internal organs among the manifold Five Agent correlations operating in nature (Rickett 1985: 158-61). To sum up, *MSV*.3 represents an early attempt at applying Five Agent theory to physiology in the context of fetal development, but its physiological correlations were not generally adopted in later medical literature except as a conventionally accepted account of gestation itself.

[1]*MWD*, vol. 4, "Transcription," fills a three-graph lacuna based on the context and on the fact that the later parallels give rice and wheat as appropriate foods for the fifth month. I bracket [rice] because it is added to the text on the basis of the later parallels. The use of brackets in the remainder of *MSV*.3 follows the same principle.

[2]*MWD*, vol. 4, "Transcription," fills the two lacunae on the basis of the later parallels.

[3]*MWD*, vol. 4, "Transcription," fills a five-graph lacuna based on the context and the later parallels; the bracketed word is based on the later parallels.

[4]Filling the lacuna is based on the later parallels.

[5]Filling the lacuna is based on the later parallels.

month Earth is bestowed on it, and [skin and hide] first form.[1] [8]. This is called 'tightening the [skin's webbed pattern].' In the ninth month [stone] is bestowed on it, and filament hairs first form.[2] [28] await it. In the tenth month the vapor spreads [2] to form [?]."

MSV.4 (lower half, C14)

Whenever attending to a birth, wash the afterbirth with clear water [?].

MSV.5 (lower half, CC15-16)

Another. You must thoroughly wash the afterbirth, and wash it again with liquor.[3] [8] {1} [13] pottery bowl, so that bugs and ants cannot enter. Then [8] a place where the sun shines. This ensures that the infant does not have scabbing, has lustrous skin, and is longlived [1].[4]

MSV.6 (lower half, C17)

Another. Bury the afterbirth beneath a mat to prevent scabby itch. Inside the inner (chamber) [4], and drink on an "establishment day."[5]

MSV.7 (lower half, CC18-19)

If when giving birth you have mostly boys and no girls, and you wish to have a girl, after [4] bury the afterbirth beneath a Yin oriented wall. If you have mostly girls and no boys, bury the afterbirth beneath a Yang oriented wall.

Another. Bind the afterbirth with the cord handle from a slotted steaming-pot,[6] and bury it.

MSV.8 (lower half, C20)

If a pregnant woman prepares boiled *bai mugou* heads[7] and she alone eats them, the child is beautiful and radiant, and also emerges

---

[1] *MWD*, vol. 4, "Transcription," fills a six-graph lacuna based on the context and the later parallels; the bracketed words are based on the later parallels.
[2] *MWD*, vol. 4, "Transcription," fills an eleven-graph lacuna based on the context and the later parallels; the bracketed words are based on the later parallels.
[3] 洒 in *MWD*, vol. 4, "Transcription," should be transcribed as *jiu* 酒 (liquor).
[4] Compare *MSIV*.23.
[5] The hemerological system underlying the designation of certain days as "establishment days" is explained in *MSI*.E.69. Perhaps the liquid drunk is water that was used to bathe the infant (see *MSV*.18).
[6] This cord is also used to string an exorcistic bow in *MSI*.E.132.
[7] *Bai mugou* 白 牡 狗 is an insect of uncertain identity (perhaps molecricket; see *MSIII*.43).

easily. If you want to make the child vigorous, at the time of [1] eat the flesh of a mother horse.

MSV.9 (lower half, C21) If a woman who is still within the third month of pregnancy swallows two *jueweng* (caterpillar cocoons), the child is a boy.

Another. If you swallow alive three blue-backed bugs from inside *jueweng* (caterpillar cocoons), you invariably give birth to a boy. Myriad perfection.[1]

MSV.10 (lower half, C22) Another. When (the fetus) is just at the stage of the "chewed mass"[2] take *hao* (artemisia), *mu*,[3] and *pixiao* (mantis egg-case)—three substances. Smith and drink them; and you invariably give birth to a boy. Already tested.

Another. Pass one half *sheng* of urine [2] is firm and has little fluid.[4]

MSV.11 (lower half, C23) Another. Take larvae from a beehive and the Yin[5] of a dog. Dry and smith them. Have the pregnant woman drink them, and she gives birth to a boy.

Another. [1] fresh fish [2] eat it.

MSV.12 (lower half, C24) [8] dry and smith them. Toss into liquor [3], and the pregnant woman gives birth to [3] the third month you cannot [1].

MSV.13 (lower half, C25) [8] {1} [14] gives birth to a boy.

MSV.14 (lower half, C26) Another. Take a black [4] the man alone eat the meat and drink the liquid. The woman sits on a mat of fine reeds [?].[6]

---

[1]Another term praising the efficacy of a medicine or treatment.

[2]I.e. the third month of pregnancy. *Guanzi* 39, 14.236, describes the fetus in the third month as resembling a *ju* 咀 (chewed mass).

[3]*MWD*, vol. 4, "Transcription," n. 2, reads *mu* 牡 as *du* 杜, citing the Guo Pu commentary in *Erya*, 8.9b, which identifies *du* as *duheng* 杜衡 (*GM*, 13.70; *ZY*: no. 2094, *Asarum forbesii* Maxim.). *SW*, 6A.4a, glosses *du* as a kind of pear. The reading is plausible, but I also suspect that the scribe might have omitted a graph or graphs following *mu*, meaning that *mu* could designate a male creature or be part of an insect name as in *MSV*.8.

[4]Perhaps the urine is drunk.

[5]I.e. the penis.

[6]*MSV*.14 must be for giving birth to a boy. Compare *MSV*.15 for giving birth to a girl.

MSV.15 (lower half, C27)

If you wish to give birth to a girl, boil a black hen; have the woman alone eat the meat and drink the liquid; and sit on a mat [?].

MSV.16 (lower half, C28)

The way to seek a child. Search for *jiuzong* herb.[1] Then the husband and wife together make liquor with it and drink it.

MSV.17 (lower half, CC29-30)

When the birth is about to take place, first take moist, clean earth from the marketplace. [1] it in a square of three to four *chi* that is three to four *cun* high. After the child is born, set it on the earth. Do not [1], and let the infant [1] on it. When its body is completely covered with earth, bathe it. This makes (the child) vigorous and strong.[2]

MSV.18 (lower half, CC31-32)

After having given birth, incinerate the straw bedding. Put it in water, and [2] the infant to prevent scabby itch.[3] In addition, have the mother drink one half cup of the water used to bathe the infant and the mother will have no further ailments.

---

[1]*Jiuzong* 九 宗 means "nine lineages," connoting fecundity. *MWD*, vol. 4, "Transcription," n. 1, suggests two interpretations of the unknown drug name. It might represent a variant of *guizong* 軌 鬷, an unidentified plant name listed in *Erya*, 8.10a. Alternatively, and less plausibly in my mind, there is a Jiu Zong Mountain 九 嵕 山 in present-day Hubei that has the alternate form 九 宗 山 (Morohashi 1957-60, vol. 1: no. 167.421).

[2]*MSV*.17 describes the preparation of a mound of earth on which the newborn infant is placed and left to move about until coated with the earth. The passage provides remarkable confirmation of Granet's thesis concerning the ritual of placing the newborn infant on the ground for a period of time immediately after birth. Granet uses Han ritual literature and related sources that describe separate rituals for boys and girls to reconstruct an original ritual in which all newborn infants, male and female, are placed on the ground to receive the Yin nurture of "mother" earth (1953: 159-202). According to the ritual literature the infant is left for three days before being taken up by the wetnurse, which Granet identifies as a type of initiatory exposure that precedes the infant's acceptance into the family. We do not know whether the ritual prescriptions were followed to the letter by elite families. However, *MSV*.17 shows that the custom of placing the newborn infant on a mound of earth was practiced; and there can be no doubt that its symbolic significance was as proposed by Granet.

[3]The infant must be bathed in the water, since the mother then drinks some of the bath water.

MSV.19 (lower half, CC33-34)

When a woman who has few children gives birth, have another person carry the [1] and leave [2] wash the afterbirth. Wrap in new cloth; seal by binding it thrice around; and put it into [1]. Have the mother hold it herself; enter a stream-gulch [3] it thrice; set it down and leave; and return home without looking back. Then have someone else bury it well.

*MS*VI.A

SHIWEN

十問

TEN QUESTIONS

*MS*VI.A.1 (SS1-7)

The Yellow Thearch asked the Heavenly Teacher:[1] "The myriad creatures, how are they able to move? Grasses and wood, how are they able to grow? The sun and moon, how are they able to glow?"

The Heavenly Teacher said: "When you examine heaven's nature, Yin and Yang are the rulers. Having lost them, the myriad creatures are discontinued; having obtained them, they thrive. Eat Yin and secure Yang; attain spirit illumination.[2]

"The way to eat Yin:[3] Empty your five depots and disperse your three malignancies,[4] as if unable to evacuate them—this being what is prized in the diet of elemental stuff.[5]

---

[1]Heavenly Teacher (*tianshi* 天師) is a title by which the Yellow Thearch's teacher Qi Bo 岐伯 is known in the *Huangdi neijing* (see *Suwen* 1, 1.1b). The title occurs elsewhere in early literature; for example, the Yellow Thearch honors a sagacious youngster as Heavenly Teacher in *Zhuangzi* 24, 361. The person addressed as Heavenly Teacher in *MS*VI.A.1 is not known (Qi Bo is an extremely unlikely candidate). In Later Han religious Daoist movements the title *tianshi* (usually translated Celestial Master) acquired added significance (Seidel 1969: 74-84, 112-14).

[2]The idea that the Yin element of the body—especially the male body—is most vulnerable to decay runs through the Mawangdui macrobiotic hygiene texts. Sexual cultivation is one, but not the only, way to ensure that the fullness of Yin is maintained (see Prolegomena, Section Four, "Body and Spirit").

[3]The Heavenly Teacher's method of eating Yin is a breath cultivation technique written in verse.

[4]"Disperse" translates *guang* 廣. I interpret the word like *kuang* 曠, meaning "abandon, discard" (see *Lüshi chunqiu*, 22. 287). The denotation of the term "three malignancies" (*sanjiu* 三咎) is not known. In *MS*VI.A.4 the "four malignancies" refer to four harmful vapors that must be avoided when practicing breath cultivation. Presumably anything harmful to physical and spiritual well-being constitutes a "malignancy."

[5]"Evacuate" translates *chu/*thjəd* 出, which rhymes with *gui/*gwjiəd* 貴 (prize) in the final phrase. I follow *MWD*, vol. 4, "Transcription," n. 2, in reading *wu/*ʔuk* 楃 as a phonetic loan for *pu/*phuk* 樸 (elemental stuff). The loan usage is confirmed by the use of 楃 to write 樸 in the first Mawangdui *Laozi* edition (*MWD*, vol. 1: 12; corresponding to *Laozi*,

"Still your spirit wind, make fast your two racks, triply pound, and let nothing escape.[1] The spirit wind then is born; the five tones then are matched.[2]

"Suck it in not more than five times, bring it to the mouth, and still it with the heart—this being what the four assistants prize.[3] The dark winepot then arrives.[4]

---

par. 28, in the received text). The interchange between a glottal/velar initial and a labial is unusual, but not unknown. For example, *SW*, 7B.17a, explains that *ba/*priat* 八 is the phonetic in *xue/*gwit* 穴. My punctuation differs from the "Transcription," which fails to recognize the rhyming between *chu/*tjkəd* and *gui/*gwjiəd*. *Pushi* 樸 食 as a term for some kind of macrobiotic diet may be related to *sushi* 素 食, which refers to a diet of plants gathered from the wild in *Mozi* 6, 1.20, and other early sources.

[1]Beginning with "spirit wind" (*shenfeng* 神 風), much of the technique is presented in metaphorical language. The spirit wind seems to refer to a quality of breath that exists internally and is at the same time linked to the external atmosphere. It is activated by forcefully holding the breath—for "triply pound" see *MS*I.A.6—so that "nothing escapes." *Zhi* 梼 (rack) is glossed in *SW*, 6A.47b, as a name for the vertical rack used for silkworm cultivation. I suspect that the "two racks" denote the ribcage.

[2]The "five tones (*wusheng* 五 聲) being matched" signifies perfect harmony in the cosmos (see the use of the synonymous *wuyin* 五 音 in *Lüshi chunqiu*, 3.33). I understand the birth of the spirit wind and the matching of the five tones to mean that there is consonance between the internal and external, and the person can begin to inhale external vapor. *Wusheng* and *wuyin* have another denotation in *MS*VI.A.3, 10; *MS*VI.B.6; and *MS*VII.B.15, 20. There they refer to signs of arousal coming from the woman's mouth during intercourse.

[3]Having inhaled vapor through the nose, it is brought to the mouth. "Still" translates *mei* 枚, which as a noun refers to a wooden bit placed in the mouth to block unwanted speech (see *Zhouli*, 34.6a, and Zheng Xuan commentary). I understand "still it with the heart" to mean that the person subjects the vapor in the mouth to the "stilling device" of the heart. *Sifu* 四 輔 (four assistants) is well attested as a term for the ruler's chief administrators; and also occurs in this sense in one of the writings preceding the second Mawangdui *Laozi* edition (*MWD*, vol. 1: 66). In *MS*VI.A.1 the term must be related to the heart's function as the ruler of the body; and I identify the "four assistants" as the four limbs. *MWD*, vol. 4, "Transcription," n. 5, interprets *mei* in the sense of "gather, collect"; giving the translation, "collect it (i.e. the vapor) in the heart." The interpretation is grammatically acceptable, but the technique at this point focuses on vapor in the mouth that is in the process of being transformed into saliva and swallowed. In my judgment the technique uses the heart/ruler to effect this transformation in the mouth, whereas the collection of vapor in the heart seems out of place in the overall progression of the technique.

[4]"Dark winepot" translates *xuanzun* 玄 尊, attested in *Lüshi chunqiu*, 5.50, and glossed in the Gao You commentary as *mingshui* 明 水 (bright water; a name for a holy water used in worship). The synonymous *xuanjiu* 玄 酒 (dark liquor) is described as the highest grade of *mingshui* in *Liji*, 26.7a, in a passage concerning various items appropriate for worshipping the *shenming* 神 明 (in this context not the physio-spiritual "spirit illumination," but the glowing manifestation of the spirits of the other world). According to the Zheng Xuan commentary, the liquid is "water obtained from the moon using the Yin mirror (a metal pan in which moon dew condenses)." Although not attested as a physiological metaphor in received literature, it is clear that "dark winepot" denotes saliva in *MS*VI.A.1. This saliva is

"Drink it not more than five times; the mouth invariably finds the taste sweet.[1] Bring it to the five depots. The form then is extremely relaxed.[2]

"Make it spread[3] to your flesh and skin, and reach to those hair tips. The hair vessels then are permeated.[4] The Yin water then arrives, drenching that Yang blaze.[5] Firm, sturdy, and undying; drink and food enter the body as guests.[6]

---

a purified concentrate produced inside the mouth from the inhaled vapor. A related term *lingzun* 靈 尊 (numinous winepot) occurs in *MS*VI.A.4. Saliva ingestion was regularly practiced in religious Daoist hygiene (Maspero 1981: 489-94; Needham 1954, vol. 5, part 5: 150-51).

There is an interesting parallel between the technique and religious worship, since the final result of swallowing the saliva is to "penetrate spirit illumination (*shenming*)," just as the final result of worship is communication with the *shenming*. The religious interaction between human and spirit worlds has become in macrobiotic hygiene an individualized internal transformation.

[1]The dark winepot/saliva is swallowed, its taste sweet like liquor. The phrase 口 必 甘 味 "the mouth invariably finds the taste sweet" also occurs in *Lüshi chunqiu*, 3.26, in a passage related to dietetics (see the discussion in the Prolegomena, Section Four, "Philosophy and Macrobiotic Hygiene").

[2]For *tui* 退 in the sense of "relaxed," see *Liji*, 10.16a, and Zheng Xuan commentary.

[3]*MWD*, vol. 4, "Transcription," transcribes 搏, read as *fu* 溥 (spread). Qiu Xigui argues that the graph is 摶, read as *zhuan* 摶 (concentrate; 1992: 535). Li Xueqin (personal communication) suggests 搏. Distinguishing between 尃 and 專 in Qin and Han manuscripts is often difficult, and there is also the possibility of the scribe having erroneously written one when the other was intended. The word *fu* 溥 best fits the context of *MS*VI.A.1, thus I follow Li Xueqin's transcription of the graph and the "Transcription" reading.

[4]The term *maomai* 毛 脈 (hair vessels) occurs in *Guoyu*, 17.8a, in a context where it seems to denote hair (hair perceived as fine thread-like extrusions of the body's vessels). *Suwen* 21, 7.2a, uses *maomai* in a more technical sense in a description of the circulation of vapor in the body; after the lungs distribute vapor to the skin and hair, the "hair vessels" transmit the vapor to a central cavity. While the concept of "hair vessels" in *Suwen* theories of vapor circulation cannot be applied directly to *MS*VI.A.1, it is evident that by "permeating the hair vessels" the vapor/saliva has been distributed to the outer limits of the body.

[5]"Yin water" (Yin *shui* 陰 水) and "Yang blaze" (Yang *fu* 陽 炥) are the complementary elements of water and fire in the body of the person practicing the technique, the latter evidently pre-existing as a kind of central forge and the former generated by the technique. According to the Duan Yucai commentary in *SW*, 10A.42b, *fu* is an orthographic variant of *fu* 燹, which refers to a conflagration. I have not found either term attested in received literature. Although their precise denotations are unknown, using the cooling Yin water to temper the Yang heat of the internal blaze is clearly the actualization of the Heavenly Teacher's instruction to "consume Yin and secure Yang." As physiological metaphors, Yang blaze and Yin water anticipate the alchemical imagery of religious Daoist hygiene.

[6]Having prepared the body according to the technique, the person now realizes the ultimate benefit: all food and drink brought into this revitalized body "enter as guests" (*bin* 賓), meaning that they provide the ideal nurture. It is possible that 賓 should be read as *shi* 實, giving the translation "drink and food fill the body." *Wanwu* contains a clear case of

"This is called the 'doubly marvelous recipe to penetrate spirit illumination.' "[1]

The way of the Heavenly Teacher to eat spirit vapor.[2]

*MS*VI.A.2 (SS8-14)

The Yellow Thearch asked Great Perfection:[3] "What do people lose so that their facial complexion is coarse and dun, blackened and dark green? What do people obtain so that the skin's webbed pattern is smooth and lustrous, freshly white and glowing?"

Great Perfection replied: "If your lordship wishes to refine a complexion that is freshly white, then examine the measuring worm. The measuring worm recipe for eating penetrates Yin and Yang. When it eats something dark green it becomes dark green; when it eats something yellow it becomes yellow. Solely on the basis of what your lordship eats you will turn into the five colors.[4]

"Your lordship must make eating Yin your constant; supplementing it with *bai* (arbor-vitae) fruit is quite excellent. By drinking running beasts' wellspring blossom[5] you can repel agedness and restore vigor, becoming lustrous and glowing.

---

scribal error in the drug name *lanbin* 蘭 賓, which should be *lanshi* 蘭 實 (eupatorium fruit; see Fuyang Han jian zhenglizu 1988: 37). *Bin* and *shi* fit the context in *MS*VI.A.1 equally well, making it difficult to judge whether scribal error has occurred.

[1]In my judgment *fuqi* 復 奇 (doubly marvelous) adds embellishment to a recipe for "penetrating spirit illumination." The compound *qifang* 奇 方 (marvelous recipe) is attested in *Shiji*, 28.31b, in connection with occult arts. Ma Jixing interprets *fuqi* to mean "recovering from irregularity" (1992: 877, n. 8); and Wei and Hu offer the interpretation "replenish Yang" (equating *qi* with Yang; 1992, vol. 2: 97, n. 25).

[2]The concluding line serves as a title for the technique described by the Heavenly Teacher. The same formula occurs in *MS*VI.A.2, 3, 5, 7, 8.

[3]Great Perfection 大 成 is attested as both an epithet and proper name in early sources. *Zhuangzi* 20, 298, attributes a teaching to the "man of Great Perfection"; and *Xinxu*, 5.71, recounts that Yu 禹 studied with Great Perfection.

[4]The measuring worm (*chihuo* 尺 蠖) is a caterpillar most often noticed for its movement—a contraction followed by a stretch that matches the ideal of *qushen* 屈 伸 (curling and stretching) in macrobiotic hygiene (see *MS*VI.A.8). There is a measuring worm exercise in the *Yinshu*; and a measuring worm sexual position in *MS*VI.B.3 and *MS*VII.B.10 (see *MS*VI.B.3). *Yanzi chunqiu*, 8.219, and *Shuoyuan*, 1.12b, record the same figurative use of the measuring worm's diet as in *MS*VI.A.2. However, the fact that its body becomes yellow and dark green when it eats yellow and dark green things serves as an analogy for court sycophants (who "eat" the ruler and become exactly like him) rather than to make the point that you are what you eat.

[5]"Wellspring blossom" translates *quanying* 泉 英. The term is attested in *Guanzi* 58, 19.312, as a technical name for a type of high mountain with a wellspring at the summit. In *MS*VI.A.7 *quanying* denotes an internal fluid (neither saliva nor semen) that the practitioner "drinks" in the course of cultivation. The usage indicates an analogy between human

"When coitus with Yin[1] is expected to be frequent, follow it with flying creatures. The spring dickeybird's round egg arouses that crowing cock. The crowing cock has an essence. If you are truly able to ingest this, the jade whip is reborn.[2] Best is engaging the member.[3] Block that jade hole.[4] When brimming then have intercourse, and bid farewell with round eggs. If the member is not engaged, conserve it with roasted-wheat meal.[5] If truly able to ingest this, you can raise the dead."[6]

Great Perfection's way to raise the dead and eat bird essence.

*MS*VI.A.3 (SS15-22)

The Yellow Thearch asked Cao Ao:[7] "What do people lose so that they die? What do people obtain so that they live?"

Cao Ao replied: "[5] and take the essence. Attend to that conjoining of vapor and lightly move her form.[8] When able to move her form and bring forth the five tones, then absorb her essence.[9] Those

---

physiology and mountain topography. *MWD*, vol. 4, "Transcription," n. 4, suggests that "running beasts' wellspring blossom" refers to cow and sheep milk. While the identification is plausible (and horse might also be added to the list of milk-producing "running beasts"), I suspect that wellspring blossom may not be restricted to milk alone. Zhou and Xiao suggest that animal semen and decoctions of male animal genitals might also be included (1988: 370, n. 8); and animal saliva is not improbable.

[1]*Jie* Yin 接 陰 (coitus with Yin) is a standard term for sexual intercourse in received literature.

[2]The jade whip is the penis (see *MS*III.38). Eating eggs and the flesh of fowl to bolster Yang vitality is described in several recipes in *MSS*III-IV; e.g. *MS*III.11, 15, 17; and *MS*IV.4, 24. Crowing cock (*mingxiong* 鳴 雄) appears to have a double reference to the rooster and to the male genitals. Rooster is the chief ingredient in *MS*III.11 for a food that increases a man's endurance during sexual encounters. At the same time, *MS*VI.A.6 teaches that the ideal diet combines eating with cultivating "penile vapor." Thus the crowing cock's essence may be that of the man's own genitals, which the man cultivates while eating dickeybird egg to revitalize the jade whip.

[3]I follow Ma Jixing (1992: 885, n. 1) in reading 埶 as *shi* 勢, and interpreting it as the male genitals (member). The usage is attested in the Han period prophecy text *Shangshu xingde fang* 尚 書 刑 德 放 (Yasui and Nakamura 1971-92, vol. 2: 65).

[4]I.e. the vagina.

[5]"Roasted-wheat meal" translates *feng* 麷, which refers to a form of *qiu* 糗 (roasted-grain meal) using wheat (see *SW*, 5B.34b, and Duan Yucai commentary). Recipes for bolstering Yang vitality that include roasted-grain meal are in *MS*III.13, 17.

[6]The limp penis is often described as "dead." Thus to "raise the dead" is to revitalize the penis.

[7]The name Cao Ao 曹 敖 is not attested in received literature.

[8]*Heqi* 合 氣 (conjoin vapor) refers to sexual intercourse; see *MS*III.89.

[9]The *wusheng* 五 聲 (five tones) and the similar *wuyin* 五 音 (five sounds) in *MS*VI.A.10 refer to sounds made by the woman during intercourse. They are probably to be identified with the *wuyin* in *MS*VI.B.6 and *MS*VII.B.15, which refer to five signs of arousal coming

who are empty can be made brimming full; the vigorous can be made to flourish lastingly; the aged can be made to live long.

"The procedure for living long is to carefully[1] employ the jade closure.[2] When at the right times the jade closure enfolds,[3] spirit illumination arrives and accumulates. Accumulating, it invariably manifests radiance. When the jade closure firms the essence, this

---

from the woman's mouth (mostly audible, but biting is included as one of the "sounds"). *MSVI.A.3* and *MSVI.A.10* both portray the man as actively stimulating the woman to produce the "five tones/sounds," which constitute positive evidence of the harmonization at work in sexual cultivation (similar to the harmonization of the "five tones" in the breath cultivation technique in *MSVI.A.1*).

[1]傎 in *MWD*, vol. 4, "Transcription," should be transcribed as *shen* 慎 (carefully).

[2]"Jade closure" translates *yubi* 玉閉. The term is not attested in received literature. *Bi*, however, is a standard term for concentrating vapor and essence inside the body by "enclosing" them. In later religious Daoist hygiene this usually involved holding one's breath according to a specified technique, followed by exhalation (Maspero 1981: 463, 495). The same verbal usage of *bi* occurs in *MSVI.A.4*, which states: "By filling what lies below and enclosing essence (*bi jing* 閉精), vapor does not leak out." The "jade closure" appears to be a physiological metaphor designating a place inside the body where vapor and essence are enclosed. The term appears again in *MSVII.B.3*: "The matter of spirit illumination lies in what is enclosed (*bi*). Vigilantly control the jade closure, and spirit illumination will arrive." As in *MSVI.A.3*, careful use of the jade closure to "enclose" facilitates the arrival of spirit illumination. In addition, both passages concern sexual cultivation as well as breath cultivation; thus there are two sources for the vapor and essence being enclosed inside the body. Wei and Hu compare the "jade closure" to the *guan* 關 (barrier; 1992, vol. 2: 102, n. 4). *Guan* is attested in *Shenjian* 3, 17, as a term for an internal barrier located near the navel where Han-time practitioners of macrobiotic hygiene stored vapor and essence; and this meaning of *guan* entered the terminology of religious Daoist physiology (Maspero 1981: 491). I agree that the idea of the "jade closure" may be similar to the later-attested "barrier," and that it is probably in the abdominal region, but I would refrain from identifying the former exactly with the latter. It is also possible that the "jade closure" is not an anatomical term, but rather designates the act of "enclosing vapor/essence." To "employ the jade closure" might then mean to practice the technique of either holding the breath or enclosing vapor in some other fashion (this is the interpretation in Ma Jixing 1992: 890, n. 2).

[3]I read *bi/*pjik* 辟 as *bi* 襞, glossed in *SW*, 8A.62a, as "fold clothing" (the use of the former graph in the sense of the latter is also attested in Han sources). The word is not attested in a physiological denotation, but I suspect that the extended meaning "enfold" is similar to *bi/*pid* 閉 (enclose; for which it cannot be a phonetic loan). *Bi* 辟 might also be understood in its sense of "wall, embankment" (as in *biyong* 辟廱, the "moated enclosure" in the ideal plan of a royal capital) to refer to the enclosing function of the jade closure. Wei and Hu understand *bi* in the sense of "open"; giving the translation, "the jade closure opens" (1992, vol. 2: 102, n. 5). However, this meaning does not best fit the context of *MSVI.A.3* or *MSVII.B.3*, which both focus on an act of "enclosing" that causes vapor and essence to accumulate and spirit illumination to arrive.

invariably ensures that the jade wellspring is not upset.[1] Then the hundred ailments do not occur; thus you can live long.

"In the way of coitus with Yin, stay the heart, settle and secure it; and the form and vapor secure one another.[2] Thus it is said: at the first arrival without emission, ears and eyes are perceptive and bright;[3] at the second arrival without emission, the voice's vapor rises high;[4] at the third arrival without emission, skin and hide glow; at the fourth arrival without emission, spine and upper side suffer no injury; at the fifth arrival without emission, buttock and ham can be squared; at the sixth arrival without emission, the hundred vessels pass clear through;[5] at the seventh arrival without emission, your entire life is without calamity; at the eighth arrival without emission, you can have a lengthy longevity; at the ninth arrival without emission, you penetrate spirit illumination."

Cao Ao's way for coitus with Yin and cultivating spirit vapor.

---

[1] *Yuquan* 玉泉 (jade wellspring) occurs again in association with the jade closure, breath cultivation, and sexual cultivation in *MS*VII.B.3. In religious Daoist hygiene *yuquan* is sometimes identified as the pool of saliva beneath the tongue and sometimes as the *bao* 胞 (the bladder or a place where essence is stored; see the Liangqiuzi commentary to the *Huangting neijing jing* in *Yunji qiqian*, 11.17a and 12.20a). *Zhenjiu jiayi jing*, 3.34b, gives *yuquan* as another name for *zhongji* 中極 (inner bourne), which it identifies as the chief acupuncture point associated with the bladder (see *MS*VI.B.8 for other denotations of *zhongji*). Based on the location of the jade wellspring inside the jade closure and the later identifications, I would identify the jade wellspring in *MS*VI.A.3 as a reservoir in the abdominal region where vapor and essence are stored. "Upsetting" the jade wellspring would result in the loss of vapor and essence.

[2] The reference to "staying the heart" is reminiscent of *Guanzi* 49, 16.270: "When a stable heart is situated inside, the ears and eyes are perceptive and bright; the four limbs are firm and solid; and you can be an abode for essence." The role of the heart (in the form of the will) in overseeing the body's needs is mentioned in *MS*VI.A.8.

[3] "Arrival" (*zhi* 至) refers to thrusting the penis inside the vagina. Parallels in *MS*VI.B.2 and *MS*VII.B.3 refer to thrusting the penis as "movement" (*dong* 動). According to *MS*VI.B.2, ten thrusts constitute one movement and there are ten movements for a total of one hundred thrusts. For every movement (ten thrusts) through the tenth (one hundred thrusts) that the man prolongs intercourse without ejaculating the benefits of sexual cultivation grow ever greater. The parallel in *MS*VII.B.3 concludes the passage concerning the jade closure, just as the listing of nine "arrivals" concludes Cao Ao's teaching.

[4] I.e. the voice has beauty and clarity.

[5] I.e. vapor passes freely through the vessels.

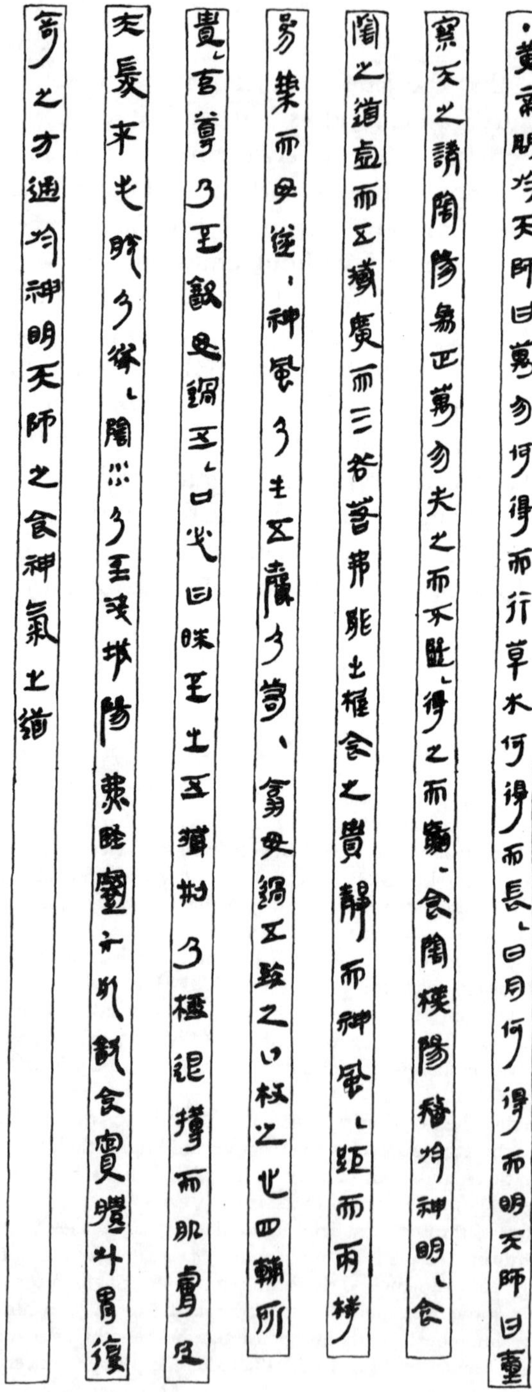

Fig. 17 Facsimile of *MS*VI.A.1

*MS*VI.A.4
(SS23–39, SS52–59)

The Yellow Thearch asked Rong Cheng:[1] "When people first dispense the purity that flows into the form, what is obtained so that life occurs?[2] When flowing into the form produces a body, what is lost so that death occurs? Among people of the age, why are some foul while others are fair; why do some die young while others are longlived? I wish to hear the reason why people's vapor thrives or shrinks, why it slackens or expands."

Rong Cheng replied: "If your lordship wishes to be longlived, then comply with and examine the way of heaven and earth. The vapor of heaven is monthly exhausted and monthly replenished; thus it is able to live long. The vapor of earth during the year is cold and hot, and the precipitous and the gentle complement one another; thus the earth endures and does not deteriorate. Your lordship must examine the nature of heaven and earth, and put it into practice with your body.[3]

"There are signs that can be known. At present it is not within the ability of even the sage. Only the person of the way knows it.[4] The culminant essence of heaven and earth is born in the signless, grows in the formless, and is perfected in the bodiless. He who ob-

---

[1]The *Liexian zhuan* identifies Rong Cheng 容成 as the Yellow Thearch's teacher; and describes his mastery of the full range of macrobiotic hygiene (Kaltenmark 1953: 55–58). Rong Cheng's role as a patron of sexual cultivation is attested in the book *Rong Cheng Yin dao* 容成陰道 (Rong Cheng's way of Yin), whose title is recorded in *Hanshu*, 30.80b.

[2]*Liuxing* 溜刑 (flow into the form) is the term for the first month of gestation in *MS*V.3. The Yellow Thearch is asking how intercourse and conception lead to the production of a life.

[3]The description of the vapor of earth is reminiscent of a passage in the *Yijing*, "Xici zhuan," 8.6a: "When coldness goes, heat comes; when heat goes, coldness comes. Cold and hot succeed one another and the year is thereby completed." For the use of *xianyi* 險易 in the sense of "precipitous and gentle (terrain)," see *Shiji*, 71.8a; for *xiangqu* 相取 in the sense of "complement one another," see *Yijing*, 8.14b.

[4]"The person of the way" (*daozhe* 道者) is mentioned again in *MS*VI.A.6 and *MS*VI.A.9. Presumably the way is the "way of macrobiotic hygiene." At the same time, the concept of Way as the ultimate quiddity was already accepted doctrine in the third century B.C., giving rise to a new form of cosmo-political thought. In referring to the *daozhe* there is a connotation of universality that extends beyond macrobiotic hygiene. The ability to achieve universality is the reason for ranking the person of the way above the sage (*sheng* 聖).

tains it has a lengthy longevity, he who loses it dies young.[1] Thus he who is skilled at cultivating vapor and concentrating essence accumulates the signless. Essence and spirit overflow like a wellspring.[2] Suck in the sweet dew and have it accumulate. Drink the blue-gem wellspring and numinous winepot and make it circulate.[3] Eliminate the foul and love the habitual,[4] and spirit then flows into the form.[5]

"The way to suck in vapor: it must be made to reach to the extremities, so that essence is generated and not deficient. Above and below are all essence; cold and warm are tranquilly generated.[6]

---

[1]*Huainanzi* often uses "formless" (*wuxing* 無形) as an epithet for Way or One (*yi* 一). For example, *Huainanzi*, 1.10: "Now then, the formless is the great ancestor of creatures"; and 1.11: "The term 'formless' refers to One; and One means that it is something without peer in Under-heaven." *Huainanzi*, 7.104, describes the person who cultivates the Way as "bodiless" (*wuti* 無體) as well as formless: "When moving he is formless; when still he is bodiless" (according to the Gao Yu commentary, "being formless and bodiless is the manner of Way"). *Guanzi* 49, 16.272, attests to the notion of Way as "signless" (*wuzheng* 無徵): "It is ever so that when a person is born heaven puts forth the essence and earth puts forth the form, and that these are conjoined to make the person. If harmonized, birth occurs; if not harmonized, it does not. Examining the way of harmonization, the essence is not visible and the signs (*zheng*) are not manifest." And *Guanzi* 49, 16.269, provides the oldest statement of obtaining Way as the key to life: "(Way) is something that when people lose it, they die; and when they obtain it, they live."

[2]The *locus classicus* for *zhuan* 摶 in the sense of "concentrate (vapor/essence)" is *Guanzi* 49, 16.271: "Concentrate vapor spirit-like, and store the myriad creatures in their entirety." *Guanzi* 49, 16.270 is the source of the wellspring as a physiological metaphor: "When essence is stored it gives birth of itself. The outside is peaceful and flourishing; inside it is deposited to form a wellspring source. Flood-like, harmonious, and even, it becomes a deep pool of vapor. When the pool does not go dry, the four limbs are solid; when the wellspring is not exhausted, the nine apertures penetrate."

[3]The *locus classicus* for "sweet dew" (*ganlu* 甘露) is *Laozi*, par. 32 (*MWD*, vol. 1: 123): "Heaven and earth conjoin and send down sweet dew." Rong Cheng's teaching demonstrates the incorporation of sweet dew into breath cultivation terminology. I suspect that sweet dew refers to a particular form of inhaled vapor (compare the "spirit wind" in *MSVI.A.1*). Once the sweet dew accumulates, saliva forms—referred to as the "blue-gem wellspring" (*yaoquan* 瑤泉) and the "numinous winepot" (*lingzun* 靈尊). The "numinous winepot" is synonymous with the "dark winepot" in *MSVI.A.1*. The "blue-gem wellspring" suggests the "blue-gem pool" (*yaochi* 瑤池) at Mount Kunlun 崑崙 where the Queen Mother of the West exchanged a toast with King Mu of the Zhou (*Mu tianzi zhuan*, 3.1a). Tang Daoist adepts also associated the mythical geography of Kunlun with breath cultivation. Schafer explains the use of the term *bijin* 碧津 (cyan exudate) to denote saliva as an allusion to the blue-gem pool at Kunlun (1981: 405, n. 110).

[4]I understand *su* 俗 (habitual) in the sense of good habits that are treated as norms and regularly cultivated (see *SW*, 8A.23b, and Duan Yucai commentary).

[5]Since "flowing into the form" is what occurs during the first month of gestation, for breath cultivation to result in "spirit flowing into the form" suggests a kind of rebirth.

[6]For cold and warm to be tranquilly (*an* 安) generated suggests the natural alternation between cold and hot that is characteristic of the vapor of earth (see above). *MWD*, vol. 4,

Breathing must be deep and long, so that the new vapor is easy to hold. The old vapor is that of agedness, the new vapor that of longevity. He who is skilled at cultivating vapor lets the old vapor disperse at night and the new vapor gather at dawn,[1] thereby penetrating the nine apertures and filling the six cavities.[2]

"When eating vapor there are prohibitions. In spring avoid Turbid Yang; in summer avoid Scalding Wind; in autumn avoid Frost Mist; in winter avoid Frozen Yin. You must eliminate the four malignancies, then breathe deeply to become longlived.[3]

"The goal of dawn breathing: during the egress, endeavor to join with heaven. During the ingress, gauge that dual-entry doorway[4] as

---

"Transcription" understands *an* as an interrogative, giving the translation "how would cold and warm occur." In my judgment the notion of cold and warm as pathogenic conditions is improbable in the present context.

[1]I.e. old vapor must be voided from the body at night in preparation for inhaling new vapor at dawn. The passage on "dawn breathing" below similarly describes "daily exhausting stale vapor" and "daily replenishing new vapor." I suspect that the technique involves a nighttime exhalation exercise followed by a morning inhalation exercise. Rong Cheng's teaching anticipates religious Daoist hygiene, which divides the day into periods of daytime "living vapor" and nighttime "dead vapor"—daytime being defined either as sunrise to sunset or as midnight to noon. Breath cultivation should only be practiced during the time of "living vapor" (Maspero 1981: 500-501). Rong Cheng's teaching also exemplifies the slogan "spit out the old and ingest the new" associated with macrobiotic hygiene in *Zhuangzi* 15, 237.

[2]The nine apertures are the mouth, ears, eyes, nostrils, genitals, and anus. The six cavities (*liufu* 六 腑) are identified in *Suwen* 4, 1.16a, as: gall bladder, stomach, large intestine, small intestine, bladder, and "triple burner" (*sanjiao* 三 焦; the only cavity that is more a theoretical construct than a readily identifiable part of the body). The *Suwen* classifies the six cavities as Yang, complementing the five depots (*wuzang*; liver, heart, spleen, lung, kidney) which are Yin. There is no evidence in the Mawangdui medical manuscripts of the physiological theories involving depots and cavities that are detailed in the *Huangdi neijing*. And while the "triple burner" is also attested in *Shiji*, 105.5b, it is doubtful that it is one of the six cavities in the Mawangdui manuscripts. A quotation from the *Hanshi waizhuan* in *Taiping yulan*, 363.2b, gives "gullet" as the sixth cavity instead of "triple burner."

[3]The four vapors to be avoided are the same vapors described in *MS*II.A.

[4]I read 誷 as *liang* 兩 (dual); and I identify the "dual-entry doorway" (*guiliang* 閨 兩) as the nostrils. *SW*, 12A.8a, glosses *gui* as follows: "It is a doorway that stands singly. The top is round and the bottom square, like the shape of the *gui* 圭 (jade tablet)." The nostrils constitute a pair of single-entry doorways of the same shape, hence the physiological metaphor *guiliang*. In addition, the etymological analysis of *liang* (originally written 兩) in *SW*, 7B.39a-b, suggests that the graph itself might be seen to depict the nose: "It is composed of 冂 (the cover), of 从 (two points of entry), and of 丨 (the divider between the two points of entry)." Received sources indicate that vapor is supposed to be inhaled through the nose during breath cultivation, and supply other metaphors for the nostrils. According to the "Heshang gong" commentary to *Laozi*, par. 10, the term *tianmen* 天 門 (heaven gate)

if storing it in a deep pool. Then the stale vapor is daily exhausted, and the new vapor is daily replenished. Then the form possesses billowing radiance and is filled with essence; thus it is able to last long. The goal of daytime breathing: exhaling and inhaling must be light, and ears and eyes are perceptive and bright. Spreading[1] vapor permeates,[2] and inside there is neither blockage[3] nor decay; thus the body is without affliction and calamity. The goal of dusk breathing: breathe deeply, long and slow, causing the ears to not hear; and when tranquil go to bed. The ethereal-spirit and earthly-spirit are at ease in the form; thus you can live long. When breathing at midnight: after awakening do not change from the sleeping posture; do it deeply and slowly, without exertion,[4] and the six cavities all open. Make long duration your ideal. If you wish to make the spirit longlived, you must breathe with the skin's webbed pattern.

"The essence[5] of cultivating vapor is to exit from death and enter into life. With zest and gusto, let the taste suckle.[6] To fill the form with this is called concentrating essence. To cultivate vapor there is a norm; the task lies in accumulating essence. When essence reaches fullness, it invariably drains; and when essence is lost, it must be replenished.[7] As for the time to replenish what drained, coordinate it with sleep.[8] Exit and enter, thereby improving the skin's webbed

---

refers both to the entrance to heaven and to the nostrils (*Daode zhenjing zhu*, 1.8a). For the role of the nose in religious Daoist breath cultivation, see Maspero 1981: 491–94.

[1]悖 in *MWD*, vol. 4, "Transcription," should be transcribed as 挚, an unattested graph. I read it as *ao* 敖, glossed in *SW*, 6B.2b, with *you* 游 (travel, drift, spread).

[2]"Permeates" translates *yinyin* 陰 陰. For use of the compound in the sense of "pervasive" (literally, something that "overshadows" everything else), see *Hanshu*, 22.20b.

[3]"Blockage" translates *hui* 薈, based on the gloss in *Guangya*, 2B.6b.

[4]執 in *MWD*, vol. 4, "Transcription," should be transcribed as 埶 and read as *shi* 勢, in the sense of "exert."

[5]This is one of the rare occasions when *jing* 精 means the "essential thing" rather than physio-spiritual essence.

[6]I read *mi/*miəd* 咪 as a phonetic loan for *wei/*mjəd* 味 (taste). *Nou* 穀 is glossed as "suckle" in *SW*, 14B.25a.

[7]The same hygienic principle of replenishment is enunciated in the *Maishu*: "When the vessels are brimful, drain them; when empty, fill them; when still, stay in attendance on them" (*MSSW*: 74). The passage in *MSVI.A.4* is also reminiscent of *Suwen* 17, 5.3b: "When replenishing and draining do not fail to be as one with heaven and earth. To grasp the nature of One is to know death and life. Therefore, tones conjoin with the Five Sounds, colors conjoin with the Five Agents, and the vessels conjoin with Yin and Yang."

[8]The end of the sentence coincides with the bottom of S39. S40 is clearly misplaced in *MWD*, vol. 4, "Transcription," and I follow Qiu Xigui in moving S40 to *MSVI.A.8* between S72 and S73 where the text fits the context perfectly (1992: 525–27). I further agree

pattern.[1] When the firm and white is perfected inside, what ailment can occur?[2]

"If there is a calamity for that life, it is invariably because Yin essence leaks out; and the hundred vessels are clogged and derelict. Joy and anger are untimely, the person is ignorant of the great way, and the vapor of life departs from him. The vulgar man lives blindly, and then relies on shaman physicians. Before reaching middle age,[3] his form invariably is buried young. To kill yourself by toiling at affairs[4] is truly a grievous and sorrowful thing.

"Wherever life and death lie, the penetrating gentleman controls it. By filling what lies below and enclosing essence, vapor does not leak out. When the heart controls death and life, who is defeated by

---

with Qiu that the text of S41 does not connect well with S39 as the conclusion to *MSVI.A.4*. Based on consideration of the overall content of *MSVI.A.4*, Qiu suggests moving SS52–59 from *MSVI.A.6* to follow S39; and moving S41 from *MSVI.A.4* to follow S51 as the conclusion to *MSVI.A.6*. Although not noted by Qiu, there is a parallel to his rearranged text of *MSVI.A.4* in *MSVII.B.3* that adds support to his argument. The parallel begins with the exact statement concerning cultivation given above: "The task lies in accumulating essence"; continues with a similar discussion of the need to drain and replenish essence; and proceeds to a description of sexual cultivation that includes the instruction to "lightly exit and lightly enter" (referring to the penis in the vagina). The instruction to "coordinate (replenishment) with sleep" at the bottom of S39 followed by "exit and enter" at the top of S52 makes the same transition to a description of sexual cultivation. In addition, S41 appears to provide a satisfactory conclusion to *MSVI.A.6*. Although the basis for the rearrangement is contextual, the diagram of the original positions of the bamboo slips when the manuscript was first excavated (in *MWD*, vol. 4: 152) does not definitely prove the sequence of the slips in *MWD*, vol. 4, nor does it disprove Qiu's rearrangement. It is also possible that the manuscript as excavated is defective, that a slip or slips with text belonging to *MSVI.A.4* or *MSVI.A.6* were missing when the bound manuscript was put into the tomb. Qiu himself regards his rearrangement of the slips as tentative, but superior to *MWD*, vol. 4; and I accept the rearrangement with the same sense of caution.

[1]美 in *MWD*, vol. 4, "Transcription," should be transcribed as *zou* 奏, read as *zou* 腠 (skin's webbed pattern). The top part of the original graph is indistinct and may have been miswritten by the scribe, but the graph itself is clearly not 美 (and is very close to the writing of *zou* in S38).

[2]*MSVI.A.10* describes the five depots as "becoming firm and white, their jade color having a renewed glow." The meaning in *MSVI.A.4* must be similar, referring to the jade-like condition of the body resulting from the cultivation of vapor and essence.

[3]桼 十 in *MWD*, vol. 4, "Transcription," should be transcribed as *weiban* 未 半 (not yet half; referring to age).

[4]"Toil at affairs" translates *songshi* 頌 事. I follow *MWD*, vol. 4, "Transcription," n. 8, in reading *song* as *yong* 庸, whose interchangeability is attested in *Yili*, 16.4a, and Zheng Xuan commentary. I understand *yong* as glossed in *Erya*, 2.3b: "toil (*lao* 勞)." The synonymous compound *laoshi* 勞 事 occurs in *Shiji*, 105.21a, where the physician Chunyu Yi warns a patient to not "toil at laborious affairs (勞 力 事)."

them? Carefully hold it and do not lose it, and long life continues across ages. For continuous ages you are peaceful and joyous, and possess longevity.

"Longevity is born of growth and accumulation. As for the fullness of that life: above it scans heaven and below it spreads over earth.[1] The person who is capable of it invariably becomes a spirit. Thus he is capable of achieving release of the form.[2] The person who perceives the great way skims the clouds as he moves. From Piled Blue-gem above,[3] like water flowing he can range far; like the dragon ascending he can rise high. Quick and untiring in strength

---

[1]The expression of universality in this sentence is reminiscent of language in the writings that precede the second Mawangdui *Laozi* edition, as well as language in *Guanzi* and *Huainanzi*. *MWD*, vol. 1: 72, has the sentence: "The explication of One scans (*cha* 察) heaven and earth." The parallel in *Huainanzi*, 1.12, is: "The explication of One reaches (*ji* 際) heaven and earth." Both sentences are anticipated in *Guanzi* 49, 16.270: "The explication of One Word, above scans (*cha*) heaven and below extends to earth." Replace "One Word" with "life" and we have the sentence in *MS*VI.A.4.

[2]"Release of the form" translates *xingjie* 形 解. The term is attested in *Shiji*, 28.10b, in a passage concerning occult specialists from the region of Yan who arrived at the court of the First Qin Thearch with recipes for "the way of transcendence (*xiandao* 僊 道)" as well as "release of the form and fluxing transformation (*xingjie xiaohua* 形 解 銷 化)." The commentary cites Fu Qian 服 虔 (second century A.D.), who equates *xingjie* with *shijie* 尸 解 (release of the corpse). *Shijie* is best known in connection with religious Daoism. For the Daoist believer, *shijie* marked the moment when a new, immortal physique was perfected and the mortal body sloughed off, leaving behind a husk-like corpse (or an object such as a sword or staff) as evidence of the adept's achievement of *shijie* (Maspero 1981: 445-48).

While *xingjie* and *shijie* are surely related, it is evident that *xingjie* in *MS*VI.A.4 does not represent the identical concept as *shijie* in religious Daoism. The occurrence of *xingjie* in *MS*VI.A.4 along with the references to "becoming a spirit" above and rising "like the dragon" below suggest cross-influences between the medical tradition of macrobiotic hygiene and the *xian*-cult, but I am uncertain what the nature of the influences is (see Prolegomena, Section Four, "Body and Spirit").

[3]*MWD*, vol. 4, "Transcription," n. 10, reads 麇 as *jun/*kwjiən* 麇, which it identifies as a phonetic loan for *qun/*gwjiən* 群 (the loan usage is attested in *Zuozhuan*, Zhao 5, 43.6b). The name Piled Blue-gem (*qunyao* 群 瑤) is similar to the Piled Jade Mountain 群 玉 之 山 mentioned in *Mu tianzi zhuan*, 2.4a, as the domain of Rong Cheng where Mu stops on his westward journey to the land of the Queen Mother of the West. While there is no evidence that Piled Blue-gem is another name for Piled Jade Mountain, the identification is plausible and adds to contextual evidence for making SS52-59 part of Rong Cheng's teaching in *MS*VI.A.4. Alternatively, Jade Mountain 玉 山 is identified as the dwelling place of the Queen Mother of the West in *Shanhaijing*, 2.19a. It is also possible that Piled Blue-gem alludes to the Blue-gem Pool at Kunlun Mountain where Mu met the Queen Mother of the West (see above).

[7] Wuchengzhao[1] [2] did not die. Wuchengzhao makes the four seasons his assistants and heaven and earth his constants. Wuchengzhao was born together with Yin and Yang. Yin and Yang do not die, and Wuchengzhao is coequal with them.[2] The gentleman who possesses the way is also like this."

*MS*VI.A.5 (SS42-47)

Yao asked Shun: "In Under-heaven what is most valuable?"

Shun replied: "Life is most valuable."

Yao said: "How can life be cultivated?"

Shun said: "Investigate Yin and Yang."

Yao said: "Man possesses nine apertures and twelve joints,[3] each one situated in its place. Why is it that the Yin is born together with a man and yet departs ahead of the body? "[4]

Shun said: "When drinking and eating it is not used; it is not utilized for counseling and thinking.[5] Its name is avoided and its

---

[1]*MWD*, vol. 4, "Transcription," n. 11, identifies the name Wuchengzhao 巫成柖 with Wuchengzhao 務成昭. According to *Xunzi* 27, 19.323, the latter was Shun's teacher. *Hanshu*, 30.81a, records the *Wuchengzi Yin dao* 務成子陰道 (Wuchengzi's way of Yin) among books on sexual cultivation; and this same Wuchengzi later gained prominence in religious Daoism. If the "Transcription" identification is accepted, one might then question whether the mention of Shun's teacher in a dialogue between the Yellow Thearch and Rong Cheng constitutes historical anachronism (assuming, that is, that the chronology of figures in old legends was a settled issue by the third century B.C.); which could cast doubt on the rearrangement of SS52-59 (there is less of a problem in *MS*VI.A.6, since tradition places Pengzu in historical proximity to Shun). In my judgment anachronism is not a significant issue. I am also skeptical of the "Transcription" identification. *Zhuangzi* 14, 219, mentions a Wuxiantiao 巫咸袑, who imparts cosmological wisdom. 咸 in the *Zhuangzi* version of the name is probably to be equated with 成 in *MS*VI.A.4; providing a second possible referent for the name (I disagree with the *Zhuangzi* commentaries which identify Wuxiantiao as the shaman Wuxian 巫咸, who is credited with the invention of divination). All three names may have some connection in legends that are only imperfectly recorded in Warring States philosophical texts.

[2]The idea of immortality expressed here is discussed in the Prolegomena, Section Four, "Body and Spirit."

[3]I follow the interpretation of the twelve joints in the Yang Shangshan commentary in *Taisu*, 3.26: "The four limbs each have three large joints" (i.e. ankle, knee, hip, wrist, elbow, and shoulder). The Wang Bing commentary in *Suwen* 3, 1.9b, identifies the twelve joints as the twelve vessels, but this denotation is clearly inapplicable to the Mawangdui medical manuscripts, which describe only eleven vessels.

[4]The Yin refers to the penis as the chief Yin component of the body. Given that Yin vitality of the body depends above all on the care of the penis, Yao is requesting instruction on how to prevent its early demise. A parallel passage occurs in *MS*VII.B.1.

[5]*MS*VI.A.6 offers further discussion of the necessity of including the penis and its vitality in an overall hygienic regimen.

body concealed, yet it is employed very frequently with neither leniency nor ritual.[1] Thus while it is born together with the body, it dies ahead of the body."

Yao said: "How can it be cultivated?"

Shun said: "You must cherish it and delight in it; instruct and counsel it; and give it drink and food. Make the prong at its tip[2] firm and strong, and employ it slackly. You must imbibe, but do not dispense;[3] you must be joyful, but do not allow emission. The stuff will accumulate and vapor grow. On reaching the age of one hundred, you will be more sterling than in the past."

Shun's way for coitus with Yin and cultivating vapor.

*MS*VI.A.6
(SS48–51, S41) Wangzi Qiaofu asked Ancestor Peng:[4] "Of man's vapor, which is the most essential?"

Ancestor Peng replied: "Of man's vapor none can compare with penile essence.[5] When the penile vapor is clogged and blocked, the hundred vessels produce illness. When the penile vapor is not perfected, you cannot procreate. Thus longevity lies entirely with the penis. When the penis is secured and cherished, its simultaneous giving becomes an aid.

---

[1]Perhaps *kuanli* 寬 禮 should be read as a compound meaning "lenient ritual" similar to *kuanzheng* 寬 政 (lenient government) in *Zuozhuan*, Zhuang 22, 9.12b.

[2]I follow *MWD*, vol. 4, "Transcription," n. 3, in reading 䘹 as *cui* 顇. The scribe probably erred in writing 衣 instead of 卒. *Cui* should be understood as *cui* 崒, in the sense of the tip of a peak (see *SW*, 9B.5b, and Duan Yucai commentary). In *MS*VI.A.5 the word serves as a euphemism for the head of the penis, hence my translation "prong." *Cui/*dzjəd* also puns with *zui/*tsuəd* 朘, which refers to the genitals or penis (see *MS*VI.A.6).

[3]I.e. the man should absorb the woman's essence during intercourse without releasing any of his own.

[4]Ancestor Peng 彭 祖 as a legendary figure in Warring States macrobiotic hygiene is discussed in the Prolegomena, Section Four, "Intellectual Background." *MWD*, vol. 4, "Transcription," n. 1, identifies the name Wangzi Qiaofu 王 子 巧 父 with Wangzi Qiao 王 子 喬, the legendary *xian*-cult adept (see Prolegomena, Section Four, "Intellectual Background"). I would treat the identification as an unverified probability rather than a proven fact.

[5]I follow *MWD*, vol. 4, "Transcription," in reading 竣 as *zui* 朘, referring to the genitals or penis (see *MS*I.E.134). *MS*VI.A.6 concerns the need to cultivate the vapor and essence of the penis by various means other than sexual intercourse. The conclusion does note that proper cultivation of the vitality of the penis permits "lasting coitus."

"For this reason, at the first light of day[1] the person of the way spits on his hands and strokes his arms. He rubs the abdomen, following the Yin and following the Yang.[2] He must first spit out the stale, then suck in the penile vapor.[3] Let penetrating breathing be together with the penis; let drinking and eating be together with the penis. Drink and food consummate the penis, like nurturing the red infant.[4] When the red infant[5] is boisterous and brash and repeatedly becomes erect, be careful to not burden it with labor.[6] Then he can have lasting coitus[7] and can travel distantly; thus he is able to have a lengthy longevity."

---

[1]"First light of day" translates *faming* 發明, which occurs again in *MS*VI.A.9 describing the time when the rooster crows. The term is attested in *Shuoyuan*, 18.6b, as the name for the call made by the mythical *feng* 鳳 bird at dawn (there are three other names for the call of the *feng* in the daytime, while in flight, and while perching). According to *SW*, 4A.40a, *faming* is one of the five spirit birds, and is associated with the east (the *feng* is the bird of the center). See Chen Mengjia 1965: 122, for other Han terms denoting the break of day in which *ming* is the second member of the compound.

[2]Yin and Yang refer to inner and outer surfaces on the body. According to *Suwen* 4, 1.16a-b, the abdomen is Yin and the back is Yang. Perhaps the rubbing motion in *MS*VI.A.6 moves between the abdomen and the back. However, I suspect that the person is supposed to stroke in a circular motion from the center of the abdomen (the Yin inner part) towards the edges (the Yang outer part).

[3]Ejecting stale vapor is discussed in *MS*VI.A.4. Perhaps sucking in penile vapor is related to the practice of contracting the anus described in *MS*VI.A.7.

[4]The *locus classicus* for the "red infant" (*chizi* 赤子; i.e. the newborn infant) is *Laozi*, par. 55, which also refers to the infant's sexual potency: "The fact that without knowing of the conjoining of female and male its penis (*zui* 朘) rises is the culmination of essence" (*MWD*, vol. 1: 105). Comparing the cultivation of the penis to nurturing the red infant suggests an analogy between macrobiotic hygiene and infant care—or, as I think is more likely, gestation. The analogy becomes a reality in the following sentence which uses "red infant" as a euphemism for the penis. In religious Daoist hygiene, "nurturing the red infant" refers to the inner cultivation of a perfected being through a process equivalent to gestation. Six Dynasties Daoist sources locate the red infant in the "cinnabar field" (*dantian* 丹田) by the navel, which functions as the womb (Schipper 1978: 370-71). The cultivation of the red infant/penis is not equivalent to the Daoist cultivation of the red infant/perfected being. But the idea of gestation prominent in the Daoist sources must also be present in *MS*VI.A.6 (the idea of cultivation as gestation is also evident in *MS*VI.A.7).

[5]Here referring to the penis itself.

[6]The injunction "be careful to not" marks the bottom of S51, followed at the top of S41 by the compound *yaoshi* 繇使, which is a standard compound meaning "corvée labor" in Han sources (see, for example, *Shiji*, 7.12b). The idea that the penis should not be "burdened with labor" parallels the idea in *MS*VI.A.5 that the penis is too often "employed without leniency."

[7]立 in *MWD*, vol. 4, "Transcription," should be transcribed as *jiao* 交 (coitus).

*MS*VI.A.7 (SS60-65)

Thearch Pan Geng asked Wizen-faced Oldster:[1] "I have heard that the Master practices coitus with Yin to become strong, and sucks in heaven's essence to achieve lengthy longevity. What might I undertake so that the way can be put into practice?"

Wizen-faced Oldster replied: "Your lordship must prize that which is born together with the body and yet grows old ahead of the body.[2] The weak, it makes them strong; the short, it makes them tall; the poor, it guarantees them abundant provisions. The regimen involves both emptying and filling, and there is a precise procedure for cultivating it.[3] First, relax the limbs, straighten the spine, and flex the buttocks; second, spread the thighs, move the Yin,[4] and contract the anus;[5] third, draw the eyelashes together, do not listen, and suck in the vapor to fill the womb;[6] fourth, contain

---

[1]*Qi* 耇 is glossed in *SW*, 8A.68a, as "face of an old man that looks frozen and blackened like refuse," hence my translation "wizen-faced." The Wizen-faced Oldster 耇老 is not attested in received literature. Pan Geng 盤庚 reigned in the middle years of the Shang period. The book *Tang Pan Geng Yin dao* 湯盤庚陰道 (Way of Yin of Tang and Pan Geng) in *Hanshu*, 30.81a, indicates his association with sexual cultivation.

[2]I.e. the penis (as in *MS*VI.A.5).

[3]The five part procedure described below is similar to the description of the "eight benefits" in *MS*VII.B.7. The "eight benefits" are eight ways to cultivate the vapor and essence associated with the genitals, some of them involving sexual intercourse. *MS*VI.A.7 differs in that the Wizen-faced Oldster appears to be describing a single technique in five linked stages, from "relaxing the limbs" to "sucking in the great illumination." The technique seems to accompany sexual intercourse, but it may also be accomplished without intercourse, as suggested by the concluding sentence that labels *MS*VI.A.7 the "Wizen-faced Oldster's way for coitus with Yin and eating spirit vapor."

[4]Presumably the Yin refers to the penis. "Move the Yin" suggests sexual stimulation, but assuming that the technique is not solely a method for intercourse some form of exercise may also be intended (like "pulling Yin" in *MS*VI.A.8).

[5]For *zhou* 州 in the sense of "anus," see *MS*I.E.153. Instead of *suo* 縮 (contract), *MS*VII.B.7 uses the verb *xi* 噏 (suck in). *Ishinpô*, 28.22b, recommends "contracting the lower region" to help stabilize the essence being generated during intercourse so that it is not lost by ejaculation of semen. The use of anal constriction in both coital and non-coital cultivation techniques is discussed in the Prolegomena, Section Four, "Techniques."

[6]The person concentrates meditatively. I read *liu/*ljəgw* 瘤 as a phonetic loan for *bao/*prəgw* 胞 (womb, uterus), which I understand to mean a "womb-like organ" where men as well as women store vapor and essence. The word occurs again in *MS*VI.A.8 in a passage that alludes to the third and fourth stages of the technique in *MS*VI.A.7. 胞 pronounced *pao* also denotes the bladder (written 脬 in *SW*, 4B.22b), but in my judgment the bladder—even though it is a receptacle for water—is not the referent of *liu/bao* (*pao* 脬 occurs in *MS*I.E.95 and *MS*I.E.101 denoting the bladder). Two *Suwen* passages support the identification of *bao* as an organ possessed by men and women in early physiological theory. *Suwen* 37, 10.10a, notes that "when the womb (*bao*) transfers heat to the bladder

(*pangguang* 膀 胱), there is urine retention and bloody urine." According to the Wang Bing commentary, "the bladder is the cavity for fluids; the womb oversees receiving and injecting." *Suwen* 48, 13.8a, attributes a certain morbid condition of the vessels to insufficient transmission of "womb essence," and Wang Bing notes that "the womb vessel is attached to the kidney." Other occurrences of *bao* in the *Huangdi neijing* denote the uterus, although it is possible that some of the statements concerning the *bao* are applicable to male as well as female anatomy. *Nanjing*, 3.30b, is the earliest source to distinguish between the left kidney, which it identifies as the location of the depot named *shen* 腎 (also a water receptacle), and the right kidney, which is the organ where vapor and essence are stored: "The right one is the gate of life (*mingmen* 命 門). The gate of life is the place where all spirit essence lodges, and where the original vapor is attached. Thus the man stores essence in it and the woman attaches it to the womb (*bao*)" (cf. Unschuld 1986b: 382). The *Nanjing* passage appears to resolve ambiguity in the *Huangdi neijing* concerning the function of the two kidneys as well as the status of the *bao*: the latter is a female organ subordinated to the right kidney which is the gate of life proper. I think that *liu/bao* in the Mawangdui manuscripts serves the function of what the *Nanjing* calls the *mingmen* (and the lack of references in the manuscripts to the kidney as a place for storing vapor and essence is probably because this function is performed by the *bao*). Significantly, *MS*VI.B.1 identifies the place where a man sends the essence generated during sexual intercourse as the *zongmen* 宗 門 (progenitive gate); and the same place is called *xuemen* 血 門 (blood gate) in *MS*VII.B.13. I suspect that both terms are related to the later *mingmen*; and I would argue for associating them with *bao* in *MS*VI.A.7-8. Although my interpretation of the manuscript evidence is contextual and circumstantial, I believe that it is sufficient to support my speculation that early macrobiotic hygiene theory included the idea that men as well as women possessed a womb/progenitive gate.

Religious Daoist hygiene makes a similar correlation between the *bao* and the *mingmen*—which is situated at the navel (the terminus of the life-cord of birth). For example, the *Lingshu ziwen*, 1.11b-12a, provides the following identifications: "The gate of life (*mingmen*) is the navel. The dark barrier (*xuanguan* 玄 關) is the passageway to the womb (*bao*) and intestines from the original time of birth. Within it there is a palace of life. . . . To replenish the fetus and return to the womb, at sunset first enclose vapor, breathing twenty-four times. . ." Robinet 1984, vol. 2: 109-110, dates this text to the original Shangqing revelations in the fourth century A.D. I am grateful to Stephen Bokenkamp for drawing my attention to this example of the pairing of *bao* and *mingmen*. For additional discussion of the significance of gestation as a model for breath cultivation and sexual cultivation in religious Daoist hygiene, see Schipper 1978: 370-71. The occurrence of *liu/bao* and the references to "nurturing the red infant" in *MS*VI.A.6 indicate that the idea of gestation was already part of early macrobiotic hygiene.

Other arguments have been made for the identification of *liu* 腳. *MWD*, vol. 4, "Transcription," n. 3, proposes reading the graph as *nao/*nagw* 腦 (brain). In Han texts examples of rhyming between Old Chinese **-əgw* and **-agw* are common (Luo and Zhou 1958: 19). Thus an argument that *liu/*ljəgw* is a loan for *nao/*nagw* is phonologically tenable. I am not persuaded by Ma Jixing's claim that 腳 is a scribal error for 腦 (1992: 937, n. 4). The flaw in the argument is, in my judgment, the a priori assumption that the passage concerns the later sexual technique of "returning the essence to replenish the brain" (*huanjing bunao* 還 精 補 腦); thus the graph in question must be the word for brain. The sequence of the technique itself belies this speculation. In the later technique, "replenishing the brain" culminates sexual cultivation. In *MS*VI.A.7 "filling the *liu*" occurs in the third stage, and cultivation (which may be non-coital as well as coital) culminates in the fifth stage when the "essence ascends." "Filling the *liu*" as the third stage in *MS*VI.A.7 cannot the five tastes and drink that wellspring blossom;[1] fifth, the mass of essence all ascends, suck in the great illumination.[2] After reaching the fifth, stop. Essence and spirit grow daily more blissful."

Wizen-faced Oldster's way for coitus with Yin and eating spirit vapor.

*MS*VI.A.8 (SS66–72, S40, S73)

Yu asked Teacher Gui:[3] "I put forth the wisdom of my ears and eyes to order Under-heaven. Above, I made the submerged land level; below, I followed the course of the Jiang River and reached Kuaiji Mountain. I have spent ten years controlling the water; and now my four limbs are useless and my household is in disorder. How can they be put into order?"[4]

Teacher Gui replied: "As a rule, the mainstay for ordering government must begin from the body.[5] When blood and vapor ought to move yet do not move, this is called the calamity of blockage; and is something that controls the six extremities.[6] So, the continu-

---

be equated with "replenishing the brain." Matters related to the culmination of sexual cultivation in the Mawangdui medical manuscripts are discussed in the Prolegomena, Section Four, "Techniques." At present the earliest attestation of *huanjing bunao* is ca. second century A.D., in the "Xianger" commentary to *Laozi*, par. 9, which condemns the practice of "lying with women without ejaculating, thinking to return the essence and replenish the brain" (Rao Zongyi 1991: 11). Based on a quotation in the *Hou Hanshu*, it has been argued that *bunao* occurred in the original version of the *Liexian zhuan* account of Rong Cheng; but Kaltenmark 1953: 58, correctly notes that the *bunao* reference belongs to the commentary and not to the text of the *Liexian zhuan*.

Ishida proposes identifying *liu/*ljəgw* as the male genitals by reading it as a phonetic loan for *gao/*kəgw* 睾 (testicle; 1991: 15). The phonological probability of the loan is good, but "sucking in vapor to fill the testicles/genitals" is an unlikely interpretation of the text.

[1]"Wellspring blossom" is obviously an internally produced fluid, unlike the "running beasts' wellspring blossom" in *MS*VI.A.2 and 10.

[2]See the parallel in *MS*VI.B.1 which also describes the ascent of essence.

[3]Teacher Gui 師癸 is not attested in received literature. Yu 禹 discusses sexual cultivation with court ladies in *MS*III.89.

[4]Descriptions of Yu's labors to tame the flood waters occur in numerous pre-Han sources, including the physical impairments that serve as the rationale for the Pace of Yu in the *Shizi* (see *MS*I.E.60). *Shiji*, 2.26a, identifies Kuaiji 會稽 as the mountain in the southeast where Yu convened his lords and then died. "Order" translates *zhi* 治, elsewhere translated as "cultivate." Yu is asking how to restore his health and bring order to his household simultaneously.

[5]I.e. to "order" (*zhi*) the state a ruler must "cultivate" (*zhi*) his body.

[6]*Liuji* 六極 (six extremities) refers to the four directions as well as up and down in *Zhuangzi* 7, 132. In *MS*VI.A.9, *liuji* appears to be equivalent to *liumo* 六末 in *MS*III.70, denoting the four limbs as well as the genital and anal regions. To say that the "calamity of

ity of vapor and blood and the meshing of muscles and vessels cannot be set aside and forgotten. As for the womb, dispense to it; as for the tastes, transmit them.[1] Guide it with the will, and use the regimen to move it. Were it not for the tastes there would be nothing filling the inside and making the joints grow. Were it not for the will there would be no means of knowing whether the inside is empty or full. Were it not for the regimen there would be no means to move the four limbs and to dispatch illness. Thus to awaken from sleep and pull Yin, this is called refining the muscles.[2] To first stretch and then curl, this is called refining the bones.[3] Movement and activity must be fitting; essence, thus, comes forth like a wellspring. By practicing this way, what age would not have perfect specimens? "[4]

Thereupon Yu drank fermented milk[5] and ate the five tastes. With the will he cultivated vapor. His eyes became bright and his ears perceptive; skin and hide glowed; the hundred vessels were full

---

blockage controls (*zong* 宗) the six extremities" means that when stagnation of blood and vapor causes internal blockage, this morbid condition affects the entire body (and by extension, the entire state). *MWD*, vol. 4, "Transcription," n. 4, proposes a different meaning for *liuji* in *MS*VI.A.8, referring to a list of six harmful things called *liuji* in *Shangshu*, "Hong fan," 12.14b. Ma Jixing cites several examples of *liuji* referring to maladies in medieval medical literature (1992: 942, n. 9). In their interpretation the translation would be, "this is called the calamity of blockage, which is the source (*zong*) of the six extremities." The interpretation is plausible, but I regard the occurrence of *liuji* in *MS*VI.A.9 as decisive.

[1]The sentence alludes to the third and fourth stages in the technique described in *MS*VI.A.7.

[2]"Pulling Yin" (*yin* Yin 引 陰) is the name for two exercises in the *Yinshu*, one a simple toe-touch and the other a procedure involving anal constriction (see the Prolegomena, Section Four, "Techniques," for details). Ma Jixing understands "pulling Yin" in *MS*VI.A.8 to refer to exercising the genitals (1992: 947, n. 1). While not impossible, this is probably not the intended meaning.

[3]*Qushen* 屈 伸 (curl and stretch) as a term connoting the ability to conform to the pattern of nature is ubiquitous in early literature. The regular occurrence of *qu* and *shen* in the exercise instructions in the *Yinshu* best illustrates the application of the concept of "curl and stretch" to macrobiotic hygiene.

[4]*Buwu* 不 物 occurs in *Zhouli*, 15.3a, in the sense of an "abnormal creature." In *MS*VI.A.8 I understand *wu* as a verb meaning "be a normal creature," embellished as "be a perfect specimen."

[5]"Fermented milk" translates *zhongjiu* 湩 酒 (*zhong* occurs at the bottom of S72, and *jiu* at the top of S40). I suspect that *zhongjiu* is a variant of *zhonglao* 湩 酪 (kumiss), the favored beverage of the Xiongnu 匈 奴 (*Shiji*, 110.15a).

and replete. The Yin then [1] born, thereby pacifying Queen Yao.[1] The household then was tranquil again.

Teacher Gui's way for cultivating spirit vapor.

*MS*VI.A.9 (SS74-93)

Wen Zhi saw King Wei of Qi.[2] King Wei asked him about the way: "The Deficient Man[3] has heard that the Master and Great Man[4] has broad knowledge of the way. Due to the sacrifices of the ancestral temple, the Deficient Man does not have the leisure to listen to all of it. I would like to hear the crux of the way in two or three words and no more."

Wen Zhi replied: "Your Servant's practice of the way consists of three hundred fascicles,[5] but sleep is foremost."

King Wei said: "Let the Master elaborate; when engaging in sleep what should be eaten?"

Wen Zhi replied: "Pure liquor and clumped *jiu* (leeks)."[6]

---

[1]I surmise from the context that Yin refers to the genitals. The lacuna may be *fu* 復, making the genitals "reborn." Queen Yao 后姚 is not attested as the name of Yu's wife. Qiu Xigui notes that the graph transcribed as *yao* 姚 is difficult to decipher and recommends further investigation (1992: 525-26). Assuming that it is *yao*, Qiu suggests that Queen Yao is equivalent to Woman Qiao 女趫, the name of Yu's wife given in *Hanshu*, 20.20b (there is phonological similarity: *yao/*dagw* and *qiao/*gjagw*).

[2]King Wei of Qi 齊威王 (r. 357-320 B.C.) is credited with establishing the Jixia 稷下 Academy, the pre-eminent center of learning of the day (Rickett 1985: 18-19; Knoblock 1988: 54-55). Wen Zhi 文摯 is identified in *Lüshi chunqiu*, 11.107, as a physician from Song 宋 who treated the illness of King Min 滑王 of Qi (r. 300-284 B.C.). The only cure was to anger the king, and once the king recovered he could not be dissuaded from executing Wen Zhi: "So they boiled Wen Zhi alive in a caldron. It cooked for three days and three nights, and his facial complexion was unchanged. Wen Zhi said, 'If you genuinely wish to kill me, why not cover it to cut off the vapor of Yin and Yang.' The king had the caldron covered, and Wen Zhi then died." *Lunheng*, "Dao xu," 7.151, presents a detailed refutation of the truth of the story in order to dismiss the popular belief that Wen Zhi was a "person of the way." The format of the exchange between master and student changes in *MS*VI.A.9-10 to the interview style characteristic of Warring States rhetoric. A specialist gains an interview with a ruler; he responds to the ruler's questions; and the ruler caps the response with the formulaic "excellent."

[3]A humilific form of self address commonly used by Warring States rulers.

[4]Master (*zi* 子) is a respectful form of address, but the additional Great Man (*dafu* 大夫) suggests that Wen Zhi was a man of rank in court hierarchy (in Song or perhaps in Qi).

[5]I read *bian* 編 as *pian* 篇, referring to a bundle of bound bamboo slips (fascicle). The statement is self-advertisement, and "three hundred fascicles" is an idealized number implying perfection. See, for example, *Shiji*, 130.12a, where the three hundred songs of the *Shijing* are referred to as the "three hundred fascicles," meaning that they are the cynosure of the moral feelings of the sages of old.

[6]"Clumped" translates *du* 毒, glossed as follows in *SW*, 1B.2a: "Thick; grass that harms people continually growing." "Harmful, poisonous" is an extended meaning. For the

King Wei said: "Why does the Master advocate *jiu* (leeks)?"

Wen Zhi replied: "When Lord Millet sowed and tilled,[1] the herb that lived a thousand years was *jiu* (leek) alone; thus, it was named for this.[2] It receives heaven's vapor early, and its receipt of earth's vapor is secure. Thus, those who are skittish, timid,[3] dispirited,[4] and frightened eat it and regain regular strength; those whose eyes do not see clearly eat it and regain regular brightness; those whose ears do not hear eat it and regain regular perceptivity. Eat it during the three months of spring and neither affliction nor illness arises; and muscle and bone grow ever stronger. For these reasons it is called king of the hundred herbs."

King Wei said: "Excellent. Why does the Master advocate liquor?"

Wen Zhi replied: "Liquor is the vapor-essence of the five grains.[5] When it enters the inside it disperses and flows; when it enters the internal network[6] it penetrates and circulates. It permeates the internal network without the need for sleep. Thus it serves as the medium for the hundred drugs."

King Wei said: "Excellent. But there is something that is not consistent with what the Master has stated. Now then, when *jiu*

---

development of the word *du* in medical usage, see Unschuld 1975. In *MSVI.A.9* it simply describes the growth of leeks in clumps.

[1]Lord Millet 后 稷 is an agricultural deity and legendary founder of the Zhou lineage. I read 半 as *ban* 拌, meaning "toss" and here used in the sense of "sow" (see *Guangya*, 1A.13a, and Wang Niansun commentary). I follow *MWD*, vol. 4, "Transcription," n. 4, in reading *rou/*njəgw* 鞣 as a phonetic loan for *you/*ʔjəgw* 耰, glossed in *SW*, 6A.43a, as "implement for tilling fields."

[2]The gloss of *jiu/*kjəgw* 韭 in *SW*, 7B.3b, also traces the origin of the name for the leek to the fact that it is *jiu/*kjəgw* 久 (long lasting): "planted once, it lives long (*jiu* 久); thus it is called *jiu*."

[3]I follow *MWD*, vol. 4, "Transcription," in reading *zhe* 聶 as *zhe* 懾 (timid). "Skittish" translates *bi* 辟, in the sense of "evasive, nervous." The "Transcription," n. 6, additionally cites the compound *zhebi* 聶 辟 as a technical term in *Suwen* 62, 17.5a, but *bi* and *zhe* are best interpreted as single descriptive words in *MSVI.A.9*.

[4]I give the pronunciation *liang/*gljang* to the unattested graph 㦒; and read it as a phonetic loan for *liang/*ljang* 悢, glossed as "dispirited" in *Guangya*, 3A.4b. The compound *kuang-liang* 懭 悢 is attested with the same meaning in *Chuci*, "Jiubian," 8.2a. *MWD*, vol. 4, "Transcription," n. 6, reads the graph as a phonetic loan for *rang/*njang* 懹 (abhor), but in my judgment *liang* "dispirited" is a better reading phonologically and semantically.

[5]I.e. it is the most refined form of the vapor of the five grains.

[6]"Internal network" translates *li* 理, here alluding to the vessels.

(leek) is offered for the spring-feast collation, why is it not together with liquor but always together with egg? "[1]

Wen Zhi replied: "Also permissible. Now then, the chicken is a Yang creature; one that at the first light of day rouses the sense of hearing, with its head extended and feathers cocked. During the three 'returned Yin' months it is combined with *jiu* (leek).[2] Thus, the person of the way eats it."

King Wei said: "Excellent. Why does the Master advocate sleep?"

---

[1]The phrase 春䟽寫人人以韭 in the first half of the sentence requires textual commentary. I read 人 as *ru* 入, a simple scribal miswriting that also occurs in the preceding paragraph. I read 䟽 as *yu* 飫, glossed in *SW*, 5B.12b, as "feast." I understand the "spring feast" to be the spring festival when the populace makes offerings of agricultural products; and I understand *xieru* 寫入 as a compound referring to the collection of offerings at an offering site, hence the translation "collation." The custom of offering the leek at the spring festival is described in *Liji*, 12.12b (which also lists the appropriate offerings for the summer, autumn, and winter festivals): "In the spring the populace offers leek, in the summer wheat, in the autumn millet, and in the winter rice. Egg accompanies leek, fish accompanies wheat, pork accompanies millet, and goose accompanies rice." King Wei's question to Wen Zhi confirms that the combination of leek and egg was a well established custom; and he wants Wen Zhi to justify the difference between medical knowledge and popular custom.

[2]I am not certain which season is specified by Wen Zhi, but I suspect summer. *Fu* Yin 復陰 (returned Yin) can be interpreted in two ways: as the time during the annual Yin Yang cycle when Yin begins to flourish while Yang recedes; or as the time when Yin "returns back" to its optimal state of fullness. There is evidence for both interpretations in received sources. *Xijing zaji*, 5.16, records a statement attributed to Dong Zhongshu 董仲舒 that understands *fu* Yin in the sense of the renewal of the Yin part of the cycle. According to Dong Zhongshu, Yang peaks in the fourth month, but it is during the same month that the latent "return to Yin" becomes manifest; and Yin continues to grow during the months after the fourth month until it peaks in the tenth month. In contrast, the Wang Bi commentary in *Yijing*, "Fu," 3.12a, understands the winter solstice to be the time of *fu* Yin, when Yin "returns back" to its origin and is at rest. The winter solstice can be equated with the eleventh month. Extrapolating from the *Xijing zaji*, Wen Zhi's three *fu* Yin months ought to be the summer months (the fourth through the sixth). Extrapolating from the Wang Bi commentary, the *fu* Yin months might be either the winter months (the tenth through the twelfth) or a combination of winter and spring months (the eleventh through the first). It is also possible that received sources fail to indicate the meaning of the term *fu* Yin as used by Wen Zhi, and that it refers idiomatically to the spring months. I am skeptical of the third possibility, and prefer to think that Wen Zhi is providing a medical rationale for the combination of leek and chicken that is based on Yin Yang classification (leek was probably also considered Yang as it was later; see *GM*, 26.40) instead of folk custom. Since spring and summer are the seasons for fresh leeks, I favor interpreting *fu* Yin as understood in the *Xijing zaji* and identifying the season as summer.

Wen Zhi replied: "Now then, sleep is not merely a matter that concerns living people. Ducks and geese, swans and *sushuang*,[1] earthworms,[2] fish and turtles, and the whole horde of mobile creatures need to eat in order to live. And having eaten, they need to sleep in order to be perfected. Now then, sleep is what causes food to disintegrate and dissolve, and what disperses drugs to flow through the form. The relation of sleep to eating is analogous to that of fire to metal. Thus, if for a single night you do not sleep, for a hundred days you do not recover. When food does not transform, you invariably become like a stuffed leather ball. This generates craving in the heart with clogging; and discomfort in the intestines with malaise.[3] Thus, the person of the way reveres sleep."

King Wei said: "Excellent. The Deficient Man is habitually fond of drinking at sunset and continuing into the night; that is, if it does not cause sickness."

Wen Zhi replied: "There is no harm. By analogy it is like birds and beasts. Those that go to sleep early rise early; those that go to sleep late rise late.[4] Heaven receives light; earth receives darkness. The person of the way does no more than investigate the matter thoroughly. Now then, when eating vapor let it sink in and spread in blackness.[5] At midnight [5] vapor, and bring it to the six ex-

---

[1]I am not certain which bird is denoted by the name *sushuang* 鷫 鷞. According to *SW*, 4A.40a, it is one of the five spirit birds, and is associated with the west. The Duan Yucai commentary cites several sources that describe the bird as goose-like with a long neck and green feathers.

[2]I follow Ma Jixing (1992: 962, n. 3) in reading *yuan* 蚖 as *wan* 蜿, and understanding *wanshan* 蜿 蟺 as a compound denoting the earthworm (see *Guangya*, 10B.9b).

[3]The phrase 桅 湯 劓 惑 in the second half of the sentence requires textual commentary. I assume that the phrase is grammatically parallel to the preceding phrase. Thus, I read 湯 as *chang* 腸 (intestine), parallel to "heart" above. I read 桅 as *nie* 臲. The compound *niewu* 臲 卼 is attested in *Yijing*, "Kun," 5.8b, with the meaning "uneasy, uncomfortable." *SW*, 6B.2b, records a variant written 槷 鼿. I understand *yi* 劓 in the sense of the compound *yiyue* 劓 刖 (literally, the mutilation punishments of cutting off the nose and the feet) in *Yijing*, "Kun," 5.8a, where it is similar in meaning to *niewu*. I suspect that *yihuo* 劓 惑 (malaise) is a variant of *yiyue*, perhaps used because *huo/*gwək* rhymes with *mo/*mək* 墨 in the compound for "clogging" in the preceding phrase.

[4]Presumably the king belongs to the latter category.

[5]"Blackness" translates *yi* 黟, glossed in *SW*, 10A.59a, as "black tree." *MWD*, vol. 4, "Transcription," reads the graph as *mei* 默 without comment, evidently regarding the former as scribal error for the latter. I prefer to interpret the original graph in the sense of the "blackness" of the body's interior.

tremities.[1] The six extremities are firm with essence, hence the inside is full and the outside even. Pustules and neck lumps have no place to lodge; not a single abscess appears. This is the culmination of the way."

King Wei said: "Excellent."

*MS*VI.A.10

(SS94–101) Wang Qi saw King Zhao of Qin, who asked him about the way:[2] "The Deficient Man has heard that the Guest[3] eats Yin to become active and strong, and sucks in vapor to achieve essence illumination.[4] What might the Deficient Man undertake so that longevity can be prolonged?"

Wang Qi replied: "You must face the sun and moon and suck in the rays of their essence; eat *song* (pine) and *bai* (arbor-vitae);[5] and drink running beasts' wellspring blossom.[6] You can repel agedness and restore vigor, becoming lustrous and glowing. In the three summer months eliminate fire and use the sun to cook and boil.[7] Then the spirit becomes keen, (the ears) perceptive, and (the eyes) bright.

---

[1]I.e. the four limbs as well as the genital and anal regions (see *MS*VI.A.8). Using breath cultivation to transport vapor to the limbs is mentioned in *MS*VI.A.4.

[2]Wang Qi 王期 is not attested in received literature. The Qin ruler is King Zhaoxiang 昭襄王 (r. 306–251 B.C.). Presumably Wang Qi was a physician who was patronized by the Qin elite.

[3]The title indicates that Wang Qi belonged to the rank of Guest (*ke* 客) in the court hierarchy.

[4]"Essence illumination" translates *jingming* 精明, which I assume to be similar in meaning to *shenming* 神明 (spirit illumination). The religious sense of the compound is attested in *Guoyu*, 18.3a: "Now as for spirits, they are what approach people with essence illumination." As a component of human physiology, *Suwen* 17, 5.1a–2b, associates essence illumination with the eyes and vision, and states that "the head is the cavity of essence illumination."

[5]See *MS*III.6, 47, 71 for dietetic use of pine rosin. Pine and arbor-vitae also figure in *xian*-cult dietetics (see Kaltenmark 1953: 54, 81).

[6]See *MS*VI.A.2.

[7]Wang Qi recommends solar cookery during the summer. There is no evidence of solar cookery in received literature or in the archaeological record. *MWD*, vol. 4, "Transcription," n. 1, speculates that "using the sun to cook" refers to using the Yang *sui* 陽燧, a kind of burning-lens that was believed to draw true Yang fire down from heaven (on the Yang *sui*, see Needham 1954–, vol. 4, part 1: 111–13). However, using a burning-lens to produce the fire is still cooking with fire. I prefer to think that a solar cooker existed, perhaps utilizing the technology of the Yang *sui*, and that food was cooked without fire in the reflected rays of the sun.

"The way of coitus with Yin uses stillness to become strong. Make the heart even like water; store the numinous dew inside.[1] Be relaxed in using the jade whip;[2] do not let the heart be nervous and flurried. The five sounds arise in response, both the short and the long.[3] Suck in the spirit mist; drink that heavenly beverage.[4] Bring it to the five depots, with the aim of storing it deeply.

"Perform dragon breathing at dawn;[5] the vapor and form, then, become hard. {1} [5] nears water. Essence and vapor are congealed,[6] hardy, and long lasting. Spirit harmony is obtained inside; ethereal-spirit and earthly-spirit are gleaming [1]. The five depots become firm and white, their jade color having a renewed glow. Your longevity forms a triad with the sun and moon; and you become the blossom of Under-heaven."

King Zhao said: "Excellent."

---

[1]Perhaps "numinous dew" (*linglu* 靈露) is similar to "sweet dew" in *MS*VI.A.4.

[2]I understand *kuan* 款 in the sense of "relaxed" as attested in *Hou Hanshu*, 24.9a. An occurrence of *kuan* in *Shiji*, 130.11b, is glossed by Ru Chun 如淳 (third century) as *kuan* 寬 (relax) and by Ying Shao 應劭 (second century) as *kou* 扣 (knock). While it is possible that Wang Qi is saying to "knock" with the jade whip (i.e. to hit the vagina with the penis), I think the meaning "relaxed" is best in this context.

[3]See *MS*VI.A.4.

[4]The vitalizing fluids must be the simultaneously generated products of sexual cultivation in combination with breath cultivation.

[5]I follow *MWD*, vol. 4, "Transcription," n. 2, in reading 龔 as *long* 龍 (dragon).

[6]"Congealed" translates *ling* 淩, which is equivalent to *ling* 凌, literally "blocks of ice" (*SW*, 11B.9a, and Duan Yucai commentary).

*MS*VI.B

HE YIN YANG

合陰陽

CONJOINING YIN AND YANG

*MS*VI.B.1

(SS102-111) The recipe for whenever you will be conjoining Yin and Yang:[1]
Grip the hands,[2] and emerge at the Yang side of the wrists;[3]
Stroke the elbow chambers;[4]
Press the side of the underarms;[5]
Ascend the stove trivet;[6]

---

[1]*He* Yin Yang 合陰陽 (conjoin Yin and Yang) is a standard term for sexual intercourse in received literature. It is synonymous with "conjoin vapor" in *MS*III.89. The "recipe for conjoining Yin and Yang" that follows is a verse composed primarily of trisyllabic phrases in which monosyllabic verbs are followed by anatomical terms referring to parts of the woman's body. The verbs tell the man what action to perform and the objects indicate where on the woman's body to perform the action. The verse, which begins with foreplay and concludes with achieving the goal of sexual cultivation, is rich in physiological metaphors.

[2]Presumably the man grips the woman's hands. However, *wo* 握 (grip) could also be interpreted as an instruction to the man to "fist" his own hands (and then stroke the woman's body with fisted hands). In religious Daoist hygiene the term *wogu* 握固 (grip the fist firmly) refers to a fist position in which the adept lays the thumb in the palm of the hand and wraps the fingers around it (see *Ishinpô*, 27.20b). The *locus classicus* for the term is *Laozi*, par. 55 (*MWD*, vol. 1: 105). It is likely that the fist position was already current in early macrobiotic hygiene.

[3]I.e. the outside of the wrists by the back of the hand. I read 土 as a scribal miswriting of *chu* 出 (emerge). The two graphs are written similarly in Qin and Han manuscripts (see Qiu Xigui 1992: 535). *Chu* is used in *MS*I.A-B to designate the place on the body where the path of a vessel first "emerges" (or "arises"; see *MS*I.A.1). In *MS*VI.B.1 *chu* indicates where the man begins his path around the woman's body.

[4]The term *rufang* 乳房 (breast chamber) is attested in *Suwen* 52, 14.4a, referring to the mammary gland. Although I have not found *fang* suffixed to other anatomical names in received sources, I suspect that *zhoufang* 肘房 (elbow chamber) refers to the elbow as a "chamber-like" joint. Alternatively, *fang* should be read as *pang* 旁 (side).

[5]"Press" translates *di* 抵, which could also be understood as "go to." The tactile and directional connotations of the word are probably both intended in the verse.

[6]"Stove trivet" translates *zaogang* 竈綱. Han tombs have yielded numerous specimens of a metal trivet used to hold a kettle over an open fire. Sun Ji (1991: 335) demonstrates that *jiong* 烓 was a contemporary name for this trivet (glossed in *SW*, 10A.44b, as "traveling

Press the neck zone;[1]
Stroke the receiving canister;[2]
Cover the encircling ring;[3]
Descend the broken basin;[4]
Cross the sweet-liquor ford;[5]

---

stove"). I suspect that *zaogang* refers to the same cooking apparatus, hence my translation of *gang* as "trivet." Applied to female anatomy, the term suggests a triangular configuration. Keeping in mind that the previous line names the underarms and the following line the neck, I would suggest identifying the "stove trivet" with the upper chest between the neck and the two breasts.

[1]"Neck zone" translates *lingxiang* 領鄉. I do not know of other examples of *xiang* suffixed to an anatomical name. *Lingxiang* may be a technical term whose nuances escape me. However, I suspect that it may be a nonce word created to fill out the third syllable with an **-ang* rhyme word.

[2]"Receiving canister" translates *chengkuang* 拯匡. The term is attested in *Yijing*, "Guimei," 5.20a; and in *Shijing*, Mao 161, 9B.1b. The *kuang* "canister" is a square basket (which adds to its earth, Yin, feminine symbolism); and both occurrences of *chengkuang* use the canister image to suggest female sexuality. The usage is consistent with other *Shijing* basket imagery in which baskets suggest the female genitals. Given the square shape of the canister, I would suggest identifying the "receiving canister" with the pelvic region—the osseous basket that holds the genitals. For further discussion, see Harper 1987b: 570-75. Having moved across her upper body, the man now touches the genital region.

[3]"Encircling ring" translates *zhouhuan* 周環, which I identify as the waist—the band that encircles the body at its midpoint. The identification is based primarily on another use of *huan* "ring" in *MSI*.C. The first Shuihudi hemerological manuscript uses *zhouhuan* to describe a road that "makes an encircling ring around a house" (an unlucky sign when siting a house; *SHD*: 210). The synonymous 周圜 occurs in *Hou Hanshu*, 88.12b, with the meaning "circumference." I suspect that the instruction to "cover the encircling ring" means that the man mounts the woman at the waist; and that there is a shift from massage-like foreplay to more direct sexual action.

[4]The clavicle (see *MSI*.A.2). Li and McMahon situate *chengkuang* at the shoulders (because the shoulders hold the head) and *zhouhuan* at the breasts (because they are round), assuming that they must be located in the vicinity of the clavicle in order for the man to touch all three in succession as part of foreplay (1992: 167-68). I find the argument unpersuasive, especially given the strong evidence for associating *chengkuang* with the genitals. Because the metaphors that follow the descent from the broken basin are geographical in their inspiration and the verbs no longer connote hand touching, I suspect that this part of the verse is intended more as a survey of the sexual topography of the woman's body than as a literal route for the man to follow with his hands (it is of course the penis that "enters the dark gate").

[5]"Sweet-liquor ford" translates *lijin* 醴津. The term is similar to *liquan* 醴泉 (sweet-liquor wellspring), which denotes saliva in religious Daoist hygiene (Maspero 1981: 508). Harper cites Han sources for the belief that the emergence of a *liquan* from the earth was an auspicious portent, a manifestation of the cosmic axis joining heaven and earth (1987b: 576-77). The terrestrial location of the cosmic axis was also conceived as a navel. According to *Shiji*, 28.9b, "heaven's navel" (*tianji* 天齊) was a spring situated at the base of a mountain in the southern suburb of Linzi 臨菑 (which accounts for the tradition that the ancient state of Qi 齊 was so named because it was the *ji* "navel" of heaven). The human navel is the

Skim the Spurting Sea;
Ascend Constancy Mountain;[1]
Enter the dark gate;[2]
Ride the coital muscle;[3]

---

corresponding axial point on the body. Perhaps the *lijin* is situated by the navel (a central location for storing vapor and essence as well). It is also possible that the term refers to the mammae. *Taipingjing*, 45.123, identifies the mammae as wellsprings (*quan*) that provide drink for a child in the same way that the wellsprings of the earth provide life-sustaining water.

[1]The Spurting Sea (Bohai 勃海) is the body of water into which the Yellow River drains. Constancy Mountain (Changshan 常山) is the sacred peak of the north, in present-day Hebei (the verse uses 常 rather than the usual *heng* 恒 in the name of Constancy Mountain to avoid the personal name of Thearch Wen 文帝). Context justifies identifying Constancy Mountain as the rise of the female genitals, the *mons veneris*. By implication, the head and upper body must be situated in the south in the verse's geography. Pondering the physiological analogue to the Spurting Sea, the Liaodong and Shandong peninsulas give this sea the appearance of an enclosure. I suspect that this enclosure is to be correlated with a location for storage of vapor in the body. If, purely for the sake of speculation, we assume that the "sweet-liquor ford" has a geographical location as "heaven's navel" in Qi, the Spurting Sea ought to be the region to the north of (beneath) the navel. If, however, the "sweet liquor ford" refers to the mammae, it would be equally plausible to situate the Spurting Sea below the breast. In my reading of the verse, I prefer situating the Spurting Sea closer to the genitals and thus I favor a location below the navel. In Tang and later religious Daoist hygiene the term *qihai* 氣海 (vapor sea) refers to a place beneath the navel (also the location of the lower cinnabar field; Maspero 1981: 459, 488). This would appear to corroborate my preference for the location of the Spurting Sea were it not for the fact that the earliest attested usage, in *Lingshu* 33, 6.5a, identifies the *qihai* as one of four "seas" in the body and situates it in the upper chest (the stomach is the location of the "water and grain sea," and the brain of the "marrow sea"). While confirming the notion of seas in the body, *qihai* in *Lingshu* might be used to justify the alternative interpretation of the "sweet liquor ford" as the mammae with the Spurting Sea underneath. In short, the physiological denotation of Spurting Sea remains uncertain.

[2]I.e. the penis penetrates the vagina. The term "dark gate" (*xuanmen* 玄門) must be derived from the "gate of the dark feminine" (玄牝之門) in *Laozi*, par. 6 (*MWD*, vol. 1: 115). The "Xianger" commentary interprets the *Laozi* phrase as a reference to the vagina (Rao 1991: 9).

[3]The "coital muscle" (*jiaojin* 交筋) is defined in the prose text below as the "coital vessel" (*jiaomai* 交脈) inside the vagina that can be stimulated by the penis, "causing both bodies to experience ecstatic excitation." Neither term is attested in received literature, but *jiaojin* also occurs in *Yinshu* (*YSSW*: 85). While it is evident that the terms refer to a physiological structure in the vagina that is probably responsible for what we call female orgasm, I would refrain from making specific correlations between the "coital muscle/vessel" as identified in *MSVI.B* and modern research on the psycho-physiological elements of female orgasm (in which the role of the vagina is generally discounted). Moreover, the concept of the woman's "coital muscle/vessel" is uniquely Chinese in that the man's penis is stimulated by it simultaneously. The *Huangdi neijing* locates both muscles and vessels in the male and female genitals. According to *Suwen* 60, 16.2a-b, the *ren* 任 and *du* 督 vessels pass through the genitals (for discussion of the role of these vessels in later sexual cultivation, see Need-

Suck the essence and spirit upward.[1]
Then you can have lasting vision[2] and exist in unison with heaven and earth.

The coital muscle is the coital vessel inside the dark gate. When you are able to rub and stroke it,[3] it causes both bodies to experience ecstatic excitation and to exude beauty that is joyful and lustrous.[4] Although desirous, do not act. Perform mutual exhalation[5] and mutual embracing, following in sequence the way of play.[6] The way of play: the first is "vapor rises and her face is flushed—slowly exhale";[7] the second is "the nipples harden and her nose sweats—

---

ham 1954–, vol. 5, part 5: 202). *Suwen* 45, 12.11a, states that the genitals are "where the manifold muscles (*zongjin* 宗 筋) are gathered"; and in *Suwen* 44, 12.9a, "manifold muscles" refers to the penis.

"Ride" translates *yu* 御, which analogizes sexual intercourse to horse-riding (see *MS*III.38, where the man's penis/jade whip contrasts with the woman's vagina/horse). The standard term for intercourse, *yunü* 御 女, has been understood to mean simply "lie with the woman" based on *Duduan*, 1.4a, which explains that *yu* refers generally to the downward-directed actions of the monarch, including his sexual relations with consorts. However, "riding the coital muscle" is clearly an act of penile horsemanship which probably reveals the original meaning of *yunü*.

[1]"Suck" translates *xia* 欱, glossed in *SW*, 8B.24b, as "drink." According to the Duan Yucai commentary *xia* is the antonym of *pen* 歕 (spout out), hence my translation "suck" for the action of drawing the sexually generated essence upward. The culmination of intercourse/cultivation for the man in *MS*VI.A.7 is similar: "the mass of essence all ascends, suck in (*xi* 噏) the great illumination." While the man obviously practices some form of essence retention, it is unclear whether orgasm occurs (see Prolegomena, Section Four, "Techniques").

[2]The earliest citation I have found for "lasting vision" (*jiushi* 久 視) is *Laozi*, par. 59 (*MWD*, vol. 1: 107), where it is paired with "extended life" (*changsheng* 長 生) in the phrase "the way of extended life and lasting vision."

[3]I.e. stimulate it with the penis.

[4]Similar language is used in *Ishinpô*, 28.7b–8a (sec. "Yang Yin"), to describe the benefits of essence retention for the woman; and in *Ishinpô*, 28.6a (sec. "Yang Yang"), for the man.

[5]*Xu* 呴 (exhalation) is one of the forms of exhalation used in breath cultivation (see *MS*II.A). Here it refers to a kiss in which the partners suck in the exhaled breath of their mate and thus mingle Yin and Yang essences. This mingling of breaths while kissing is referred to in the Gao You commentary in *Huainanzi*, 2.24. For the phrase "that into which Yin and Yang exhale," the commentary notes, "the word *xu* is read like the word *xu* 吁 as in mouths exhaling into each other." *Ishinpô*, 28.8b (sec. "Hezhi"), provides a detailed description of the kissing technique (cf. Wile 1992: 108).

[6]The five stage "way of play" detailed below (also called the "signs of the five desires") concerns foreplay. There is a parallel text in *MS*VII.B.17. The language of a passage on the "five signs" in *Ishinpô*, 28.12b (sec. "Wuzheng"), is clearly related to the manuscript, but the actions performed by the man in response to the signs exhibited by the woman are not limited to foreplay (cf. Wile 1992: 87).

[7]I.e. kiss.

slowly embrace"; the third is "the tongue spreads and becomes slippery—slowly press";[1] the fourth is "the fluid flows below and her thighs are damp—slowly rub";[2] the fifth is "her throat is dry, swallowing saliva—slowly rock." These are the "signs of the five desires." When the signs are complete, ascend. Jab upward but do not penetrate inside, thereby bringing the vapor. When the vapor arrives penetrate deeply inside and thrust it upward, thereby dispensing the heat.[3] Then once again bring it back down. Do not let the vapor spill out, lest the woman become greatly parched.[4] Afterward practice the ten movements;[5] conjoin in the ten postures;[6] and intersperse the ten refinements.[7] Conjoin forms after sunset; and send the vapor to the progenitive gate.[8] Then observe the eight movements;[9] listen to the five sounds;[10] and examine the signs of the ten pauses.[11]

---

[1]I translate *tun* 屯 as "press" primarily on the basis of the parallel *fu* 傅 in *MS*VII.B.17. I suspect that *tun* in the sense of "press" is an extension from the meaning "amass" (see *Guangya*, 3B.4a). The actions denoted by "press" as well as by "rub" and "rock" below probably involve the man's hands against the woman's body, but whole body action and penile action are also possible. In any case, penetration does not occur.

[2]For other occurrences of *cao* 操 in the meaning "rub," see *MS*I.E.242, 251; *MS*III.38, 43. *Xi* 汐 and the parallel *xi* 夕 in *MS*VII.B.17 probably refer to tidal flow, a meaning first attested in received literature in Guo Pu's 郭 樸 (276-324) "Jiang fu" 江 賦, *Wenxuan*, 12.6b. *Xi* denotes the evening or neap tide in contrast to *chao* 潮, the morning or spring tide (Needham 1954-, vol. 3: 484-85). In *MS*VI.B.1 the "fluid flowing" is vaginal secretion (compare *MS*V.3 where menstrual blood is associated with spring tide). *MWD*, vol. 4, "Transcription," n. 6, reads *xi/*rjiak* 汐 as a phonetic loan for *ye/*rag* 液 (fluid), which is phonologically and semantically plausible. However, I think the analogy between vaginal secretion and tidal flow favors reading the graph as written (the fact that the first attestation of this meaning of *xi* in received literature is post-Han is not in itself cause for rejecting the graph as written).

[3]Having completed foreplay, the man jabs at the vagina with the penis until he "brings the vapor", and then penetrates after "the vapor arrives." The vapor referred to might be the woman's, but in my interpretation it is the vapor of the penis. *MS*VII.B.2 and *MS*VII.B.18 describe the penis' "three arrivals": to become large, flesh or skin must arrive first; to become hard, muscle must arrive next; and to become hot, vapor must arrive before the penis can finally enter the vagina. The references to "bringing the vapor" and "dispensing the heat" in *MS*VI.B.1 indicate the same concern for achieving full arousal of the male organ before penetration.

[4]I.e. the penis must still block the vaginal opening in order to seal the sexually generated essence inside.

[5]The "ten movements" refers to the technique of thrusting the penis without ejaculating. See *MS*VI.B.2.

[6]The ten positions for intercourse are listed in *MS*VI.B.3.

[7]The "ten refinements" refers to the ways to move the penis in the vagina. See *MS*VI.B.4.

[8]*MS*VII.B.13 provides a parallel to this sentence in which the words *yihun* 以 昏 (in the evening) appear in place of *yimo* 已 沒. The parallel leads me to interpret *mo* as elliptical

MSVI.B.2 (SS112-15)

The ten movements: commence with ten, followed by twenty, thirty, forty, fifty, sixty, seventy, eighty, ninety, and one hundred—exiting and entering without spilling.[1] At the first movement with-

---

for *rimo* 日没 (sunset; *yimo* could mean "at sunset" rather than "after sunset"). Without the parallel, *mo* might easily be understood as "finish", giving the translation "after finishing the conjoining of forms." For me the statement in *MS*VI.B.7 that the man's essence flourishes in the evening while the woman's essence accumulates in the morning is decisive confirmation of evening as the recommended time for the man to practice sexual cultivation. In addition, *Yinshu*, "Seasonal Regimen," recommends evening hours for intercourse (translated at the beginning of Section Four in the Prolegomena).

For *zongmen* 宗門 (progenitive gate), *MS*VII.B.13 has *xuemen* 血門 (blood gate). In my judgment both terms refer to a place where the man stores vapor and essence; perhaps related to the *mingmen* 命門 (gate of life) in received literature, and to the womb in *MS*VI.A.7. And I suspect that "filling the womb" in *MS*VI.A.7 and "dispensing to the womb" in *MS*VI.A.8 correspond to "sending the vapor to the progenitive gate" in *MS*VI.B.1. Li and McMahon translate the sentence differently as the vapor "passing through the master gate (*zongmen*)" of the woman after intercourse is finished (*sui* 遂 in intransitive usage means "pass through" and in transitive usage means "send"); and further claim that both this sentence and the parallel in *MS*VII.B.13 are descriptions of "sexual climax in the woman" (1992: 178). While the *zongmen* was surely a part of female anatomy as well, the sentence occurs at the conclusion of a series of actions performed by the man for his own benefit. It is clearly the man who is the focus of attention; and it is his *zongmen* that receives vapor.

[9]The "eight movements" refer to body movements made by the woman that indicate to the man what she wants him to do in order to satisfy her sexually. See *MS*VI.B.5. Similarly, the "five sounds" and "ten intermissions" below concern the woman's state of arousal, something that the man must carefully monitor if he is to bring her to orgasm (and then store the sexually generated essence in his body). Their placement at the end of the passage is simply a matter of describing a technique in a text: those items concerning the man himself are listed first, including essence retention when "vapor is sent to the progenitive gate"; and those concerning the woman are appended at the end. During actual intercourse the man's observation of the woman's reactions would be part of process leading up to the moment of successful sexual cultivation.

[10]Signs of arousal coming from the woman's mouth. See *MS*VI.B.6.

[11]The "ten pauses" refers to stages of transformation as the woman moves toward orgasm. See *MS*VI.B.8.

[1]"Movement" refers to thrusting the penis inside the vagina. As detailed in *MS*VI.B.2, ten thrusts constitute one movement and there are ten movements for a total of one hundred thrusts. There are text parallels in *MS*VII.B.3 and *MS*VI.A.3. The latter refers to "nine arrivals" rather than "ten movements"; and *MS*VI.B.2 is the only passage to explicitly state that each movement consists of ten thrusts. None of the passages on penile "movements" specify whether the man should finally reach orgasm. I reject the argument in Li and McMahon (1992: 175) that the numbers ten and one hundred should be understood figuratively as signifying fullness and not as a literal count of the number of thrusts. To be sure, one hundred is an ideal number, but ideal numbers can be counted and often were in religious Daoist hygiene. There is no reason to assume that early macrobiotic hygiene was different. The longer intercourse continues without ejaculation, the greater the benefit for

out spilling, ears and eyes are perceptive and bright; at the second, the voice's sound is brilliant; at the third, skin and hide glow; at the fourth, spine and side are strong; at the fifth, buttock and ham are squared; at the sixth, the waterway passes through;[1] at the seventh, you achieve culminant firmness and strength; at the eighth, the skin's webbed pattern glows; at the ninth, you penetrate spirit illumination; at the tenth, the body achieves constancy. These are the ten movements.

*MS*VI.B.3 (SS116-17)

The ten postures:[2] the first is "tiger roving";[3] the second is "cicada clinging";[4] the third is "measuring worm";[5] the fourth is "river deer butting";[6] the fifth is "locust splayed"; the sixth is "gibbon grabbing";[7] the seventh is "toad"; the eighth is "rabbit bolting";[8] the ninth is "dragonfly"; the tenth is "fish gobbling."[9]

---

the man. *Ishinpô*, 28.22a (sec. "Huanjing"), describes a sequence of ten movements without ejaculation (the number of thrusts in a movement is not specified) with benefits similar to those identified in the Mawangdui texts (cf. Wile 1992: 92).

[1]For "waterway" (*shuidao* 水 道), *MS*VI.A.3 has "hundred vessels." *Huangdi neijing* also uses *shuidao* to refer to the course followed by fluids in the body (not necessarily just the vapor and blood in the vessels); see, for example, *Suwen* 8, 3.1b. There is an obvious analogy between waterways through the earth and through the body.

[2]There are parallel lists of sexual positions in *MS*VII.B.10 and *MS*III.88. Li and McMahon discuss each position and its possible correlation with positions in later sexual literature (1992: 170).

[3]"Tiger roving" (*huyou* 虎 游) may be related to "tiger pace" (*hubu* 虎 步) in *Ishinpô*, 28.14b (sec. "Jiufa"). In the latter position the woman bends over on all fours, buttocks raised and head lowered; the man kneels and performs rear entry (cf. Wile 1992: 89).

[4]"Cicada clinging" (*chanfu* 蟬 附) appears as a sexual position in *Ishinpô*, 28.15a (sec. "Jiufa"). The woman lies prone; the man lies on top of her and enters from the rear (cf. Wile 1992: 89).

[5]"Measuring worm" (*chihuo* 尺 蠖) is the name of an exercise in the *Yinshu*. The person extends his lower leg and curls his toes thirty times (*YSSW*: 82). As a sexual position, measuring worm must involve bending and stretching.

[6]I follow *MWD*, vol. 4, "Transcription," n. 2, in reading 桷 as *jue* 角. Perhaps the man and woman face one another in "river deer butting" (*junjue* 麇 角). There may be a connection with the sport known as *juedi* 角 抵 (horn butting; see Lewis 1990: 157-60), but it should be noted that the water deer lacks antlers in both sexes (Tate 1947: 331).

[7]"Gibbon grabbing" (*yuanju* 猨 據) may be related to "gibbon striking" (*yuanbo* 猿 搏) in *Ishinpô*, 28.15a (sec. "Jiufa"). In the latter position the woman lies supine; the man raises her legs over his shoulders until her buttocks and back are raised off the ground, and performs front entry (cf. Wile 1992: 89).

[8]"Rabbit bolting" (*tuwu* 兔 鶩) may be related to "rabbit licking hair" (*tu shunhao* 兔 吮 豪) in *Ishinpô*, 28.15b (sec. "Jiufa"). In the latter position the man lies supine; the woman straddles him facing his feet, and he enters from the rear (cf. Wile 1992: 89).

MSVI.B.4 (SS118-19)

The ten refinements:[1] the first is "go up"; the second is "go down"; the third is "go to the left"; the fourth is "go to the right"; the fifth is "thrust rapidly"; the sixth is "thrust slowly"; the seventh is "thrust rarely"; the eighth is "thrust frequently"; the ninth is "enter shallowly"; the tenth is "enter deeply."

MSVI.B.5 (SS120-24)

The eight movements:[2] the first is "clasping hands"; the second is "extending elbows"; the third is "straightening heels"; the fourth is "hooking the flanks"; the fifth is "hooking up above"; the sixth is "crossing thighs"; the seventh is "level upspring"; the eighth is "shaking." When she clasps hands, she wants her abdomen pressed; when she extends elbows, she wants the upper part rubbed and scratched;[3] when she straightens heels, entry is insufficiently deep; when she hooks the flanks, she wants the sides rubbed; when she hooks up above, she wants the lower part rubbed; when she crosses thighs, penetration is excessive; when she makes a level upspring, she wants shallow entry; when she shakes, she wants the man to continue holding for a long time.

MSVI.B.6 (SS125-26)

When there is convulsive breathing, the inside is tense;[4] when there is panting, she feels culminant delight; when there is continual

---

[9]"Fish gobbling" (*yuzuo* 魚 噣) may be related to "fish touching scales" (*yu jielin* 魚 接 鱗) in *Ishinpô*, 28.15b (sec. "Jiufa"). In the latter position, the man lies supine; the woman straddles him facing his head, and after he inserts his penis she alone makes a rocking movement (cf. Wile 1992: 89).

[1]There are parallels for the ways a man moves his penis in the vagina in *MS*VII.B.12 and *MS*III.88. A related passage in *Ishinpô*, 28.18a-b (sec. "Jiuzhuang"), is more descriptive, often comparing the thrusting of the penis to the actions of various creatures with indications like "rapidly" and "slowly" incorporated into the description (cf. Wile 1992: 111).

[2]For parallels see *MS*VII.B.14, 16; and *MS*III.88. According to *MS*VII.B.15, the man observes the woman's movements during intercourse in order to "know what gives her pleasure and gets through to her." There is a related passage in *Ishinpô*, 28.13a-b (sec. "Shidong"; cf. Wile 1992: 88).

[3]From "extend elbows" through "level upspring" the woman's movements communicate to the man how he should stimulate her vagina with his penis.

[4]*MS*VI.B.6 concerns the "five sounds"—signs emanating from the woman's mouth that are indicative of her state of arousal during intercourse. For parallels see *MS*VII.B.15, 20; and *MS*III.88. Judging from the descriptions of what each sound indicates in *MS*VI.B.6 and *MS*VII.B.20, the sequence of the five sounds reflects the progressive intensification of her passion. There is nothing comparable in received sexual literature. "Convulsive breathing" translates *chixi* 瘛 息. I understand the breathing to be like the description of the ailment

moaning,[1] the jade whip has entered and excitation then commences; when there is blowing, rapturous craving is intense;[2] when there is biting, her body shakes and she wants the man to continue for a long time.

*MS*VI.B.7
(SS127-28)[3] In the evening the man's essence flourishes; in the morning the woman's essence accumulates. By nurturing the woman's essence with my essence, muscles and vessels[4] both move; skin, vapor, and blood are all activated. Thus, you are able to open blockage and penetrate obstruction. The central cavity receives the transmission and is filled.[5]

*MS*VI.B.8 (SS129-33)
The signs of the ten pauses:[6] at the first pause, clear coolness emerges; at the second pause, the odor is like burning bones; at the

---

chi "convulsions" in *MS*I.E.27 ("the breath is quick and shrill"). The parallels in *MS*VII.B.15 and 20 give the first sound as "throaty breathing."

[1]I follow *MWD*, vol. 4, "Transcription," n. 2, in reading *ji/*kjəd* 濺 as a phonetic loan for *ai/*ʔəd* 哀 (moan; the latter graph occurs in the *MS*VII.B parallels).

[2]"Blowing" translates *he* 吙, literally denoting a kind of hot exhalation. The word is also used for chanting incantations in *MS*I.E.56 and *MS*I.E.59. "Rapturous craving" translates *yangan* 鹽 甘. For *gan* in the sense of craving see *MS*III.24. *Yan* occurs in *Liji*, 25.14b, where it is glossed as *yan* 艷 (rapturous) in the Zheng Xuan commentary.

[3]*MWD*, vol. 4, "Transcription," n. 2, indicates that SS127-28 may belong to the end of the text, after *MS*VI.B.8.

[4]前 in *MWD*, vol. 4, "Transcription," should be transcribed as *jin* 筋 (muscle). The top part of the graph looks like 艹 (the significs 艹 and ⺮ are sometimes used interchangeably in the manuscripts); but the graph is otherwise similar to *jin* in S104 and S105, and is clearly unlike other occurrences of 前. Because of the transcription error Li and McMahon incorrectly identify *qianmai* 前 脈 as a term for genitals (translated "front artery"; 1992: 163).

[5]*Zhongfu* 中 府 occurs in a plural sense in *Suwen* 27, 8.11b, referring to the internal organs in general. *MS*VI.B.7 concerns the man's achievement in sexual cultivation. While it is possible that the sexually generated essence goes to the "inner cavities," I think the reference is to a "central cavity" inside both the male and female body where vapor and essence are stored (like the "progenitive gate" in *MS*VI.B.1 and the "central bourne" in *MS*VI.B.8).

[6]"Pause" translates *yi* 已. The conclusion of *MS*VI.B.8 describes female orgasm and successful sexual cultivation. At each of the "ten pauses" a transformation occurs, and the cyclical return to the condition of the first pause corresponds to female orgasm. I think the transformation involves the fused essence of the man and woman generated through intercourse. There are parallels in *MS*VII.B.18-19. The parallel for the sixth pause in *MS*VII.B.18 explicitly refers to "the essence being like choice glutinous millet" (in *MS*VI.B.8 the characteristic is "slippery"). Alternatively, Li and McMahon interpret the pauses as corresponding to sensations that accompany states of arousal rather than to the transformation of essence (1992: 177-78; this is also the interpretation in Ma Jixing 1992:

third pause, it is freshened;[1] at the fourth pause, it is viscid; at the fifth pause, it is fragrant; at the sixth pause, it is slippery; at the seventh pause, it is congealed;[2] at the eighth pause, it is tallowy; at the ninth pause, it is gelatinous; at the tenth pause, it clusters.[3] After clustering it becomes slippery again, and the clear coolness emerges once again. This is called "great completion."[4] The signs of great completion: the nose sweats and the lips are white; the hands and feet all twitch; the buttocks do not adhere to the bedmat, but rise up and away.[5] When she becomes corpse-like, there is spreading.[6]

1000, n. 2). Wile misunderstands the meaning of *yi* and mistranslates all three passages (1992: 79, 82–83). The parallel in *MS*VII.B.19 adds a crucial piece of evidence concerning the ten pauses. Following a description of female orgasm similar to *MS*VI.B.8, the text states "the count has already reached one hundred." One hundred is, of course, the ideal number of penile thrusts in the "ten movements." Thus the "ten pauses" are correlated with the "ten movements"; and the man's completion of the movements coincides with female orgasm (the "great completion" that occurs when the cycle of pauses is complete). I would argue that the words *dong* 動 (movement) and *yi* 已 (pause) should be understood as relating sexual intercourse to the process of *dongjing* 動 靜 (movement and stillness) in nature as described in the opening of *Yijing*, "Xici zhuan," 7.1b: "When movement and stillness have constancy, hard and pliant will be determined." In intercourse it is the Yang man who favors movement and the Yin woman who favors stillness; it is his hard penis that encounters her pliant vagina. *MS*VII.B.20 elaborates on precisely these kinds of correlations, which are called "the calculation of Yin and Yang." The same passage states that in order to delight a woman, intercourse "must be slow and prolonged . . . *as if pausing but not pausing* (如 已 不 已)." Pausing is to female arousal what movement is to male arousal. The cycle of the "ten pauses" formalizes the value attached to female arousal in sexual cultivation technique.

[1]"Freshened" translates *zao* 澡. I reject *MWD*, vol. 4, "Transcription," which reads *zao* 燥 (scorched, dry).

[2]遅 in *MWD*, vol. 4, "Transcription," should be transcribed as 遲, pronounced *chi/*drid*. The parallel graph in *MS*VII.B.18 is *di/*drjad* 懘, which the "Transcription" reads as *zhi/*drjad* 滯 (congealed; see *SW*, 11A-2.27b). I suspect that *chi/*drid* is a phonetic loan for *zhi/*drjad* (see Luo and Zhou 1958: 253, for examples of rhyming between *-*id* and *-*ad* in the *Huainanzi*); hence the translation "congealed."

[3]緛 in *MWD*, vol. 4, "Transcription," should be transcribed as *qiu* 𦃇, which is attested as an orthographic variant of 緧 (Morohashi 1957–60, vol. 8: no. 27661). I read the graph as *jiu* 揂, glossed in *SW*, 12A.39a, as "cluster."

[4]I understand *zu* 卒 (completion) to signify completing a cycle, like in the idiomatic phrase 卒 其 時 (leave for one whole day; see *MS*I.E.200; and *MS*III.40, 74).

[5]Similar physiological changes during female orgasm are noted in Kinsey 1953: 613–23; and Masters and Johnson 1966: 128–34.

[6]The sentence 成 死 爲 薄 is difficult to interpret. The parallel in *MS*VII.B.19 is 成 死 有 薄. I am convinced that the sentence concludes the physiological description of the woman. I understand *si* 死 to be equivalent to *shi* 屍 (corpse). The usage is attested in *Hanshu*, 70.7a, as well as in the Shuihudi *Fengzhen shi* (*SHD*: 157–58). I suspect that "corpse-like" describes the relaxed state following orgasm rather than the muscle tension that accompanies it (Kinsey 1953: 627; Masters and Johnson 1966: 276–77). A description

Precisely at this time vapor expands in the central bourne. Essence and spirit enter and are deposited, then engendering spirit illumination.[1]

---

of female arousal in *Sunü miaolun*, 128–29, concludes with: "When her body is hot and soaked with sweat, her feet are relaxed, and her hands are languid—it is a sign that her feelings have culminated and her desires are satisfied" (cf. Wile 1992: 128). If I may be allowed the conjecture that "corpse-like" refers to this relaxed state, *pu* 溥 seems to refer to the subsequent "spreading" of the sexually generated essence in the same way that the breath cultivation technique in *MSVI*.A.1 describes the transformed vapor "spreading (*pu*) to your flesh and skin, and reaching to those hair tips." In the *MSVII*.B.19 parallel the spreading is further described as "racing to the internal network hairs and settling in the waist and heart." The parallel leads me to reject translating the sentence as "spread out like a corpse," which might otherwise seem as plausible as the translation I offer. I also reject Ma Jixing's interpretation that *si* refers to the penis gone limp (1992: 1002, n. 14). Ma understands the last several sentences to mean something like: ". . . the buttocks do not adhere to the bedmat. (The man) should withdraw (his penis) and leave. When (the penis) dies there is injury." *Si* has this meaning, as indicated in *Ishinpô*, 28.11b (sec. "Linyu"): "When the woman's fluids are overflowing, the man must retreat (i.e. withdraw his penis). He cannot come back dead (*si*), but must return alive (i.e. with the penis still erect). Exiting dead does great injury to a man." This meaning does not fit the context of *MSVI*.B.8 well, and Ma's interpretation is forced. The passage is an integrated description of female orgasm that concludes below with the successful completion of sexual cultivation. *MSVII*.B.19 concludes similarly with the man achieving a count of one hundred thrusts of the penis.

[1]I understand the conclusion to be a description of the man successfully completing sexual cultivation when the woman reaches orgasm. I also assume that spirit illumination occurs when the essence and spirit are concentrated in a location like the "progenitive gate" (*MSVI*.B.1) or the "central cavity" (*MSVI*.B.7). Thus I translate 藏 verbally as *cang* "deposit" rather than adopting the translation "essence and spirit enter the depot(s)." I suspect that *zhongji* 中 極 (central bourne) denotes this storage location in the man's body. *Suwen* 60, 16.2a, gives *zhongji* as the name of an acupuncture point, and locates the origin of the *ren* vessel (see *MSVI*.B.1) beneath it. In religious Daoist hygiene *zhongji* is one of the names for the navel region, which links it to the lower cinnabar field and the womb (see *MSVI*.A.7). The earlist citation is in *Laozi zhongjing*, par. 14 (*Yunji qiqian*, 18.10b). If *zhongji* in *MSVI*.B.8 refers to a location in the man's body, the phrase "vapor expands in the central bourne" probably means that his *zhongji* opens to receive the inflow of sexually generated essence. Alternatively, *zhongji* may belong to female physiology. *Zhongji* is attested as the name of a point inside the vagina in *Ishinpô*, 28.14b (sec. "Jiufa"); and it is not implausible for the term to have been applied to the vagina itself. Perhaps "vapor expanding in the central bourne" refers to the release of sexually generated essence from her *zhongji*, which is then absorbed by the man. I favor the first interpretation, but in either case it is the man who receives the benefit of sexual cultivation. My interpretation is at odds with Li and McMahon, who understand this passage as a description of the woman achieving spirit illumination (1992: 178).

*MS*VII.A

ZAJIN FANG

雜禁方

RECIPES FOR VARIOUS CHARMS

*MS*VII.A.1 (SS1–5)

When there is a dog that likes to bark in the courtyard and gate, daub mud on the well in a rectangular band five *chi* long.[1] When husband and wife dislike one another, daub mud on the doorway [1][2] in a rectangular band five *chi* long. When you wish to seduce a noble person, daub mud on the left and right sides of the gate in a rectangular band five *chi* long.[3] When you have frequent foul dreams, daub mud beneath the bed in a rectangular band seven *chi* long. When the husband's mother and his wife like to fight, daub mud on the doorway in a rectangular band five *chi* long. When an infant likes to cry, daub mud on the window in a rectangular band five *chi* long.

*MS*VII.A.2 (S6)

When involved in a suit with another person, write the person's name and set it inside a shoe.[4]

---

[1]*Tu* 塗 alone means to "daub something with mud." *MS*VII.A.1 indicates that daubing mud at specified locations in the house was an all-purpose magical act. I assume that the phrase 方 五 尺 refers to daubing a rectangular band of mud that is one *chi* wide and five *chi* long, rather than to daubing an area of five square *chi*. The medieval demonography *Baizetu* 白 澤 圖 includes examples of the same type of magic. The following is representative: "Whenever a rat causes a prodigy it is called Yin murder. [2] blend with yellow earth and daub it inside the chamber on the ground near the bed in a rectangular band three *chi* long. Make a six *cun* high dog of yellow earth and set it on the (band of) earth. On an Earth day (in the cycle of the Five Agents), take the dog and throw it in a crossroad. The calamity will be eliminated" (Rao Zongyi 1969: pl. 6; Matsumoto 1956: 147, no. 27). A second example is simpler: "When a person's clothing shines at night, daub the wall of the inner chamber with mud in a rectangular band three *chi* long, and whatever you are searching for will be obtained" (Rao Zongyi 1969: pl. 7; Matsumoto 1956: 147, no. 59)

[2]Based on the remaining traces of the graph, *MWD*, vol. 4, "Transcription," n. 2, suggests that it might be *mei* 楣 (lintel).

[3]These two applications of daubing mud are related to the examples of love magic below.

[4]The expectation is that by treading on your opponent's name in your shoe, you will magically emerge the winner in the suit. The same type of agonistic magic is attested in the

*MS*VII.A.3 (S8)

Take *quantou* that faces east-west. Incinerate and smith. Give it to the husband and wife to drink, and they will be driven apart.[1]

*MS*VII.A.4 (S7)

Incinerate and smith the tails of two female doves. Drink it yourself, and seduction will occur.[2]

*MS*VII.A.5 (SS9-10)

Take four nails from the left claw of a male dove and four nails from the left hand of a young girl. Scorch in a saucepan, combine, and smith. Apply it to the person and the person will be obtained.[3]

*MS*VII.A.6 (S11)

Put the person's left eyebrow in liquor and drink it.[4] You invariably obtain the person.

Greek magical papyri (Betz 1986: 142-43). A similar charm used for seduction occurs in *Ishinpô*, 26.19b (sec. "Xiang'ai"): "On a *wuzi* 戊子 day write the person's surname and name and set it beneath your foot. The person is invariably obtained."

[1]*Quantou* 犬頭 (dog head) must be the name of an herbal drug. Choosing the part that grows east-west has the magical effect of sending husband and wife in opposite directions. *Ishinpô*, 26.19b (sec. "Xiang'ai"), states that placing horsehair and dog fur in the husband's and wife's bed will make them dislike one another. I agree with Qiu Xigui that the sequence of the wooden slips as given in *MWD*, vol. 4, "Transcription," is incorrect (1992: 527-29). We both agree that S8 should follow S6, and that the text following S6 is concerned with love magic (the "Transcription" misinterprets S7 as related to the suit in S6). I place S7 after S8. Both *MS*VII.A.3 (S8) and *MS*VII.A.4 (S7) involve drinking a potion. There is a clear contextual relation between surreptitiously giving a potion to the husband and wife in order to separate them in *MS*VII.A.3 and drinking a potion yourself in order to magically seduce the object of desire in *MS*VII.A.4. Qiu interprets the context differently and places S7 at the end of the text.

[2]In *MS*VII.A.1, *MWD*, vol. 4, "Transcription," n. 3, reads *wei/*mjəd* 微 as a phonetic loan for *mei/*mjiəd* 媚 (seduce). The reading is the same in *MS*VII.A.4 (the "Transcription" understands the graph differently here because of the error in the sequence of the wooden slips).

[3]There is a similar philter recipe in *Ishinpô*, 26.19b (sec. "Xiang'ai"): "Take the nails from the left claw of a rooster and the nail from the middle finger of the right hand of a never married woman. Burn to ash and apply it to that person's clothing." The result, of course, is that the object of desire will be obtained.

[4]*Mei* 麋 (eyebrow; usually written 眉) and *mei* 媚 (seduction) are etymologically related (eyebrows are literally bewitching in early religious belief; see Shirakawa 1974: 443-57). Ingesting the left eyebrow of the object of desire gives you a magical hold on the person.

*MS*VII.B

TIANXIA ZHIDAO TAN

天下至道談

DISCUSSION OF THE CULMINANT WAY IN UNDER-HEAVEN

*MS*VII.B.1 (SS12–14)

The Yellow Spirit asked the Left Spirit:[1] "Why is it that the Yin is born together with the nine apertures and twelve joints, yet it alone dies first?"[2]

The Left Spirit replied:[3] "It is not utilized in strenuous activity; when there is sorrow and joy it is not used; it does not assist when drinking and eating.[4] It dwells in deepest Yin and does not see Yang.[5] Suddenly it is violently employed[6] without waiting for it to become vigorous. It cannot withstand the double hotness,[7] and therefore is severely injured. Its name is avoided and its body concealed, yet it engages frequently in violent activity without ritual. Therefore it is born together with the body, yet it alone dies first."

*MS*VII.B.2 (SS15–16)

When it is angered yet not large, flesh has not arrived; when large yet not firm, muscle has not arrived; when firm yet not hot, vapor

---

[1]The Yellow Spirit 黄神 is the Yellow Thearch (see *MS*I.E.178). Ma Jixing cites an argument identifying Left Spirit 左神 as a name for Goumang 句芒, the spirit who presides over the east (associated with left and Wood; 1992: 1012, n. 1). I doubt the identification is correct. In the absence of positive evidence, I simply treat Left Spirit as another of the Yellow Thearch's teachers in the Mawangdui medical manuscripts. The Left Spirit named in *Huangting neijing jing*, par. 17 (*Yunji qiqian*, 11.42a), cannot be related.

[2]The Yin is the penis. Yao asks the same question of Shun in *MS*VI.A.5.

[3]Much of the content of the Left Spirit's reply also occurs in *MS*VI.A.5.

[4]See *MS*VI.A.5-6 on the necessity of "feeding" the penis. I am uncertain why the penis is not involved in situations of sorrow and joy, unless formal, ritual occasions of sorrow and joy are intended (funerals, births, etc.).

[5]I.e. the penis is kept hidden and not exposed to view.

[6]*Yong* 用 (employ) refers specifically to engaging in intercourse as in *MS*VII.B.2.

[7]I.e. the hotness emanating from the man and the woman.

has not arrived.[1] If you engage in intercourse[2] when flesh has not arrived, it collapses.[3] If you engage in intercourse when vapor has not arrived, it retreats.[4] When all three arrive this is called "triple coming."

*MS*VII.B.3 (SS17-24)

Discussion of the Culminant Way in Under-heaven[5]

Like bubbles in the water's torrent, like the vapor of spring and autumn—what has passed by I do not see, and I do not obtain its benefits; I do not espy what is coming, yet I enjoy its fruits.[6] O be careful indeed! The matter of spirit illumination lies in what is enclosed. Vigilently control the jade closure, and spirit illumination will arrive.[7] As a rule, to cultivate the body the task lies in accumulating essence. When essence reaches fullness, it invariably is lost; when essence is deficient, it must be replenished. As for the time to replenish a loss, do it when essence is deficient. To do it, conjoin in a sitting position; tailbone, buttocks, nose, and mouth each partici-

---

[1]The "it" is the penis. *MS*VII.B.2 describes three stages necessary for the penis to become fully aroused and ready for intercourse. There is a parallel in *MS*III.88 (*MS*VII.B.18 also includes a brief parallel). *Ishinpô*, 28.13b (sec. "Sizhi"), discusss four stages of arousing the penis in similar terms, and the stage when the penis is "hot" marks the arrival of "spirit vapor" (cf. Wile 1992: 88).

[2]For the use of *yong* 用 to mean "engage in intercourse," see *MS*III.23.

[3]遀 in *MWD*, vol. 4, "Transcription," should be transcribed as 遀, equivalent to *duo* 隋 (collapse) in *MS*III.88 (where it describes the consequence of attempting intercourse when vapor has not arrived).

[4]The text omits reference to the consequence of engaging in intercourse when muscle has not arrived.

[5]This heading is written at the top of S17; the text begins in S18. A dot mark • appears above the graphs of the heading in S17. Each new entry in *MS*VII.B is marked with a dot in this fashion. It is probable, therefore, that the heading in S17 serves as a title for *MS*VII.B.3. *MWD*, vol. 4, "Transcription," n. 1, argues that the dot at the top of S17 represents scribal error; and that the heading should be understood as the general title for the remainder of *MS*VII.B.

[6]The thought is reminiscent of *Zhuangzi* 20, 297, which concerns the spontaneity of a bell-maker: "Clustering! Billowing! Such is his sending off what passes by and his greeting what is coming. What is coming, do not bar; what passes by, do not stay." The point is that a person must plunge unreservedly into the activity at hand without dwelling on opportunities already lost and ever aware of the shape of things to come. In *MS*VII.B.3 the activity is sexual cultivation; and the remainder of the passage concerns what to do so that when "the culminant essence is about to be lost" the techniques of sexual cultivation can be used to "stay it."

[7]On the jade closure, see *MS*VI.A.3.

pate at the proper time.[1] Passing by fleetingly and coming momentarily, the culminant essence is about to be lost. How can I stay it? Emptiness and fullness have a constant; carefully employ it without negligence. Do not thwart, do not deplete; muscle and bone are bulging and strong.[2] Move the jade wellspring and eat the fragrant aroma.[3] Lightly exit and lightly enter; await fullness—this is the constant.[4] When the three harmonious vapors arrive you become firm, vigorous, and strong.[5] When you wish to cultivate it, you must avoid verbalization.[6] Move the jade closure, and you can unite with the changes.[7] At the first movement, ears and eyes are perceptive and bright;[8] at the second movement, the voice's sound is brilliant; at the third movement, skin and hide glow; at the fourth movement, the spine is strong; at the fifth movement, buttock and ham are squared; at the sixth movement, the waterway passes through; at the seventh movement, you achieve culminant firmness and strength; at the eighth movement, the will soars boisterously; at the ninth movement, you conform to that heavenly blossom;[9] at the tenth movement, spirit illumination is engendered.

---

[1]I.e. engage in sexual intercourse. The statements concerning accumulating essence and replenishing loss through sexual cultivation are paralleled in *MS*VI.A.4.

[2]淩 in *MWD*, vol. 4, "Transcription," should be transcribed as 浲. Qiu Xigui reads the graph as *long* 隆, citing the compound *longqiang* 隆 彊 (bulging and strong; 1992: 535). *Longqiang* is attested in *Shiming*, 7.232, as a name for the braces of a carriage canopy.

[3]On the jade wellspring, see *MS*VI.A.3.

[4]Exiting and entering refers to penile action.

[5]I am uncertain of the referents for the "three harmonious vapors."

[6]The meaning of the phrase *hai qi yan* 害 其 言 is uncertain. My "avoid verbalization" assumes that the instruction is related to the idea of being spontaneous expressed above. *MWD*, vol. 4, "Transcription," n. 4. suspects that 害 is scribal error for *shen* 審 (examine), which would give the translation "examine the words (of the sexual cultivation technique?)."

[7]"Unite with the changes" translates *yiqian* 一 遷. Sima Tan's assessment of the Daoists in *Shiji*, 130.4a, praises their ability to "change and shift (*qianyi* 遷 移) with the times." *Yijing*, "Xici zhuan," 8.11a, also refers to "repeated changing" (*lüqian* 屢 遷) as a characteristic of the hexagrams. Management of the jade closure is evidently the key to success in sexual cultivation; and the "ten movements" described below (matched by the "ten pauses" in *MS*VII.B.18) represent a specific technique that enable a person to "unite with the changes." *MWD*, vol. 4, "Transcription" reads 遷 as *xian* 僊 (transcendent), which I reject. Nothing in *MS*VII.B.3 suggests a connection with the concept of *xian* or with any practices associated with the *xian* cult.

[8]On the ten movements, see *MS*VI.B.2.

[9]I do not know the referent of "heavenly blossom" (*tianying* 天 英).

*MS*VII.B.4 (SS25-30)

Vapor has eight benefits and also has seven detriments.[1] If you are unable to utilize the eight benefits and eliminate the seven detriments, at the age of forty, Yin vapor has halved itself;[2] at fifty, mobility deteriorates; at sixty, ears and eyes are not perceptive and bright; at seventy, the lower body withers and the upper body shrinks, the Yin's vapor is useless, and effluvia and tears flow out.[3] There is a way to restore its vigor. Eliminate the seven detriments, thereby shaking off its ailments. Utilize the eight benefits, thereby assisting its vapor. Therefore, the aged are restored to vigor, and the vigor does not deteriorate.[4]

---

[1]The "eight benefits" (*bayi* 八 益) and "seven detriments" (*qisun* 七 損) all concern the man. They are listed in *MS*VII.B.5-6, and are further described in *MS*VII.B.7-8. While the emphasis is on sexual intercourse, the first two benefits described in *MS*VII.B.7 concern cultivation practices similar to the cultivation of "penile essence" in *MS*VI.A.6 and the five-stage technique described in *MS*VI.A.7. The detriments described in *MS*VII.B.8 concern conditions that must be avoided lest intercourse be injurious to health. *Ishinpô*, 28.19a-21b (secs. "Bayi" and "Qisun"), also describes a system of "eight benefits" and "seven detriments" related to intercourse. Each benefit or detriment involves practicing a specific sexual technique to either achieve the benefit or eliminate the detriment (cf. Wile 1992: 89-91). The eight benefits in *MS*VII.B and in the *Ishinpô* are dissimilar. The names and characteristics of the seven detriments in the two sources bear comparison, but *MS*VII.B does not mention sexual techniques to alleviate the detriments. *Suwen* 5, 2.7a-b, discusses the "seven detriments and eight benefits" without listing their names or describing their nature. Given the general absence of references to sexual cultivation in the *Huangdi neijing*, I suspect that these detriments and benefits concern some other aspect of hygiene. The *Suwen* passage is notable for its parallel account of the decade by decade aging process described immediately below in *MS*VII.B.4. To sum up, *MS*VII.B provides the earliest documentation of the idea of "eight benefits" and "seven detriments" as part of sexual cultivation theory, which continues in a different form in later sexual literature. The *Suwen* parallel suggests that a more general notion of cultivating "eight benefits" and eliminating "seven detriments" was also current in Han medicine.

[2]Yin vapor is the essential complement to Yang vapor. The connection between loss of Yin vapor and aging is mentioned in *MS*VI.A.4.

[3]The description of the body at seventy is similar to the description of the body at sixty in *Suwen* 5, 2.7b. In the *Suwen* it is the Yin (i.e. penis) that becomes impotent, hence 陰 氣 in *MS*VII.B.4 must refer to the penis and its vapor and not to Yin vapor in general. *Guan* 浘 (usually written 祼) refers to the ritual of pouring liquor on the ground after it has been offered to the impersonator of the dead in ancestral worship (*SW*, 1A.11b, and Duan Yucai commentary). The word as used in *MS*VII.B.4 probably refers to the spent vapor or fluid given off by the aging body, hence my impressionistic translation "effluvia." The parallel word in the *Suwen* is *ti* 涕 (snot).

[4]According to *MWD*, vol. 4, "Transcription," n. 3, the context requires adding 者 to the text following 壯 and the emendation is made in the transcription, which would give the translation "the vigorous do not deteriorate." From the standpoint of grammar and mean-

The gentleman dwells in peace and happiness. Drinking and eating as he pleases, the skin's webbed pattern is lustrous and taut; vapor and blood are replete; and the body is light and lithe. But if he has intercourse impulsively,[1] he is unable to effect the passage (of vapor) and becomes ill. Sweating and panting, the inside is feverish and the vapor disordered. When not treated, internal hotness is produced. He drinks medicine and undergoes cauterization to bring forth the vapor; and he practices dietetics[2] to bolster his exterior. If he forces intercourse,[3] he is unable to effect the passage (of vapor), producing pustules and swollen scrotum.[4] Vapor and blood are replete while the nine apertures are not clear; the upper and lower body are useless, producing pustules and *ju* abscesses.[5] Thus, when you are skilled at utilizing the eight benefits and eliminating the seven detriments, the five ailments do not arise.

*MS*VII.B.5 (S31)

The eight benefits:[6] first is "cultivate vapor"; second is "bring the fluid";[7] third is "know timing"; fourth is "gather vapor"; fifth is "harmonize the fluid"; sixth is "steal vapor"; seventh is "await fullness"; eighth is "secure against upset."[8]

---

ing there is no reason to assume that the phrase necessarily contrasts "the vigorous" with "the aged" above, and I reject the emendation.

[1]I understand *shinei* 使 内 to be similar to *jinnei* 近 内, which refers to sexual intercourse in *MS*III.34.

[2]I read 司 as *si* 飼 (also written 飤), meaning "feed" (*SW*, 5B.10a, and Duan Yucai commentary). The compound 服 飼 refers to dietetics.

[3]"Forcing intercourse" refers to having intercourse when the condition of the penis is unfit, as when impulsive intercourse results in illness.

[4]橐 in *MWD*, vol. 4, "Transcription," should be transcribed as *gao* 櫜, attested as a word for a "large sack" in *SW*, 6B.9b. Qiu Xigui argues that *gao* is equivalent to *gao* 睾, still in use in the compound *gaowan* 睾 丸 (testicles; 1992: 536). The same graph is used for the scrotum in *Maishu*, "Ailment List" (*MSSW*: 72). On the ailment "swollen scrotum," see *MS*I.E.117.

[5]For *ju* 疽 as a type of abscess, see *MS*I.E.157.

[6]The names of some of the benefits are similar to the "ten refinements" in *MS*VII.B.11, however the latter are all concerned with sexual intercourse.

[7]"Fluid" translates *mo* 沫, which is primarily the word for water bubbles (see *MS*VII.B.3). Association with saliva is indicated in *Zhuangzi* 6, 109; and 18, 277. The descriptions of the second and fifth benefits in *MS*VII.B.7 associate *mo* with fluids generated in the lower body rather than the mouth.

[8]*Guoyu*, 21.1a, gives "securing against upset" (*dingqing* 定 傾) as one of a state's three central concerns.

*MS*VII.B.6 (S32)

The seven detriments: first is "blockage"; second is "leakage"; third is "parching"; fourth is "incapacity"; fifth is "feverishness"; sixth is "curtailment"; seventh is "wastage."

*MS*VII.B.7 (SS33-36)

Cultivation of the eight benefits. To rise at dawn, sit upright, straighten the spine, open the buttocks, suck in the anus, and press it down is "cultivating vapor."[1] When drinking and eating, to relax the buttocks, straighten the spine, suck in the anus, and let the vapor pass through is "bringing the fluid."[2] To first play until each is delighted and to have intercourse when both are desirous is "knowing timing."[3] While having intercourse, to relax the spine, suck in the anus, and press it down is "gathering vapor." While having intercourse, to not hurry and not be hasty,[4] and to exit and enter with harmonious control is "harmonizing the fluid." When getting out of bed, to have the other person make it erect and let it subside when angered is "accumulating vapor."[5] When nearly finished, to not let the inner spine move,[6] to suck in the vapor and

[1]"Cultivating vapor" appears to be a kind of morning exercise routine whereby vapor is generated and sent to an internal storage area using anal constriction. The description is reminiscent of *MS*VI.A.7, which describes "contracting the anus" (equivalent to "sucking in the anus") and "sucking in the vapor to fill the womb." *Yi* 抑 refers literally to "pressing (something) with the hand"; and *yi* is the verb used for pressing behind the scrotum with the middle fingers to block the urethra in the description of "returning the essence to replenish the brain" in *Ishinpô*, 28.22b (sec. "Huanjing bunao"). Although "returning the essence" in later sexual cultivation made use of both anal constriction and pressure applied to the urethra (Wile 1992: 59), I think the three occurrences of the phrase 抑下之 (press it down) in *MS*VII.B.7 are best understood as referring to pressure applied by means of anal constriction to force vapor to flow toward its destination inside the body. The "it" in each case is, then, vapor. In short, the practice of applying pressure to the urethra at the moment of male orgasm is not mentioned in the Mawangdui medical manuscripts (and in any case, the first benefit is not directly concerned with sexual intercourse).

[2]"Bringing the fluid" appears to represent a technique for "drinking and eating together with the penis" as recommended in *MS*VI.A.6.

[3]For the use of 爲之 to mean "have intercourse," see *MS*III.39.

[4]"Hasty" translates *shu* 數, glossed in *Erya*, 2.2b, as "rapid."

[5]The "it" is clearly the penis. I am uncertain whether the phrase "get out of bed" (出臥) refers to getting up in the morning or to rising from bed after intercourse. In either case, the female partner is supposed to stimulate the penis until erect in order to invigorate the man's vapor. In *MS*VII.B.5 this benefit is called "stealing vapor," implying that the man's gain is the woman's loss.

[6]"Inner spine" translates *neiji* 内脊. I think the phrase refers to the cessation of movement on the side of the spine where the man's genitals lie as the climax of intercourse approaches, presumably in order to delay or prevent ejaculation. It is also possible that *nei*

press it down, and to still the body while waiting for it is "awaiting fullness."[1] To wash it after finishing and let go of it after becoming angered is "securing against upset."[2] These are the eight benefits.

*MS*VII.B.8 (SS37-39)

The seven detriments. To have acute pain during intercourse is "internal blockage."[3] To sweat during intercourse is "external leakage."[4] To have intercourse without pausing is "parching."[5] To desire it but to be unable is "incapacity."[6] To pant and suffer internal disorder during intercourse is "feverishness."[7] To force it when desire is lacking is "curtailment."[8] To become ill from intercourse is "wastage."[9] These are the seven detriments. Thus, when you are

---

should be understood as a verb with spine as the direct object, but I am not satisfied by the possible verbal renderings of *nei* in this context.

[1]"Fullness" (*ying* 贏) is, of course, the goal of sexual cultivation. The seventh benefit concerns the critical stage of intercourse when the woman reaches orgasm and the man absorbs the sexually generated essence. This is the point at which the man "sends the vapor to the blood gate" in *MS*VII.B.13. The descriptions of the "ten pauses" and female orgasm in *MS*VII.B.18-19 are also related.

[2]Washing the penis is done to bring about detumescence. *MS*III.5 describes washing the penis after ejaculation when an aphrodisiac has been used to induce an erection; and *MS*IV.3 similarly describes washing the penis to cause detumescence. The eighth benefit appears to equate this post-coital washing (which returns the penis to its ordinary condition) with the principle of preventing ejaculation during intercourse by allowing the erect penis to subside each time it is "angered"—thereby "securing against upset." Li and McMahon mistranslate the eighth benefit as "finally to ejaculate" (*qing* 傾 does not denote ejaculation as claimed); and misinterpret the seventh and eighth benefits as referring to the man's sexual climax and ejaculation respectively (1992: 173). The text itself does not mention whether ejaculation occurs.

[3]The first detriment in *MS*VII.B is related to the sixth in the *Ishinpô*—"hundred blockages."

[4]Related to the fourth detriment in the *Ishinpô*—"leakage of vapor."

[5]"Parching" (*jie* 渴; my reading for text 楬) refers to the desiccation of vapor that occurs when intercourse is practiced immoderately. The phenomenon of parching is mentioned in *MS*VI.B.1, which warns the man to not let vapor leak out after the penis enters the vagina, "lest the woman become greatly parched (*jie*)"; and is alluded to in *MS*VII.B.1, which warns of the damage done when the penis is unprepared for intercourse and "cannot withstand the double hotness" generated by the man and woman. The seventh detriment in the *Ishinpô* is "blood parching."

[6]I.e. impotence. This is probably related to the third detriment in the *Ishinpô*—"vessel disarmament" (which also concerns impotence).

[7]Probably related to the second detriment in the *Ishinpô*—"overflowing essence."

[8]The first detriment in the *Ishinpô* is "curtailment of vapor," referring to "forcing intercourse when the heart and thoughts are not desirous." Compare *MS*VII.B.4, which describes the consequences of "forcing intercourse" when the penis is unfit.

[9]Related to the fifth detriment in the *Ishinpô*—"reversal and injury of the vital joints" (which concerns illness arising from intercourse).

skilled at utilizing the eight benefits and eliminating the seven detriments, ears and eyes are perceptive and bright; the body is light and lithe; Yin vapor grows increasingly strong; your years are extended and longevity increased; and you dwell in continuing happiness.

*MS*VII.B.9 (SS40-41)

When a person is born there are two things that do not need to be learned: the first is to breathe and the second is to eat. Except for these two, there is nothing that is not the result of learning and habit. Thus, what assists life is eating; what injures life is lust. Therefore, the sage when conjoining male and female invariably possesses a model. Thus.[1]

*MS*VII.B.10

(SS42-43) The first is "tiger roving";[2] the second is "cicada clinging"—focus on the outside;[3] the third is "measuring worm"; the fourth is "river deer butting";[4] the fifth is "locust splayed"—breath on the inside; the sixth is "gibbon grabbing"[5]—focus on the outside; the seventh is "toad"; the eighth is "rabbit bolting"; the ninth is "dragonfly"—focus on the outside; the tenth is "fish gobbling." These are the ten positions.

---

[1]The eight graphs written on S41, concluding with *gu* 故 (thus), occupy only the top one fourth of the bamboo slip. *MWD*, vol. 4, "Transcription," places a colon after *gu*, evidently regarding the word as introducing the lists of sexual procedures that follow in subsequent sections of *MS*VII.B. I suspect that having written 故, the scribe omitted the text for what should have been a conclusion for *MS*VII.B.9.

[2]See *MS*VI.B.3 for the sexual positions listed in *MS*VII.B.10.

[3]I am uncertain of the meaning of the added instruction to "focus on the outside" (*siwai* 思外), which occurs again following "gibbon grabbing" and "dragonfly." The related instruction "breath on the inside" (*xinei* 息 内) follows "locust splayed." Wei and Hu conjecture that *siwai* refers to the man positioning himself behind the woman (the interpretation involves reading 思 as *si* 司); and *xinei* to the man and woman positioned face to face (1992, vol. 2: 153, n. 6). Li and McMahon conjecture differently, associating *siwai* with meditation during intercourse and *xinei* with breathing methods (1992: 171). The content of *MS*VII.B.10 does not provide enough evidence to reach a definite conclusion. I am partial to the idea that *siwai* is related to the man's mental state, but it might simply mean that he should pay attention to external matters; and in contrast, *xinei* might mean that he should pay attention to internal matters. Whether or not the interpretation in Wei and Hu is correct, the idea that the two terms specify how the man and woman are positioned also has merit. It would be logical for a list of sexual positions to include details of this sort, whereas references to the man's mental state when using certain positions for intercourse are less easily explained.

[4]I read *ju/*kjug* 椇 as a phonetic loan for *jue/*kruk* 角 (butt; see *MS*VI.B.3).

[5]I read 居 as *ju* 据 (grab).

*MS*VII.B.11 (SS44-45)

The first is "bring vapor";[1] the second is "secure the taste";[2] the third is "control the joints";[3] the fourth is "exercise the fruit";[4] the fifth is "perfect timing"; the sixth is "transport material";[5] the seventh is "move lightly"; the eighth is "await fullness";[6] the ninth is "equalize life";[7] the tenth is "rest the form."[8] These are the ten refinements.

*MS*VII.B.12 (S46)

The first is "go up";[9] the second is "go down"; the third is "go to the left"; the fourth is "go to the right"; the fifth is "enter deeply"; the sixth is "enter shallowly"; the seventh is "thrust rapidly"; the eighth is "thrust slowly." These are the eight ways.

*MS*VII.B.13 (SS47-48)

The ten refinements have already been completed, the ten positions displayed in advance, and the eight ways interspersed. Conjoin forms in the evening. Sweat should not begin to flow; and send the vapor to the blood gate.[10] Suck in and swallow the blue-gem wellspring to penetrate the vessels and benefit the muscles.[11] Then ex-

---

[1]The "ten refinements" listed in *MS*VII.B.11 concern the actions that the man must accomplish during intercourse. *MS*VII.B provides only the names of these actions without detailing their exact nature. The names reflect a system similar to but not identical with the eight benefits. Perhaps the action of "bringing vapor" is related to *MS*VI.B.1, where the penis jabs at the entrance to the vagina without penetrating in order to "bring the vapor." However, it just as likely refers to breath cultivation, one form of which is kissing.

[2]Perhaps a reference to swallowing saliva or storing sexually generated fluids internally. The fourth stage in the five-stage cultivation technique described in *MS*VI.A.7 is "contain the five tastes and drink that wellspring blossom."

[3]Perhaps a reference to skill in moving the body during intercourse.

[4]The "fruit" (*shi* 實) probably refers to a point inside the vagina, as it does in *Ishinpô*, 28.15b (sec. "Jiufa").

[5]I read 才 as *cai* 材 (material). Since the seventh refinement is to have the penis "move lightly," the material that is transported may be the penis being brought into the vagina.

[6]Compare the seventh benefit in *MS*VII.B.7.

[7]Perhaps a reference to the successful accomplishment of sexual cultivation.

[8]Perhaps similar to the eighth benefit in *MS*VII.B.7, which concerns refraining from ejaculation and post-coital conduct.

[9]See *MS*VI.B.4 for a list of ten ways to move the penis ("thrust rarely" and "thrust frequently" are not included in *MS*VII.B.12).

[10]Compare the parallel passage in *MS*VI.B.1.

[11]I read 榣 as *yao* 瑤 (blue-gem); and *qian/*dzian* 前 as a phonetic loan for *quan/*dzjuan* 泉 (wellspring). The loan usage is comparable to the standard Qin and Han use of *qian/*dzjan* 錢 for *quan/*dzjuan* in the sense of "currency" (*SW*, 14A.10b, and Duan Yucai commentary). The "blue-gem wellspring" occurs as a metaphor for saliva in the description of breath cultivation in *MS*VI.A.4 ("Drink the blue-gem wellspring and numi-

amine the eight movements, and observe where vapor lies. Then know the five sounds,[1] both the later and the earlier.[2]

*MS*VII.B.14 (S49)

The eight movements:[3] the first is "clasping hands"; the second is "extending elbows"; the third is "level upspring"; the fourth is "straightening heels"; the fifth is "crossing thighs"; the sixth is "shaking"; the seventh is "hooking the flanks"; the eighth is "hooking up above."

*MS*VII.B.15 (SS50-51)

The five sounds:[4] the first is "throaty breathing";[5] the second is "panting"; the third is "continual moaning"; the fourth is "blowing"; the fifth is "biting." Examine the five sounds to know her heart; investigate the eight movements to know what delights and affects her.

*MS*VII.B.16 (SS52-53)

When she clasps hands, she wants her abdomen pressed;[6] when she extends elbows, she wants the upper part rubbed and scratched;[7] when she hooks the flanks, she wants the sides rubbed; when she crosses thighs, penetration is excessive; when she straightens heels,

---

nous winepot and make it circulate"). In my interpretation, swallowing saliva coincides with sending vapor to the blood gate; and both actions have the effect of invigorating the man's body. The combining of sexual intercourse with breath cultivation in *MS*VI.A.10 is comparable. Alternatively, *qian* may refer to the female genitals (see *MS*IV.8), making "blue-gem front" an elegant term for the vagina. However, there is no other attestation of this usage in the Mawangdui medical manuscripts; and I cannot explain what it would mean in sexual cultivation technique to have the man "suck in and swallow the blue-gem front." It makes better sense for him to be swallowing the same "blue-gem wellspring" attested in *MS*VI.A.4. *MWD*, vol. 4, "Transcription," reads 榣 as *yao* 搖 (shake, wave), which I reject (the "Transcription" reads the same graph as *yao* 瑤 in *MS*VI.A.4). And I do not accept the interpretation of Li and McMahon, which errs in treating *MS*VII.B.13 as a description of sexual climax for the woman rather than for the man; and understands 搖前 as the woman who "sways her vagina" (1992: 178).

[1]音 in *MWD*, vol. 4, "Transcription," should be transcribed as 言; however, the latter graph is a scribal error for the former (the same scribal error occurs in *MS*VII.B.15).

[2]Compare *MS*VI.A.10, which includes the sentence, "The five sounds arise in response, both the short and the long."

[3]These are movements made by the woman during intercourse that indicate what she wants the man to do. See *MS*VI.B.5.

[4]I.e. signs that emanate from the woman's mouth. See *MS*VI.B.6.

[5]The parallel in *MS*VI.B.6 is "convulsive breathing."

[6]This continues the discussion of the eight movements from *MS*VII.B.14 (see *MS*VI.B.5).

[7]From "extend elbows" through "level upspring" the woman's movements communicate to the man how he should stimulate her vagina with his penis.

entry is insufficiently deep; when she hooks up above, the lower part is not reaching the heart;[1] when she makes a level upspring, she wants shallow entry; when she shakes, superbness is culminant. These are the eight observations.[2]

*MS*VII.B.17

Vapor rises and her face is flushed—slowly exhale. The nipples (SS54-55)
harden and her nose sweats—slowly embrace. The tongue spreads and becomes slippery—slowly press. The fluid flows below and her thighs are damp—slowly rub. Her throat is dry, swallowing saliva—slowly rock. These are the "five signs"; these are the "five desires." When the signs are complete, ascend.[3]

*MS*VII.B.18

When it is angered yet not large, skin has not arrived; when large (SS56-58)
yet not firm, muscle has not arrived; when firm yet not hot, vapor has not arrived. When the three arrive, enter.[4] At the first pause, clear coolness emerges;[5] at the second pause, the odor is like rotting bones; at the third pause, it is freshened; at the fourth pause, it is viscid; at the fifth pause, it is fragrant; at the sixth pause, the essence is like choice glutinous millet; at the seventh pause, it is congealed; at the eighth pause, it is tallowy; at the ninth pause, it is pasty;[6] at the tenth pause, it matures.[7] After maturing it becomes slippery again, and dawn vapor then emerges.[8]

---

[1]The parallel in *MS*VI.B.5 is "she wants the lower part rubbed," referring to the lower part of the vagina. "The lower part is not reaching the heart" must mean that she wants that part to be stimulated by the penis.

[2]Another name for the "eight movements" based on the fact that it is the man who must "observe" the movements and react appropriately.

[3]The "five signs" constitute stages to be followed in foreplay (see the parallel in *MS*VI.B.1).

[4]The "it" is the penis (see the parallels in *MS*VII.B.2 and *MS*III.88).

[5]The remainder of *MS*VII.B.18 concerns the "ten pauses" that lead up to female orgasm. *MS*VII.B.19 concludes with a description of female orgasm. The pauses and description of female orgasm are combined in the parallel in *MS*VI.B.8.

[6]"Pasty" translates *li* 黎, glossed in *SW*, 7A.57b, as the paste used to glue shoes. The parallel graph in *MS*VI.B.8 is *jiao* 膠 (gelatinous).

[7]I read 滊 as *kai* 愾 in the sense of "full, mature" (*Guangya*, 1A.10a). The parallel graph in *MS*VI.B.8 is *jiu* 揂 (cluster).

[8]The reference to the emergence of dawn vapor must be related to the statement in *MS*VI.B.7 that "in the morning the woman's essence accumulates." After the tenth pause in *MS*VI.B.8 there is a return to the condition of the first pause, "clear coolness."

*MS*VII.B.19

(SS59-61) The first is "hairpin light";[1] the second is "sealing cord";[2] the third is "dry gourd";[3] the fourth is "rat wife"; the fifth is "grain fruit"; the sixth is "wheat teeth";[4] the seventh is "infant girl";[5] the eighth is "depart to return";[6] the ninth is "why remain";[7] the tenth is "red thread";[8] the eleventh is "red bead";[9] the twelfth is "*zao* stone."[10] Obtain it and do not release it.[11] When she becomes corpse-like, there is spreading that races to the internal network hairs and settles in the waist and heart.[12] The lips are completely

---

[1]*MS*VII.B.19 lists twelve names for parts of the female genitals, both external and internal. Some of the names also occur in *MS*III.91; and some may be related to names in *MS*III.88. The names in *MS*VII.B.19 do not follow an identifiable sequence from the exterior to the interior of the vagina. See *MS*III.91 for discussion of the problems involved in associating the names with later sexual literature. *Jiguang* 笄 光 (hairpin light) occurs in *MS*III.91 as the name of a point inside the vagina. I am unsure of its location. *MWD*, vol. 4, "Transcription," n. 1, notes that the scribe of *MS*VII.B writes *mai* 辰 in a style that is indistinguishable from *guang* 光. It is possible that the graph in *MS*VII.B.19 should be identified as 辰 and read as *mai* 脈 (vessel; see the occurrence of 辰 for 脈 in *MS*VII.B.13). The graph transcribed as 光 in *MS*III.91 is fragmentary, and the scribe of *MS*III may have followed the same calligraphic convention as the scribe of *MS*VII.B.

[2]*Fengji* 封 紀. The name occurs again in *MS*VII.B.20, but the latter occurrence does not help to identify the part of the vagina denoted by the name. I assume that *feng* refers to the "sealing" of documents and letters, however I do not know of the use of a sealing cord.

[3]讕 in *MWD*, vol. 4, "Transcription," should be transcribed as *jian* 澗. *Jianhu* 澗瓠 may be related to *kuhu* 枯 瓠 (dry gourd) in *MS*III.88, which leads me to suspect that *jian/*krian* may be a phonetic loan for *gan/*kan* 乾 (dry).

[4]See *MS*III.91 for the names "grain fruit" and "wheat teeth" and their identification in later sexual literature.

[5]*Yingnü* 嬰 女. The name is attested in later sexual literature as a point inside the vagina between "wheat teeth" and "grain fruit" (see the table in Li and McMahon 1992: 164).

[6]A literal rendering of *fanqu* 反 去. Perhaps it identifies a point inside the vagina beyond which the penis should not penetrate.

[7]A literal rendering of *heyu* 何 寓, perhaps so named because the penis should not be there.

[8]I read 婁 as *lü* 縷 (thread). "Red thread" may refer to a part of the external genitals (the name for the clitoris follows).

[9]I.e. the clitoris (see *MS*III.91).

[10]*Zaoshi* 磲 石. Perhaps related to *yunshi* 云 石 in *MS*III.88. The name *kunshi* 昆 石 occurs in later sexual literature for a point deep inside the vagina (Li and McMahon 1992: 164).

[11]I understand this line to mean that the man's penis should continually stimulate the inside of the vagina to bring about female orgasm. Compare the passage concerning the "coital muscle" in *MS*VI.B.1.

[12]See the parallel description of female orgasm in *MS*VI.B.8. For *li* 理 in the sense of the "internal network" of vessels in the body, see *MS*VI.A.9. *Mao* 毛 (hair) is probably related to the idea of *maomai* 毛 脈 (hair vessels) in *MS*VI.A.1. I understand the sentence to mean that the woman's vapor and essence circulate to the outer limits of her body (compare the breath cultivation technique in *MS*VI.A.1) and then return to concentrate in the midsection of her body.

white; sweat flows down to the hollow at the back of the knees;[1] and the count has already reached one hundred.[2]

*MS*VII.B.20 (SS62-67)

What all men enjoy without exception is women. Possessing a woman, the skilled man alone is capable.[3] Do not give, but do not control;[4] do not initiate, but do not hesitate.[5] It must be slow and prolonged, and must be light and sustained—as if pausing but not pausing. The woman then is greatly delighted.

When there is throaty breathing, the lower body is stimulated, spitting Yin and radiating Yang.[6] When there is panting, the vapors ascend to touch one another, expanding out from the palace.[7] When there is continual moaning, she quickens her buttocks and he has moved the sealing cord.[8] When there is blowing, rapturous craving is intense and excitation then commences. When there is

---

[1]*Guo* 膕 is the standard anatomical term for the popliteal space behind the knee (see *Suwen* 60, 16.4a, and Wang Bing commentary).

[2]I.e. when the woman reaches orgasm the man simultaneously completes the count of the "ten movements" (see *MS*VI.B.8).

[3]*MWD*, vol. 4, "Transcription," n. 1, suspects that there are errors and perhaps omitted text in the above sentences, but I think the text is intelligible as written. There is a play on the word *shan* 善, which in its first occurrence refers to what all men "enjoy" and in its second occurrence refers to the man who is "skilled" at sexual cultivation.

[4]Even though the man's goal is to retain the sexually generated essence for his own benefit, he should not be domineering.

[5]Undoubtedly an exhortation to the man to proceed with intercourse based on his observations of the woman's responses.

[6]The "five sounds" are reprised in order to underscore the need for the man to observe the woman. I follow *MWD*, vol. 4, "Transcription," in reading 土 as *tu* 吐 (spit). I understand *guang* 光 to have a parallel meaning, hence my translation "radiating." The description of what the first sound indicates about the woman's state of arousal is different in the parallel in *MS*VI.B.6, which states that "the inside is tense" (the sound is also different, "convulsive breathing"). Subsequent descriptions in *MS*VII.B.20 tend to give more physiological detail than *MS*VI.B.6.

[7]I.e. Yin and Yang vapors begin to fuse. I read 宮 as *gong* 宮 (palace), which *MWD*, vol. 4, "Transcription," n. 3, gives as an alternative reading to its preferred reading *rong* 容 (perhaps "contain" or "absorb"). I suspect that *gong* refers to the vagina. The best evidence I can adduce for this meaning is the term *rugong* 入宮 (enter the palace), which denotes sexual intercourse in *Yinshu*, "Seasonal Regimen" (*YSSW*: 82; Prolegomena, Section Four). I am unable to find early attestation of the term *zigong* 子宮 for the womb.

[8]In the phrase 尻彼疾, I understand *kao* 尻 (buttocks) as the object of *ji* 疾 (quicken), and *bi* 彼 as an emphatic demonstrative marking the exposed placement of *kao* at the head of the phrase. The grammar pattern is noted in Yang Shuda 1986: 5. For "sealing cord" as a name for a part of the vagina, see *MS*VII.B.19.

biting, her body shakes[1] and he times pausing to continue for a long time.

Therefore, what is masculine belongs to the category male and is Yang; and what is Yang is external. What is feminine belongs to the category female and is Yin; and what is Yin is internal. Everything belonging to the category male is rubbed outside; everything belonging to the category female is rubbed inside. This is called the calculation of Yin and Yang, and the intrinsic pattern of female and male.[2] If when having intercourse he is unsuccessful, the blame can be placed entirely on haste.[3] The essential task in the pleasures of play is to be slow and prolonged. If only he can be slow and prolonged, the woman then is greatly pleased. She treats him with the closeness she feels for her brothers, and loves him like her father and mother. Whoever is capable of this way is designated "heaven's gentleman."[4]

---

[1]While the term *zhenhan* 振寒 (shaking with cold) might refer to shivering from sexual arousal, I follow *MWD*, vol. 4, "Transcription," n. 5, in reading 寒 as a scribal error for *dong* 動. The parallel graph in *MS*VI.B.6 is 動.

[2]See *MS*III.42 for an example of *pin* 牝 (female) denoting the female genitals.

[3]There is a play on the word *shu* 數, which in the previous sentence is the "calculation" of Yin and Yang and here is "haste" (the latter meaning is also attested in *MS*VII.B.7).

[4]*Tianshi* 天士 (heaven's gentleman) is attested in *Shiji*, 28.25b, as part of the honorary title inscribed on a seal granted to the recipe gentleman Luan Da 欒大 by Thearch Wu: "At his waist he wore the seals of the General who is Heaven's Gentleman, the General who is Earth's Gentleman, and the General of Great Penetration." *Tianshi* is also used as a title for an astrological specialist in *Hanshu*, 75.24a.

APPENDIX I
TRANSCRIPTION OF *MSI*.B, *MSI*.C, *MSI*.D

The transcription of *MSI*.B, *MSI*.C, and *MSI*.D given below is based on the reproduction and transcription of the three texts in *MWD*, vol. 4, and on the revised transcription of *MSI*.C appended to *MSSW*. In place of the emendations of lacunae in the *MWD*, vol. 4, transcription, which does not take account of the Zhangjiashan *Maishu* editions of the three texts ("Eleven Vessels," "Vessels and Vapor," and "Five Signs of Death" respectively), my transcription fills lacunae using *MSSW* whenever possible. *MSSW* transcribes *Maishu* in simplified graphs, which I write with modern *kaishu* 楷書 graphs. A reproduction of *Maishu* has not yet been published, and I have seen neither the original manuscript nor photographs (several of the bamboo slips are reproduced in Zhangjiashan Han mu zhujian zhengli xiaozu 1985). There are errors in the identification of the original slips in *MSSW*, which does not compromise its general reliability. More serious are several mistranscribed graphs in *MSSW*. Li Xueqin, who participated in the preparation of the *MSSW* transcription, kindly reviewed his own handwritten transcription of *Maishu* and checked photographs of the original manuscript kept at the Bureau of Cultural Relics in Beijing in order to confirm the correct identification of slips and of graphs (the errors occurred at the stage of typesetting, and the editorial committee was not able to correct them before publication). I have confidence in the accuracy of *MSSW* as corrected by Professor Li, but a reproduction of *Maishu* needs to be published before this confidence can be completely justified.

Lacunae due to damaged silk and illegible graphs are extensive: two columns of text are missing at the beginning of *MSI*.B, and significant gaps occur throughout; much of *MSI*.C was unreadable before the *Maishu* edition came to light; *MSI*.D, the shortest text, suffered the least. The *MWD*, vol. 4, transcription emends *MSI*.B using the *MSII*.B edition and parallels in *Lingshu* 10 (*MSII*.B is moderately damaged); little could be done for lacunae in *MSI*.C and *MSI*.D. Comparison of *MSI*.B and *MSII*.B with *Maishu*, "Eleven Vessels," reveals a closer correspondence between *MSI*.B and

"Eleven Vessels." Both editions arrange the vessels in the same order, whereas *MS*II.B differs by placing the foot Minor Yin vessel ahead of the foot Ceasing Yin vessel. Occasional differences in wording also separate *MS*I.B and "Eleven Vessels" from *MS*II.B. Comparing *MS*I.B to "Eleven Vessels," the latter shows signs of being a younger edition. Most obvious is the addition of ailments at the end of certain vessel entries in "Eleven Vessels" using the formula "and also including (*ji* 及) ailment X." My judgment that *MS*I.B and "Eleven Vessels" are more closely related editions is the basis for my decision to emend lacunae in *MS*I.B using "Eleven Vessels" whenever possible. I have not collated the two editions; "Eleven Vessels" is used only to emend lacunae in *MS*I.B. I make two exceptions where it is obvious that the scribe of *MS*I.B omitted graphs that occur in "Eleven Vessels." And because of lacunae in "Eleven Vessels" six emendations rely on *MS*II.B. The result is a reasonable approximation of *MS*I.B in its original condition.

Like "Eleven Vessels," the *Maishu* "Vessels and Vapor" and "Five Signs of Death" give evidence of being younger editions of *MS*I.C and *MS*I.D. For example, "Vessels and Vapor" uses *gu* 故 (thus) several times to accentuate the discursive tone of a passage; the same passage without *gu* in *MS*I.C is older. For the *MS*I.C phrase 氣出 ("if vapor emerges") "Vessels and Vapor" writes 氣一上一下 ("if vapor now ascends and now descends"), the latter a paraphrase of the former. Similarly, *gu* 滑 (smooth) in "Vessels and Vapor" is a *lectio facilior* for *gu* 汩 (flow evenly) in *MS*I.C. "Vessels and Vapor" being the younger edition, I refrain from emendation of *MS*I.C other than to fill lacunae (in one case using a parallel in *Taisu* when a lacuna also occurs in "Vessels and Vapor"). There are few lacunae in *MS*I.D; "Five Signs of Death" is worded somewhat differently, but the only significant difference is its reversing of the signs of death associated with vapor and with blood.

The transcription does not include the three text markers used in the original manuscripts. Graphs followed by the double-bar repeat sign are written twice. For convenience I add periods corresponding to the periods in the sentences of the Translation. Emended lacunae are indicated with brackets. When emendation is not possible, the number of graphs estimated to be missing is enclosed in the brackets. The source of bracketed emendations (mostly *MSSW*) is given parenthetically following the emendation. Notes on emendations (including several exceptions to the standard emendation of lacunae) are provided separately as needed. Additional textual notes are in the Translation.

The transcription uses modern ***kaishu*** graphs, adopting the conventions of the *MWD*, vol. 4, transcription. For example, 穜 is written 種 (however, I retain 穜 if it is used in the *MWD*, vol. 4, transcription). Graphs in emendations are not changed to reflect the orthography of *MS*I.B, *MS*I.C, and *MS*I.D. For example, all three *MS*I texts write 脈 for *mai* "vessel"; *Maishu* writes 脈, and this graph is used directly in emendations. Graphs that are not attested for the appropriate word and meaning in received literature (including graphs the scribe miswrote) are followed by a standard attested graph placed in parentheses in the form (:). Any mistranscribed graphs in the *MSSW* transcription (see above) are written as corrected by Li Xueqin and noted. In some cases a barely legible graph in one of the three *MS*I texts is mistranscribed in the *MWD*, vol. 4, transcription. Based on the reproduction of *MS*I and on *MSSW* it is possible to determine the correct graph (the revised transcription of *MS*I.C appended to *MSSW* supplies a number of such corrections). My transcription records the correct graph without note.

*MS*I .B

CC 35-36

[鉅陽之脈。毄(:繫)於踵外踝中。出胎衷。上穿臀出𩩲(:厭)中夾脊。出於項上頭角下顏夾頞毄(:繫)目内廉。是動則病沖頭目以(:似)脱項以(:似)伐胸痛要以(:似)折脾(:髀)不可以運胠

C 37

如結] (*MSSW*)腨如[裂。此] (*MSSW*) 爲踵蹶(:厥)。是鉅陽脈(:脈)[主治。其所之(:產)病頭痛耳聾項痛灊

C 38

强] (*MSSW*) 瘧北(:背)痛要痛尻痛時(:痔)胠[1] 痛腨痛[足小指踝(:痹)爲十] (*MSSW*) 二病。

C 39

[少](*MSSW*) 陽脈(:脈)。毄(:繫)於外踝之前廉。上出魚股之[外出脅。] (*MSSW*) 上[出耳前。] (*MSSW*)是動則病[心與脅痛

C 40

不] (*MSSW*) 可以反稷(:側)甚則无膏足外反。此爲陽[厥。](*MSSW*) 是少陽[脈主] (*MS*II. B)治。其所産病[3] [痛

C 41

項] (*MSSW*)痛脅痛瘧汗出節盡痛脾(:髀) 廉[痛](*MSSW*) 魚股痛[厀外廉] (*MSSW*)痛振寒[足中指] (*MSSW*)

C 42

踝(:痹)爲十二病。

C 43

陽明脈(:脈)。[毄(:繫)](*MSSW*) 於骭骨外廉循骭而上。穿臏出魚股[之廉。上] (*MSSW*) 穿[乳](*MSSW*) 穿頰[出目外] (*MSSW*)

C 44

廉環[顏。](*MSSW*) 是動則病洒洒病寒喜龍婁(:數)吹(:欠)顏[墨(:黑)病種(:腫)至則惡人與火聞] (*MSSW*)

C 45

木音則僫(:惕)然驚心腸(:惕)欲獨閉户牖而處[病甚] (*MSSW*)則欲[乘高而歌棄] (*MSSW*)衣[而走。此爲] (*MSSW*)

---

[1] See *MS*I.B.1, p. 205, n. 1.

C 46
骭蹶(:厥)。是陽明眽(:脈)主治。其所產病顏痛鼻肍(:鼽)
領[疢(:痛)乳痛脊痛](*MSSW*)心與胠痛

C 47
腹外穜(:腫)陽(:腸)痛厀跳付(:跗)[上踝(:痹)爲](*MSSW*)十
[病。](*MSSW*)

C 48
肩眽(:脈)。起於耳後下肩出肘[内廉。](*MSSW*) 出[3]乘
手北(:背)。是[動則病領穜(:腫)痛](*MSSW*)不可以顧肩

C 49
以(:似)脱臑以(:似)折。是肩眽(:脈)主治。[其所產病]
(*MSSW*) 領[痛脥(:喉)踝(:痹)肩痛肘外](*MSSW*) 痛爲四
病。

C 50
耳眽(:脈)。起於手北(:背)出臂外兩骨之間[上骨](*MSSW*)
下廉。[出肘中](*MSSW*)入耳中。是動則病耳聾

C 51
煇煇脖脖嗌穜(:腫)。是耳眽(:脈)主治。其所產病目外漬
(:眥)痛頰[痛](*MSSW*)耳聾爲三病。

C 52
齒眽(:脈)。起於次指與大指上出臂上廉入肘中乘
臑。[穿](*MSSW*)頰入齒中夾鼻。是[動](*MSSW*)

C 53
則病齒痛朏(:䪼)穜(:腫)。是齒眽(:脈)主治。其所產病齒
痛朏(:䪼)穜(:腫)目黄口乾臑痛爲五[病。](*MSSW*)

C 54
大陰眽(:脈)。是胃眽(:脈)殹。彼(:披)胃出魚股陰下廉腨
上廉出[内](*MSSW*)踝之上廉。是動則病上[1]

C 55
走心使復(:腹)張(:脹)善噫食欲歐(:嘔)得後與氣則怢然
衰。是鉅陰眽(:脈)主治。其所[產

C 56
病獨](*MSSW*)心煩死心痛與復(:腹)張(:脹)死不能食不能
卧强吹(:欠)三者同則死唐(:溏)泄死[水與](*MSSW*)

C 57
閉同則死爲十病。

C 58

厥陰脈(:脈)。毄(:繫)於足大指菆(:叢)[毛](*MSSW*)之上。乘足[柎(:跗)上廉](*MSSW*)去内腂(:踝)一寸。上[腂(:踝)](*MS*II. B)五寸而[出於大陰之後。](*MS*II. B)

C 59

上出魚股内廉觸少腹夾瀆(:背)旁。是動則[病丈](*MSSW*)夫隤(:癩)[山(:疝)婦人則少腹種(:腫)要痛](*MSSW*)

C 60

不可以印(:仰)甚則嗌乾面疵。是厥陰脈(:脈)主治。[其](*MSSW*)所産病熱中[痒穨扁(:偏)山(:疝)爲五病。五病](*MSSW*)

C 61

有而心煩死勿治殹。有陽脈(:脈)與之[俱](*MSSW*)病可治殹。

C 62

少陰脈(:脈)。毄(:繫)於内腂(:踝)外廉穿腨出胎[中](*MSSW*)央。上穿脊之[内](*MSSW*)廉毄(:繫)於腎夾舌。[是動即(:則)病](*MSSW*)

C 63

悔(:喝)悔(:喝)如喘坐而起則目瞙(:眊)如毋見心如縣(:懸)病飢氣[不足](*MSSW*)善怒心腸(:惕)恐[人將捕之](*MSSW*)

C 64

不欲食面黭若灺(:炧)色欬則有血。此爲骨蹷(:厥)。是少[陰](*MSSW*)脈(:脈)主[治。](*MSSW*)[1] 其[所産病口熱](*MSSW*)

C 65

舌柝(:坼)嗌乾上氣饐(:噎)嗌中痛癉耆(:嗜)卧欬音(:瘖)爲十病。[少](*MSSW*)陰之脈(:脈)[久(:灸)則强食産肉緩帶](*MSSW*)

C 66

皮(:被)髮大丈(:杖)重履而步。久(:灸)幾息則病已矣。

C 67

臂鉅陰脈(:脈)。在於手掌中出内陰兩骨之間上骨下廉筋之上。出臂[内陰入心中。](*MS*II. B)

---

[1] The scribe of *MS*I. B omitted 治.

C 68
是動則病心滂滂如痛缺盆痛甚[則] (*MS*II. B) 交兩手而戰。此爲臂蹶(:厥)。[是臂巨陰脈主] (*MS*II. B)
C 69
治。其所産病脑(:胸)痛瘛(:脘)痛[心痛] (*MSSW*)[1] 四末痛叚(:瘕)爲五病。
C 70
臂少陰眽(:脈)。起於臂兩骨之間之間[2]之下骨上廉筋之下。[出] (*MSSW*)臑内陰[入心中。是動則病心] (*MSSW*)
C 71
痛益(:嗌)渴欲飲。此爲臂蹶(:厥)。是臂少陰眽(:脈)主治。其所産[病脅] (*MSSW*)痛爲[一病。] (*MSSW*)

*MS*I. C
C 72
以眽(:脈)法明教下。眽(:脈)亦聽(:聖)人之所貴殹。氣殹者到下而[害] (*MSSW*) 上[從煖而去清] (*MSSW*)
C 73
焉。聽(:聖)人寒頭而煖足。治病者取有餘而益不足殹。[氣] (*MSSW*)上而不下[則視有] (*MSSW*)
C 74
過之眽(:脈)當環而久(:灸)之。病甚陽上於環二寸而益爲一久(:灸)。氣出胳與肘之眽(:脈)而[砭之。] (*MSSW*)
C 75
用碧(:砭)啓眽(:脈)者必如式。壅(:癰)穜(:腫)有膿(:膿)則稱其小大而[爲] (*MSSW*) 之[砭。砭] (*MSSW*) 有四[害。] (*MSSW*) 膿(:膿)深[而] (*MSSW*)
C 76
碧(:砭)輚(:淺)謂上(:之)不遝 一害。膿(:膿)輚(:淺)而碧(:砭)深胃(:謂)之過二害。膿(:膿)大[而砭小胃(:謂)之澰澰者惡
C 77
不畢] (*MSSW*) 三[害。農(:膿)] (*MSSW*) 小而碧(:砭)大胃(:謂)之碧(:泛)碧(:泛)者傷良肉殹四害。膿(:膿)[多而深者上黑] (*MSSW*)而大。[農(:膿)

[1] The scribe of *MS*I. B omitted 心痛. See *MS*I. B. 10, p. 212, n. 2.

[2] The scribe of *MS*I. B wrote 之間 twice; the second occurence is excrescent.

C 78
少而深者上黑而小。農(:膿)多而淺者上白而大。](*MSSW*) 膿(:膿)少[而](*MSSW*)輚(:淺)[者上白而小。此不可不](*MSSW*)察殹。[有](*MSSW*)
C 79
膿(:膿)者不[可久(:灸)殹。相脈之道。左](*MSSW*)[手上去踝五寸](*Taisu*)案之。右[手直踝而簟(:撣)之。它脈](*MSSW*)盈此
C 80
獨虛則主病。它脈(:脈)汩此獨[衛(:率)](*MSSW*)則主[病。](*MSSW*) 它脈(:脈)[靜此獨動則生(:主)病。夫脈固有動者骭](*MSSW*)
C 81
之少陰臂之大陰少陰。氏(:是)主[動疾](*MSSW*)則[病。](*MSSW*) 此[所以論有過之脈殹。其餘謹視當脈之過。](*MSSW*)
C 82
脈(:脈)之縣書而熟學之。季子忠謹。學[4]見於爲人[6]
C 83
言不可不察殹。

MSI. D
C 84
凡三陽天氣殹。其病唯折骨列(:裂)膚一死。凡三陰地氣殹死脈(:脈)殹。[陰](*MSSW*)病而亂則[不](*MSSW*)
C 85
過十日而死。三陰𦚔(:腐)臧(:臟)煉(:爛)腸而主殺。[2]五死。唇反人盈則肉[先死。齦齊齒長則](*MSSW*)
C 86
骨先死。面黑目環(:睘)視衺(:衺)則氣先死。汗出如絲傅而不流則血先死。舌捆(:梱)橐(:卵)卷[則筋](*MSSW*)
C 87
先死。五者扁(:徧)有則不沽(:活)矣。

APPENDIX 2
REVISIONS TO THE TRANSCRIPTION OF GRAPHS IN *MWD*, VOL. 4

The revisions are based on Qiu Xigui (1992), my own research, and consultation with Li Xueqin, who is responsible for the final editing of the transcription in *MWD*, vol. 4. I am indebted to Professor Li for personally checking the revisions and indicating his general agreement with them. In several instances the correct transcription remains open to argument; I bear sole responsibility for the revisions proposed in the list below (each revision is also noted in the Translation). Because the transcription of *MSI*.B, *MSI*.C, and *MSI*.D in Appendix 1 replaces the transcription in *MWD*, vol. 4, revisions are not given for those texts.

	MWD	Qiu	Harper	Revision
MSI.A.1				
C1	⿰月谷		⿰谷月	⿰谷月
C3	脽		⿰月隼	⿰月隼
C4	⿺尢壬	⿺尢生		⿺尢生
MSI.A.3				
C11	⿺尢壬	⿺尢生		⿺尢生
MSI.A.4				
C13	⿰月谷		⿰谷月	⿰谷月
MSI.A.5				
C16	陽	陰		陰

	MWD	Qiu	Harper	Revision
C16	循	揗		揗
*MS*I.E.58 C94	食	金		金
*MS*I.E.107 C183	⿷匚畐	虒		虒
*MS*I.E.117 C193	橐	囊		囊
*MS*I.E.118 C196	潼	穜		穜
*MS*I.E.120 C200	九	亢		亢
*MS*I.E.125 C206	九	亢		亢
*MS*I.E.138 C230	己	已		已
*MS*I.E.139 C232	灸	炙		炙
*MS*I.E.151 C260	以		爲	爲
*MS*I.E.162 C281	灸	炙		炙
C282	己	已		已

	MWD	Qiu	Harper	Revision
*MS*I.E.164 C284	灸	炙		炙
*MS*I.E.175 C305	灸	炙		炙
*MS*I.E.188 C318	月		日	日
C319	己	已		已
*MS*I.E.222 C361	脩	滫		滫
*MS*I.E.227 C366	潼	穜		穜
*MS*I.E.229 C369	自	曰		曰
C369	取	敢		敢
C370	桯	柱		柱
C370	肉		今	今
*MS*I.E.252 C412	後	后		后
*MS*I.E.276 C442	倡	儈		儈
*MS*II.C.35	熱		炅[1]	炅

[1] See *MS*II.C.35, p·315, n. 2.

	MWD	Qiu	Harper	Revision
*MS*III.2 C3	醬	漿		漿
*MS*III.6 C18	蕑		閒	閒
*MS*III.11 C30	以	取		取
*MS*III.38 C84	菽	赦		?
*MS*III.44 C96	玩	抏		抏
*MS*III.62 C128	止	已		已
*MS*III.71 C152	各	吞		吞
*MS*III.88 C197	無	无		无
*MS*III.89 C214	也	虖		虖
*MS*V.5 C15	洒	酒		酒
*MS*VI.A.1 S5	搏	摶		摶 [1]

[1] See *MS*VI.A.1, p.387, n.3.

	MWD	Qiu	Harper	Revision
*MS*VI.A.3				
S17	偵		慎	慎
*MS*VI.A.4				
S35	桲	挬		挬
S37	執	埶		埶
*MS*VI.A.6				
S41	立	交		交
*MS*VI.A.4				
S52	美	奏		奏
S53	桼十	未半		未半
*MS*VI.B.7				
S127	前		筋	筋
*MS*VI.B.8				
S130	遲	遟		遟
S131	緓	綬		綬
*MS*VII.B.2				
S16	遭	逍		逍
*MS*VII.B.3				
S21	淩	洚		洚
*MS*VII.B.4				
S29	槖	橐		橐

	MWD	Qiu	Harper	Revision
MS VII.B.13 S48	音	言		言
MS VII.B.19 S59	調		潤	潤

HAN WEIGHTS AND MEASURES

EQUIVALENTS*

Length:			
1 *cun* 寸		2.31	centimeters
1 *chi* 尺	(10 *cun*)	23.1	centimeters
1 *zhang* 丈	(10 *chi*)	2.31	meters
1 *li* 里		.415	kilometer
Capacity:			
1 *ge* 合		19.968	cubic centimeters
1 *sheng* 升	(10 *ge*)	199.687	cubic centimeters
1 *dou* 斗	(10 *sheng*)	1.996	liters
Weight:			
1 *liang* 两		15.36	grams
1 *jin* 斤	(16 *liang*)	245	grams

*See Twitchett and Loewe 1986: xxxviii. Only those weights and measures that occur in the Prolegomena and Translation are included.

BIBLIOGRAPHY

Only works cited are included. Abbreviated titles appear at the appropriate alphabetic position. Traditional works in Chinese and Japanese are listed by title. Authors or compilers are identified following the title when possible; dates are often approximate (detailed information on Han and pre-Han works may be found in Loewe 1993). In addition, commentaries to which specific reference is made are identified.

Andersen, P. 1989-90. "The Practice of *Bugang*." *Cahiers d'Extrême-Asie* 5. 15-53.

Akahori, Akira 赤堀昭. 1978. "Bu-i Kandai ikan ni tsuite" 武威漢代醫簡について. *Tôhô gakuhô* 東方學報 50. 75-107.

———. 1985. "Yahô o meguru mondai" 冶法をめぐろ問題. *KGS*, vol. 2. 123-65.

———. 1989. "The Interpretation of Classical Chinese Medical Texts in Contemporary Japan: Achievements, Approaches, and Problems." *Approaches to Traditional Chinese Medical Literature*. Ed. P. Unschuld. Dordrecht: Kluwer Academic Publishers. 19-27.

Akizuki, Kan'ei 秋月觀暎, ed. 1987. *Dôkyô to shûkyô bunka* 道教と宗教文化. Tokyo: Hirakawa shuppansha.

BC. *Shennong bencaojing* 神農本草經. First to second centuries A.D. References are to citations of *BC* in *GM*.

BL. *Mingyi bielu* 名醫別錄. Ca. sixth century. References are to citations of *BL* in *GM*.

Baopuzi 抱朴子. Ge Hong 葛洪 (283-343). *Zhuzi jicheng* ed.

Bencaojing jizhu 本草經集注. Tao Hongjing (456-536). References are to *Honzôkyô shûchû* 本草經集注. Ed. Mori Risshi 森立之 (between 1849 and 1852) and Okanishi Tameto 岡西爲人. Osaka: Minami Ôsaka insatsu sentâ, 1972.

Betz, H., ed. 1986. *The Greek Magical Papyri in Translation*. Chicago: University of Chicago Press.

Biji xiaoshuo daguan 筆記小說大觀. Taibei: Xinxing shuju, 1973.

Biji xiaoshuo daguan xubian 筆記小說大觀續編. Taibei: Xinxing shuju, 1973.

Bodde, D. 1975. *Festivals in Classical China: New Year and Other Annual Observances during the Han Dynasty 206 B.C.-A.D. 220.* Princeton: Princeton University Press.

Bokenkamp, S. 1983. "Sources of the *Ling-pao* Scriptures." *Tantric and Taoist Studies in Honour of R.A. Stein*, vol. 2 (*Mélanges chinois et bouddhiques* 21). Ed. M. Strickmann. 434-86.

Bowuzhi 博物志. Zhang Hua 張華 (232-300). *Sibu beiyao* ed.

Brashear, W. 1992. "Magical Papyri: Magic in Bookform." *Das Buch als magisches und als Repräsentationsobjekt*. Ed. P. Ganz. Wiesbaden: Harrassowitz. 25-57.

Bridgman, R. 1952-55. "La medicine dans la Chine antique." *Mélanges chinois et bouddhiques* 10. 1-213.

Chaoshi zhubing yuanhoulun 巢氏諸病源候論. Chao Yuanfang 巢元方 (fl. 610). *Siku quanshu* ed.

Chen, Banghuai 陳邦懷. 1982. "Zhanguo 'Xingqi yuming' kaoshi" 戰國行氣玉銘考釋. *Guwenzi yanjiu* 古文字研究 7. 187-93.

Chen, Mengjia 陳夢家. 1936. "Shang dai de shenhua yu wushu" 商代的神話與巫術. *Yanjing xuebao* 燕京學報 20. 485-576.

———. 1965. "Han jian nianli biaoxu" 漢簡年曆表敘. *Kaogu xuebao* 考古學報 1965.2. 103-49.

Chen, Pan 陳槃. 1948. "Zhanguo Qin Han jian fangshi kaolun" 戰國秦漢間方士考論. *Zhongyang yanjiuyuan lishi yuyan yanjiusuo jikan* 中央研究院歷史語言研究所集刊 17. 7-57.

Chen, Songchang 陳松長. 1994. "Mawangdui sanhao Han mu mudu sanlun" 馬王堆三號漢墓木牘散論. *Wenwu* 文物 1994.6. 64-70.

Chen, Xiangchun. 1942. "Examples of Charm against Epidemics with Short Explanations." *Folklore Studies* 1. 37-54.

Chuci 楚辭. Contents of various dates, from late fourth century B.C. to second century A.D. *Sibu beiyao* ed. Commentaries cited: Wang Yi 王逸 (ca. 89-ca. 158).

Chuogenglu 輟耕錄. Tao Zongyi 陶宗儀 (ca. 1316–ca. 1402). *Congshu jicheng* ed.

Congshu jicheng 叢書集成. Shanghai: Shangwu yinshuguan, 1935–37.

Daode zhenjing zhu 道德真經註 (with the Heshang gong 河上公 commentary). *Daozang* ed. (*HY* 682).

Daozang 道藏. Taibei: Yiwen yinshuguan, 1977 (reprint of the 1926 Hanfenlou reproduction of the woodblock ed. housed in the Baiyunguan, Beijing; the latter based on eds. of 1444–45 and 1607).

Dubs, H. 1938–55. *The History of the Former Han Dynasty*. 3 vols. Baltimore: Waverly Press.

Duduan 獨斷. Cai Yong 蔡邕 (133–92). *Han Wei congshu* 漢魏叢書 ed. Shanghai: Hanfen lou, 1925 (reproduction of 1592 woodblock ed.).

Eamon, W. 1985. "Science and Popular Culture in Sixteenth Century Italy: The 'Professors of Secrets' and Their Books." *The Sixteenth Century Journal* 16. 471–85.

———. 1990. "From Secrets of Nature to Public Knowledge." *Reappraisals of the Scientific Revolution*. Ed. D. Lindberg and R. Westman. Cambridge: Cambridge University Press. 333–65.

Eberhard, W. 1968. *The Local Cultures of South and East China*. Trans. A. Eberhard. Leiden: E.J. Brill.

Edelstein, L. 1987. *Ancient Medicine: Selected Papers of Ludwig Edelstein*. Ed. O. Temkin and C. Temkin. Baltimore: Johns Hopkins University Press.

Eis, G. 1967. *Mittelalterliche Fachliteratur*. Stuttgart: Sammlung Metzler.

Emura, Haruki 江村治樹 et al., eds. 1987. *Ma-ô-tai shutsudo isho jikei bunrui sakuin* 馬王堆出土醫書字形分類索引. Private publication.

Epler, D. 1980. "Bloodletting in Early Chinese Medicine and Its Relation to the Origin of Acupuncture." *Bulletin of the History of Medicine* 54. 337–67.

Erya 爾雅. Ca. third century B.C. *Shisanjing zhushu* ed. Commentaries cited: Guo Pu 郭璞 (276–324).

Fangyan 方言. Yang Xiong 揚雄 (58 B.C.–A.D. 18). *Sibu beiyao* ed.

Fantianlu conglu 梵天廬叢錄. Chai E 柴萼 (1892-?). Author's preface dated 1925, n.p.

Faraone, C. 1991. "The Agonistic Context of Early Greek Binding Spells." Faraone and Obbink 1991. 3-32.

Faraone, C. and D. Obbink, eds. 1991. *Magika Hiera: Ancient Greek Magic and Religion*. Oxford: Oxford University Press.

Fayan 法言. Yang Xiong 揚雄 (58 B.C.-A.D. 18). *Zhuji jicheng* ed.

Fengsu tongyi 風俗通義. Ying Shao 應劭 (ca. 140-ca. 200). *Sibu beiyao* ed.

Follon, J. 1968. "Manuscripts of Ortolf von Bayerlants 'Arzneibuch'. Their Contents, Exemplifying German Mediaeval Artes Literature." Keil et al. 1968. 31-52.

Fu, Juyou 傅舉有. 1983. "Guanyu Changsha Mawangdui sanhao Han mu de muzhu wenti" 關於長沙馬王堆三號漢墓的墓主問題. *Kaogu* 考古 1983.2. 165-72.

Fu, Juyou 傅舉有 and Chen Songchang 陳松長. 1992. *Mawangdui Han mu wenwu* 馬王堆漢墓文物. Changsha: Hunan chubanshe.

Fuyang Han jian zhenglizu 阜陽漢簡整理組. 1983. "Fuyang Han jian jianjie" 阜陽漢簡簡介. *Wenwu* 文物 1983.2. 21-23.

———. 1988. "Fuyang Han jian *Wanwu*" 阜陽漢簡萬物. *Wenwu* 文物 1988.4. 36-47.

GM. Bencao gangmu 本草綱目. Li Shizhen 李時珍 (1518-93). Taibei: Hongye shuju, 1985.

Gansu sheng wenwu kaogu yanjiusuo 甘肅省文物考古研究所. 1989. *Qin Han jiandu lunwenji* 秦漢簡牘論文集. Lanzhou: Gansu renmin chubanshe.

Goodrich, C. 1966. "Two Chapters in the Life of an Empress of the Later Han (II)." *Harvard Journal of Asiatic Studies* 26. 187-210.

Graham, A. 1981. *Chuang Tzu: The Inner Chapters*. London: George Allen and Unwin.

———. 1986. *Yin-Yang and the Nature of Correlative Thinking*. Singapore: Institute of East Asian Philosophies.

———. 1989. *Disputers of the Tao*. La Salle: Open Court.

Granet, M. 1925. "Remarques sur le taoisme ancien." *Asia Major* 2. 146-51.

———. 1953. "Le dépôt de l'enfant sur le sol: rites anciens et ordalies mythiques." *Études sociologiques sur la Chine*. By M. Granet. Paris: Presses Universitaires de France. 159–202.

de Groot, J. 1892–1910. *The Religious System of China*. 6 vols. Leiden: E.J. Brill.

Gu, Shi 顧實. 1924. *Hanshu yiwenzhi jiangshu* 漢書藝文志講疏. Shanghai: Shangwu yinshuguan.

Guangya 廣雅. Zhang Yi 張揖 (fl. 227–32). References are to the *Sibu beiyao* ed. of *Guangya shuzheng* 廣雅疏證. Ed. Wang Niansun 王念孫 (1742–1832). Commentaries cited: Wang Niansun.

Guanzi 管子. Fourth to first centuries B.C. *Zhuzi jicheng* ed.

Gujin xiaoshuo 古今小說. Feng Menglong 馮夢龍 (1574–1645). Taibei: Shijie shuju, 1958.

Gujinzhu 古今注. Cui Bao 催豹 (fl. 290–306). *Sibu beiyao* ed.

van Gulik, R. 1961. *Sexual Life in Ancient China*. Leiden: E.J. Brill.

Guoyu 國語. Ca. third century B.C. *Sibu beiyao* ed.

HY. *Daozang zimu yinde* 道藏子目引得. Harvard-Yenching Institute Sinological Index Series, no. 25. Taibei: Chengwen Publishing Company, 1966. Works in the *Daozang* are further identified by their *HY* number.

Han, Zhongmin 韓仲民 (see also Xiao Han). 1992. *Bo Yi shuolüe* 帛易說略. Beijing: Beijing Shifan daxue chubanshe.

Hanfeizi 韓非子. Han Fei 韓非 (d. 233 B.C.) and others. *Zhuzi jicheng* ed.

Hanshu 漢書. Ban Gu 班固 (32–92). References are to *Hanshu buzhu* 漢書補注. Ed. Wang Xianqian 王先謙 (1842–1918). Taibei: Xinwenfeng chuban gongsi, 1975 (reproduction of 1900 woodblock ed.). Commentaries cited: Yan Shigu 顏師古 (581–645); Wang Xianqian.

Harper, D. (see also Xia De'an). 1978–79. "The Han Cosmic Board." *Early China* 4. 1–10.

———. 1982. "The *Wu Shih Erh Ping Fang*: Translation and Prolegomena." Diss. University of California, Berkeley. Ann Arbor: University Microfilms International. 8312837.

———. 1985. "A Chinese Demonography of the Third Century B.C." *Harvard Journal of Asiatic Studies* 45. 459–98.

———. 1987a. "Wang Yen-shou's Nightmare Poem." *Harvard Journal of Asiatic Studies* 47. 239–83.

———. 1987b. "The Sexual Arts of Ancient China as Described in a Manuscript of the Second Century B.C." *Harvard Journal of Asiatic Studies* 47. 539–93.

———. 1988. "A Note on Nightmare Magic in Ancient and Medieval China." *T'ang Studies* 6. 69–76.

———. 1990. "The Conception of Illness in Early Chinese Medicine, as Documented in Newly Discovered 3rd and 2nd Century B.C. Manuscripts." *Sudhoffs Archiv* 74. 210–35.

———. 1994. "Resurrection in Warring States Popular Religion." *Taoist Resources* 5.2. 13–28.

———. 1995. "Warring States, Ch'in and Han Periods." In "Chinese Religions: The State of the Field." Ed. D. Overmyer. *Journal of Asian Studies* 51.1. 152–60.

———. Forthcoming. "Warring States, Qin, and Han Manuscripts Related to Natural Philosophy and the Occult." Shaughnessy forthcoming.

Hawkes, D. 1985. *The Songs of the South: An Anthology of Ancient Chinese Poems by Qu Yuan and Other Poets*. Harmondsworth: Penguin Books.

Hayashi, Minao 林巳奈夫. 1975. "Kandai no inshoku" 漢代の飲食. *Tôhô gakuhô* 東方學報 48. 1–98.

———. 1976. *Kandai no bunbutsu* 漢代の文物. Kyoto: Kyôto daigaku jinbun kagaku kenkyûjo.

He, Linyi 何琳儀. 1989. *Zhanguo wenzi tonglun* 戰國文字通論. Beijing: Zhonghua shuju.

He, Shuangquan 何雙全. 1989a. "Tianshui Fangmatan Qin jian zongshu" 天水放馬灘秦簡綜述. *Wenwu* 文物 1989.2. 23–31.

———. 1989b. "Tianshui Fangmatan Qin jian jiazhong *Rishu* kaoshu" 天水放馬灘秦簡甲種日書考述. Gansu sheng wenwu kaogu yanjiusuo 1989. 7–28.

Heywood, V. and S. Chant, eds. 1982. *Popular Encyclopedia of Plants*. Cambridge: Cambridge University Press.

Horiike, Nobuo 堀池信夫. 1988. "Kandai no shinsen yôsei-setsu, igaku to chishikijin" 漢代の神仙養生説醫學と知識人. Sakade 1988. 296–321.

Hou Hanshu 後 漢 書. Fan Ye 范 曄 (398-446) and others. References are to *Hou Hanshu jijie* 後 漢 書 集 解. Ed. Wang Xianqian 王 先 謙 (1842-1918). Taibei: Xinwenfeng chuban gongsi, 1975 (reproduction of 1915 woodblock ed.).

Hu, Houxuan 胡 厚 宣. 1984. "Lun Yin ren zhiliao jibing zhi fangfa" 論殷人治療疾病之方法. *Zhongyuan wenwu* 中原文物 1984.4. 27-30.

Hu, Pingsheng 胡 平 生 and Han Ziqiang 韓 自 强. 1988. "*Wanwu lüeshuo*" 萬 物 略 說. *Wenwu* 文 物 1988.4. 48-54.

Huainan wanbishu 淮 南 萬 畢 術. Ca. first century B.C. References are to the reconstructed text in *Guangutang suo zhushu* 觀 古 堂 所 著 書. Ed. Ye Dehui 葉 德 輝 (1864-1927). *Congshu jicheng xubian* 叢 書 集 成 續 編. Taibei: Yiwen yinshuguan, 1970 (reproduction of the 1902 woodblock ed. of *Guangutang suo zhushu*).

Huainanzi 淮 南 子. Liu An 劉 安 (179-122 B.C.) and others. *Zhuzi jicheng* ed. Commentaries cited: Gao You 高 誘 (ca. 160-220).

Huangdi neijing 黄 帝 内 經. Ca. first century B.C. See *Lingshu*, *Suwen*, *Taisu*.

Huangting neijing jing 黄 庭 内 景 經. Fourth to sixth centuries A.D. References are to the edition in *Yunji qiqian*. Commentaries cited: Liangqiuzi 梁 丘 子 (Tang period).

Huangting waijing jing 黄 庭 外 景 經. Ca. third century. References are to the edition in *Yunji qiqian*.

Hubei sheng Jing Sha tielu kaogudui 湖 北 省 荆 沙 鐵 路 考 古 隊. 1991. *Baoshan Chu jian* 包 山 楚 簡. Beijing: Wenwu chubanshe.

Hudson, R. 1993. "Concepts of Disease in the West." Kiple 1993. 45-52.

Hulsewé, A. 1985. *Remnants of Ch'in Law: An Annotated Translation of the Ch'in Legal and Administrative Rules of the 3rd Century B.C. Discovered in Yün-meng Prefecture, Hu-pei Province, in 1975*. Leiden: E.J. Brill.

Hunan nongxueyuan 湖 南 農 學 院 et al., eds. 1978. *Changsha Mawangdui yihao Han mu chutu dongzhiwu biaoben de yanjiu* 長沙馬王堆一號漢墓出土動植物標本的研究. Beijing: Wenwu chubanshe.

Hunan sheng bowuguan 湖南省博物館 and Zhongguo kexueyuan kaogu yanjiusuo 中國科學院考古研究所. 1973. *Changsha Mawangdui yihao Han mu* 長沙馬王堆一號漢墓. 2 vols. Beijing: Wenwu chubanshe.

———. 1974. "Mawangdui er, san hao Han mu fajue jianbao" 馬王堆二三號漢墓發掘簡報. *Wenwu* 文物 1974.7. 39-48, 63.

Hunan yixueyuan 湖南醫學院. 1980. *Changsha Mawangdui yihao Han mu gushi yanjiu* 長沙馬王堆一號漢墓古尸研究. Beijing: Wenwu chubanshe.

Ishida, Hidemi 石田秀實. 1981. "Chûgoku kodai ni okeru seishin shippei kan" 中國古代における精神疾病觀. *Nihon Chûgoku gakkai hô* 日本中國學會報 33. 29-42.

———. 1991. "Shoki no bôchû yôsei shisô to sensetsu" 初期の房中養生思想と僊說. *Tôhô shûkyô* 東方宗教 77. 1-21.

Ishinpô 醫心方. Tanba Yasuyori 丹波康賴 (912-995). Tokyo: Kôdansha, 1973 (reproduction of 1854 Japanese woodblock ed.).

Jackson, R. 1988. *Doctors and Diseases in the Roman Empire*. London: British Museum Publications.

Jianhu guangji 堅瓠廣集. Chu Jiaxuan 褚稼軒 (fl. 1695). *Biji xiaoshuo daguan xubian* ed.

Jing Chu suishi ji 荊楚歲時記. Zong Lin 宗懍 (sixth century). References are to the edition in Moriya 1963.

KGS. Shin hatsugen Chûgoku kagakushi shiryô no kenkyû 新發現中國科學史資料の研究. Ed. Yamada Keiji 山田慶兒. 2 vols. (vol. 1, *Yakuchû hen* 譯注篇; vol. 2, *Ronkô hen* 論考篇). Kyoto: Kyôto daigaku jinbun kagaku kenkyûjo, 1985.

Kalinowski, M. 1983. "Les instruments astro-calendériques des Han et la méthode *liuren*." *Bulletin de l'École Française d'Extrême-Orient* 72. 309-419.

———. 1985. "La transmission du dispositif des neuf palais sous les Six Dynasties." *Tantric and Taoist Studies in Honour of R.A. Stein*, vol. 3 (*Mélanges chinois et bouddhiques* 22). Ed. M. Strickmann. 773-811.

———. 1986. "Les traités de Shuihudi et l'hémérologie chinoise à la fin des Royaumes Combattants." *T'oung Pao* 72. 175-228.

———. 1991. *Cosmologie et divination dans la Chine ancienne*. Paris: École Française d'Extrême-Orient.

Kaltenmark, M. 1953. *Le Lie-sien tchouan*. Bejing: Université de Paris, Centre d'Etudes sinologiques de Pekin.

Karlgren, B. 1957. *Grammata Serica Recensa*. Stockholm: Museum of Far Eastern Antiquities.

Kechuang xianhua xuji 客窗閒話續集. Wu Xianghan 吳薌厈 (fl. 1875-1908). *Biji xiaoshuo daguan* ed.

Keegan, D. 1988. "The 'Huang-ti Nei-ching': The Structure of the Compilations; The Significance of the Structure." Diss. University of California, Berkeley. Ann Arbor: University Microfilms International. 8916728.

Keil, G., ed. 1982. *Fachprosa-Studien: Beiträge zur mittelalterlichen Wissenschafts- und Geistesgeschichte*. Berlin: Erich Schmidt Verlag.

Keil, G. and P. Assion, eds. 1974. *Fachprosaforschung: Acht Vorträge zur mittelalterlichen Artesliteratur*. Berlin: Erich Schmidt Verlag.

Keil, G. et al., eds. 1968. *Fachliteratur des Mittelalters: Festschrift für Gerhard Eis*. Stuttgart: J.B. Metzlersche Verlagsbuchhandlung.

Kinsey, A. 1953. *Sexual Behavior in the Human Female*. Philadelphia: Saunders.

Kiple, K., ed. 1993. *The Cambridge World History of Human Disease*. Cambridge: Cambridge University Press.

Knoblock, J. 1988. *Xunzi: A Translation and Study of the Complete Works*, vol. 1. Stanford: Stanford University Press.

Kotansky, R. 1991. "Incantations and Prayers for Salvation on Inscribed Greek Amulets." Faraone and Obbink 1991. 107-37.

Kudô, Motoo 工藤元男. 1990. "Un-bô Sui-ko-chi Shin bo chikukan nissho to dôkyô teki shûzoku" 雲夢睡虎地秦墓竹簡日書と道教的習俗. *Tôhô shûkyô* 東方宗教 76. 43-61.

Kusuyama, Haruki 楠山春樹. 1987. "*Enan chûhen* to *Enan man-hitsu*" 淮南中篇と淮南萬畢. Akizuki 1987. 27-44.

Laozi 老子. Ca. third century B.C. References are to various editions as cited.

Laozi zhongjing 老子中經. Second to third centuries A.D. References are to the edition in *Yunji qiqian*.

Lewis, M. 1990. *Sanctioned Violence in Early China*. Albany: State University of New York Press.

Li, Hui-lin. 1979. *Nan-fang ts'ao-mu chuang: A Fourth Century Flora of Southeast Asia*. Hong Kong: Chinese University Press.

Li, Ling 李零. 1985. *Changsha Zidanku Zhanguo Chu boshu yanjiu* 長沙子彈庫戰國楚帛書研究. Beijing: Zhonghua shuju.

———. 1990. "Formulaic Structure of the Chu Divinatory Bamboo Slips." *Early China* 15. 71-86.

———. 1991. "Mawangdui Han mu 'Shenqi tu' ying shu bibing tu" 馬王堆漢墓神祇圖應屬辟兵圖. *Kaogu* 考古 1991.10. 940-42.

———. 1993. *Zhongguo fangshu kao* 中國方術考. Beijing: Renmin Zhongguo chubanshe.

Li, Ling and K. McMahon. 1992. "The Contents and Terminology of the Mawangdui Texts on the Arts of the Bedchamber." *Early China* 17. 145-85.

Li, Xueqin 李學勤. 1981. "Xin chu jianbo yu Chu wenhua" 新出簡帛與楚文化. *Chu wenhua xintan* 楚文化新探. Ed. Hubei sheng shehui kexueyuan lishi yanjiusuo 湖北省社會科學院歷史研究所. Wuhan: Hubei renmin chubanshe. 28-39.

———. 1990. "Fangmatan jianzhong de zhiguai gushi" 放馬灘簡中的志怪故事. *Wenwu* 文物 1990.4. 43-47.

———. 1991. "*Yinshu* yu *Daoyin tu*" 引書與導引圖. *Wenwu tiandi* 文物天地 1991.2. 7-9.

Li, Zhongwen 李鐘文. 1980. "*Wushier bingfang* zhong gaozhi lei yaowu de tantao" 五十二病方中膏脂類藥物的探討. *Mawangdui yishu yanjiu zhuankan* 馬王堆醫書研究專刊 1. 43-48.

Lian, Shaoming 連劭名. 1989. "Jiangling Zhangjiashan Han jian *Maishu* chutan" 江陵張家山漢 簡脈書初探. *Wenwu* 文物 1989.7. 75-81.

Liao, Yuqun 廖育群. 1989. "*Yin Yang shiyi mai jiujing* yanjiu: jianlun jingluo tixi de xingcheng yu fazhan" 陰陽十一脈灸經研究兼論經絡體系的形成與發展. *Zhonghua yishi zazhi* 中華醫史雜志 1989.1. 20-24.

———. 1991. "Qin Han zhi ji zhenjiu liaofa lilun de jianli" 秦漢之際鍼灸療法理論的建立. *Ziran kexue yanjiu* 自然科學研究 10. 272-79.

Liexian zhuan 列仙傳. Ca. second century A.D. References are to Kaltenmark 1953.

Liji 禮記. Han period. *Shisanjing zhushu* ed. Commentaries cited: Zheng Xuan 鄭玄 (127-200).

Lindberg, D. 1992. *The Beginnings of Western Science: The European Scientific Tradition in Philosophical, Religious, and Institutional Context, 600 B.C. to A.D. 1450*. Chicago: University of Chicago Press.

Lingshu 靈樞. Tang period recension of Han period *Huangdi neijing*. *Sibu beiyao* ed.

Lingshu ziwen 靈書紫文. Fourth century. *Daozang* ed. (*HY* 639).

Liu, Junzheng 劉均正. 1989. "*Wushier bingfang* 'zhe' kao" 五十二病方庶考. *Zhonghua yishi zazhi* 中華醫史雜志 1989.2. 75.

Liu, Xiaolu 劉曉路. 1994. "Cong Mawangdui sanhao mu chutu ditu kan muzhu guanzhi" 從馬王堆三號墓出土地圖看墓主官職. *Wenwu* 文物 1994.6. 59-62.

Liu, Zhiwan 劉枝萬. 1974. *Zhongguo minjian xinyang lunji* 中國民間信仰論集. Taibei: Zhongyang yanjiuyuan minzuxue yanjiusuo.

Liu, Zonghan 劉宗漢. 1992a. "Changsha Mawangdui chutu boshu *Jingmai shu* yanjiu zhi yi" 長沙馬王堆出土帛書經脈書研究之一. *Wenshi* 文史 36. 91-100.

———. 1992b. "Changsha Mawangdui chutu boshu *Jingmai shu* yanjiu zhi er" 長沙馬王堆出土帛書經脈書研究之二. *Yazhou wenming* 亞洲文明 2. 249-54.

Lloyd, G. 1979. *Magic, Reason and Experience*. Cambridge: Cambridge University Press.

———, ed. 1983. *Hippocratic Writings*. Harmondsworth: Penguin Books.

Loewe, M. 1967. *Records of Han Administration*. 2 vols. Cambridge: Cambridge University Press.

———. 1974. *Crisis and Conflict in Han China*. London: George Allen and Unwin.

———. 1977. "Manuscripts Found Recently in China: A Preliminary Survey." *T'oung Pao* 63. 99-136.

———, ed. 1993. *Early Chinese Texts: A Bibliographic Guide*. Berkeley: Society for the Study of Early China and Institute of East Asian Studies, University of California, Berkeley.

Lu, G. and J. Needham. 1967. "Records of Diseases in Ancient China." *Diseases in Antiquity*. Ed. D. Brothwell and A. Sandison. Springfield: Charles C Thomas. 222-37.

———. 1980. *Celestial Lancets: A History and Rationale of Acupuncture and Moxa*. Cambridge: Cambridge University Press.

Lunheng 論衡. Wang Chong 王充 (A.D. 27-ca. 100). References are to *Lunheng jijie* 論衡集解. Ed. Liu Pansui 劉盼遂. Beijing: Guji chubanshe, 1957.

Luo, Changpei 羅常培 and Zhou Zumo 周祖謨. 1958. *Han Wei Jin Nan Bei chao yunbu yanbian yanjiu* 漢魏晉南北朝韻部演變研究. Beijing: Kexue chubanshe.

Lüshi chunqiu 呂氏春秋. Lü Buwei 呂不韋 (d. 235 B.C.) and others. *Zhuzi jicheng* ed. Commentaries cited: Gao You 高誘 (ca. 160-220).

MSSW. Jiangling Zhangjiashan Han jian zhengli xiaozu 江陵張家山漢簡整理小組. "Jiangling Zhangjiashan Han jian *Maishu* shiwen" 江陵張家山漢簡脈書釋文. *Wenwu* 文物 1989.7: 72-74.

MWD. *Mawangdui Han mu boshu* 馬王堆漢墓帛書. Ed. Mawangdui Han mu boshu zhengli xiaozu 馬王堆漢墓帛書整理小組. 3 vols. to date. Beijing: Wenwu chubanshe. Vol. 1, 1980 (philosophical texts); vol. 3, 1983 (historical and anecdotal texts); vol. 4, 1985 (medical texts).

Ma, Jixing 馬繼興 (see also Zhong Yiyan). 1980. "*Maifa* kaoshi" 脈法考釋. *Mawangdui yishu yanjiu zhuankan* 馬王堆醫書研究專刊 1. 21-26.

———. 1992. *Mawangdui gu yishu kaoshi* 馬王堆古醫書考釋. Changsha: Hunan kexue jishu chubanshe.

Ma, Jixing 馬繼興 and Zhou Shirong 周世榮. 1978. "Kaogu fajuezhong suo jian bianshi de chubu tantao" 考古發掘中所見砭石的初步探討. *Wenwu* 文物 1978.11. 80–82.

Mair, V. 1990. "Old Sinitic **Myag*, Old Persian *Magus*, and English 'Magician.'" *Early China* 15. 27–47.

Mansvelt Beck, B. 1987. "The First Emperor's Taboo Character and the Three Day Reign of King Xiaowen." *T'oung Pao* 73. 68–85.

Maspero, H. 1981. *Taoism and Chinese Religion*. Trans. F. Kierman. Amherst: University of Massachusetts Press.

Masters, W. and V. Johnson. 1966. *Human Sexual Response*. Boston: Little, Brown and Company.

Matsumoto, Eiichi 松本榮一. 1956. "Tonkô hon *Haku-taku seikai zu* kan" 敦煌本白澤精怪圖卷. *Kokka* 國華 770. 135–47.

Mawangdui Han mu boshu zhengli xiaozu 馬王堆漢墓帛書整理小組, ed. 1979. *Daoyin tu* 導引圖. Beijing: Wenwu chubanshe.

Mengzi 孟子. Meng Ke 孟軻 (ca. 372–ca. 289 B.C.) and others. *Zhuzi jicheng* ed.

Miyashita, Saburo 宮下三郎. 1959. "Chûgoku kodai no shippei-kan to ryôhô" 中國古代の疾病觀と療法. *Tôhô gakuhô* 東方學報 30. 227–52.

Mizukami, Shizuo 水上靜夫. 1977. *Chûgoku kodai no shokubutsugaku no kenkyû* 中國古代の植物學の研究. Tokyo: Kadokawa shoten.

Morimura, Ken-ichi 森村謙一. 1981. "Shin shutsudo iyaku shiryô ni okeru shizen himmoku no tankyû" 新出土醫藥資料における自然品目の探究. *Tôhô gakuhô* 東方學報 53. 341–85.

Moriya, Mitsuo 守屋美都雄. 1963. *Chûgoku ko saijiki no kenkyû* 中國古歲時記の研究. Tokyo: Teikoku shoin.

Morohashi, Tetsuji 諸橋轍次. 1957–60. *Dai Kan-Wa jiten* 大漢和辭典. 13 vols. Tokyo: Taishûkan shoten.

Mozi 墨 子. Mo Di 墨 翟 (ca. 479-ca. 381 B.C.) and others. *Zhuzi jicheng* ed.

Mu tianzi zhuan 穆天子傳. Ca. fourth century B.C. *Sibu beiyao* ed.

Murakami, Yoshimi 村 上 嘉 實. 1985. "*Gojûni byôhô* no jinbuyaku" 五 十 二 病 方 の 人 部 藥. *KGS*, vol. 2. 167-223.

Nanjing 難 經. First century A.D. *Sibu beiyao* ed.

Nanshi 南 史. Li Yanshou 李 延 壽 (600-680) and others. Taibei: Xinwenfeng chuban gongsi, 1975 (reproduction of 1739 Palace woodblock ed.).

Needham, J. 1954-. *Science and Civilisation in China*. 6 vols. to date. Cambridge: Cambridge University Press.

Ngo, Van Xuyet. 1976. *Divination, magie et politique dans la Chine ancienne*. Paris: Presses Universitaires de France.

Onozawa, Sei-ichi 小 野 沢 精 一 et al., eds. 1978. *Ki no shisô: Chûgoku ni okeru shizenkan to ningenkan no tenkai* 氣の思想: 中國における自然觀と人間觀の展開. Tokyo: Tôkyô daigaku shuppankai.

Peng, Hao 彭 浩. 1990. "Zhangjiashan Han jian *Yinshu* chutan" 張家山漢簡引書初探. *Wenwu* 文 物 1990.10. 87-91.

Phillips, C. 1991. "*Nullum Crimen sine Lege*: Socioreligious Sanctions on Magic." Faraone and Obbink 1991. 260-76.

Qianjin yaofang 千 金 藥 方. Sun Simo 孫 思 邈 (seventh century). *Daozang* ed. (*HY* 1155).

Qianjin yifang 千 金 翼 方. Sun Simo 孫 思 邈 (seventh century). Taibei: Guoli Zhongguo yiyao yanjiusuo, 1965 (reproduction of 1829 Japanese woodblock ed.).

Qimin yaoshu 齊民要術. Jia Sixie 賈思勰 (sixth century). References are to *Qimin yaoshu jiaoshi* 齊 民 要 術 校 釋. Ed. Miao Qiyu 繆 啓 愉. Beijing: Nongye chubanshe, 1982.

Qin jian zhengli xiaozu 秦 簡 整 理 小 組. 1989. "Tianshui Fangmatan Qin jian jiazhong *Rishu* shiwen" 天 水 放 馬 灘 秦 簡甲種日書釋文. Gansu sheng wenwu kaogu yanjiusuo 1989. 1-6.

Qingbai leichao 清 稗 類 鈔. Xu Ke 徐 珂 (1869-1928). Taibei: Shangwu yinshuguan, 1966 (reprint of 1917 ed.).

Qinjing 禽 經. Ca. tenth century. *Tang Song congshu* 唐 宋 叢 書. Jingde tang 經 德 堂 woodblock ed. (n.p., n.d).

Qiu, Long 邱隆 et al., ed. 1984. *Zhongguo gudai du liang heng tuji* 中國古代度量衡圖集. Beijing: Wenwu chubanshe.

Qiu, Xigui 裘錫圭. 1990. *Wenzixue gaiyao* 文字學概要. Beijing: Shangwu yinshuguan.

———. 1992. "Mawangdui yishu shidu suoyi" 馬王堆醫書釋讀瑣議. *Gu wenzi lunji* 古文字論集. By Qiu Xigui. Beijing: Zhonghua shuju.

Rao, Zongyi 饒宗頤. 1969. "Ba Dunhuang ben *Baize jingguai tu* liang canjuan" 跋敦煌本白澤精怪圖兩殘卷. *Zhongyang yanjiuyuan lishi yuyan yanjiusuo jikan* 中央研究院歷史語言研究所集刊 41. 539-43.

———. 1991. *Laozi "Xianger zhu" jiaozheng* 老子想爾注校證. Shanghai: Guji chubanshe.

Rickett, A. 1985. *Guanzi: Political, Economic, and Philosophical Essays from Early China; A Study and Translation*. Princeton: Princeton University Press.

Riegel, J. 1975. "A Summary of Some Recent *Wenwu* and *Kaogu* Articles on Mawangdui Tombs Two and Three." *Early China* 1. 10-15.

———. 1976. "Mawangdui Tomb Three: Documents, II. The Maps." *Early China* 2. 69-72.

———. 1989-90. "Kou-mang and Ju-shou." *Cahiers d'Extrême-Asie* 5. 55-83.

Robinet, I. 1984. *La révelation du Shangqing dans l'histoire du taoisme*. 2 vols. Paris: École Française d'Extrême-Orient.

de Romilly, J. 1975. *Magic and Rhetoric in Ancient Greece*. Cambridge: Harvard University Press.

Roth, H. 1991. "Psychology and Self-cultivation in Early Taoistic Thought." *Harvard Journal of Asiatic Studies* 51. 599-650.

———. 1992. *The Textual History of the Huai-nan Tzu*. Ann Arbor: Association for Asian Studies.

———. 1993. "Text and Edition in Early Chinese Philosophical Literature." *Journal of the American Oriental Society* 113. 214-27.

Ryan, W. and C. Schmitt, eds. 1982. *Pseudo-Aristotle The Secret of Secrets: Sources and Influences*. London: Warburg Institute.

SHD. *Shuihudi Qin mu zhujian* 睡虎地秦墓竹簡. Ed. Shuihudi Qin mu zhujian zhengli xiaozu 睡虎地秦墓竹簡整理小組. Beijing: Wenwu chubanshe, 1990.

SW. *Shuowen jiezi* 說文解字. Xu Shen 許慎 (d. A.D. 146). References are to *Shuowen jiezi zhu* 說文解字注. Ed. Duan Yucai 段玉裁 (1735-1815). Shanghai: Guji chubanshe (reproduction of 1872 woodblock ed.).

Sakade, Yoshinobu 坂出祥伸. 1980. "Dô-in kô" 導引考. *Ikeda Suetoshi hakuse koki kinen tôyôgaku ronshû* 池田末利博士古稀記念東洋學論集. Hiroshima: Ikeda Suetoshi hakuse koki kinen jigyôkai. 225-39.

———. 1985. "Hôso densetsu to *Hôso kei*" 彭祖傳説と彭祖經. *KGS*, vol. 2. 405-62.

———, ed. 1988. *Chûgoku kodai yôsei shisô no sôgôteki kenkyû* 中國古代養生思想の総合的研究. Tokyo: Hirakawa shuppansha.

Scarborough, J. 1988. "Hermetic and Related Texts in Classical Antiquity." *Hermetisicm and the Renaissance: Intellectual History and the Occult in Early Modern Europe*. Ed. I. Merkal and A. Debus. Cranbury: Associated University Presses. 19-44.

———. "The Pharmacology of Sacred Plants, Herbs, and Roots." Faraone and Obbink 1991. 138-74.

Schafer, E. 1955. "Notes on Mica in Medieval China." *T'oung Pao* 43. 265-86.

———. 1967. *The Vermilion Bird: T'ang Images of the South*. Berkeley: University of California Press.

———. 1981. "Wu Yün's 'Cantos on Pacing the Void.' " *Harvard Journal of Asiatic Studies* 41. 377-415.

———. 1987. *Consolidated Supplements to Mathews*. Berkeley: private publication.

Schipper, K. 1965. *L'empereur Wou des Han dans la légende taoiste: Han Wou-ti Nei-tchouan*. Paris: École Française d'Extrême-Orient.

———. 1969. "Science, Magic, and the Mystique of the Body." *The Clouds and the Rain: The Art of Love in China*. Ed. M. Beurdeley. London: Hammond and Hammond. 14-20.

———, ed. 1975. *Concordance du Houang-t'ing king*. Paris: École Française d'Extrême-Orient.

———. 1978. "The Taoist Body." *History of Religions* 17. 355-86.

Schuessler, A. 1987. *A Dictionary of Early Zhou Chinese*. Honolulu: University of Hawaii Press.

Seidel, A. 1969. *La divinisation de Lao Tseu dans le taoisme des Han*. Paris: École Française d'Extrême-Orient.

———. 1987. "Traces of Han Religion in Funeral Texts Found in Tombs." Akizuki 1987. 21-57.

Shangshu 尚書. Contents of various dates, from the early Zhou period to the fourth century A.D. (the forged sections). *Shisanjing zhushu* ed.

Shanhaijing 山海經. Contents of various dates, from ca. fourth century B.C. to ca. first century A.D. *Sibu beiyao* ed. Commentaries cited: Guo Pu 郭璞 (276-324).

Shanshenmiao Pei Du huan dai 山神廟裴度還帶. Yuan period. *Quan Yuan zaju chubian* 全元雜劇初編. Ed. Yang Jialuo 楊家駱. Taibei: Shijie shuju, 1962.

Shaughnessy, E., ed. Forthcoming. *New Sources of Early Chinese History: An Introduction to Reading Inscriptions and Manuscripts*. Berkeley: Society for the Study of Early China.

Shen, Shou 沈壽. 1980. "Xi Han bohua *Daoyin tu* jiexi" 西漢帛畫導引圖解析. *Wenwu* 文物 1980.9. 70-76.

Shenjian 申鑒. Xun Yue 荀悦 (148-209). *Zhuzi jicheng* ed.

Shibata, Kiyotsugu 柴田清繼. 1984. "*Kanshi* shihen ni okeru shin to dô" 管子四篇における神と道. *Nihon Chûgoku gakkai hô* 日本中國學會報 36. 12-24.

Shiji 史記. Sima Qian 司馬遷 (ca. 145-ca. 86 B.C.). Taibei: Xinwenfeng chuban gongsi, 1975 (reproduction of 1739 Palace woodblock ed.).

Shijing 詩經. Contents of various dates, from ca. 1000 to ca. 600 B.C. *Shisanjing zhushu* ed. Commentaries cited: Kong Yingda 孔穎達 (574-648).

Shiming 釋名. Liu Xi 劉熙 (fl. 200). *Congshu jicheng* ed.

Shirakawa, Shizuka 白川靜. 1974. *Kôkotsu kinbungaku ronshû* 甲骨金文學論集. Kyoto: Hôyû shoten.

———. 1976. *Kanji no sekai* 漢字の世界. 2 vols. Tokyo: Heibonsha.

Shisanjing zhushu 十 三 經 注 疏. Ed. Ruan Yuan 阮 元 (1764–1849). Shanghai: Zhonghua shuju, 1957 (reprint of *Sibu beiyao* ed.).

Shizi 尸 子. Ca. third to first centuries B.C. *Sibu beiyao* ed.

Shuoyuan 說 苑. Liu Xiang 劉 向 (79–8 B.C.). *Sibu beiyao* ed.

Sibu beiyao 四部備要. Shanghai: Zhonghua shuju, 1927–35.

Sibu congkan 四 部 叢 刊. 3 ser. Shanghai: Shangwu yinshuguan, 1920–36.

Siku quanshu 四 庫 全 書. Taibei: Shangwu yinshuguan (reproduction of 1782 Wenyuange woodblock ed.).

Sivin, N. 1987. *Traditional Medicine in Contemporary China*. Ann Arbor: University of Michigan Center for Chinese Studies.

———. 1992. "Ruminations on the Tao and Its Disputers" (rev. of Graham 1989). *Philosophy East and West* 42. 21–29.

———. 1993. "*Huang ti nei ching.*" Loewe 1993. 196–215.

Sun, Ji 孫 機. 1991. *Han dai wuzhi wenhua ziliao tushuo* 漢 代 物 質 文 化 資 料 圖 說. Beijing: Wenwu chubanshe.

Sunü miaolun 素 女 妙 論. Ming period. References are to the edition in R. van Gulik, *Erotic Colour Prints of the Ming Period, with an Essay on Chinese Sexual Life from the Han to the Ch'ing Dynasty, B.C. 206–A.D. 1644*. 3 vols. Tokyo: private publication, 1951. Vol. 2. 115–39.

Suwen 素 問. Tang period recension of Han period *Huangdi neijing*. *Sibu beiyao* ed. Commentaries cited: Wang Bing 王 冰 (eighth century).

Taiping yulan 太平御覽. Li Fang 李 昉 (925–96) and others. Beijing: Zhonghua shuju, 1960 (reproduction of Song woodblock ed.).

Taipingjing 太 平 經. Ca. second century A.D. References are to *Taipingjing hejiao* 太 平 經 合 校. Ed. Wang Ming 王 明. Beijing: Zhonghua shuju, 1979.

Taisu 太 素. Sui period recension of Han period *Huangdi neijing*. *Congshu jicheng* ed. Commentaries cited: Yang Shangshan 楊 上 善 (fl. 610).

Tambiah, S. 1990. *Magic, Science, Religion, and the Scope of Rationality*. Cambridge: Cambridge University Press.

Tang, Lan 唐蘭. 1979. "Shilun Mawangdui sanhao Han mu chutu *Daoyin tu*" 試論馬王堆三號漢墓出土導引圖. Mawangdui Han mu boshu zhengli xiaozu 1979. 1–10.

Tate, G. 1947. *Mammals of Eastern Asia*. New York: Macmillan Company.

Tsien, T. 1962. *Written on Bamboo and Silk: The Beginnings of Chinese Books and Inscriptions*. Chicago: University of Chicago Press.

Twitchett, D. and M. Loewe, eds. 1986. *The Cambridge History of China*, vol. 1 (The Ch'in and Han Empires, 221 B.C.–A.D. 220). Cambridge: Cambridge University Press.

Unschuld, P. 1975. "Zur Bedeutung des Terminus *tu* in der traditionellen medizinisch-pharmazeutischen Literatur Chinas." *Sudhoffs Archiv* 57. 165–83.

———. 1982a. "Der Wind als Ursache des Krankseins: Einige Gedanken zu Yamada Keijis Analyse der *Shao-shih* Texte des *Huang-ti nei-ching*." *T'oung Pao* 68. 91–131.

———. 1982b. "Ma-wang-tui *Materia Medica*: A Comparative Analysis of Early Chinese Pharmaceutical Knowledge." *Zinbun: Memoirs of the Research Institute for Humanistic Studies, Kyoto University* 18. 11–63.

———. 1985. *Medicine in China: A History of Ideas*. Berkeley: University of California Press.

———. 1986a. *Medicine in China: A History of Pharmaceutics*. Berkeley: University of California Press.

———, trans. 1986b. *Nan-ching: The Classic of Difficult Issues*. Berkeley: University of California Press.

———. 1987. "Traditional Chinese Medicine: Some Historical and Epistemological Reflections." *Social Science and Medicine* 24. 1023–29.

———. 1993. "History of Chinese Medicine." Kiple 1993. 20–27.

Vickers, B. 1984. Introduction. *Occult and Scientific Mentalities in the Renaissance*. Ed. B. Vickers. Cambridge: Cambridge University Press.

WWYJ. *Wuwei Handai yijian* 武威漢代醫簡. Ed. Gansu sheng bowuguan 甘肅省博物館 and Wuwei xian wenhuaguan 武威縣文化館. Beijing: Wenwu chubanshe, 1975.

Waitai biyaofang 外臺秘要方. Wang Tao 王燾 (eighth century). *Siku quanshu* ed.

Wang, Shimin 王世民. 1986. "Mawangdui boshu" 馬王堆帛書. *Zhongguo da baike quanshu: kaoguxue* 中國大百科全書:考古學. Beijing: Zhongguo da baike quanshu chubanshe. 307–309.

Wang, Yucheng 王育成. 1991. "Dong Han daofu shili" 東漢道符釋例. *Kaogu xuebao* 考古學報 1991.1. 45–56.

Wei, Qipeng 魏啓鵬 and Hu Xianghua 胡翔驊. 1992. *Mawangdui Han mu yishu jiaoshi* 馬王堆漢墓醫書校釋. 2 vols. Chengdu: Chengdu chubanshe.

Wenxuan 文選. Xiao Tong 蕭統 (501–31). *Sibu beiyao* ed.

Wile, D. 1992. *Art of the Bedchamber: The Chinese Sexual Yoga Classics Including Women's Solo Meditation Texts*. Albany: State University of New York Press.

Wuzazu 五雜組. Xie Zhaozhe 謝肇淛 (1567–1624). 1795 Japanese woodblock ed.

Xia, De'an 夏德安 (D. Harper). 1994. "*Wushier bingfang* yu Yue fang" 五十二病方與越方. *Mawangdui Han mu yanjiu wenji* 馬王堆漢墓研究文集. Ed. Hunan sheng bowuguan 湖南省博物館. Changsha: Hunan chubanshe. 118–24.

Xiao Han 曉菡 (pen name for Han Zhongmin, which also see). 1974. "Changsha Mawangdui Han mu boshu gaishu" 長沙馬王堆漢墓帛書概述. *Wenwu* 文物 1974.9. 40–44.

Xijing zaji 西京雜記. Ca. fourth century. *Sibu congkan* ed.

Xinxu 新序. Liu Xiang 劉向 (79–8 B.C.). *Congshu jicheng* ed.

Xinyu 新語. Lu Jia 陸賈 (fl. 200–180 B.C.). *Sibu beiyao* ed.

Xunzi 荀子. Xun Qing 荀卿 (ca. 298–ca. 238 B.C.). *Zhuzi jicheng* ed.

YSSW. Zhangjiashan Han jian zhenglizu 張家山漢簡整理組. "Zhangjiashan Han jian *Yinshu* shiwen" 張家山漢簡引書釋文. *Wenwu* 文物 1990.10. 82–86.

Yamada, Keiji 山田慶兒. 1979. "The Formation of the *Huang-ti Nei-ching*." *Acta Asiatica* 36. 67–89.

———. 1980. "Kyû-ku hachi-fu setsu to shôshiha no tachiba" 九宮八風説と少師派の立場. *Tôhô gakuhô* 東方學報 52. 199–242.

———. 1985a. "Shinkyû to tôeki no kigen" 鍼灸と湯液の起源. *KGS*, vol. 2. 3-122.

———. 1985b. "Ma-o-tai Kan bo shutsudo isho sansoku" 馬王堆漢墓出土醫書三則. *KGS*, vol. 2. 225-62.

———. 1988. "Hen Shaku densetsu" 扁鵲傳説. *Tôhô gakuhô* 東方學報 60. 73-158.

———. 1990. "Igaku no denju" 醫學の傳授. *Ya naku tori: igaku, jujutsu, densetsu* 夜鳴く鳥: 醫學呪術傳説. By Yamada Keiji. Tokyo: Iwanami shoten. 55-96.

Yang, Shuda 楊樹達. 1986. *Ciquan* 詞詮. Shanghai: Guji chubanshe.

Yanzi chunqiu 晏子春秋. Ca. fourth century B.C. *Zhuzi jicheng* ed.

Yasui, Kôzan 安居香山 and Nakamura Shôhachi 中村璋八. 1971-92. *Jûshû isho shûsei* 重修緯書集成. 6 vols. Tokyo: Meitoku shuppansha.

Yijing 易經. Zhou period. *Shisanjing zhushu* ed. Commentaries cited: Wang Bi 王弼 (226-49).

Yili 儀禮. Ca. third to second centuries B.C. *Shisanjing zhushu* ed. Commentaries cited: Zheng Xuan 鄭玄 (127-200).

Yoneda, Kaisuke 米田該典. 1988. "Chûgoku kodai isho chû no yakubutsu no bussanshi teki kôsatsu" 中國古代醫書中の藥物の物産誌的考察. Sakade 1988. 45-63.

Yu, Yan 余嚴. 1972. *Gudai jibing minghou shuyi* 古代疾病名候疏義. Taibei: Ziyou chubanshe.

Yu, Ying-shih. 1977. "Han." *Food in Chinese Culture: Anthropological and Historical Perspectives*. Ed. K. Chang. New Haven: Yale University Press. 55-83.

Yunji qiqian 雲笈七籤. Zhang Junfang 張君房 (fl. first quarter of the eleventh century). *Daozang* ed. (*HY* 1026).

ZY. *Zhongyao dacidian* 中藥大辭典. Ed. Jiangsu xin yixueyuan 江蘇新醫學院. 3 vols. Shanghai: Shanghai kexue jishu chubanshe, 1977-79.

Zhang, Peiyu 張培瑜. 1989. "Chutu Han jian boshu shang de li zhu" 出土漢簡帛書上的曆注. *Chutu wenxian yanjiu xuji* 出土文獻研究續集. Ed. Guojia wenwuju guwenxian yanjiushi 國家文物局古文獻研究室. Beijing: Wenwu chubanshe.

Zhangjiashan Han mu zhujian zhengli xiaozu 張家山漢墓竹簡整理小組. 1985. "Jiangling Zhangjiashan Han jian gaishu" 江陵張家山漢簡概述. *Wenwu* 文物 1985.1. 9-15.

Zhanguoce 戰國策. Third century B.C. *Sibu beiyao* ed.

Zhao, Pushan 趙璞珊. 1986. "*Shanhaijing* jizai de yaowu, jibing he wuyi" 山海經記載的藥物疾病和巫醫. *Shanhaijing xintan* 山海經新探. Ed. Zhongguo *Shanhaijing* xueshu taolunhui 中國山海經學術討論會. Chengdu: Sichuan sheng shehui kexueyuan chubanshe.

Zhao, Youchen 趙有臣. 1981. "*Wushier bingfang* zhong 'duo' zi de kaoshi" 五十二病方中隋字的考釋. *Wenwu* 文物 1981.3. 22.

Zhenjiu jiayi jing 鍼灸甲乙經. Huangfu Mi 皇甫謐 (third century). *Siku quanshu* ed.

Zhong, Yiyan 鐘依研 (pen name for Ma Jixing, which also see). 1972. "Xi Han Liu Sheng mu chutu de yiliao qiju" 西漢劉勝墓出土的醫療器具. *Kaogu* 考古 1972.3. 49-53.

Zhou, Yao 周堯. 1957. *Zhongguo zaoqi kunchongxue yanjiushi* 中國早期昆蟲學研究史. Beijing: Kexue chubanshe.

Zhou, Yimou 周一謀 and Xiao Zuotao 蕭佐桃, eds. 1988. *Mawangdui yishu kaozhu* 馬王堆醫書考注. Tianjin: Tianjin kexue jishu chubanshe.

Zhouli 周禮. Third to second centuries B.C. *Shisanjing zhushu* ed. Commentaries cited: Zheng Xuan 鄭玄 (127-200); Zheng Sinong 鄭司農 (d. A.D. 83).

Zhuangzi 莊子. Zhuang Zhou 莊周 and others, fourth to second centuries B.C. References are to *Zhuangzi jishi* 莊子集釋. Ed. Guo Qingfan 郭慶藩 (1844-96). *Zhuzi jicheng* ed. Commentaries cited: Cheng Xuanying 成玄英 (fl. 631).

Zhuzi jicheng 諸子集成. Beijing: Zhonghua shuju, 1954.

Zunsheng bajian 遵生八箋. Gao Lian 高濂 (fl. 1570-91). Chengdu: Ba Shu shushe, 1992.

Zuozhuan 左傳. Fourth century B.C. *Shisanjing zhushu* ed.

INDEX OF MATERIA MEDICA

Materia medica is indexed by entry in the Translation. The name of a substance may occur more than once in the same entry; the index does not provide a lexical count of the total number of occurrences of a given name in the manuscripts. Materia medica is defined broadly to include nearly everything that forms part of the treatment of ailments or the execution of techniques; cooking pots, dishes, and sundry utensils used solely in the preparation of drugs are excluded. A few fragmentary drug names have been omitted. An asterisk following an entry indicates further discussion in a footnote in that entry. If the names of plants, animals, and minerals can be identified with a high degree of certainty, relevant citations to *GM* and *ZY* are provided (those occurring in *BC* are also noted; reference to *ZY* is omitted for some common animals and minerals). If the identification is uncertain, likely identifications are often discussed in the footnotes. Citations to *ZY* are to the entry that provides the basic description of the plant, animal, or mineral, which may be the source of several drugs having separate *ZY* entries; the *ZY* entry cited may not correspond to the specific drug in the manuscripts. Similarly, the index does not correlate every drug in the manuscripts (e.g. the various parts of a plant or animal) with a corresponding drug in *BC* or *GM*; most *GM* citations are to the main entry for a plant, animal, or mineral, not to the individual drugs listed after the main entry in *GM* (see also the index of materia medica in Ma Jixing 1992: 1073-98, which notes likely correlations between the Mawangdui medical manuscripts and later materia medica). Some headings in the index provide subheadings for the parts of a substance used as drugs in the manuscripts. However, occasional references in the manuscripts to the root, fruit, leaf, stalk, or other parts of many substances are not specified in the index. Chinese graphs are provided selectively; they often represent a standard graph in received literature, not the graph written on the original manuscripts.

INDEX OF PHYSIOLOGICAL TERMS

Physiological terms are indexed by entry in the Translation. A term may occur more than once in the same entry; the index does not provide a lexical count of the total number of occurrences of a given term in the manuscripts. When the same English translation is used for several Chinese terms, the Chinese terms are recorded separately under the main heading (there are exceptions; e.g. the heading **body**, in which the two Chinese terms occasionally occur in compound form in the manuscripts). Some headings in the index list related terms as subheadings. The graphs for the Chinese terms often represent a standard graph in received literature, not the graph written on the original manuscripts. An asterisk following an entry indicates that the term is discussed in a footnote in that entry.

INDEX OF AILMENTS

Ailments are indexed by entry in the Translation. An ailment name may occur more than once in the same entry; entries known to treat a given ailment, yet in which the ailment name is not written in the text, are also included (e.g. recipes arranged by category of ailment in *MS*I.E). Note that "ailment" is understood to refer broadly to "a condition warranting medical attention." Ailments which focus on parts of the body (back pain, cheekbone swelling, throat numbness, etc.) are arranged under the appropriate part. Some headings in the index bring together several related ailments under one category. Graphs are provided selectively; they often represent a standard graph in received literature, not the graph written on the original manuscripts. An asterisk following an entry indicates that the ailment is discussed in a footnote in that entry.

GENERAL INDEX

Important terms, subjects, persons, and books mentioned in the Prolegomena are indexed.